Workbook for

Fordney's Medical Insurance

Workbook for

Fordney's Medical Insurance

Fifteenth Edition

Linda M. Smith, CPC, CPC-I, CEMC, CMBS
Training and Consulting
MedOffice Resources
Greene, New York

ELSEVIER

Notice

Practitioners and researchers must always rely on their own experience and knowledge in evaluating and using any information, methods, compounds or experiments described herein. Because of rapid advances in the medical sciences, in particular, independent verification of diagnoses and drug dosages should be made. To the fullest extent of the law, no responsibility is assumed by Elsevier, authors, editors or contributors for any injury and/or damage to persons or property as a matter of products liability, negligence or otherwise, or from any use or operation of any methods, products, instructions, or ideas contained in the material herein.

Previous editions copyrighted 2016, 2014, and 2012.

International Standard Book Number: 978-0-323-59441-7

Publishing Director: Kristin Wilhelm
Senior Content Strategist: Linda Woodard
Senior Content Development Manager: Ellen Wurm-Cutter
Senior Content Development Specialist: Maria Broeker
Publishing Services Manager: Shereen Jameel
Project Manager: Aparna Venkatachalam

Printed in the United States of America

Last digit is the print number: 9 8 7 6 5 4 3 2 1

ELSEVIER

3251 Riverport Lane
St. Louis, Missouri 63043

Working together
to grow libraries in
developing countries

www.elsevier.com • www.bookaid.org

Contributors

CONTRIBUTORS

Rachael D'Andrea, MS, RHIA, CPHQ, CDIP, CHTS-TR
Professor, Health Information Management
Lake Sumter State College
Leesburg, Florida

Professor, Health Information Management and Health
Care Administration
Charter Oak State College
New Britain, Connecticut

Cheryl Fassett, CPC, CPB, CPPM, CPC-I
Educator
Practice Manager
Riverside Associates in Anesthesia, PC
Binghamton, New York

**Nanette Sayles, EdD, RHIA, CCS, CHPS, CHDA, CPHI,
CPHIMS, FAHIMA**
Associate Professor, Health Information Management
East Central College
Union, Missouri

Contents

Instruction Guide to the Workbook

LEARNING OBJECTIVES

The student will be able to:

- Define and spell key terms and key abbreviations for each chapter.
- Answer review questions for each chapter of *Fordney's Medical Insurance*.
- Complete assignments to enhance and develop better critical thinking skills.
- Define abbreviations as they appear on a patient record.
- Abstract subjective and objective data from patient records.
- Review documentation on patient records.
- Code professional services properly, using the *Current Procedural Terminology* (CPT) Code Book.
- Select diagnostic code numbers, using the *International Classification of Diseases*, Tenth Revision, Clinical Modifications (ICD-10-CM).
- Locate errors on insurance claims before submission to insurance companies.
- Locate errors on returned insurance claims.
- Carry out collection procedures on delinquent accounts.
- Execute financial management procedures for tracing managed care plans.
- Extract information necessary to complete insurance claim forms from patient records and billing statements/ledger cards.
- Post payments, adjustments, and balances to patients' statements/ledger cards when submitting insurance claims.
- Compute mathematic calculations for Medicare and TRICARE cases.
- Analyze insurance claims for errors in both hospital inpatient and outpatient settings.
- Answer questions about the insurance verification process using patients' health insurance cards.
- Study case scenarios and explain how these violate security and confidentiality and give solutions to prevent the breaches.
- List important activities in each stage of the life cycle of an insurance claim.
- Prepare a cover letter, résumé, job application, and follow-up letter to search for employment.
- Access the Internet and visit websites to research and/or obtain data.

INSTRUCTIONS TO THE STUDENT

The 15th edition of *Workbook for Fordney's Medical Insurance* has been prepared for those who use the textbook, *Fordney's Medical Insurance*. It is designed to assist the learner in a practical approach to doing insurance billing and coding.

The key terms and key abbreviations are repeated for quick reference when studying. Each chapter's outline serves as a lecture guide to use for note taking. The review questions in the form of short answer, true/false, multiple choice, and matching are presented to reinforce learning of key concepts for each topic.

Some assignments give students hands-on experience in completing claim forms using National Uniform Claim Committee (NUCC) guidelines. Insurance claim forms and other sample documents that are easily removable are included for practice.

Current procedural and diagnostic code exercises are used throughout to facilitate and enhance coding skills for submitting a claim or making an itemized billing statement.

Self-study assignments encompass important points from each chapter and allow you to study at your own pace.

Critical thinking assignments require skills that help prepare you for real-world scenarios encountered in insurance billing.

KEY TERMS AND KEY ABBREVIATIONS

Key terms and key abbreviations are presented for each chapter, and definitions may be located in the glossary at the end of *Fordney's Medical Insurance*. It is suggested that you make up 3- by 5-inch index cards for each term or abbreviation and write in the definitions as you encounter them while reading each chapter in the *Fordney's Medical Insurance*. Doing this will reinforce your knowledge and help you learn the words and abbreviations. Your instructor may wish to select certain words for you to study for pop quizzes.

NOTE TAKING

Taking notes is an important key to success in studying and learning. Note taking helps an individual pay attention during class and retain information. Each chapter has a study outline for organizational purposes, and the outline may be used as a guide for writing down key points during lectures or when studying or reviewing from *Fordney's Medical Insurance* for tests. Use file cards, notepads, notebooks, computers, or tablets for taking notes. Underline or highlight important words or phrases. To improve the usefulness of notes, try the following format:

1. Using a tablet note-taking app, notepad sheet, or file card, draw a margin 3 inches from the left.
2. Use the left side for topic headings and the right side for notes.
3. Skip a few lines when the topic changes.
4. Write numbers or letters to indicate sub-ideas under a heading.
5. Be brief; do not write down every word except when emphasizing a quotation, rule, or law. Write notes in your own words because that is what you will understand.
6. Use abbreviations that you know how to translate.
7. Listen carefully to the lecture.
8. After the lecture, reread your notes. Highlight the word(s) on the left side of the page to identify the topic of the notes on the right.
9. For study purposes, cover the right side and see if you can explain to yourself or someone else the topic or word.
10. Remember: learning is by doing, and doing is up to you. So take notes for better understanding.

REVIEW QUESTION ASSIGNMENTS

Review questions have been designed to encompass important points for each chapter to assist you in studying insurance billing and coding theory.

SIMULATION ASSIGNMENTS

Assume that you have been hired as an insurance billing specialist and that you are working in a clinic setting for an incorporated group of medical doctors, other allied health specialists, and a podiatrist. You will be asked to complete various assignments. These doctors will be on the staff of a nearby hospital. Appendix A details this clinic's policies and procedures, which you must read completely before beginning the competency-based assignments. Within each chapter, the simulation assignments progress from easy to more complex. Some assignments are given with critical thinking problems, which the instructor may use for class discussion.

Always read the assignment entirely before starting.

MEDICAL TERMINOLOGY AND ABBREVIATIONS

A list of abbreviations is provided in Appendix A to help you learn how to abstract and read physicians' notes. Decode any abbreviations that you do not understand or that are unfamiliar to you. To reinforce learning these abbreviations, write their meanings on the assignment pages. If you do not have a background in medical terminology, it may be wise to use a good medical dictionary as a reference or, better yet, enroll in a terminology course to master that skill.

PATIENT RECORDS

Patient records, financial accounting records (ledgers), and encounter forms are presented, so the learner may have the tools needed to extract information to complete claim forms.

Patient records have been abbreviated because of space and page constraints. The records contain pertinent data for each type of case, but it has been necessary to omit a lengthy physical examination. Because detailed documentation is encouraged in medical practices, the records all appear typewritten rather than in handwritten notes. The physician's signature appears after each dated entry on the record.

All the materials included in the assignments have been altered to prevent identification of the cases or parties involved. The names and addresses are fictitious, and no reference to any person living or dead is intended. No evaluation of medical practice or medical advice is to be inferred from the patient records, nor is any recommendation made toward alternative treatment methods or prescribed medications.

FINANCIAL RECORDS

Financial accounting record statements (ledgers) are included for practice in posting, totaling fees, and properly recording appropriate information when an insurance claim is submitted. Refer to Appendix A to obtain information about the Mock Fee Schedule and the physicians' fees for posting to the statements.

CMS-1500 CLAIM FORM

If you have access to a computer, use the practice management software that accompanies the *Workbook* to complete each assignment and print it out for evaluation. To complete the CMS-1500 claim form properly for each type of program, refer to the section in Chapter 14 of *Fordney's Medical Insurance* that describes in detail the correct information to be put in each block.

Do's and don'ts for claim completion and NUCC guidelines are mentioned in Chapter 14. If you do not have access to a computer, type or neatly write in the information on the insurance form as you abstract it from the patient record.

PERFORMANCE EVALUATION CHECKLIST

The 15th edition features a competency-based format for each assignment indicating performance objectives to let you know what is to be accomplished. The task (job assignment), conditions (elements needed to perform and complete the task), and standards (time management), as well as directions for the specific task, are included.

A two-part performance evaluation checklist used when completing a CMS-1500 claim form is depicted in Figures I.1 and I.2. Reproduce these sheets only for the assignments that involve completing the CMS-1500 claim form. Your instructor will give you the number of points to be assigned for each step.

STUDENT REFERENCE NOTEBOOK

A student reference notebook is recommended so that you can access information quickly to help you complete the *Workbook* assignments. Before beginning the assignments, tear out Appendix A and place it in a three-ring binder with the chapter indexes. Appendix A includes the clinic policies and guidelines, data about the clinic staff, medical and laboratory abbreviations, and the Mock Fee Schedule used while working as an insurance billing specialist for the College Clinic.

Besides these suggestions, you may wish to either tear out or make photocopies of other sections of *Fordney's Medical Insurance* for your personal use. In addition, your instructor may give you handouts from time to time, pertaining to regional insurance program policies and procedures, to place in your notebook.

TESTS

Tests appear at the end of the *Workbook* to provide a complete, competency-based educational program.

REFERENCE MATERIAL

To do the assignments in this *Workbook* and gain expertise in coding and insurance claims completion, an individual must have access to the books listed here. Addresses for obtaining these materials are given in parentheses. Additional books and booklets on these topics, as well as on Medicaid, Medicare, TRICARE, and more, can be found at bookstores or online retailers.

Dictionary

Dorland's Illustrated Medical Dictionary, 32nd edition, Elsevier, 2012 (6277 Sea Harbor Drive, Orlando, FL 32821-9989; 1-800-545-2522).

Code Books

Current Procedural Terminology, American Medical Association, published annually (515 North State Street, Chicago, IL 60610; 1-800-621-8335).

International Classification of Diseases, Tenth Revision, Clinical Modification, Elsevier, published annually (6277 Sea Harbor Drive, Orlando, FL 32821-9989; 1-800-545-2522).

Word Book

Sloane's Medical Word Book, 5th edition, by Ellen Drake, CMT, FAAMT, Elsevier (6277 Sea Harbor Drive, Orlando, FL 32821-9989; 1-800-545-2522).

Pharmaceutical Book

Optional publications for drug names and descriptions might be either drug books used by nurses (e.g., *Mosby's Gen RX*, Elsevier, published annually [3251 Riverport Lane, St. Louis, MO 63043; 1-800-325-4177; www.elsevier.com]) or ones used by physicians (e.g., *Physician's Desk Reference* [PDR], Medical Economics Company, published annually [5 Paragon Drive, Montvale, NJ, 07645; 1-800-432-4570]).

PERFORMANCE EVALUATION CHECKLIST

Assignment No. _____

Name: _____ Date: _____

Performance Objective

Task: Given access to all necessary equipment and information, the student will complete a CMS-1500 health insurance claim form.

Standards: Claim Productivity Management
Time _____ minutes
Note: Time element may be given by instructor.

Directions: See assignment.

NOTE TIME BEGAN _____ **NOTE TIME COMPLETED** _____

PROCEDURE STEPS	ASSIGNED POINTS	STEP PERFORMED SATISFACTORY	COMMENTS
1. Assembled CMS-1500 claim form, patient record, E/M code slip, ledger card, computer, pen or pencil, and code books.	_____	_____	_____
2. Posted ledger card correctly.	_____	_____	_____
3. Proofread form for spelling and typographical errors while form remained on computer screen.	_____	_____	_____
4. Points earned for correct completion of CMS-1500 block-by-block data.	_____	_____	_____

Figure I-1

PERFORMANCE EVALUATION CHECKLIST

BLOCK	INCORRECT	MISSING	NOT NEEDED	REMARKS	BLOCK	INCORRECT	MISSING	NOT NEEDED	REMARKS
					18				
1A					19				
2					20				
3					21				
4									
5					22				
6					23				
7					24A				
8					24B				
					24C				
9					24D				
9A									
9B									
9C					24E				
9D									
					24F				
10A					24G				
10B					24H, 24I				
10C					24J				
10D									
11					25, 26				
11A					27				
11B					28				
11C					29				
11D									
12					30				
13									
14					31				
15									
16					32				
17									
17A					33				
					Reference Initials				

TOTAL POINTS EARNED: _____

Evaluator's signature _____

TOTAL POINTS POSSIBLE: _____

NEED TO REPEAT: _____

Figure I-2

Instruction Guide to the Workbook

EMPLOYEE INSURANCE PROCEDURAL MANUAL

If you currently work in a health care office, you may custom design an insurance manual for your organization's practice as you complete insurance claims in this *Workbook*. Obtain a three-ring binder with indexes and label them "Group Plans," "Private Plans," "Medicaid," "Medicare," "Managed Care Plans," "State Disability," "TRICARE," and "Workers' Compensation." If many of your patients have group plans, complete an insurance data or fact sheet for each plan and organize them alphabetically by group plan (Figure I.3).

An insurance manual with fact sheets listing benefits can keep you up to date on policy changes and ensure maximum reimbursement. Fact sheets can be prepared from information obtained when patients bring in their benefit booklets. Obtain and insert a list of the procedures that must be performed as an outpatient and those that must have second opinions for each of the insurance plans.

As you complete the assignments in this *Workbook*, place them in the insurance manual as examples of completed claims for each particular program.

INSURANCE DATA

1. Employer's name _____

2. Address _____ Telephone Number _____

3. Insurance Company Contact Person _____

4. Insurance Carrier _____

5. Address _____ Telephone Number to Call for Benefits _____

6. Group Policy Number _____

7. Group Account Manager _____ Telephone Number _____

8. **Insurance Coverage:**

   Annual Deductible _____ Patient Copayment Percentage _____

   Noncovered Procedures _____

   Maximum Benefits _____

9. **Diagnostic Coverage:**

   Limited Benefits _____

   Maximum Benefits _____

   Noncovered Procedures _____

10. **Major Medical:**

    Annual Deductible _____ Patient Copayment Percentage _____

    Limited Benefits _____

    Maximum Benefits _____

    Noncovered Procedures _____

Mandatory Outpatient Surgeries _____

Second Surgical Opinions _____

Preadmission Certification   Yes _____ No _____   Authorized Labs _____

Payment Plan:

UCR _____ Schedule of Benefits _____ CPT _____ RVS _____

Send claims to: _____

_____

Date Entered _____ Date Updated _____

Figure I-3

Role of an Insurance Billing Specialist

Linda M. Smith

KEY TERMS

Your instructor may wish to select some specific words pertinent to this chapter for a test. For definitions of the terms, further study, and/or reference, the words, phrases, and abbreviations may be found in the glossary at the end of the Textbook. *Key terms for this chapter follow.*

American Medical Association
cash flow
claims assistance professional
claims examiner
cycle
electronic mail
errors and omissions insurance
ethics
etiquette
facility billing

independent contractor
insurance billing specialist
list service
medical billing representative
professional billing
reimbursement specialist
respondeat superior
revenue
self-pay patient
senior billing representative

KEY ABBREVIATIONS

See how many abbreviations and acronyms you can translate and then use this as a handy reference list. Definitions for the key abbreviations are located near the back of the Textbook *in the glossary.*

AAMA _____

_____

_____

AMA _____

ASHD _____

CAP _____

e-mail _____

listserv _____

MSO _____

NPP _____

PERFORMANCE OBJECTIVES

The student will be able to:

- Define and spell the key terms and key abbreviations for this chapter, given the information from the *Textbook* glossary, within a reasonable time period and with enough accuracy to obtain a satisfactory evaluation.
- Answer the fill-in-the-blank, multiple choice, and true/false review questions after reading the chapter, with enough accuracy to obtain a satisfactory evaluation.

- Use critical thinking to write one or two grammatically correct paragraphs with sufficient information to obtain a satisfactory evaluation.
- Visit websites and site-search information via the Evolve website at http://evolve.elsevier.com/Smith/Fordneys/, with sufficient information to obtain a satisfactory evaluation.

1

STUDY OUTLINE

Background of Insurance Claims, Coding, and Billing
Role of the Insurance Billing Specialist
    Job Responsibilities
    Educational and Training Requirements
    Career Advantages
    Self-Employment or Independent Contracting
    Flexible Hours
    Disabled Workers
    Qualifications and Attributes
    Skills

    Personal Image
    Behavior
Medical Etiquette
Professional Ethics
Scope of Practice and Liability
    Employer Liability
    Employee Liability
    Independent Contractor Liability
    Claims Assistant Professional Liability
Future Challenges

ASSIGNMENT 1.1 REVIEW QUESTIONS

Part I Fill in the Blank

Review the objectives, key terms, and chapter information before completing the following review questions.

1. Name some of the settings where facility billing is used.

   a. _____

   b. _____

   c. _____

   d. _____

   e. _____

2. Name some of the various types of providers who use professional billing.

   a. _____

   b. _____

   c. _____

   d. _____

   e. _____

3. Name examples of non-physician practitioners (NPPs).

   a. _____

   b. _____

   c. _____

   d. _____

   e. _____

   f. _____

   g. _____

   h. _____

4. Name several job titles associated with medical billing personnel in both small and large health care organizations.

   a. _____

   b. _____

   c. _____

5. List some of the responsibilities and duties an insurance billing specialist might perform generally, as well as when acting as a collection manager. Refer to the section on "Job Responsibilities" in Fig. 1.1 of the text.

a. _____

b. _____

c. _____

d. _____

e. _____

f. _____

g. _____

6. List the duties of a claims-assistance professional.

a. _____

b. _____

c. _____

7. Insurance claims must be promptly submitted within _____ business days to ensure continuous cash flow.

8. Define *cash flow*.

_____

9. An individual who takes a patient to a private area before their visit with the provider to discuss the practice's financial policies and review the patient's insurance coverage.

_____

10. Reasons for a medical practice's large accounts receivable are:

a. _____

b. _____

c. _____

d. _____

11. Skills required for an insurance billing specialist are:

a. _____

b. _____

c. _____

d. _____

e. _____

f. _____

g. _____

h. _____

i. _____

j. _____

12. Standards of conduct by which an insurance billing specialist determines the propriety

   of his or her behavior in a relationship are known as _____.

13. Complete these statements with either the word *illegal* or *unethical*.

   a. To make critical remarks about another health care organization or physician is _____.

   b. To report incorrect information to a Medicare fiscal intermediary is _____.

14. To treat a patient with a lack of courtesy is _____. When a physician is legally

   responsible for an employee's conduct during employment, it is known as _____.

15. A claims assistance professional neglects to submit an insurance claim to a Medicare
   supplemental insurance carrier within the proper time limit. What type of insurance is
   needed for protection against this loss for the client?

   _____

Part II Multiple Choice

Choose the best answer.

16. Two billing components are facility billing and professional billing. Professional billing is done for:
   a. hospitals.
   b. skilled nursing facilities.
   c. ambulatory surgical centers.
   d. physicians.

17. *Physician extenders* are health care personnel trained
   to provide medical care under the direct or indirect
   supervision of a physician, are also referred to as:
   a. independent contractors.
   b. claims assistance professionals (CAPs).
   c. non-physician practitioners (NPPs).
   d. insurance billing specialists.

18. The individual responsible for documenting the patient's clinical notes and assigning a diagnosis code
   and procedure code for medical services rendered is
   a/an:
   a. physician.
   b. insurance biller.
   c. office manager.
   d. financial accounting clerk.

19. Insurance payers that require the provider to submit
   insurance claims for the patient are:
   a. federal and state programs.
   b. private insurance plans.
   c. managed care programs.
   d. health care insurance plans.

20. Facility billing is charging for services done by:
   a. hospitals.
   b. physicians.
   c. ambulatory surgical centers.
   d. both a and c.

5

Part III True/False

Write "T" or "F" in the blank to indicate whether you think the statement is true or false.

_____ 21. Insurance billing specialists have a well-defined scope of practice.

_____ 22. If you knowingly submit a false claim or allow such a claim to be submitted, you can be liable for a civil violation.

_____ 23. It is the coder's responsibility to inform administration or his or her immediate supervisor if unethical or illegal coding practices are occurring.

_____ 24. A claims assistant professional (CAP) can interpret insurance policies for patients.

_____ 25. Independent contractors are covered under the health care organization's professional liability insurance whom they provide services to.

CRITICAL THINKING

To enhance your critical thinking skills, problems will be interspersed throughout the *Workbook*. Thinking is the goal of instruction and a student's responsibility. When trying to solve a problem by critical thinking, it is desirable to have more than one solution and to take time to think out answers. Remember that an answer may be changed when additional information is provided in a classroom setting.

Performance Objective

Task: Describe why you are training to become an insurance billing specialist.

Conditions: Use one or two sheets of white typing paper and pen or pencil.

Standards: Time: _____ minutes

               Accuracy: _____

               (Note: The time element and accuracy criteria may be given by your instructor.)

Directions: Write one or two paragraphs describing why you are training to become an insurance billing specialist. Or, if enrolled in a class that is part of a medical assisting course, explain why you are motivated to seek a career as a medical assistant. Make sure grammar, punctuation, and spelling are correct.

Performance Objective

Task: Access the Internet and visit several websites.

Conditions: Use a computer with printer and/or pen or pencil to make notes.

Standards: Time: _____ minutes

                Accuracy: _____

                (Note: The time element and accuracy criteria may be given by your instructor.)

Directions: Use a computer and use a browser to access the Internet. Go to some search engines to locate job opportunities.

1. Access the Internet and find one of the web search engines (Yahoo, Google, Bing). Begin a web search (e.g., key in "insurance billers") to search for information about insurance billers. List three to five websites found. Go to one or more of those resources and list the benefits that those sites might have for a student in locating job opportunities or networking with others for professional growth and knowledge. Bring the website addresses to share with the class.

2. Site-search information on standards of ethical coding by visiting the website of the American Health Information Management Association (AHIMA). Download and print a hard copy of this code of ethics developed by the AHIMA. Next, obtain information on the eHealth code of ethics, and respond to the following:

   A. Write a brief definition for each of the following terms: health information, health products, and health services.

       health information: _____

       health products: _____

       health services: _____

   B. State the eight guiding principles of organizations and individuals who provide health information over the Internet.

   _____

   _____

ASSIGNMENT 1.4 COMPOSE EMAIL MESSAGES

Performance Objective

Task: Compose brief messages for electronic mail transmission after reading each scenario.

Conditions: List of scenarios, one sheet of 8½- × 11-inch plain typing paper, and a computer or a pen.

Standards: Time: _____ minutes

             Accuracy: _____

             (Note: The time element and accuracy criteria may be given by your instructor.)

Directions: Read each scenario. Compose polite, effective, and brief messages that, on the job, would be transmitted via e-mail. Use the guidelines for e-mail presented on the Evolve website. Be sure to list a descriptive subject line as the first item in each composition. Single-space the message. Insert a short signature at the end of the message to include your name and affiliation, and create an e-mail address for yourself if you do not have one. Print hard copies of e-mail messages for Scenarios 1 through 5 to give to your instructor. After the instructor has returned your work, either make the necessary corrections and place your work in a three-ring notebook for future reference or, if you received a high score, place it in your portfolio for use when applying for a job.

Scenario 1:

Ask an insurance biller, Mary Davis, in a satellite office to locate and fax you a copy of the billing done on account number 43500 for services rendered to Margarita Sylva on March 2, 20xx. Explain that you must telephone the patient about her account. Mary Davis' e-mail address is mdavis@aal.com.

Scenario 2:

Patient Ellen Worth was recently hospitalized; her hospital number is 20-9870-11. Compose an e-mail message to the medical record department at College Hospital (collegehospmedrecords@rrv.net) for her final diagnosis and the assigned diagnostic code needed to complete the insurance claim form.

Scenario 3:

You are working for a billing service and receive an encounter form that is missing the information about the patient's professional service received on August 2, 20xx. The patient's account number is 45098. You have the diagnosis data. Compose an e-mail message to Dr. Mason (pmason@email.mc.com) explaining what you must obtain to complete the billing portion of the insurance claim form.

Scenario 4:

A new patient, John Phillips, has e-mailed your office to ask what the outstanding balance is on his account. The account number is 42990. You look up the financial record and note the service was for an office visit on June 14, 20xx. The charge was $106.11. Compose an e-mail response to Mr. Phillips, whose e-mail address is jphillips@hotmail.com.

Scenario 5:

You are having difficulty deciding whether the codes 13101, 13102, and 13132 with modifier 51 selected for a case are appropriate. Compose an e-mail message that will be posted on the American Academy of Professional Coders (AAPC)'s list service (listserv) (www.aapc.com) asking for comments. The case involves a 12-year-old boy who fell against a bicycle, lacerating the left side of his chest to the pectoralis muscle through a 12-cm gaping wound. He also sustained a 5-cm laceration to his left cheek. Complex repairs were required for these two wounds and totaled 17 cm. Find out whether modifier 51 should be appended to the second code or to the third code.

For each message, check for concise composition, single-spaced message, closing signature, and accuracy and effectiveness of message in terms of scenario presented. E-mail may contain abbreviations. On the job, a biller would compose a message quickly, so the instructor might want to award additional points for the speed with which this assignment is done.

2 Privacy, Security, and HIPAA

Cheryl Fassett

KEY TERMS

Your instructor may wish to select some specific words pertinent to this chapter for a test. For definitions of the terms, further study, and/or reference, the words, phrases, and abbreviations may be found in the glossary at the end of the Textbook. *Key terms for this chapter follow.*

American Recovery and Reinvestment Act
authorization
authorization form
breach of confidential communication
business associate
clearinghouse
confidential communication
confidentiality
consent
covered entity
designated record sets
disclosure
electronic media
health care organization
Health Information Technology for Economic and Clinical Health Act
HIPAA Omnibus Rule
Incidental use and disclosure

individually identifiable health information
Minimum Necessary Rule
mitigation
National Provider Identifier
nonprivileged information
Notice of Privacy Practices
Patient Protection and Affordable Care Act
portability
preexisting condition
privacy
privacy officer, privacy official
privileged information
protected health information
psychotherapy notes
security officer
Security Rule
transaction
use

KEY ABBREVIATIONS

See how many abbreviations and acronyms you can translate, and then use this as a handy reference list. Definitions for the key abbreviations are located near the back of the Textbook *in the glossary.*

ARRA _____

DHHS _____

EIN _____

ePHI _____

FBI _____

FTP _____

HIPAA _____

HITECH _____

IIHI _____

NPI _____

NPP _____

OCR _____

OIG _____

P&P _____

PHI _____

PO _____

PPACA _____

TPO _____

PERFORMANCE OBJECTIVES

The student will be able to:

- Define and spell the key terms and key abbreviations for this chapter, given the information from the Textbook glossary, within a reasonable time period and with enough accuracy to obtain a satisfactory evaluation.
- Answer the fill in the blank, multiple choice, and true/false review questions after reading the chapter, with enough accuracy to obtain a satisfactory evaluation.
- Decide when a situation is an incidental disclosure, HIPAA violation, or neither, with sufficient information to obtain a satisfactory evaluation.
- Visit websites and site-search information via the Evolve website, with sufficient information to obtain a satisfactory evaluation.

STUDY OUTLINE

Health Information Portability and Accountability Act
Title I: Health Insurance Reform
Title II: Administrative Simplification
Defining HIPAA Roles, Relationships, and Key Terms
Transaction and Code Set Regulations
National Identifiers
The Privacy Rule: Confidentiality and Protected Health Information
Privileged and Nonprivileged Information
Patients' Rights
Obligations of the Health Care Organization
The Security Rule: Administrative, Physical, and Technical Safeguards

Health Information Technology for Economic and Clinical Health Act
Business Associates
Notification of Breach
HIPAA Compliance Audits
Increased Penalties for Noncompliance With the Provisions of HIPAA
HIPAA Omnibus Rule
Consequences of Noncompliance With HIPAA and the HITECH Act
Application to the Health Care Setting
Organization and Staff Responsibilities in Protecting Patient Rights
Best Practices to Avoid Common HIPAA Violations

Part I Fill in the Blank

Review the objectives, key terms, and chapter information before completing the following review questions.

1. What is the primary purpose of HIPAA Title I: Insurance Reform?

   _____

   _____

2. The focus on the health care practice setting and reduction of administrative costs and burdens are the goals of which part of HIPAA?

   _____

3. An independent organization that receives insurance claims from the physician's office, performs edits, and transmits claims to insurance carriers is known as a/an

   _____.

4. Name the standard code sets used for the following:

   a. Drugs and supplies _____

   b. Inpatient procedures _____

   c. Diagnosis coding _____

5. Under HIPAA guidelines, a health care coverage carrier, such as Blue Cross/Blue Shield, that transmits health information in electronic form in connection with a

   transaction is called a/an _____.

6. Dr. John Doe contracts with an outside billing company to manage claims and accounts receivable. Under HIPAA guidelines, the billing company is considered

   a/an _____ of the provider.

7. An individual designated to assist the provider by putting compliance policies and

   procedures in place and training office staff is known as a/an _____ under HIPAA guidelines.

8. If you give, release, or transfer information to another entity, it is known as

   _____.

9. Define *protected health information* (PHI).

   _____

   _____

   _____

10. Unauthorized release of a patient's health information is called _____.

11. A confidential communication related to the patient's treatment and progress that may be disclosed only with the patient's permission is known as

_____.

12. Under HIPAA, exceptions to the right of privacy are those records involving

a. _____

b. _____

c. _____

d. _____

e. _____

f. _____

g. _____

h. _____

i. _____

13. At a patient's first visit under HIPAA guidelines, the document that must be given so the patient acknowledges the provider's confidentiality of his or her PHI is the

_____.

14. If a breach of privacy is discovered, the health care provider is required to take affirmative action to respond to the breach and alleviate the severity of it. This is known as

_____.

15. Name the three main sections of the HIPAA Security Rule for protecting electronic health information.

a. _____

b. _____

c. _____

16. Name the three specific areas of significant change that resulted from the Health Information Technology for Economic and Clinical Health (HITECH) Act.

a. _____

b. _____

c. _____

Part II Multiple Choice

Choose the best answer.

17. HIPAA transaction standards apply to the following, which are called *covered entities*:
    a. health care third-party payers.
    b. health care providers.
    c. health care clearinghouses.
    d. all of the above.

18. Enforcement of the privacy standards of HIPAA is the responsibility of the:
    a. Health Care Fraud and Abuse Control Program (HCFAP).
    b. National Committee on Vital and Health Statistics (NCVHS).
    c. Office for Civil Rights (OCR).
    d. Federal Bureau of Investigation (FBI).

19. Verbal or written agreement that gives approval to some action, situation, or statement is called:
    a. authorization.
    b. consent.
    c. disclosure.
    d. release.

20. An individual's formal written permission to use or disclose his or her personally identifiable health information for purposes other than treatment, payment, or health care operations is called:
    a. authorization.
    b. disclosure.
    c. release.
    d. consent.

21. The Notice of Privacy Practices (NPP) document is given to patients:
    a. at the first visit to the practice.
    b. at every visit to the practice.
    c. on an annual basis.
    d. only on request of the patient.

22. Privacy regulations allow patients the right to obtain a copy of PHI:
    a. under all circumstances.
    b. if they have a court order.
    c. only if the health care provider has determined that it would be appropriate and would not endanger the patient or any other person.
    d. only if the patient can pay the associated fee for the copies.

23. Under HIPAA, patient sign-in sheets:
    a. are never permissible.
    b. are permissible.
    c. are permissible but limit the information that is requested.
    d. are permissible but require the practice to give the patient a number to be used when calling the patient.

24. Which section of the HIPAA Security Rule recommends unique usernames and passwords to log on to any computer with access to PHI?
    a. Administrative safeguards
    b. Technical safeguards
    c. Physical safeguards

25. Which section of the HIPAA Security Rule recommends use of screensavers that will activate after 1 to 60 minutes of inactivity?
    a. Administrative safeguards
    b. Technical safeguards
    c. Physical safeguards

26. Under HITECH, if a breach occurs, the covered entity:
    a. does not have to notify the affected party.
    b. only has to notify the affected party if they feel it is reasonable.
    c. must notify the affected party no later than 30 calendar days after the discovery of the breach.
    d. must notify the affected party no later than 60 calendar days after the discovery of the breach.

27. The HIPAA Omnibus Rule enhanced:
    a. patients' privacy rights.
    b. patients' rights to restrict immunization records to schools.
    c. health care providers' rights limiting access to patient records.
    d. business associates' rights to use and disclose patient records.

28. Measurable solutions that have been taken, based on accepted standards, and are periodically monitored to demonstrate that an office is in compliance with HIPAA privacy rules are referred to as:
    a. reasonable safeguards.
    b. privacy safeguards.
    c. security safeguards.
    d. standards.

29. A person or organization that performs a function for a covered entity but is not employed by them is a/an:
    a. business associate.
    b. clearinghouse.
    c. provider.
    d. employee.

30. Health information that does not identify the patient is called:
    a. confidential communication.
    b. nonprivileged information.
    c. de-identified health information.
    d. protected health information.

Part III True/False

Write "T" or "F" in the blank to indicate whether you think the statement is true or false.

_____ 31. Individually identifiable health information (IIHI) is any part of a person's health data (e.g., demographic information, address, date of birth) obtained from the patient that is created or received by a covered entity.

_____ 32. HIPAA requirements protect disclosure of PHI outside of the organization but do not protect against internal use of health information.

_____ 33. Under HIPAA, patients may request confidential communications and may restrict certain disclosures of PHI.

_____ 34. It is not necessary to turn documents over or lock them in a secure drawer if you are only leaving your desk for a few moments.

_____ 35. Deleting files or formatting the hard drive is sufficient to keep electronic protected health information from being accessed.

_____ 36. Under HIPAA privacy regulations, patients do not have the right to access psychotherapy notes.

_____ 37. The HITECH Act requires that business associates comply with the HIPAA Security Rule in the same manner that a covered entity would.

_____ 38. Under HITECH, civil penalties for HIPAA violations are $100 for each violation with a maximum penalty of $25,000 for all violations of the same provision in a calendar year.

_____ 39. The Federal Register publishes regulations pertaining to health care regulations.

_____ 40. The penalty for violating HIPAA and HITECH can be $100 to $50,000 or more per violation.

Performance Objective

Task: Make a decision using your best judgment after reading each case study regarding whether it should be considered an incidental disclosure, a HIPAA violation, or neither.

Conditions: Use pen or pencil.

Standards: Time: _____ minutes

                    Accuracy: _____

                    (Note: The time element and accuracy criteria may be given by your instructor.)

Directions: Read through each case study. Use your best judgment and circle whether you think it is an incidental disclosure issue (ID), a HIPAA violation (V), or neither (N). Briefly explain the answer that you selected.

Scenarios

1. Dr. Practon's office sign-in sheets ask patients to fill in their names, appointment times, and physicians' names.

    ID   V   N

    Explain:

    _____

    _____

2. It is Monday morning and you are inundated with work that needs to be done. You receive a telephone call and give patient information without confirming who is on the line.

    ID   V   N

    Explain:

    _____

    _____

3. You send a fax, but accidentally you switch the last two digits of the fax number and the patient's billing information is received in the wrong location.

    ID   V   N

    Explain:

    _____

    _____

4. You are in a high-traffic area where patients might overhear PHI, and you are careful to keep your voice down.

    ID   V   N

    Explain:

    _____

    _____

5. It is 10:30 AM, and you go on a coffee break, leaving two patients' charts on the checkout counter.

ID   V   N

Explain:

_____

_____

6. In the reception room, a patient, Martha Havasi, overhears your telephone conversation, even though you spoke quietly and shut the glass window.

ID   V   N

Explain:

_____

_____

7. You telephone a patient, Alex Massey, to remind him of tomorrow's appointment and leave a voicemail message on his answering machine.

ID   V   N

Explain:

_____

_____

8. Three patients near the reception area of the office overhear you telling another staff member that Daisy Dotson is scheduled for a Pap smear tomorrow at 4:00 PM.

ID   V   N

Explain:

_____

_____

9. You telephone a patient, Janet Hudson. She is not home, so you leave a message on her answering machine that her breast cancer biopsy results came back negative.

ID   V   N

Explain:

_____

_____

10. You call out Fran O'Donnell's complete name in the waiting room where other patients are sitting.

ID   V   N

Explain:

_____

_____

11. You do not close the glass window to the reception room when talking on the telephone with your sister.

ID   V   N

Explain:

_____

_____

12. The office nurse tells a patient, Hugo Wells, his test results in front of his relatives in a treatment area.

ID   V   N

Explain:

_____

_____

13. You leave Katy Zontag's medical chart open at the receptionist's counter.

ID   V   N

Explain:

_____

_____

14. You telephone a patient, José Ramirez, and leave your name, the physician's name, and your telephone number on his answering machine.

ID   V   N

Explain:

_____

_____

15. A patient, Kim Lee, is in the examination room and overhears a conversation concerning blood test results of another patient in an adjoining room.

ID   V   N

Explain:

_____

_____

16. While waiting in the reception room, a patient, Xavier Gomez, overhears a receptionist talking with another patient on the telephone about a colonoscopy appointment.

ID   V   N

Explain:

_____

_____

17. Betty Burton, a patient who is being weighed on the office scale by the medical assistant, overhears a conversation between an insurance billing specialist and an insurance company representative in which the billing specialist is trying to obtain preauthorization for another patient's medical procedure.

    ID   V   N

    Explain:

    _____

    _____

18. In a restaurant, a waitress overhears an insurance biller talking to a friend and telling her about a famous actress who visited her physician's office yesterday.

    ID   V   N

    Explain:

    _____

    _____

    _____

    _____

Performance Objective

Task: Access the Internet and visit several websites.

Conditions: Use a computer with printer and/or pen or pencil to make notes.

Standards: Time: _____ minutes

               Accuracy: _____

               (Note: The time element and accuracy criteria may be given by your instructor.)

Directions: Use a computer and use a browser to access the Internet. Go to some search engines to locate information.

1. Site-search information on patient confidentiality by visiting the website of the American Medical Association (www.ama-assn.org). At top of menu, click on Resources/Legal Issues and then click the link physician/hospital engagement issues. Site-search information on patient confidentiality in health care by visiting the Google search engine. Key in *patient confidentiality in health care*. Locate an article and print a hard copy to share and discuss with the class.

2. Site-search information of settled HIPAA investigations by visiting the website for the Department of Human Services/Office of Civil Rights (https://www.hhs.gov/hipaa/for-professionals/index.html). Print out a press release to share and discuss with the class.

Compliance, Fraud, and Abuse

Cheryl Fassett

KEY TERMS

Your instructor may wish to select some specific words pertinent to this chapter for a test. For definitions of the terms, further study, and/or reference, the words, phrases, and abbreviations may be found in the glossary at the end of the Textbook. *Key terms for this chapter follow.*

abuse
assumption coding
auditing
Civil False Claims Act
Civil Monetary Penalty
Clinical Laboratory Improvement Amendments
clustering
compliance
compliance plan
Comprehensive Error Rate Testing
corrective action plan
cost reports
Criminal False Claims Act
DRG creep
embezzlement
Emergency Medical Treatment and Labor Act
Federal Deposit Insurance Corporation
fraud

Fraud Enforcement and Recovery Act
Health Care Fraud Prevention and Enforcement Action Team
Health Care Fraud and Abuse Control
medical necessity
Medicare Administrative Contractor
Medicare Integrity Program
monitoring
Occupational Safety and Health Administration
Office of Inspector General
Operation Restore Trust
patient dumping
phantom bills
qui tam
Recovery Audit Contractor
Self-Disclosure Protocol
upcoding
Zone Program Integrity Contractor

KEY ABBREVIATIONS

See how many abbreviations and acronyms you can translate and then use this as a handy reference list. Definitions for the key abbreviations are located near the back of the Textbook *in the glossary.*

CERT _____

CLIA _____

CMP _____

CMS _____

DHHS _____

DOJ _____

EMTALA _____

FCA _____

FDIC _____

FERA _____

HCFAC _____

HEAT _____

MAC _____

MIP _____

OCR _____

OIG _____

ORT _____

OSHA _____

RAC _____

SDP _____

ZPIC _____

21

PERFORMANCE OBJECTIVES

The student will be able to:

■ Define and spell the key terms and key abbreviations for this chapter, given the information from the *Textbook* glossary, within a reasonable time period and with enough accuracy to obtain a satisfactory evaluation.

■ Answer the fill-in-the-blank, multiple choice, and true/false review questions after reading the chapter, with enough accuracy to obtain a satisfactory evaluation.

■ Make decisions after reading scenarios regarding whether the situations are considered fraud, abuse, or neither, with sufficient information to obtain a satisfactory evaluation.

■ Visit websites and site-search information via the Evolve website, with sufficient information to obtain a satisfactory evaluation.

STUDY OUTLINE

Compliance Defined

Fraud and Abuse Laws

    Defining Fraud and Abuse Roles, Responsibilities, and Key Terms

    Criminal False Claims Act (18 US Code §287)

    Civil False Claims Act (31 US Code §3729-3733)

    Qui Tam Provision

    Exclusion Statute (42 US Code §1320a-7)

    Stark Laws (42 US Code §1395nn)

    Anti-Kickback Statute (42 US Code §1320a-7b[b])

    Civil Monetary Penalties Law (41 US Code §1320a-7a)

    Safe Harbors

    Operation Restore Trust

    Additional Laws and Compliance

    Compliance Audits and Oversight

    Special Alerts, Bulletins, and Guidance Documents

Compliance Programs

    Increased Productivity and Decreased Penalties With Compliance Plan

    Seven Basic Components of a Compliance Plan

    Written Policies, Procedures, and Standards of Conduct

    Compliance Program Oversight

    Training and Education

    Open Lines of Communication

    Auditing, Monitoring, and Disclosure

    Consistent Discipline

    Corrective Actions

OIG Compliance Program Guidelines

    Individual and Small Group Practices

    Third-Party Medical Billing Companies

    Hospitals

Compliance as a Career

What to Expect From Your Health Care Organization

Part I Fill in the Blank

Review the objectives, key terms, and chapter information before completing the following review questions.

1. *Compliance* is the process of

   _____

   _____

2. What is the first step health insurance specialists should take toward achieving compliance so they do not violate laws, which may result in penalties or fines?

   _____

3. Indicate whether each of the following situations is one of fraud or abuse.

   a. Under the FCA, billing a claim for services not medically necessary _____

   b. Changing a figure on an insurance claim form to get increased payment _____

   c. Dismissing the copayment owed by a Medicare patient _____

   d. Neglecting to refund an overpayment to the patient _____

   e. Billing for a complex fracture when the patient suffered a simple break _____

4. The OIG publication that lists guidelines for compliance programs is the

   _____

5. CLIA certifies _____.

6. The law that prohibits self-referrals is the _____.

7. The term for providing appropriate care for the diagnosis is _____.

8. Accepting a gift for referring a patient to a specific physical therapy group is a

   _____

9. According to the Affordable Care Act, the seven steps required for an effective compliance program are:

   1) _____

   2) _____

   3) _____

   4) _____

   5) _____

   6) _____

   7) _____

10. The statute that requires the OIG to exclude individuals, providers, and health care organizations from participating in federal health care programs if they are found

    guilty of fraud or abuse is _____.

23

Part II Multiple Choice

Choose the best answer.

11. One of the agencies charged with enforcing laws that regulate the health care industry is the:
    a. Drug Enforcement Agency (DEA).
    b. Office of Inspector General (OIG).
    c. National Committee on Vital and Health Statistics (NCVHS).
    d. Department of Internal Affairs (DIA).

12. Stealing money that has been entrusted in one's care is referred to as:
    a. fraud.
    b. abuse
    c. embezzlement.
    d. obstruction.

13. Under the Criminal False Claims Act, fines and imprisonment penalties for making a false claim in connection with payment for health care benefits can be imposed on:
    a. the physician who provided the services.
    b. the health care billing specialist who prepared the claim.
    c. the health care administrator who oversees the practice or organization.
    d. anyone who knowingly and willfully participated in the scheme.

14. The FCA provision that allows a private citizen to bring civil action for a violation on behalf of the federal government and share in any money recovered is referred to as:
    a. minimum necessary.
    b. qui tam.
    c. privileged information.
    d. exclusion statute.

15. The initiative that established hotlines for the public to report issues that might indicate fraud, abuse, or waste is:
    a. Operation Restore Trust (ORT).
    b. Civil Monetary Penalty (CMP).
    c. Health Care Fraud Prevention and Enforcement Action Team (HEAT).
    d. Recovery Audit Contractor (RAC).

16. Health care providers who determine that they have submitted false claims should resolve the issue by seeking the Department of Health and Human Services (HHS) and OIG guidance established in 2006 and referred to as:
    a. Operation Restore Trust.
    b. Stark I and II.
    c. Self-Disclosure Protocol.
    d. Safe Harbor.

17. The OIG recommends that health care staff should attend trainings in "general" compliance:
    a. as part of their initial orientation.
    b. at least annually.
    c. every 6 months.
    d. every 6 years.

18. When faced with the discovery of an offense or an error, health insurance specialists should immediately report concerns:
    a. using the established chain of command outlined in their compliance plan.
    b. to the OIG through their telephone hotline.
    c. to the OIG through their e-mail address directly to the HHS.
    d. directly to the HHS.

19. Compliance is the responsibility of:
    a. physicians.
    b. coders.
    c. everyone.
    d. the compliance officer.

20. The following are parts of a well-rounded compliance program except:
    a. policies and procedures.
    b. staff education.
    c. open lines of communication.
    d. practice management software.

21. The OIG has published compliance guidelines for all of the following except:
    a. hospitals.
    b. private physician groups.
    c. patients.
    d. billing companies.

22. The law that states that emergency rooms must evaluate and stabilize patients regardless of ability to pay is called:
    a. EMTALA.
    b. The Stark Law.
    c. Anti-Kickback Statute.
    d. False Claims Act.

23. Fraudulent claims may include:
    a. multiple modifiers.
    b. unbundled codes.
    c. more than one diagnosis code.
    d. place of service codes.

24. Penalties of noncompliance may include:
    a. jail time.
    b. monetary penalties.
    c. termination.
    d. all of the above.

25. The purpose of an RAC audit is to:
    a. recoup overpayments.
    b. determine if a provider is clinically sound.
    c. investigate discrimination.
    d. all of the above.

Part III True/False

Write "T" or "F" in the blank to indicate whether you think the statement is true or false.

_____ 26. Every compliance program should include a method for employees to report issues anonymously.

_____ 27. To submit an insurance claim for medical services that were not medically necessary is a violation of the FCA.

_____ 28. Organizations who hire or contract with individuals who have been convicted of a misdemeanor or criminal offense and are on the OIG's list of excluded individuals may be subject to civil monetary penalties.

_____ 29. In the federal health care program, accepting discounts, rebates, or other types of reductions in price is encouraged.

_____ 30. Recovery audit contractors are highly motivated to find claim errors, as they are paid a percentage of the money they recover.

_____ 31. If fraud and abuse are detected, Zone Program Integrity Contractors (ZPICs) report to the Department of Justice (DOJ) for further investigation.

_____ 32. In the event of an OIG audit, the presence of an OIG compliance program will prevent any penalties and fines from being imposed.

_____ 33. Disciplinary standards for situations involving misconduct may result in termination of employment.

_____ 34. Private medical groups are exempt from CMS fraud audits.

_____ 35. In a qui tam lawsuit, the whistleblower shares in penalty money.

_____ 36. Reporting multiple codes instead of one combination code is an example of up-coding.

_____ 37. A coding or billing specialist cannot be found guilty of fraud.

_____ 38. It is fraudulent to always adjust off deductibles and coinsurance.

_____ 39. If a health care organization receives an overpayment from a third-party payer, it is compliant to apply the amount to another patient's balance.

_____ 40. When a patient is transferred from one hospital to another, it is fraudulent for the first hospital to bill for a discharge.

Performance Objective

Task: Make a decision after reading each case study regarding whether it is considered fraud, abuse, or neither.

Conditions: Use pen or pencil.

Standards: Time: _____ minutes

                 Accuracy: _____

                 (Note: The time element and accuracy criteria may be given by your instructor.)

Directions: Read through each scenario and circle whether it is a fraud (F) issue, practice of abuse (A), or neither (N). To distinguish the difference between fraud and abuse situations, remember that under the Medicare program, abuse relates to incidents or practices that are inconsistent with accepted sound business practices, whereas fraud is intentional deception that an individual knows, or should know, to be false, and the individual knows the deception could result in some unauthorized benefit to himself or herself or to some other person(s). Briefly explain the answer you selected.

Scenarios

1. Dr. Pedro Atrics has a friend whose child needs elective surgery. He agrees to perform the surgery and bill as an "insurance only" case.

     F   A   N

     Explain:

     _____

     _____

2. A patient, Carl Skinner, calls the office repeatedly about his prescriptions. When seen in the office the next time, Dr. Input bills a higher level of evaluation and management service to allow for the additional time.

     F   A   N

     Explain:

     _____

     _____

3. Dr. Skeleton sets a simple fracture and puts a cast on Mr. Davis. He bills for a complex fracture.

     F   A   N

     Explain:

     _____

     _____

4. A patient, Maria Gomez, asks a friendly staff member to change the dates on the insurance claim form. The medical assistant complies with the request.

     F   A   N

     Explain:

     _____

     _____

5. A patient, Roberto Loren, asks the physician to restate a diagnosis so the insurance company will pay because payment would be denied based on the present statement. The physician complies with the request.

F   A   N

Explain:

_____

_____

6. Dr. Rumsey sees a patient twice on the same day but bills as though the patient was seen on two different dates.

F   A   N

Explain:

_____

_____

7. A Medicare patient, Joan O'Connor, is seen by Dr. Practon, and the insurance claim shows a charge to the Medicare fiscal intermediary at a fee schedule rate higher than and different from that of non-Medicare patients.

F   A   N

Explain:

_____

_____

8. A patient, Hazel Plunkett, receives a service that is not medically necessary to the extent rendered, and an insurance claim is submitted.

F   A   N

Explain:

_____

_____

9. A patient, Sun Cho, paid for services that were subsequently declared not medically necessary, and Dr. Cardi failed to refund the payment to the patient.

F   A   N

Explain:

_____

_____

10. Dr. Ulibarri tells the insurance biller not to collect the deductible and copayments from Mrs. Gerry Coleman.

F   A   N

Explain:

_____

_____

ASSIGNMENT 3.3 VISIT WEBSITES

Performance Objective

Task: Access the Internet and visit several websites.

Conditions: Use a computer with printer and/or pen or pencil to make notes.

Standards: Time: _____ minutes

Accuracy: _____

(Note: The time element and accuracy criteria may be given by your instructor.)

Directions: Use a computer and use a browser to access the Internet. Go to some search engines to locate information.

1. Site-search for information on fraud and abuse by visiting one or more of the federal websites. See what you can discover and either print out or take notes and bring back information to share with the class for discussion.

2. Search the AAPC site (http://www.aapc.com) for their Code of Ethics. How will this support your health care organization's compliance goals?

4 Basics of Health Insurance

Cheryl Fassett

KEY TERMS

Your instructor may wish to select some words pertinent to this chapter for a test. For definitions of the terms, further study, and/or reference, the words, phrases, and abbreviations may be found in the glossary at the end of the Textbook. *Key terms for this chapter follow.*

accounts receivable management
assignment
cancelable
Civilian Health and Medical Program of the Department
    of Veterans Affairs
claim
coinsurance
competitive medical plan
conditionally renewable
Consumer Directed Health Plan
contract
coordination of benefits
copayment (copay)
daysheet
deductible
disability income insurance
emancipated minor
Exchanges
exclusions
exclusive provider organization
expressed contract
foundation for medical care
guaranteed renewable
guarantor
health maintenance organization
implied contract
Indemnity Health Insurance

independent or individual practice association
major medical
mandated benefits
Maternal and Child Health Program
Medicaid
medically necessary
Medicare
Medicare/Medicaid
noncancelable policy
nonparticipating health care organization or provider
optionally renewable
participating health care organization or provider
point-of-service plan
preauthorization
precertification
predetermination
preexisting conditions
preferred provider organization
premium
running balance
State Children's Health Insurance Program
State Disability Insurance
TRICARE
unemployment compensation disability
Veterans Health Administration (CHAMPVA)
Veterans Affairs outpatient clinic
workers' compensation insurance

29

KEY ABBREVIATIONS

See how many abbreviations and acronyms you can translate and then use this as a handy reference list. Definitions for the key abbreviations are located near the back of the Textbook *in the glossary.*

ACA _____

A/R _____

CDHP _____

CHAMPVA _____

CMP _____

COB _____

COBRA _____

DOS _____

EPO _____

FMC _____

FSA _____

HCERA _____

HDHP _____

HMO _____

HRA _____

HSA _____

IPA _____

MCHP _____

Medi-Medi _____

MSA _____

nonpar _____

NPP _____

par _____

PMS _____

POS plan _____

PPACA _____

PPO _____

ROA _____

SCHIP _____

SDHP _____

SDI _____

SHOP _____

SOF _____

UCD _____

VA _____

WC _____

PERFORMANCE OBJECTIVES

The student will be able to:

- Define and spell the key terms and key abbreviations for this chapter, given the information from the *Textbook* glossary, within a reasonable time period and with enough accuracy to obtain a satisfactory evaluation.
- Answer the fill in the blank, multiple choice, and true/false review questions after reading the chapter, with enough accuracy to obtain a satisfactory evaluation.
- Arrange 18 administrative processing steps of an insurance claim in proper sequence, given data from the textbook, within a reasonable time period and with enough accuracy to obtain a satisfactory evaluation.

- Use critical thinking to explain some of the differences in insurance key terms, given data from the textbook, within a reasonable time period and with enough accuracy to obtain a satisfactory evaluation.
- Prepare a financial accounting record, given data from the textbook, within a reasonable time period and with enough accuracy to obtain a satisfactory evaluation.
- Abstract data from some insurance identification cards, given data from the textbook, within a reasonable time period and with enough accuracy to obtain a satisfactory evaluation.

STUDY OUTLINE

Part I Fill in the Blank

Review the objectives, key terms, glossary definitions to key terms, chapter information, and figures before completing the following review questions.

1. A/an _____ is a legally enforceable agreement or contract.

2. An individual promising to pay for medical services rendered is known as a/an

   _____.

3. List five health insurance policy renewal provisions.

   a. _____

   b. _____

   c. _____

   d. _____

   e. _____

4. Insurance reimbursement or payment is also called _____.

5. Name two examples of services that are typically excluded in general health insurance policies.

   a. _____

   b. _____

6. Under PPACA, health plans must allow employees to keep their children on their

   plans until the children are _____ years old.

7. The act of determining whether treatment is covered under an individual's health

   insurance policy is called _____.

8. The procedure to obtain permission for a procedure before it is done, to determine whether the insurance program agrees it is medically necessary, is termed

   _____.

9. Determining the maximum dollar amount the insurance company will pay for a

   procedure before it is done is known as _____.

10. Name two ways an individual may obtain health insurance.

    a. _____

    b. _____

11. List four methods a health care organization may use to submit insurance claims to insurance companies.

    a. _____

    b. _____

    c. _____

    d. _____

12. A document signed by the insured directing the insurance company to pay benefits

    directly to the health care organization is known as a/an _____.

13. A patient service slip personalized to the health care organization and used as a communications/billing tool during routing of the patient, can also be referred to as the following terms.

    a. _____

    b. _____

    c. _____

    d. _____

    e. _____

    f. _____

14. For electronic access to computer data, computerized signatures may consist of the following verification or access methods:

    a. _____

    b. _____

    c. _____

    d. _____

    e. _____

    f. _____

    g. _____

15. A method of making an automatic deposit of funds from the payer into the provider's bank account and used in place of a mailed paper check is referred to as

    _____.

Part II Mix and Match

16. Match the following insurance terms in the right column with their descriptions, and fill in the blank with the appropriate letter.

_____ An insurance company considering benefits payable by another carrier in determining its own liability

_____ Transfer of one's right to collect an amount payable under an insurance contract

_____ Time that must elapse before benefits for sickness or accident become payable

_____ Acts for insurance company or insured in settlement of claims

_____ Periodic payment to keep insurance policy in force

_____ Amount insured person must pay before policy will pay

_____ Time period in which a claim must be filed

_____ Certain illnesses or injuries listed in a policy that the insurance company will not cover

_____ Insurance company that carries the insurance

_____ One who belongs to an insurance plan

a. Adjuster

b. Assignment

c. Carrier

d. Coordination of benefits (COB)

e. Deductible

f. Exclusions

g. Premium

h. Subscriber

i. Time limit

j. Waiting period

Part III Multiple Choice

Choose the best answer.

17. When a patient goes to a health care organization seeking medical services, the health care organization accepts the patient and agrees to render treatment, and both parties agree. This contract is known as a/an:
    a. expressed contract.
    b. agreed contract.
    c. implied contract.
    d. written contract.

18. The process of checking and confirming that a patient is covered under an insurance plan is known as:
    a. precertification.
    b. eligibility verification.
    c. COB.
    d. predetermination.

19. A provision that allows the policyholder the right to refuse to renew the insurance policy on a premium due date is called:
    a. conditionally renewable.
    b. guaranteed renewable.
    c. optionally renewable.
    d. noncancelable.

20. A provision in a health insurance policy in which two insurance carriers work together for payment so that there is no duplication of benefits paid between the primary insurance carrier and the secondary insurance carrier is called:
    a. copayment.
    b. coinsurance.
    c. COB.
    d. cost-share rider.

21. A type of tax-free savings account that allows individuals and their employers to set aside money to pay for health care expenses is known as:
    a. a health savings account.
    b. a medical savings account.
    c. a flexible spending account.
    d. all of the above.

22. Time limits for filing insurance claims to a commercial carrier may have a range of:
    a. 10 days from the date medical service is received to 1 year.
    b. 30 days from the date of service to 1½ years.
    c. 60 days from the date of service.
    d. no time limit.

Part IV True/False

Write "T" or "F" in the blank to indicate whether you think the statement is true or false.

_____ 23. If a health care organization belongs to a preferred provider organization (PPO) and does not follow his or her contract with the PPO, the patient is liable for the bill.

_____ 24. The birthday rule is a change in the order of determination of COB regarding primary and secondary insurance carriers for dependent children.

_____ 25. The Consolidated Omnibus Budget Reconciliation Act of 1985 (COBRA) mandates that when an employee is laid off from a company, the group health insurance coverage must continue at group rates for up to 18 months.

_____ 26. A group policy usually provides better benefits; however, the premiums are generally higher than an individual contract would be.

_____ 27. A signature stamp is acceptable by all insurances as proof of the provider's signature on a CMS-1500 claim form.

ASSIGNMENT 4.2 CRITICAL THINKING: ADMINISTRATIVE SEQUENCE OF PROCESSING AN INSURANCE CLAIM

Performance Objective

Task: Number from 1 to 18 the proper sequence of processing an insurance claim.

Conditions: Use given data and pen or pencil.

Standards: Time: _____ minutes

                 Accuracy: _____

                 (Note: The time element and accuracy criteria may be given by your instructor.)

Directions: Arrange the listed steps 1 through 18 in proper sequence by placing the correct number to the left of the statement. (Note: Each medical practice has its own order of the way office procedures are carried out; thus, these steps may vary slightly from practice to practice.)

_____ Bank deposit made and unpaid claims followed up

_____ Patient's financial account is pulled

_____ Insurance information (obtained and verified)

_____ Payer processing/payment received with explanation of benefits (EOB) document

_____ Patient's financial data posted and patient checkout

_____ Patient appointment and preregistration

_____ CMS-1500 paper claim forms submitted

_____ Provider's signature is obtained

_____ Electronic (Health Insurance Portability and Accountability Act [HIPAA] X12 837) claims transmitted

_____ Insurance claims preparation

_____ HIPAA Notice of Privacy is reviewed and signed

_____ Balance due statement mailed to patient

_____ Track pending insurance claims

_____ All required patient's signatures are obtained

_____ Assignment of benefits

_____ Medical services performed and encounter form completed

_____ Insurance identification card photocopied

_____ Full payment received and financial records retained

ASSIGNMENT 4.3 CRITICAL THINKING: DIFFERENCES IN INSURANCE KEY TERMS

Performance Objective

Task: Describe and/or explain your response to five questions.

Conditions: Use one or two sheets of white paper and pen or pencil.

Standards: Time: _____ minutes

Accuracy: _____

(Note: The time element and accuracy criteria may be given by your instructor.)

Directions: Respond verbally or in writing to these questions or statements.

1. Explain the difference between the following:

Blanket contract _____

Individual contract _____

2. Explain the difference between a participating health care organization and a nonparticipating health care organization for the following:

Commercial insurance company or managed care plan participating health care organization:

_____

Commercial insurance company or managed care plan nonparticipating health care organization:

_____

Medicare participating health care organization:

_____

Medicare nonparticipating health care organization:

_____

3. State the difference between the following:

Implied contract: _____

Expressed contract: _____

4. Explain the birthday law (rule) and when it is used.

_____

ASSIGNMENT 4.4 ABSTRACT DATA FROM AN INSURANCE IDENTIFICATION CARD

Performance Objective

Task: Answer questions in reference to an insurance identification card for Case A.

Conditions: Use an insurance identification card (Fig. 4.1), the questions presented, and pen or pencil.

Standards: Time: _____ minutes

Accuracy: _____

(Note: The time element and accuracy criteria may be given by your instructor.)

Directions: An identification card provides much of the information needed to establish a patient's insurance coverage. You have photocopied the front and back sides of three patients' cards and placed copies in their patient records, returning the originals to the patients. Answer the questions by abstracting or obtaining the data from the cards.

CASE A

1. Name of patient covered by the policy. _____

2. Provide the insurance policy's effective date. _____

3. List the telephone number for preauthorization. _____

4. State name and address of insurance company. _____

5. List the telephone number to call for provider access. _____

6. Name the type of insurance plan. _____

7. List the insurance identification number (e.g., subscriber, certificate, or member numbers) _____

_____.

8. Furnish the group number. _____ Plan or coverage code. _____

9. State the copay requirements. _____

10. Does the card indicate the patient has hospital coverage?

_____

Fig. 4.1

ASSIGNMENT 4.5 ABSTRACT DATA FROM AN INSURANCE IDENTIFICATION CARD

Performance Objective

Task: Answer questions in reference to the insurance identification card for Case B.

Conditions: Use an insurance identification card (Fig. 4.2), the questions presented, and pen or pencil.

Standards: Time: _____ minutes

                  Accuracy: _____

                  (Note: The time element and accuracy criteria may be given by your instructor.)

CASE B

1. Name of patient covered by the policy. _____

2. Provide the insurance policy's effective date. _____

3. List the telephone number for preauthorization. _____

4. State name of insurance company. _____

5. List the telephone number to call for patient benefits and eligibility. _____

6. Name the type of insurance plan. _____

7. List the insurance identification number (e.g., subscriber, certificate, or member numbers). _____
_____

8. Furnish the group number. _____ Plan or coverage code. _____

9. State the copay requirements, if any. _____

10. List the Blue Shield website. _____

Preferred Plan

PPO

SUBSCRIBER NAME:

M T FORDHAM

EFFECTIVE DATE:

010120XX

SUBSCRIBER ID NUMBER

AJC557469969

GROUP NUMBER

00P1901

PLAN CODE

542

CUSTOMER SERVICE

(800) 331-2001

07/16/20XX

Use Blue Shield of California Preferred Physicians and Hospitals to receive maximum benefits.

Carry the Blue Shield Identification Card with you at all times and present it whenever you or one of your covered dependents receives medical services. Read your employee booklet/Health Services Agreement which summarizes the benefits, provisions, limitations and exclusions of your plan. Your health plan may require prior notification of any hospitalization and notification, within one business day, of an emergency admission. Review of selected procedures may be required before some services are performed. To receive hospital pre-admission and pre-service reviews, call 1-800-343-1691. Your failure to call may result in a reduction of benefits.

For questions, including those related to benefits, and eligibility, call the customer service number listed on the front of this card.

The PPO logo on the front of this ID Card identifies you to preferred providers outside the state of California as a member of the Blue Card PPO Program.

When you are outside of California call 1-800-810-2583 to locate the nearest PPO Provider. Remember, any services you receive are subject to the policies and provisions of your group plan.

ID-23200-PPO REVERSE   www.blueshieldca.com

Fig. 4.2

Performance Objective

Task: Answer questions in reference to the insurance identification card for Case C.

Conditions: Use an insurance identification card (Fig. 4.3), the questions presented, and pen or pencil.

Standards: Time: _____ minutes

Accuracy: _____

(Note: The time element and accuracy criteria may be given by your instructor.)

CASE C

1. Name of patient covered by the policy. _____

2. Provide the insurance policy's effective date, if there is one. _____

3. List the number to call for out-of-network preauthorization. _____

4. State name and address of insurance company. _____

5. List the telephone number to call for member inquiries. _____

6. Name the type of insurance plan. _____

7. List the insurance identification number (e.g., subscriber, certificate, or member numbers). _____

8. Furnish the group number. _____

9. State the copay requirements, if any. _____

10. Who is the patient's primary care physician? _____

UNITEDhealthcare

LINDA L. FLORES
Member # 52170-5172

CALMAT

Group # 176422
COPAY: Office Visit $10 ER $50
   Urgent $35

Electronic Claims Payor ID 87726

Call 800-842-5751 for Member Inquiries

POS PCP Plan
WITH RX D - UHC
and MH/CD
PCP: G. LOMAN
805-643-9973

MTH

This identification card is not proof of membership nor does it guarantee coverage. Persons with coverage that remains in force are entitled to benefits under the terms and conditions of this group health benefit plan as detailed in your benefit description.

IMPORTANT MEMBER INFORMATION
In non-emergencies, call your Primary Care Physician to receive the highest level of benefits. If you have an emergency and are admitted to a hospital, you are required to call your Primary Care Physician within two working days.
For out of network services that require authorization, call the Member Inquiries 800 number on the front of this card.

Claim Address: P.O. Box 30990, Salt Lake City, UT 84130-0990

Fig. 4.3

5 The Blue Plans, Private Insurance, and Managed Care Plans

Linda M. Smith

KEY TERMS

Your instructor may wish to select some words pertinent to this chapter for a test. For definitions of the terms, further study, and/or reference, the words, phrases, and abbreviations may be found in the glossary at the end of the Textbook. *Key terms for this chapter follow.*

ancillary services
Blue Cross/Blue Shield Association
buffing
capitation
churning
coinsurance
copayment
deductible
direct referral
disenrollment
exclusive provider organization
fee-for-service
formal referral
gatekeeper
group practice model
health maintenance organization
indemnity insurance plan
independent (or individual) practice association

managed care
participating physician
per capita
physician provider group
point-of-service plan
preferred provider organization
prepaid group practice model
primary care physician
private health insurance
self-referral
staff model
stop-loss
tertiary care
traditional insurance plan
turfing
utilization review
verbal referral
withhold

KEY ABBREVIATIONS

See how many abbreviations and acronyms you can translate and then use this as a handy reference list. Definitions for the key abbreviations are located near the back of the Textbook *in the glossary.*

BCBSA _____

copay _____

_____

EPO _____

_____

_____

HMO _____

IPA _____

MCO _____

NCQA _____

PCP _____

POS _____

PPG _____

PPO _____

_____

QISMC _____

UR _____

PERFORMANCE OBJECTIVES

The student will be able to:

- Define and spell the key terms and key abbreviations for this chapter, given the information from the *Textbook* glossary, within a reasonable time period and with enough accuracy to obtain a satisfactory evaluation.
- After reading the chapter, answer the fill in the blank, multiple choice, and true/false review questions with enough accuracy to obtain a satisfactory evaluation.

- Complete treatment authorization forms of managed care plans, given completed new patient information forms, within a reasonable time period and with enough accuracy to obtain a satisfactory evaluation.

STUDY OUTLINE

Private Health Insurance
    Blue Cross and Blue Shield Plans
    Fee-for-Service Plans
Managed Care
Managed Care Systems
    Health Maintenance Organizations
    Preferred Provider Organizations
    Exclusive Provider Organizations
    Point-of-Service Plans
    Physician Provider Groups
    Triple-Option Health Plans
    Provider-Sponsored Organization
    Consumer Directed Health Plans
Medical Review
    Quality Improvement System for Managed Care
    Utilization Review of Management

Management of Plans
    Contracts
Plan Administration
    Patient Information Letter
    Preauthorization or Prior Approval
    Diagnostic Tests
    Managed Care Guide
Financial Management
    Payment
    Statement of Remittance
    Accounting
    Fee-for-Service
    Year-End Evaluation
    Bankruptcy

Part I Fill in the Blank

Review the objectives, key terms, glossary definitions of key terms, figures, and chapter information before completing the following review questions.

1. An insurance plan requires the insured to pay a fixed monthly premium. The insurance that will pay the health care organization for services each time the service is rendered is referred to as

   _____.

2. A group of techniques used by insurance companies to reduce the cost of providing health care while improving access to care and the quality of care is referred to as

   _____.

3. What type of medical insurance provides coverage of health services for a prepaid fixed annual fee and requires enrollees to seek services through a panel of providers

   contracted with the insurance company? _____.

4. A not-for-profit organization that has built a set of standards to which health plans attest that they have met key elements required by state and federal laws allowing

   them to participate in managed care programs is called _____.

5. In a managed care setting, a primary care physician who controls patient access to

   specialists and diagnostic testing services is known as a/an _____.

6. Name four types of health maintenance organization (HMO) models.

   a. _____

   b. _____

   c. _____

   d. _____

7. If a physician or hospital in a managed care plan is paid a fixed, per capita amount for each patient enrolled, regardless of the type and number of services rendered, this is a payment system known as

   _____.

8. A health benefit program in which enrollees may choose any physician or hospital for services but obtain a higher level of benefits if preferred providers are used is known

   as a/an _____.

9. HMOs and preferred provider organizations (PPOs) consisting of a network of physicians and hospitals that provide an insurance company or employer with discounts

   on their services are referred to collectively as a/an _____.

10. To control health care costs, the process of reviewing and establishing medical necessity

    for services and providers' use of medical care resources is termed _____

    _____.

11. Explain the meaning of a "stop-loss" provision that might appear in a managed care contract.

_____

_____

12. When a certain percentage of the monthly capitation payment or a percentage of the allowable charges to physicians is set aside to operate a managed care plan, it is known as a/an

_____.

Part II Multiple Choice

Choose the best answer.

13. A specified dollar amount that the patient must pay annually before an insurance plan begins covering health care costs is called:
    a. coinsurance.
    b. copayment.
    c. deductible.
    d. withhold.

14. A type of managed care plan regulated under insurance statutes that combines features of HMOs and PPOs and requires that employers agree not to contract with any other plan is known as a/an:
    a. independent practice association (IPA).
    b. exclusive provider organization (EPO).
    c. physician provider group (PPG).
    d. point-of-service (POS) plan.

15. Which of the following is a term used in utilization review when the sickest high-cost patients are transferred to other physicians?
    a. Churning
    b. Turfing
    c. Buffing
    d. Carving

16. Medical services that are not included in a managed care contract's capitation rate but that may be contracted for separately are referred to as:
    a. carve outs.
    b. stop-loss limits.
    c. payment mechanisms.
    d. copayments.

17. When the primary care physician informs the patient and telephones the referring physician that the patient is being referred for an appointment, it is called a:
    a. direct referral.
    b. formal referral.
    c. self-referral.
    d. verbal referral.

18. Plan-specified facilities listed in managed care plan contracts where patients are required to have laboratory and radiology tests performed are called:
    a. hospital facilities.
    b. medical facilities.
    c. network facilities.
    d. outside facilities.

19. A type of payment model in which the patient pays a monthly or annual fee to the physician is known as:
    a. capitation.
    b. cash only practice.
    c. concierge medicine.
    d. copayment.

20. A value-based reimbursement model in which providers receive performance-based incentives to share cost savings combined with disincentives to share the excess costs of health care delivery is called:
    a. shared risk.
    b. shared savings.
    c. one-sided risk.
    d. full risk.

Part III True/False

Write "T" or "F" in the blank to indicate whether you think the statement is true or false.

_____ 21. Private health insurances are government-sponsored programs.

_____ 22. Blue Cross plans provide health care coverage for hospital expenses.

_____ 23. All managed care plans are alike.

_____ 24. A provider-sponsored organization is a managed care plan that can be owned and operated by a hospital rather than an insurance company.

_____ 25. Consumer-driven health plans (CDHP) are referred to as low deductible plans.

_____ 26. The Quality Improvement System for Managed Care (QISMC) provides oversight and ensures accountability of managed care programs.

_____ 27. Obtaining preapproval for services always ensures payment of a claim by the insurance company.

_____ 28. Value-based reimbursement programs reward health care providers with incentive payments for the quality of care they provide.

_____ 29. When a health care organization agrees to accept a single negotiated fee to deliver all medical services related a patient's hip replacement surgery, it is referred to as *pay for performance.*

ASSIGNMENT 5.2 OBTAIN AUTHORIZATION FOR A CONSULTATION FROM A MANAGED CARE PLAN

Performance Objective

Task: Complete a treatment authorization form to obtain permission for an office consultation for a patient covered by a managed care plan.

Conditions: Use a treatment authorization form (Fig. 5.1), a new patient information form (Fig. 5.2), a computer, and a printer.

Standards: Time: _____ minutes

Accuracy: _____

(Note: The time element and accuracy criteria may be given by your instructor.)

Directions: Complete a treatment authorization form (see Fig. 5.1) for Mrs. Cohn's managed care plan to obtain permission for the office consultation and date it August 2 of the current year. To obtain information, refer to the New Patient Information form completed by Mrs. Cohn when she came into the office for her visit with Dr. Practon (see Fig. 5.2). Dr. Practon's Family Health Plan provider number is FHP C01402X.

Scenario: Meriweather B. Cohn's primary care physician, Dr. Gerald Practon, took her clinical history. Physical examination revealed a normal blood pressure (120/80); however, abnormal heart sounds were heard, and a diagnosis of a heart murmur was made. Dr. Practon decided to make a semiurgent request to refer Mrs. Cohn for a cardiac consultation (other service) to Dr. Victor M. Salazar, whose office is located at 20 Excalibur Street, Woodland Hills, XY 12345, and whose office telephone number is 555-625-7344. Dr. Salazar will take a detailed history, perform a detailed examination, and make low-complexity medical decisions to evaluate Mrs. Cohn's heart murmur.

After the instructor has returned your work to you, either make the necessary corrections and place your work in a three-ring notebook for future reference or, if you receive a high score, place it in your portfolio for reference when applying for a job.

IPA TREATMENT AUTHORIZATION FORM

FHP® HEALTH CARE

____ Referral
____ Participating
____ Nonparticipating
____ Commercial
____ Senior

For Billing Instructions, Patient and Nonaffiliated Providers, and Consultants please see reverse side for instructions

THIS PORTION COMPLETED BY PHYSICIAN

Patient Name _____ Date _____ / _____ / _____

M _____ F _____ Age _____ FHP # _____ Home Phone _____

Address _____

Primary Care MD_____ Primary Care MD's FHP # _____

Referring MD _____ Referring MD's FHP # _____

Referred To _____ Address _____

_____ Office Phone _____

Type of Service: ☐ In-Patient ☐ Out-Patient Services ☐ Initial Visit ☐ Return Visit ☐ Other

Clinical History and Findings _____

_____

_____

Diagnosis _____

ICD-10-CM CODE

Evaluation and Treatment to Date _____

_____

_____

Procedure _____

RVS CPT-4 CODE

Reason for Referral/Consultation/Procedure _____

_____

Accident: ☐ Yes ☐ No   Where Occurred: ☐ Home ☐ Work ☐ Auto ☐ Other
☐ Urgent ☐ Semi-Urgent ☐ Elective

Facility to be Used: _____ Estimated Length of Stay _____
☐ Office ☐ Out-Patient ☐ In-Patient

THIS PORTION COMPLETED BY FHP UR

THIS AUTHORIZATION GOOD FOR 60 DAYS ONLY

Type of Contract: ☐ Capitation ☐ Fee For Service ☐ Per Diem

Projected Cost of Procedure _____ Projected Cost of Facility _____

HMO Verification: Effective _____ Group # _____

Benefits: Co-Pay Per Visit _____ Hospital _____

Limitations: _____

_____ Authorized   Date _____ Initials _____ Reason _____ Authorization #_____

_____ Deferred   Date _____ Initials _____ Reason _____

_____ Denied   Date _____ Initials _____ Reason _____

_____ Modified   Date _____ Initials _____ Reason _____

WHITE – UR Copy   CANARY – Hospital Copy   PINK – Physician Copy   GOLDENROD – Claims Copy

Fig. 5.1

49

Welcome To Our Office

NEW PATIENT INFORMATION

DATE ___8-2-20xx___

PATIENT'S NAME (PLEASE PRINT) Meriweather B. Cohn	S.S. # 430-XX-0261	MARITAL STATUS S [X]M W D SEP	SEX M [X]	BIRTH DATE 11-14-65	AGE	RELIGION (optional)

STREET ADDRESS PERMANENT TEMPORARY 267 Blake Street	CITY AND STATE Woodland Hills XY	ZIP CODE 12345	HOME PHONE # 555-263-0911

PATIENT'S OR PARENT'S EMPLOYER Sun Corporation	OCCUPATION (INDICATE IF STUDENT) sales representative	HOW LONG EMPLOYED 5 yrs	BUS. PHONE # EXT # 555-263-0099

EMPLOYER'S STREET ADDRESS 74 Rain Street	CITY AND STATE Woodland Hills XY	ZIP CODE 12345

DRUG ALLERGIES, IF ANY
Penicillin

SPOUSE OR PARENT'S NAME Starkweather L. Cohn	S.S. # 273-XX-9961	BIRTH DATE 7-9-63

SPOUSE OR PARENT'S EMPLOYER B & L Stormdrain Co.	OCCUPATION (INDICATE IF STUDENT) accountant	HOW LONG EMPLOYED 10 yrs	BUS. PHONE # 555-421-0091

EMPLOYER'S STREET ADDRESS 20 South Wind Road	CITY AND STATE Woodland Hills XY	ZIP CODE 12345

*SPOUSE'S STREET ADDRESS, IF DIVORCED OR SEPARATED	CITY AND STATE	ZIP CODE	HOME PHONE #

PLEASE READ: ALL CHARGES ARE DUE AT THE TIME OF SERVICES. IF HOSPITALIZATION IS INDICATED, THE PATIENT IS RESPONSIBLE FOR FURNISHING INSURANCE CLAIM FORMS TO THE OFFICE PRIOR TO HOSPITALIZATION.

PERSON RESPONSIBLE FOR PAYMENT, IF NOT ABOVE	STREET ADDRESS, CITY, STATE	ZIP CODE	HOME PHONE #

BLUE SHIELD (GIVE NAME OF POLICYHOLDER) [ ]	EFFECTIVE DATE	CERTIFICATE #	GROUP #	COVERAGE CODE

OTHER (WRITE IN NAME OF INSURANCE COMPANY) [ ] FHP Healthcare	EFFECTIVE DATE 1-1-8X	POLICY # FHP # A4932

OTHER (WRITE IN NAME OF INSURANCE COMPANY) [ ]	EFFECTIVE DATE	POLICY #

MEDICARE (PLEASE GIVE NUMBER) [ ]	RAILROAD RETIREMENT (PLEASE GIVE NUMBER) [ ]

MEDICAID [ ]	EFFECTIVE DATE	PROGRAM #	COUNTY #	CASE #	ACCOUNT #

INDUSTRIAL [ ]	WERE YOU INJURED ON THE JOB? [ ] YES [X] NO	DATE OF INJURY	INDUSTRIAL CLAIM #

ACCIDENT [ ]	WAS AN AUTOMOBILE INVOLVED? [ ] YES [X] NO	DATE OF ACCIDENT	NAME OF ATTORNEY

WERE X-RAYS TAKEN OF THIS INJURY OR PROBLEM? [ ] YES [X] NO	IF YES, WHERE WERE X-RAYS TAKEN? (HOSPITAL, ETC)	DATE X-RAYS TAKEN

HAS ANY MEMBER OF YOUR IMMEDIATE FAMILY BEEN TREATED BY OUR PHYSICIAN(S) BEFORE? INCLUDE NAME OF PHYSICIAN AND FAMILY MEMBER
No

REFERRED BY BREEZIE N. CLOUD	STREET ADDRESS, CITY, STATE 521 N. Wind Rd, Woodland Hills XY	ZIP CODE 12345	PHONE # 555-721-9641

ALL PROFESSIONAL SERVICES RENDERED ARE CHARGED TO THE PATIENT. NECESSARY FORMS WILL BE COMPLETED TO HELP EXPEDITE INSURANCE CARRIER PAYMENTS. HOWEVER, THE PATIENT IS RESPONSIBLE FOR ALL FEES, REGARDLESS OF INSURANCE COVERAGE. IT IS ALSO CUSTOMARY TO PAY FOR SERVICES WHEN RENDERED UNLESS OTHER ARRANGEMENTS HAVE BEEN MADE IN ADVANCE WITH OUR OFFICE BOOKKEEPER.

INSURANCE AUTHORIZATION AND ASSIGNMENT

Name of Policy Holder ___Meriweather B. Cohn___   HC Number _____

I request that payment of authorized Medicare/Other Insurance company benefits be made either to me or on my behalf to ___College Clinic___ for any services furnished me by that party who accepts assignment/physician. Regulations pertaining to Medicare assignment of benefits apply.

I authorize any holder of medical or other information about me to release to the Social Security Administration and Health Care Financing Administration or its intermediaries or carrier or any other insurance company any information needed for this or a related Medicare/Other Insurance company claim.

I understand my signature requests that payment be made and authorizes release of medical information necessary to pay the claim. If item 9 of the HCFA-1500 claim form is completed, my signature authorizes releasing of the information to the insurer or agency shown. In Medicare/Other Insurance company assigned cases, the physician or supplier agrees to accept the charge determination of the Medicare/Other Insurance company as the full charge, and the patient is responsible only for the deductible, coinsurance, and noncovered services. Coinsurance and the deductible are based upon the charge determination of the Medicare/Other Insurance company.

Signature ___Meriweather B. Cohn___   Date ___8-2-20XX___

NEW PATIENT INFORMATION

Fig. 5.2

ASSIGNMENT 5.3 OBTAIN AUTHORIZATION FOR PHYSICAL THERAPY FROM A MANAGED CARE PLAN

Performance Objective

Task: Complete a treatment authorization form to obtain permission for physical therapy for a patient covered by a managed care plan.

Conditions: Use a treatment authorization form (Fig. 5.3), computer, and printer.

Standards: Time: _____ minutes

                   Accuracy: _____

                   (Note: The time element and accuracy criteria may be given by your instructor.)

Directions: Complete the treatment authorization form for this patient (see Fig. 5.3), date it July 7 of the current year, and submit it to the managed care plan. Refer to Fig. 5.2 in the *Textbook* for visual guidance.

Scenario: Mrs. Rosario Jimenez comes into Dr. Gerald Practon's office complaining of neck pain. Mrs. Jimenez is a member of the managed care program HealthNet, and Dr. Practon is her primary care physician. Mrs. Jimenez lives at 350 South Carib Street, Woodland Hills, XY 12345-0003. Her telephone number is 555-450-9987, and she was born April 6, 1960. Her plan identification number is JIM40896, and the effective date is January 1, 20xx. After taking a history, completing a physical examination, and taking and reviewing radiographs, Dr. Practon makes a diagnosis of cervical radiculitis. He gives Mrs. Jimenez a prescription for some medication and says it is necessary to order outpatient physical therapy (one area, for 15 minutes; therapeutic exercises to develop strength, motion, and flexibility) twice a week for 6 weeks at College Hospital. Authorization must be obtained for this treatment. Dr. Practon's HealthNet provider number is HN C01402X.

After the instructor has returned your work to you, either make the necessary corrections and place your work in a three-ring notebook for future reference or, if you receive a high score, place it in your portfolio for reference when applying for a job.

College Clinic
4567 Broad Avenue
Woodland Hills, XY 12345-0001
Telephone No. (555) 487-8976
Fax No. (555) 487-8976

MANAGED CARE PLAN AUTHORIZATION REQUEST

❑ Health Net   ❑ Met Life
❑ Pacificare   ❑ Travelers
❑ Secure Horizons   ❑ Pru Care
❑ Other

Member/Group No.

TO BE COMPLETED BY PRIMARY CARE PHYSICIAN OR OUTSIDE PROVIDER

Patient Name_____ Date_____

❑ Male ❑ Female Birthdate_____ Home Telephone Number _____

Address _____

Primary Care Physician _____ NPI_____

Referring Physician _____ NPI_____

Referred to _____ NPI_____

Address _____ Telephone No. _____

Diagnosis Code _____ Diagnosis _____

Diagnosis Code _____ Diagnosis _____

Treatment Plan _____

Authorization Requested for: ❑ Consult Only   ❑ Treatment Only   ❑ Consult/Treatment
                              ❑ Consult/Procedure/Surgery   ❑ Diagnostic Tests

Procedure Code: _____ Description: _____

Procedure Code: _____ Description: _____

Place of Service ❑ Office ❑ Outpatient ❑ Inpatient ❑ Other   Number of Visits:_____

Facility: _____ Length of Stay:_____

Physician's Signature: _____

TO BE COMPLETED BY PRIMARY CARE PHYSICIAN

PCP Recommendations: _____ PCP Initials: _____

Date Eligibility Checked: _____

TO BE COMPLETED BY UTILIZATION MANAGEMENT

Authorized: _____ Auth. No:_____ Not Authorized _____

Deferred: _____ Modified: _____

Effective Date: _____ Expiration Date: _____ No. of Visits: _____

Fig. 5.3

ASSIGNMENT 5.4 OBTAIN AUTHORIZATION FOR DIAGNOSTIC ARTHROSCOPY FROM A MANAGED CARE PLAN

Performance Objective

Task: Complete a treatment authorization form to obtain permission for diagnostic arthroscopy with debridement for a patient covered by a managed care plan.

Conditions: Use a treatment authorization form (Fig. 5.4), computer, and printer.

Standards: Time: _____ minutes

Accuracy: _____

(Note: The time element and accuracy criteria may be given by your instructor.)

Directions: Complete the treatment authorization form for this patient (see Fig. 5.4), date it August 12 of the current year, and submit it to the managed care plan. Refer to Fig. 5.2 in the *Textbook* for visual guidance.

Scenario: Daniel Chan has been referred by his primary care physician, Dr. Gerald Practon, to an orthopedic surgeon, Dr. Raymond Skeleton. Both physicians are members of his managed care plan, Metropolitan Life. The patient comes into Dr. Skeleton's office complaining of pain, swelling, and crepitus of the right knee. The patient is having difficulty walking but indicates no recent injury to the knee.

Mr. Chan lives at 226 West Olive Avenue, Woodland Hills, XY 12345-0001, and his telephone number is 555-540-6700. His plan identification number is FTW90876, effective February 1, 20xx, and he was born February 23, 1971.

After taking a history, completing a physical examination, and taking and reviewing radiographs, Dr. Skeleton suspects the patient has a tear of the medial meniscus and may require débridement of articular cartilage. This procedure will be performed on an outpatient basis at College Hospital. Authorization must be obtained for the surgical arthroscopy with débridement of articular cartilage. Dr. Practon's Metropolitan Life provider number is ML C01402X and Dr. Skeleton's Metropolitan Life provider number is ML C4561X.

After the instructor has returned your work to you, either make the necessary corrections and place your work in a three-ring notebook for future reference or, if you received a high score, place it in your portfolio for reference when applying for a job.

College Clinic
4567 Broad Avenue
Woodland Hills, XY 12345-0001
Telephone No. (555) 487-8976
Fax No. (555) 487-8976

MANAGED CARE PLAN AUTHORIZATION REQUEST

❑ Health Net	❑ Met Life
❑ Pacificare	❑ Travelers
❑ Secure Horizons	❑ Pru Care
❑ Other	

Member/Group No. _____

TO BE COMPLETED BY PRIMARY CARE PHYSICIAN OR OUTSIDE PROVIDER

Patient Name _____ Date _____

❑ Male ❑ Female   Birthdate _____ Home Telephone Number _____

Address _____

Primary Care Physician _____ NPI _____

Referring Physician _____ NPI _____

Referred to _____ NPI _____

Address _____ Telephone No. _____

Diagnosis Code _____ Diagnosis _____

Diagnosis Code _____ Diagnosis _____

Treatment Plan _____

Authorization Requested for: ❑ Consult Only   ❑ Treatment Only   ❑ Consult/Treatment
                               ❑ Consult/Procedure/Surgery   ❑ Diagnostic Tests

Procedure Code: _____ Description: _____

Procedure Code: _____ Description: _____

Place of Service ❑ Office ❑ Outpatient ❑ Inpatient ❑ Other   Number of Visits: _____

Facility: _____ Length of Stay: _____

Physician's Signature: _____

TO BE COMPLETED BY PRIMARY CARE PHYSICIAN

PCP Recommendations: _____ PCP Initials: _____

Date Eligibility Checked: _____

TO BE COMPLETED BY UTILIZATION MANAGEMENT

Authorized: _____ Auth. No: _____ Not Authorized _____

Deferred: _____ Modified: _____

Effective Date: _____ Expiration Date: _____ No. of Visits: _____

Fig. 5.4

ASSIGNMENT 5.5 OBTAIN AUTHORIZATION FOR CONSULTATION FROM A MANAGED CARE PLAN

Performance Objective

Task: Complete a treatment authorization form to obtain permission for consultation for a patient from a managed care plan.

Conditions: Use a treatment authorization form (Fig. 5.5), computer, and printer.

Standards: Time: _____ minutes

Accuracy: _____

(Note: The time element and accuracy criteria may be given by your instructor.)

Directions: Complete the treatment authorization form for this patient (see Fig. 5.5), date it September 3 of the current year, and submit it to the managed care plan. Refer to Fig. 5.2 in the *Textbook* for visual guidance.

Scenario: Frederico Fellini, with a history of getting up four times during the night with a slow urinary stream, was seen by his primary care physician, Dr. Gerald Practon. An intravenous pyelogram yielded negative results except for distention of the urinary bladder. Physical examination of the prostate showed an enlargement. The preliminary diagnosis is benign prostatic hypertrophy (BPH).

The patient will be referred to Dr. Douglas Lee, a urologist, for consultation (Level 4) and cystoscopy. Transurethral resection of the prostate is possible at a future date. Dr. Lee's address is 4300 Cyber Street, Woodland Hills, XY 12345, and his office telephone number is 555-675-3322. His National Provider Identifier (NPI) is 55026717XX.

Dr. Practon's managed care contract is with PruCare, identification number PC C01402X, of which this patient is a member.

Mr. Fellini lives at 476 Miner Street, Woodland Hills, XY 12345, and his telephone number is 555-679-0098. His PruCare plan identification number is VRG87655, effective January 1, 20xx. His birth date is May 24, 1944.

After the instructor has returned your work to you, either make the necessary corrections and place your work in a three-ring notebook for future reference or, if you received a high score, place it in your portfolio for reference when applying for a job.

College Clinic
4567 Broad Avenue
Woodland Hills, XY 12345-0001
Telephone No. (555) 487-8976
Fax No. (555) 487-8976

MANAGED CARE PLAN AUTHORIZATION REQUEST

❑ Health Net	❑ Met Life
❑ Pacificare	❑ Travelers
❑ Secure Horizons	❑ Pru Care
❑ Other	

Member/Group No.

TO BE COMPLETED BY PRIMARY CARE PHYSICIAN OR OUTSIDE PROVIDER

Patient Name_____ Date_____

❑ Male ❑ Female Birthdate_____ Home Telephone Number _____

Address _____

Primary Care Physician _____ NPI_____

Referring Physician _____ NPI_____

Referred to _____ NPI_____

Address _____ Telephone No. _____

Diagnosis Code _____ Diagnosis _____

Diagnosis Code _____ Diagnosis _____

Treatment Plan _____

Authorization Requested for: ❑ Consult Only ❑ Treatment Only ❑ Consult/Treatment

❑ Consult/Procedure/Surgery ❑ Diagnostic Tests

Procedure Code: _____ Description: _____

Procedure Code: _____ Description: _____

Place of Service ❑ Office ❑ Outpatient ❑ Inpatient ❑ Other   Number of Visits: _____

Facility: _____ Length of Stay: _____

Physician's Signature: _____

TO BE COMPLETED BY PRIMARY CARE PHYSICIAN

PCP Recommendations: _____ PCP Initials: _____

Date Eligibility Checked: _____

TO BE COMPLETED BY UTILIZATION MANAGEMENT

Authorized: _____ Auth. No:_____ Not Authorized _____

Deferred: _____ Modified: _____

Effective Date: _____ Expiration Date: _____ No. of Visits: _____

Fig. 5.5

ASSIGNMENT 5.6 OBTAIN AUTHORIZATION FOR DIAGNOSTIC BODY SCAN FROM A MANAGED CARE PLAN

Performance Objective

Task: Complete a treatment authorization form to obtain permission for diagnostic complete body bone scan and mammogram for a patient covered by a managed care plan.

Conditions: Use a treatment authorization form (Fig. 5.6), computer, and printer.

Standards: Time: _____ minutes

Accuracy: _____

(Note: The time element and accuracy criteria may be given by your instructor.)

Directions: Complete the treatment authorization form for this patient (see Fig. 5.6), date it October 23 of the current year, and submit it to the managed care plan. Refer to Fig. 5.2 in the *Textbook* for visual guidance.

Scenario: A patient, Debbie Dye, sees her primary care physician, Dr. Gerald Practon, for complaint of midback pain. She underwent a lumpectomy 2 years ago for a malignant neoplasm of the lower left breast; thus she has a history of breast cancer. She has been referred by Dr. Practon (PacifiCare identification number PC C01402X) to Dr. Donald Patos, an oncologist, for a complete workup. He finds that her complaint of midback pain warrants the need to refer her to XYZ Radiology for bilateral diagnostic mammography and a complete body bone scan.

Dr. Patos' address is 4466 East Canter Drive, Woodland Hills, XY 12345, and his office telephone number is 555-980-5566. Dr. Patos' PacifiCare identification number is PC 5673X. His NPI is 6520101678XX.

Ms. Dye lives at 6700 Flora Road, Woodland Hills, XY 12345, and her telephone number is 555-433-6755. Her PacifiCare plan identification number is SR45380, effective January 1, 20xx. Her birth date is August 6, 1952.

XYZ Radiology's address is 4767 Broad Avenue, Woodland Hills, XY 12345-0001, and the office telephone number is 555-486-9162.

After the instructor has returned your work to you, either make the necessary corrections and place your work in a three-ring notebook for future reference or, if you received a high score, place it in your portfolio for reference when applying for a job.

College Clinic
4567 Broad Avenue
Woodland Hills, XY 12345-0001
Telephone No. (555) 487-8976
Fax No. (555) 487-8976

MANAGED CARE PLAN AUTHORIZATION REQUEST

❑ Health Net	❑ Met Life
❑ Pacificare	❑ Travelers
❑ Secure Horizons	❑ Pru Care
❑ Other	

Member/Group No.

TO BE COMPLETED BY PRIMARY CARE PHYSICIAN OR OUTSIDE PROVIDER

Patient Name_____ Date_____

❑ Male ❑ Female Birthdate_____ Home Telephone Number _____

Address _____

Primary Care Physician _____ NPI_____

Referring Physician _____ NPI_____

Referred to _____ NPI_____

Address _____ Telephone No. _____

Diagnosis Code _____ Diagnosis_____

Diagnosis Code _____ Diagnosis_____

Treatment Plan _____

Authorization Requested for: ❑ Consult Only   ❑ Treatment Only   ❑ Consult/Treatment

❑ Consult/Procedure/Surgery   ❑ Diagnostic Tests

Procedure Code: _____ Description: _____

Procedure Code: _____ Description: _____

Place of Service ❑ Office ❑ Outpatient ❑ Inpatient ❑ Other   Number of Visits: _____

Facility: _____ Length of Stay: _____

Physician's Signature: _____

TO BE COMPLETED BY PRIMARY CARE PHYSICIAN

PCP Recommendations: _____ PCP Initials: _____

Date Eligibility Checked: _____

TO BE COMPLETED BY UTILIZATION MANAGEMENT

Authorized: _____ Auth. No:_____ Not Authorized _____

Deferred: _____ Modified: _____

Effective Date: _____ Expiration Date: _____ No. of Visits: _____

Fig. 5.6

6 Medicare

Linda M. Smith

KEY TERMS

Your instructor may wish to select some words pertinent to this chapter for a test. For definitions of the terms, further study, and/or reference, the words, phrases, and abbreviations may be found in the glossary at the end of the Textbook. *Key terms for this chapter follow.*

adjudication
adjustment
Advance Beneficiary Notice of Noncoverage
Advanced Alternative Payment Model
approved charges
assignment
beneficiaries
benefit period
Centers for Medicare and Medicaid Services
Correct Coding Initiative
crossover claim
disabled
donut hole
durable medical equipment
end-stage renal disease
formulary
hospice
hospital insurance
jurisdiction
limiting charge
Local Coverage Determination
medical necessity
Medicaid
Medicare
Medicare administrative contractor
Medicare Access and CHIP Reauthorization Act of 2015
Medicare Advantage Plan
Medicare Beneficiary Identifier

Medicare Claims Processing Manual—Internet Only Manual
Medicare Improvements for Patients and Providers Act
Medicare/Medicaid
Medicare Part A
Medicare Part B
Medicare Part C
Medicare Part D
Medicare secondary payer
Medicare Summary Notice
Medigap
Merit-based Incentive Payment System
National Coverage Determination
national health insurance
national provider identifier
nonparticipating provider
nursing facility
participating provider
premium
prepayment screen
prospective payment system
Quality Improvement Organization
Recovery Audit Contractor Initiative
remittance advice
resource-based relative value scale
respite care
Supplemental Security Income
value-based programs

KEY ABBREVIATIONS

See how many abbreviations and acronyms you can translate and then use this as a handy reference list. Definitions for the key abbreviations are located near the back of the Text-book *in the glossary.*

ABN _____

APM _____

CCI _____

_____

CMS _____

DC _____

DHHS _____

DME _____

ERA _____

ESRD _____

GPCIs _____

ICU _____

LCDs _____

LGHP _____

66

MA Plan _____	NF _____
MAC _____	nonpar _____
MACRA _____	NPI _____
MBI _____	par _____
Medi-Medi _____	PFFS plan _____
MIPAA _____	PPS _____
MIPS _____	PSO _____
MG _____	QIO _____
MMA _____	RA _____
MSA _____	RAC Initiative _____
MSN _____	RBRVS _____
MSP _____	SSI _____
NCDs _____	

PERFORMANCE OBJECTIVES

The student will be able to:

- Define and spell the key terms and key abbreviations for this chapter, given the information from the *Textbook* glossary, within a reasonable time period and with enough accuracy to obtain a satisfactory evaluation.
- After reading the chapter, answer the fill in the blank, multiple choice, and true/false review questions, with enough accuracy to obtain a satisfactory evaluation.
- Compute mathematical calculations, given Medicare problem situations, within a reasonable time period and with enough accuracy to obtain a satisfactory evaluation.
- Complete an ABN form.

STUDY OUTLINE

Background
Policies and Regulations
  Eligibility Requirements
  Medicare Enrollment
  Health Insurance Card
  Benefits
Additional Insurance Programs
  Medicare/Medicaid
  Medicare/Medigap
  Medicare Secondary Payer
  Automobile or Liability Insurance Coverage
Utilization and Quality Control
  Quality Improvement Organizations
  Medicare Billing Compliance Issues
Program Fundamentals
  Provider
  Prior Authorization

National and Local Coverage Determinations
  Prepayment Screens
Medicare Reimbursement
  Medicare Fee Schedule
  Prospective Payment System
  Value-Based Programs
  Medicare Improvements for Patients and Providers Act
  Medicare Access and CHIIP Reauthorization Act of 2015
Claim Submission
  Medicare Administrative Contractors
  Provider Identification Numbers
After Claim Submission
  Remittance Advice
  Medicare Summary Notice
  Posting Payments
  Medicare Overpayments

Part I Fill in the Blank

Review the objectives, key terms, glossary definitions of key terms, chapter information, and figures before completing the following review questions.

1. Medicare is administered by the federal agency _____.

2. Medicare Part A is _____ coverage, and Medicare Part B is _____ coverage.

3. A program designed to provide pain relief, symptom management, and supportive services to terminally ill individuals and their families is known as _____ _____.

4. An individual becomes eligible for Medicare Parts A and B at age _____.

5. The program of income support for low-income, aged, blind, and disabled persons established by the Social Security Act is called a/an _____.

6. An individual who is not a citizen of the United States is called a/an _____.

7. Patients who are entitled to received Medicare benefits are referred to as _____ _____.

8. The number that will replace social security numbers on Medicare insurance cards is referred to as the _____.

9. Define a Medicare Part A hospital benefit period.

   _____

   _____

   _____

10. Short-term inpatient medical care for terminally ill individuals to give temporary relief to the caregiver is known as _____.

11. The frequency of Pap tests for Medicare patients is _____, and that for mammograms is _____.

12. Medicare coverage plans offered by private insurance companies to Medicare beneficiaries are known as _____.

13. _____is a temporary limit on what a Medicare drug plan will cover.

14. A list of covered drugs kept by each Medicare drug plan is called a/an _____ _____.

15. A document by Medicare explaining the decision made on a claim for services that were paid is called a/an _____

16. Some third-party payers offer policies that fall under guidelines issued by the federal government and may cover prescription costs, Medicare deductibles, and copayments; these secondary or supplemental policies are known as _____ _____ insurance policies.

17. The amount that a nonparticipating provider can charge the Medicare beneficiary is referred to as _____ _____.

18. If a Medicare beneficiary is injured in an automobile accident, the physician submits the claim form to _____.

Part II Multiple Choice

Choose the best answer.

19. The fee that Medicare decides a medical service is worth, is referred to as the:
    a. reasonable charge for services.
    b. assigned amount.
    c. approved amount.
    d. paid amount.

20. Physicians who are nonparticipating with the Medicare program are only allowed to bill the limiting charge to the patient, which is:
    a. the provider's usual fee.
    b. 80% of the provider's fee schedule.
    c. 20% of the Medicare fee schedule allowed amount.
    d. 115% of the Medicare fee schedule allowed amount.

21. National Coverage Determinations are coverage guidelines that are mandated:
    a. at the federal level.
    b. at the Medicare contractor level.
    c. at the Medicare Advantage Plan level.
    d. by Recovery Audit Contractors Initiative.

22. A decision by a Medicare administrative contractor (MAC) whether to cover (pay) a particular medical service on a contractor-wide basis in accordance with whether it is reasonable and necessary is known as a/an:
    a. Local Coverage Determination.
    b. Correct Coding Initiative edit.
    c. prepayment screen.
    d. redetermination process.

23. A Medicare prepayment screen which would suspend a claim for the excision of an appendix performed by an audiologist would be referred to as:
    a. diagnosis to procedure edits.
    b. procedure to procedure edits.
    c. procedure to specialty code edits.
    d. procedure to place of service edits.

24. The resource-based relative value scale establishes fees, taking into account:
    a. physician's specialty, work value, and overhead expense.
    b. work value, overhead expense, and malpractice expense.
    c. work value, physician's specialty, and malpractice expense.
    d. physician's specialty, overhead expense, and malpractice expense.

25. The prospective payment system is a method of reimbursement to:
    a. physicians.
    b. ambulance services.
    c. hospitals.
    d. pharmacies.

26. The number of Medicare administrative contractors that currently process claims for DME suppliers is:
    a. 1.
    b. 4.
    c. 12.
    d. 50.

27. The 10-digit identification number required on a claim form to identify a service provider is the:
   a. SSN.
   b. MBI.
   c. NPI.
   d. PIP.

28. According to regulations, a Medicare patient must be billed for a copayment:
   a. at least once before a balance is adjusted off as uncollectible.
   b. at least two times before a balance is adjusted off as uncollectible.
   c. at least three times before a balance is adjusted off as uncollectible.
   d. no more than four times before a balance is adjusted off as uncollectible.

Part III True/False

Write "T" or "F" in the blank to indicate whether you think the statement is true or false.

_____ 29. All patients who have a Medicare health insurance card have Part A hospital and Part B medical coverage.

_____ 30. Prescription drug plans refer to the drugs in their formularies by tier numbers.

_____ 31. Nonparticipating physicians may decide on a case-by-case basis whether to accept assignment when providing medical services to Medicare patients.

_____ 32. Medicare's Correct Coding Initiative was implemented by the Centers for Medicare and Medicaid Services to identify procedures that are usually described by a single code or are inherent to another procedure.

_____ 33. A Medicare/Medigap claim is not called a crossover claim.

_____ 34. A Medicare preventive health benefit is an annual mammogram screening.

_____ 35. Medicare patients must pay for diabetes screening.

_____ 36. Obesity screening and counseling are Medicare preventive health benefits.

_____ 37. Pneumococcal pneumonia vaccine may be administered annually to Medicare patients.

_____ 38. Glaucoma screening is a covered screening for Medicare patients when performed every 6 months.

ASSIGNMENT 6.2 CALCULATE MATHEMATICAL PROBLEMS

Performance Objective

Task: Calculate and insert the correct amounts for nine Medicare scenarios.

Conditions: Use a pen or pencil and the description of the problem.

Standards: Time: _____ minutes

Accuracy: _____

(Note: The time element and accuracy criteria may be given by your instructor.)

Directions: Submitting insurance claims, particularly Medicare claims, involves a bit of arithmetic. Several problems are given here so that you will gain experience with situations encountered daily in your work. The Medicare deductible is always subtracted from the allowed amount first before mathematical computations continue.

Problem 1: Mr. Doolittle has Medicare Parts A and B coverage. He was well during the entire past year. On January 1, Mr. Doolittle is rushed to the hospital, where Dr. Input performs an emergency gastric resection. The hospital bills Medicare under the Part A coverage, and under the Part B coverage, the physician bills $450 for surgical services. The doctor agrees to accept assignment. The patient has not met any of his deductible for 2017 which is $183. Complete the following statements by putting in the correct amounts.

Original Bill

   a. Medicare allows $400. Medicare payment: _____

   b. Patient owes Dr. Input: _____

   c. Dr. Input's courtesy adjustment: _____

   Mathematical computations:

Problem 2: Mrs. James has Medicare Parts A and B coverage. She met her deductible when she was ill in March of this year. On November 1, Dr. Caesar performs a bilateral salpingo-oophorectomy. The hospital bills Medicare under the Part A coverage, and under Part B coverage, the physician bills $300 for surgical services. The doctor agrees to accept a Medicare assignment.

Original Bill

   a. Medicare allows $275. Medicare payment: _____

   b. Patient owes Dr. Caesar: _____

   c. Dr. Caesar's courtesy adjustment: _____

   Mathematical computations for surgeon:

The assistant surgeon charged Mrs. James $60 (the Medicare limiting charge) and does not accept assignment. After receiving her check from Medicare, Mrs. James sends the surgeon his $60. Medicare has allowed $55 for the fee.

  a. How much of the money was from Mrs. James' private funds? $ _____

  b. How much did Medicare pay? _____

   Mathematical computations:

Problem 3: You work for Dr. Coccidioides. He does not accept assignment. He is treating Mr. Robinson for allergies. Mr. Robinson has Medicare Part A. You send in a bill to Medicare for the $135 that Mr. Robinson owes you. What portion of the bill will Medicare pay?

Problem 4: In June, Mr. Fay has an illness that incurs $89 in medical bills. He asks you to bill Medicare, and the physician does not accept assignment. He has paid the deductible at another physician's office.
  a. If Medicare allows the entire amount of your fees, the Medicare check to the

   patient is $_____ (which comes to you).

  b. The patient's part of the bill to you is_____.

   Mathematical computations:

Problem 5: Mr. Iba, a Medicare patient with a Medigap insurance policy, is seen for an office visit, and the fee is $80. The Medicare-approved amount is $54.44. The patient has met his deductible for the year.

  a. The Medicare payment check is $ _____.
  b. After the claim is submitted to the Medigap insurance, the Medigap payment check

   is $ _____.

  c. To zero out the balance, the Medicare courtesy adjustment is _____.

   Mathematical computations:

Problem 6: Mrs. Smith, a Medicare patient, had surgery, and the participating physician's fee is $1250. This patient is working part-time, and her employer group health plan (primary insurance) allowed $1100, applied $500 to the deductible, and paid 80% of $600.

   a. Amount paid by this plan: $_____

   b. The spouse's employer group health plan (secondary insurance) is billed for the balance, which is $ _____. This program also has a $500 deductible. This plan pays 100% of the fee billed, minus the deductible.

   c. The spouse's employer group plan makes a payment of _____.

   You send copies of the remittance advice from the two group health plans and submit a claim to Medicare (the third insurance) for $1250. The balance at this point is $ _____.

   Mathematical computations:

Problem 7: Beverly James has Medicare Part B coverage. She has $242 in medical bills and has met $100 of the $183 (2017 deductible). Dr. Practon agrees to accept assignment.

Original Bill

   a. Medicare allows $200. Medicare payment: _____

   b. Beverly James owes Dr. Practon: _____

   c. Dr. Practon's courtesy adjustment: _____

   Mathematical computations:

73

Problem 8: Oliver Mills has Medicare Part B coverage. He fell at home and suffered a sprain and Dr. Skeleton treated him. His medical bill totaled $370, and he has met $60 of the $183 (2017 deductible). Dr. Skeleton agrees to accept assignment.

Original Bill

    a. Medicare allows $280. Medicare payment: _____

    b. Oliver Mills owes Dr. Skeleton: _____

    c. Dr. Skeleton's courtesy adjustment: _____

    Mathematical computations:

Problem 9: Maria Sanchez has Medicare Part B coverage. She has $565 in medical bills at Dr. Cardi's office and met $45 of the $183 (2017 deductible) at another physician's office. Dr. Cardi agrees to accept assignment.

Original Bill

    a. Medicare allows $480. Medicare payment: _____

    b. Maria Sanchez owes Dr. Cardi: _____

    c. Dr. Cardi's courtesy adjustment: _____

    Mathematical computations:

ASSIGNMENT 6.3 COMPLETE A MEDICARE ADVANCE BENEFICIARY NOTICE OF NONCOVERAGE

Performance Objective

Task: Complete Medicare ABN.

Conditions: Use the ABN form (Fig. 6.1)

Standards: ABN Completion Productivity Measurement

Time: _____ minutes

Accuracy: _____

(Note: The time element and accuracy criteria may be given by your instructor.)

Directions:

1. Complete an ABN form using the information provided below.

2. Patient: Raymond Fay (Medicare ID # A887661235A)
   a. Procedure performed: nystagmus test (CPT 92531) is a noncovered service and requires that an ABN be on file.
   b. The estimated cost of the nystagmus test is $26.00.
   c. After review of the ABN with the patient, the patient would like to proceed with the test and understands that they may be responsible for payment of the service.
   d. Provider of Services: Concha Antrum, MD; College Clinic; 4567 Broad Ave., Woodland Hills, XY 12345

A. Notifier:

B. Patient Name:

C. Identification Number:

Advance Beneficiary Notice of Noncoverage (ABN)

NOTE: If Medicare doesn't pay for **D.** _____ below, you may have to pay.
Medicare does not pay for everything, even some care that you or your health care provider have good reason to think you need. We expect Medicare may not pay for the **D.** _____ below.

D.	E. Reason Medicare May Not Pay:	F. Estimated Cost

WHAT YOU NEED TO DO NOW:
- Read this notice, so you can make an informed decision about your care.
- Ask us any questions that you may have after you finish reading.
- Choose an option below about whether to receive the **D.** _____ listed above.
   Note: If you choose Option 1 or 2, we may help you to use any other insurance that you might have, but Medicare cannot require us to do this.

G. OPTIONS: Check only one box. We cannot choose a box for you.

☐ **OPTION 1.** I want the **D.** _____ listed above. You may ask to be paid now, but I also want Medicare billed for an official decision on payment, which is sent to me on a Medicare Summary Notice (MSN). I understand that if Medicare doesn't pay, I am responsible for payment, but **I can appeal to Medicare** by following the directions on the MSN. If Medicare does pay, you will refund any payments I made to you, less co-pays or deductibles.

☐ **OPTION 2.** I want the **D.** _____ listed above, but do not bill Medicare. You may ask to be paid now as I am responsible for payment. **I cannot appeal if Medicare is not billed.**

☐ **OPTION 3.** I don't want the **D.** _____ listed above. I understand with this choice I am **not** responsible for payment, and **I cannot appeal to see if Medicare would pay.**

H. Additional Information:

This notice gives our opinion, not an official Medicare decision. If you have other questions on this notice or Medicare billing, call **1-800-MEDICARE** (1-800-633-4227/**TTY:** 1-877-486-2048).
Signing below means that you have received and understand this notice. You also receive a copy.

I. Signature:	J. Date:

Form CMS-R-131 (03/11)   Form Approved OMB No. 0938-0566

Fig. 6.1

7 Medicaid and Other State Programs

Linda M. Smith

KEY TERMS

Your instructor may wish to select some words pertinent to this chapter for a test. For definitions of the terms, further study, and/or reference, the words, phrases, and abbreviations may be found in the glossary at the end of the Textbook. *Key terms for this chapter follow.*

categorically needy
coinsurance
copayment
covered services
Early and Periodic Screening, Diagnosis, and Treatment
federal poverty level
fiscal agent
Medicaid
Medi-Cal

medically needy
Medicare Savings Programs
payer of last resort
prior approval
recipient
share of cost
Children's Health Insurance Program
Supplemental Security Income

KEY ABBREVIATIONS

See how many abbreviations and acronyms you can translate and then use this as a handy reference list. Definitions for the key abbreviations are located near the back of the Textbook *in the glossary.*

CHIP _____

DEFRA _____

EPSDT _____

FPL _____

MN _____

MSP _____

OBRA _____

OOY claims _____

POS machine _____

QI program _____

QMB _____

RA _____

SLMB _____

SSI _____

TANF _____

PERFORMANCE OBJECTIVES

The student will be able to:

- Define and spell the key terms and key abbreviations for this chapter, given the information from the *Textbook* glossary, within a reasonable time period and with enough accuracy to obtain a satisfactory evaluation.

- After reading the chapter, answer the fill in the blank, multiple choice, and true/false review questions with enough accuracy to obtain a satisfactory evaluation.
- Determine if prior authorization is required for a specific scenario.

Part I Fill in the Blank

Review the objectives, key terms, glossary definitions of key terms, chapter information, and figures before completing the following review questions.

1. Medicaid is not considered an insurance program. It is a/an _____ program.

2. The Medicaid program is jointly funded by the _____ and _____ governments.

3. Because the federal government sets minimum requirements, states are free to enhance the Medicaid program. Name two ways in which Medicaid programs vary from state to state.

   a. _____

   b. _____

4. Title XIX of the Social Security Act became federal law and created Medicaid in the year _____.

5. Health care reform legislation passed in 2010, known as _____ affected the Medicaid program by expanding access for childless adults and nonelderly and nonpregnant individuals.

6. To help compensate for budget cuts, many Medicaid programs instituted required specific dollar amounts, known as _____, to be collected at each office visit from the individual seeking medical services.

7. The measure of income issued every year by HHS and used to determine Medicaid eligibility is known as _____.

8. In all other states, the program is known as *Medicaid*, but in California the program is called _____.

9. Name the four Medicare Savings Programs for low-income Medicare patients.

   a. _____

   b. _____

   c. _____

   d. _____

10. Medicare beneficiaries who are disabled but have annual incomes below the federal poverty level may be eligible for the _____ program.

11. _____ is the portion the patient pays of the Medicare allowed amount.

12. States have the option to cover nonimmigrant and unauthorized aliens who are pregnant or who are children and can meet the definition of _____ in the U.S.

13. When health care services are rendered, the Medicaid identification card or electronic verification must show eligibility for the _____.

14. Name two broad classifications of people eligible for Medicaid assistance.

    a. _____

    b. _____

15. A _____ is an individual certified by the local welfare department to receive benefits of Medicaid.

16. The name of the program for the prevention, early detection, and treatment of conditions of children receiving welfare is known as _____.

    It is abbreviated as _____.

17. Your Medicaid patient seen today needs long-term hemodialysis services. You telephone for authorization to get verbal approval. Four important items to obtain are:

    a. _____

    b. _____

    c. _____

    d. _____

18. The time limit for submitting a Medicaid claim varies from _____

    to _____
    from the date the service is rendered.

19. The insurance claim form for submitting Medicaid claims in all states is

    _____.

20. Your Medicaid patient also has TRICARE. What billing procedure do you follow? Be exact in your steps for a dependant of an active military person.

    a. _____

    b. _____

21. Five categories of adjudicated claims that may appear on a Medicaid remittance advice document are:

    a. _____

    b. _____

    c. _____

    d. _____

    e. _____

22. Name three levels of Medicaid appeals.

    a. _____

    b. _____

    c. _____

23. _____ is the processing of an insurance claim through a series of edits for final determination of coverage (benefits) for possible payment.

Part II Multiple Choice

Choose the best answer.

24. An organization under contract with the state to process claims for a state Medicaid program is a/the:
    a. Medicaid administrative contractor.
    b. Department of Social Services.
    c. Center for Medicare and Medicaid Services.
    d. fiscal agent.

25. A patient's Medicaid eligibility may be verified by:
    a. touch-tone telephone.
    b. modem.
    c. special Medicaid terminal equipment.
    d. all of the above.

26. When a Medicaid patient requires a piece of durable medical equipment, the physician must:
    a. write a prescription.
    b. obtain prior authorization, preferably written.
    c. instruct the patient on how to use the equipment.
    d. give the name and address of where to purchase the equipment.

27. Which of the following services are mandated Medicaid basic benefits?
    a. Ambulance services
    b. Podiatric care
    c. Immunizations
    d. Dental care

28. If a patient is eligible for group health insurance coverage through an employer and they are also eligible for Medicaid benefits, Medicaid is referred to as the:
    a. payer of last resort.
    b. primary payer.
    c. co-insurance.
    d. fiscal agent.

29. If a patient is eligible for Medicare and Medicaid, Medicare is referred to as the:
    a. payer of last resort.
    b. primary payer.
    c. co-insurance.
    d. fiscal agent.

Part III True/False

Write "T" or "F" in the blank to indicate whether you think the statement is true or false.

_____ 30. Hospital-acquired conditions are payable by the Medicaid program.

_____ 31. All states have a Medicaid time limit of 12 months from the date of service for filing claims.

_____ 32. Medicaid spend down eligibility is determined annually to find out the patient's monthly copayment amount.

_____ 33. In some states, the phrase *prior approval* may be referred to as *prior authorization*.

_____ 34. There is only one type of copayment requirement in the Medicaid program.

_____ 35. Providers must enroll for participation in the Medicaid program with the fiscal agent for their region.

_____ 36. A state agency that investigates complaints of mistreatment in long-term care facilities is the Medicaid Fraud Control Unit (MFCU).

_____ 37. If a Medicaid patient requires medical care while out of state, the claim for services should be filed with the patient's home state Medicaid program.

_____ 38. If a Medicaid managed care patient requires medical care, the claim for services should be filed with the state Medicaid's fiscal agent.

Performance Objective

Task: After reading the scenario, answer the following questions, using critical thinking skills.

Conditions: Use a pen or pencil.

Standards: Time: _____ minutes

             Accuracy: _____

             (Note: The time element and accuracy criteria may be given by your instructor.)

Directions: After reading the scenario, answer the question, using your critical thinking skills. Record your answers on the blank lines.

Scenario: Mrs. Ho suddenly experiences a pain in her right lower abdominal area and rushes to a local hospital for emergency care. Laboratory work verifies that she has a ruptured appendix, and immediate surgery is recommended. Is prior authorization required in a bona fide emergency situation like this?

1. _____

   Reason: _____

8 TRICARE and Veterans' Health Care

Linda M. Smith

KEY TERMS

Your instructor may wish to select some words pertinent to this chapter for a test. For definitions of the terms, further study, and/or reference, the words, phrases, and abbreviations may be found in the glossary at the end of the Textbook. *Key terms for this chapter follow.*

active duty service member
allowable charge
authorized provider
beneficiary
catastrophic cap
catchment area
Civilian Health and Medical Program of the Uniformed Services
cooperative care
coordination of benefits
cost share
Defense Enrollment Eligibility Reporting System
Department of Veterans Affairs
emergency
health benefits advisor
health care finder
medically (or psychologically) necessary
Military Treatment Facility
Non-Availability Statement
nonparticipating provider
other health insurance
participating provider

partnership program
point-of-service option
preauthorization
primary care manager
regional contractor
service benefit program
service-connected injury
service retiree (military retiree)
sponsor
summary payment voucher
total, permanent, service-connected disability
TRICARE
TRICARE Extra
TRICARE for Life
TRICARE Prime
TRICARE service center
TRICARE Select
TRICARE Standard
urgent care
veteran
Veterans Health Administration

KEY ABBREVIATIONS

See how many abbreviations and acronyms you can translate and then use this as a handy reference list. Definitions for the key abbreviations are located near the back of the Text-book *in the glossary.*

ADSM _____

CHAMPUS _____

CHAMPVA _____

DEERS _____

HBA _____

HCF _____

MHS _____

MTF _____

NAS _____

nonpar _____

OHI _____

par _____

PCM _____

POS _____

SHCP _____

TFL _____

TMA _____

TPR _____

TSC _____

VA _____

84

PERFORMANCE OBJECTIVES

The student will be able to:

- Define and spell the key terms and key abbreviations for this chapter, given the information from the *Textbook* glossary, within a reasonable time period and with enough accuracy to obtain a satisfactory evaluation.

- After reading the chapter, answer the fill in the blank, multiple choice, and true/false review questions with enough accuracy to obtain a satisfactory evaluation.

STUDY OUTLINE

TRICARE
History of TRICARE
   Eligibility
   Nonavailability Statement
Health Plans
   TRICARE Select
   TRICARE Prime
   TRICARE Prime Remote
   TRICARE Prime Overseas
   U.S. Family Health Plan
   TRICARE Reserve Select
   TRICARE Retired Reserve
   TRICARE Young Adult
   TRICARE for Life
   TRICARE Plus
   Supplemental Health Care Program
   TRICARE Hospice Program

Veterans Health Administration Program
   Eligibility
   Enrollment
   Identification Card
   Benefits
   Provider
   Preauthorization
Claims Procedure
   Regional Contractor
   TRICARE Select and Veterans Health Administration (CHAMPVA)
   Access to Health Records
   Computer Matching and Privacy Protection Act of 1988
After Claims Submission
   TRICARE Summary Payment Voucher

Part I Fill in the Blank

Review the objectives, key terms, glossary definitions of key terms, chapter information, and figures before completing the following review questions.

1. CHAMPUS, the acronym for Civilian Health and Medical Program of the Uniformed Services, is now called _____ and was organized to control escalating medical costs and to standardize benefits for active duty families and military retirees.

2. The regional contractor for TRICARE East is _____.

3. An active duty service member is known as a/an _____; once retired, this former member is called a/an _____.

4. An individual who qualifies for TRICARE is known as a/an _____.

5. A system for verifying an individual's TRICARE eligibility is called

   _____.

6. Mrs. Hancock, a TRICARE beneficiary, lives 2 miles from a Uniformed Services Medical Treatment Facility but needs to be hospitalized for mental health care services at Orlando Medical Center, a civilian hospital. What type of certification does she require to receive care from a civilian hospital?

   _____

7. Active duty uniformed service personnel are issued a/an _____ to be used for standard identification.

8. Military family members and retirees are issued a/an _____to access health care benefits.

9. The maximum dollar amount that a TRICARE member has to pay in any fiscal year for covered medical benefits is referred to as the _____, after which TRICARE pays 100% of the allowable charges for the rest of the year.

10. The two primary TRICARE programs are _____and_____.

11. Programs that allow TRICARE Standard beneficiaries to receive treatment, services, or supplies from civilian providers are called _____ and

    _____.

12. An individual who is located at TRICARE service centers who can help TRICARE beneficiaries and providers with preauthorization of medical services is a/an _____.

    _____

13. A voluntary TRICARE health maintenance organization type of option is known as

    _____.

14. A physician who is responsible for coordinating and managing all of the TRICARE Prime beneficiary's health care unless there is an emergency is a/an _____.

15. TRICARE Prime provides the same covered services as TRICARE Select beneficiaries, plus there are additional _____ and _____ services.

16. A _____ is an individual at military hospitals or clinics who is available to assist TRICARE beneficiaries to obtain medical care through the military and through TRICARE.

17. TRICARE Young Adult enrollees must be a dependant of an eligible uniformed service sponsor, unmarried, at least age _____, and not eligible to enroll in an employer-sponsored health plan.

18. TRICARE for Life is a program for TRICARE-eligible beneficiaries who are age _____.

19. The TRICARE _____ program is designed to provide care and comfort to patients who are terminally ill.

20. CHAMPVA is the acronym for _____ now known as the _____.

21. Those individuals who serve in the United States Armed Forces, finish their service, and are honorably discharged are known as _____.

22. Veterans Health Administration (CHAMPVA) is not an insurance program but is considered as a/an _____ program.

23. Which individuals are entitled to Veterans Health Administration (CHAMPVA) medical benefits?

    a. _____

    b. _____

       _____

    c. _____

       _____

24. The public law establishing a person's right to review and contest inaccuracies in personal medical records is known as the _____.

25. An organization that contracts with the government to process TRICARE and Veterans Health Administration (CHAMPVA) health insurance claims is known as a/an _____.

26. The time limit for submitting a TRICARE Standard or CHAMPVA claim for outpatient service is _____; for inpatient service, it is _____.

Part II Multiple Choice

Choose the best answer.

27. Effective January 1, 2018, the two TRICARE regions are designated as:
    a. Region West and Region South.
    b. Region North and Region South.
    c. Region East and Region West.
    d. Region South and Region East.

28. The catchment area for a specific geographic region is defined by zip code and is based on an area surrounding each Medical Treatment Facility in the U.S. of approximate radius:
    a. 30 miles.
    b. 40 miles.
    c. 50 miles.
    d. 100 miles.

29. An authorized civilian provider who has not signed a contract with a regional TRICARE contractor to give medical care to TRICARE beneficiaries but agrees to accept assignment on a case-by-case basis is known as a/an:
    a. authorized provider.
    b. network provider.
    c. nonnetwork participating provider.
    d. nonnetwork notparticipating provider.

30. The TRICARE fiscal year:
    a. begins January 1 and ends December 31.
    b. begins April 1 and ends March 30.
    c. begins June 1 and ends May 30.
    d. begins October 1 and ends September 30.

31. A health care professional who helps a patient who is under the TRICARE program obtain preauthorization for care is called a:
    a. primary care physician (PCP).
    b. health care finder (HCF).
    c. health benefits advisor (HBA).
    d. participating provider.

32. TRICARE Prime Remote is a managed plan that can only be used if the distance from both the sponsor's home and work addresses to a military hospital or clinic is more than:
    a. 30 miles.
    b. 40 miles.
    c. 50 miles.
    d. 100 miles.

33. TRICARE Prime Remote Overseas is an HMO-style managed care plan available in the designated remote overseas locations of:
    a. Europe-Australia, and Canada.
    b. Africa, Canada, and the Pacific.
    c. Latin America, Australia, and Canada.
    d. Eurasia-Africa, Latin America, Canada, and the Pacific.

34. Under the U.S. Family Health Plan, the designated provider for Upstate New York is:
    a. Johns Hopkins Medicine.
    b. Martin's Point Health Care.
    c. Brighton Marine Health Center.
    d. St. Vincent Catholic Medical Centers.

35. To qualify for TRICARE for Life (TFL), a beneficiary must be:
    a. a TRICARE beneficiary.
    b. eligible for Medicare Part A.
    c. enrolled in Medicare Part B.
    d. all of the above.

Part III True/False

Write "T" or "F" in the blank to indicate whether you think the statement is true or false.

_____ 36. TRICARE is funded by both the state and federal governments.

_____ 37. A Nonavailability Statement is for individuals who are seeking any type of emergency care service.

_____ 38. TRICARE beneficiaries who use nonauthorized providers and receive medical services may be responsible for their entire bill.

_____ 39. The catastrophic cap does not apply to noncovered TRICARE services.

_____ 40. The TRICARE Select program became effective January 1, 2017.

_____ 41. Referrals are not required for the TRICARE Select program.

_____ 42. TRICARE Prime Remote (TPR) is a program designed for military retirees and their families.

_____ 43. Beneficiaries of the Veterans Health Administration (CHAMPVA) program have complete freedom of choice in selecting their civilian health care providers.

_____ 44. A patient enrolled in the Veterans Health Administration (CHAMPVA) program does not need preauthorization for hospice services.

_____ 45. Service members move often, so it is prudent to ask beneficiaries enrolled in TRICARE to update their information during each office visit.

_____ 46. When transmitting a TRICARE claim, always send it to the TRICARE claims office nearest to the residence of the military sponsor.

_____ 47. TRICARE is considered primary to Medicare for persons younger than age 65 who have Medicare Part A as a result of a disability and who have enrolled in Medicare Part B.

_____ 48. CHAMPVA is considered primary to Medicare for persons younger than age 65 who are enrolled in Medicare Parts A and B.

_____ 49. TRICARE is considered primary to Worker's Compensation if the beneficiary is injured on the job or becomes ill because of his or her work.

_____ 50. If a provider participates with TRICARE, accepts assignment, and receives payment directly from the regional contractor, the patient will receive a copy of the voucher.

Performance Objective

Task: After reading the scenarios, answer the following questions, using critical thinking skills.

Conditions: Use a pen or pencil.

Standards: Time: _____ minutes

                Accuracy: _____

                (Note: The time element and accuracy criteria may be given by your instructor.)

Directions: After reading the scenarios, answer the following questions, using your critical thinking skills. Record your answers on the blank lines.

1. If Bertha Evans is seen for an office visit and has other insurance besides TRICARE, and she is the dependant of an active military person, whom do you bill first?

   _____

   Reason: _____

2. If Jason Williams, a TRICARE beneficiary who became disabled at age 10 years and who is also receiving Medicare Part A and Medicare Part B benefits, is seen for a consultation, whom do you bill first?

   _____

   Reason: _____

3. If Tanner Vine, a Veterans Health Administration (CHAMPVA) and Medicaid beneficiary, is seen on an emergency basis in the office, whom do you bill first?

   _____

   Reason: _____

9 Workers' Compensation

Linda M. Smith

KEY TERMS

Your instructor may wish to select some words pertinent to this chapter for a test. For definitions of the terms, further study, and/or reference, the words, phrases, and abbreviations may be found in the glossary at the end of the Textbook. *Key terms for this chapter follow.*

accident
adjudication
claims examiner
compromise and release
deposition
ergonomic
extraterritorial
Federal Employees' Compensation Act
injury
insurance adjuster
lien
medical service order
nondisability claim
occupational illness or disease
Occupational Safety and Health Administration
Office of Workers' Compensation Programs

permanent and stationary
permanent disability
petition
reexamination report
second-injury fund
sequelae
state-run program
sub rosa films
subsequent-injury fund
temporary disability
third-party liability
third-party subrogation
waiting period
work hardening
Workers' Compensation Appeals Board
workers' compensation insurance

KEY ABBREVIATIONS

See how many abbreviations and acronyms you can translate and then use this as a handy reference list. Definitions for the key abbreviations are located near the back of the Text-book *in the glossary.*

AME _____

C and R _____

ERISA _____

FECA _____

IME _____

LHWCA _____

OSHA _____

OWCP _____

P and S _____

PD _____

QME _____

ROM _____

SIF _____

TD _____

WCAB _____

WP _____

PERFORMANCE OBJECTIVES

The student will be able to:

- Define and spell the key terms and key abbreviations for this chapter, given the information from the *Textbook* glossary, within a reasonable time period and with enough accuracy to obtain a satisfactory evaluation.
- After reading the chapter, answer the fill in the blank, multiple choice, and true/false review questions with enough accuracy to obtain a satisfactory evaluation.
- Given a list of common medical abbreviations and symbols that appear in chart notes, fill in the correct meaning of each abbreviation within a reasonable time period and with enough accuracy to obtain a satisfactory evaluation. Students may use a medical dictionary or internet resource.
- Given the patients' medical chart notes and blank workers' compensation forms, complete each workers' compensation form related to billing within a reasonable time period and with enough accuracy to obtain a satisfactory evaluation.

STUDY OUTLINE

History
  Workers' Compensation Statutes
  Workers' Compensation Reform
Workers' Compensation Laws and Insurance
  Purposes of Workers' Compensation Laws
  Program Funding
  Self-Insurance
  Managed Care
Eligibility
  Work-Related Accident
  Occupational Illness
Coverage
  Federal Laws
  State Laws
Types of State Compensation Benefits
Types of State Workers' Compensation Claims
  Nondisability Claim
  Temporary Disability Claim
  Permanent Disability Claim
Fraud and Abuse
Legal Situations
  Medical Evaluator

  Depositions
  Medical Testimony
  Liens
  Third-Party Subrogation
Medical Reports
  Health Information Record Keeping
  Terminology
Reporting Requirements
  Employer's Report
  Medical Service Order
  Physician's First Report
  Progress or Supplemental Report
  Final Report
Claim Submission
  Financial Responsibility
  Fee Schedules
  Helpful Billing Tips
  Billing Claims
  Out-of-State Claims
  Delinquent or Slow Pay Claims

Part I Fill in the Blank

Review the objectives, key terms, glossary definitions of key terms, chapter information, and figures before completing the following review questions.

1. Individuals who are paid by someone in exchange for labor or services are referred to as

   _____.

2. Name two kinds of statutes under workers' compensation.

   a. _____

   b. _____

3. List five reasons that workers' compensation laws were developed.

   a. _____

   b. _____

   c. _____

   d. _____

   e. _____

4. _____ pays the workers' compensation insurance premiums.

5. State three methods used for funding workers' compensation.

   a. _____

   b. _____

   c. _____

6. Self-insured employers are governed by _____, a federal law that sets minimum requirements for group health plans.

7. A form of self-insurance that is owned by its policyholders and serves smaller or mid-size companies is known as _____.

8. When an employee with a preexisting condition is injured at work and the injury produces a disability greater than what would have been caused by the second injury alone, the benefits are drawn from a/an

   _____.

9. An unexpected, unintended event that occurs at a particular time and place, causing injury to an individual not of his or her own making, is called a/an

   _____.

10. Maria Cardoza works in a plastics manufacturing company and inhales some fumes that cause bronchitis. Because this condition is associated with her employment, it is called a/an

    _____.

93

11. Name the federal workers' compensation acts that cover workers.

a. _____

b. _____

c. _____

d. _____

12. Federal law mandates that states set up laws to meet _____ requirements.

13. State compensation laws that require each employer to accept its provisions and to provide for specialized benefits for employees who are injured at work are called

_____.

14. State compensation laws that may be accepted or rejected by the employer are known

as _____

_____.

15. When billing for an injury of a patient who lives out-of-state, the insurance billing specialist should follow the rules and fee schedule of the state in which the workers'

compensation claim was _____ filed.

16. The waiting period for income and medical benefits in your state is _____.

17. List five types of workers' compensation benefits.

a. _____

b. _____

c. _____

d. _____

e. _____

18. Who can treat an industrial injury?

_____

_____

19. What are three types of workers' compensation claims and the differences among them?

a. _____

b. _____

c. _____

20. Weekly temporary disability payments are based on

_____.

21. After suffering an industrial injury, Mr. Fields is in a treatment program in which he is given real work tasks for building strength and endurance. This form of therapy is

called _____.

22. When an industrial case reaches the time for rating the disability, this is accomplished by what state agency? _____

23. May an injured person appeal his or her case if he or she is not satisfied with the rating? _____ If so, to whom does he or she appeal? _____ or _____

24. When fraud or abuse is suspected in a workers' compensation case, the physician should report the situation to _____.

25. Physicians who conduct medical–legal evaluations of injured workers must pass a complex medical examination to become certified by the _____ Council.

26. A proceeding that generally takes place in an attorney's office in which an attorney asks a witness questions about a case and the witness answers under oath is referred to as a/an _____.

27. In a workers' compensation case, when a claim is made against a separate person or company, but not the employer, it is referred to as a _____ liability.

28. Explain third-party subrogation.

_____

_____

29. When an individual suffers a work-related injury or illness, the employer must complete and send a form called a/an _____ to the insurance company and workers' compensation state offices, and if the employee is sent to a physician's office for medical care, the employer must complete a form called a/an _____, which authorizes the physician to treat the employee.

30. Temporary disability ends when the patient is able to return to work or if the disability lasts longer than _____ months.

Part II Multiple Choice

Choose the best answer.

31. Employers are required to meet health and safety standards for their employees under federal and state statutes known as the:
    a. Occupational Safety and Health Administration (OSHA) Act of 1970.
    b. Health Insurance Portability and Accountability Act (HIPAA).
    c. Clinical Laboratory Improvement Amendment (CLIA).
    d. Employee Retirement Income Security Act (ERISA).

32. The process of carrying on a lawsuit is called:
    a. lien.
    b. litigation.
    c. deposition.
    d. adjudication.

33. A proceeding during which an attorney questions a witness who answers under oath but not in open court is called a:
    a. subpoena.
    b. subrogation.
    c. petition.
    d. deposition.

34. The legal claim on the property of another for payment of a debt is termed a:
    a. medical service order.
    b. subpoena.
    c. lien.
    d. promissory note.

35. The contract for treatment and the financial responsibility in a workers' compensation case is between:
    a. the health care organization and the patient.
    b. the health care organization and the employer.
    c. the health care organization and the workers' compensation insurance carrier.
    d. the employer and the workers' compensation insurance carrier.

36. Workers' compensation fee schedules that consider the time, skills, and extent of the service provided by the physician are:
    a. maximum fee schedules.
    b. relative value scale fee schedules.
    c. Medicare-based fee schedules.
    d. compulsory fee schedules.

Part III True/False

Write "T" or "F" in the blank to indicate whether you think the statement is true or false.

_____ 37. When working for the ABC Machining Company, an employee cuts his finger off while using a lathe. He is covered under workers' compensation.

_____ 38. A roofer takes his girlfriend to a roofing job and she is injured. She is covered under workers' compensation insurance.

_____ 39. A private duty nurse employed by the XYZ homecare service is injured while moving a patient. She is covered under workers' compensation insurance.

_____ 40. A Department of Energy subcontractor diagnosed with a disease resulting from exposure to radiation is covered under workers' compensation.

_____ 41. A postal worker twists his ankle while delivering mail. He is covered under workers' compensation.

_____ 42. An employee who is at an official company retreat suffers from a concussion due to a fall. The injury would be covered under workers' compensation.

_____ 43. An independent contractor is injured while working for a local construction company. The construction company's workers' compensation would cover the related medical bills.

_____ 44. If an individual seeks medical care for a workers' compensation injury from another state, the state's regulations are followed in which the injured person's claim was originally filed.

_____ 45. When a patient arrives at a medical office and says he or she was hurt at work, you should verify insurance information with the benefits coordinator for the employer.

_____ 46. A stamped physician's signature is acceptable on the Doctor's First Report of Occupational Injury or Illness form.

ASSIGNMENT 9.2 COMPLETE A DOCTOR'S FIRST REPORT OF OCCUPATIONAL INJURY OR ILLNESS FORM FOR A WORKERS' COMPENSATION CASE

Performance Objective

Task: Complete a Doctor's First Report of Occupational Injury or Illness form and define patient record abbreviations.

Conditions: Use the patient's record (Fig. 9.1), a Doctor's First Report of Occupational Injury or Illness form (Fig. 9.2), and a computer.

Standards: Claim Productivity Measurement

Time: _____ minutes

Accuracy: _____

(Note: The time element and accuracy criteria may be given by your instructor.)

Directions:

1. Complete the Doctor's First Report of Occupational Injury or Illness form (see Fig. 9.2) for this nondisability type of claim.

2. Using a medical dictionary or an internet resource, define abbreviations found in the patient's medical record.

After the instructor has returned your work to you, either make the necessary corrections and place your work in a three-ring notebook for future reference or, if you received a high score, place it in your portfolio for reference when applying for a job.

Abbreviations pertinent to this record:

apt	_____	CT	_____
lt	_____	neg	_____
pt	_____	MC	_____
ED	_____	MDM	_____
hosp	_____	DC	_____
ER	_____	PD	_____
C	_____	FU	_____
HX	_____	wks	_____
PX	_____	approx	_____
c/o	_____	RTW	_____
L	_____	WC	_____

PATIENT RECORD NO. 15-2-3

Hiranuma	Glen	M.	12-24-55	M	555-467-3383
LAST NAME	FIRST NAME	MIDDLE NAME	BIRTH DATE	SEX	HOME PHONE

4372 Hanley Avenue	Woodland Hills	XY	12345
ADDRESS	CITY	STATE	ZIP CODE

555-908-3433		555-467-3383		hiranuma@wb.net
CELL PHONE	PAGER NO.	FAX NO.		E-MAIL ADDRESS

558-XX-9960	U3402189
PATIENT'S SOC. SEC. NO.	DRIVER'S LICENSE

house painter	Pittsburgh Paint Company (commercial painting company)
PATIENT'S OCCUPATION	NAME OF COMPANY

3725 Bonfeld Avenue, Woodland Hills, XY 12345	555-486-9070
ADDRESS OF EMPLOYER	PHONE

Esme M. Hiranuma	homemaker
SPOUSE OR PARENT	OCCUPATION

EMPLOYER	ADDRESS	PHONE

State Compensation Insurance Fund, 14156 Magnolia Boulevard, Torres, XY 12349
NAME OF INSURANCE

016-2432-211
POLICY/CERTIFICATE NO.   GROUP NO.

REFERRED BY: Pittsburgh Paint Company

DATE	PROGRESS NOTES
5-22-xx	At 9:30 a.m. this ♂ house painter was painting an apt ceiling (apt located at 3540 W. 87th Street, Woodland Hills, XY 12345, County of Woodland Hills) when he slipped and fell from a tall ladder landing on his head and lt side of body; brief unconsciousness for approximately 15 minutes. Employer was notified by coworker and pt was sent to College Hosp ED. I was called to the hosp at request of employer and saw pt in ER at 5 PM (performed a C HX/PX). Pt c/o L shoulder pain and swelling; L leg and hip pain; neck and head pain. X-rays were taken of lt hip (complete), lt femur (2 views), and cervical spine (3 views) as well as CT of brain (without contrast)—all neg. I admitted pt for overnight stay in hosp for concussion. Applied sling for L shoulder sprain. Cleaned and dressed L hip and leg abrasions (MC/MDM). Plan to DC 5/23/xx. No PD expected. Pt to FU in 2 wks. Approx. RTW 6/6 xx. Prepared WC report.
	GP/llf *Gerald Practon, MD*
5-23-xx	Pt's HA gone. Vital signs normal. Discharged home. RTO 1 wk.
	GP/llf *Gerald Practon, MD*

Fig. 9.1

STATE OF CALIFORNIA

DOCTOR'S FIRST REPORT OF OCCUPATIONAL INJURY OR ILLNESS

Within 5 days of your initial examination, for every occupational injury or illness, send two copies of this report to the employer's workers' compensation insurance carrier or the insured employer. Failure to file a timely doctor's report may result in assessment of a civil penalty. In the case of diagnosed or suspected pesticide poisoning, send a copy of the report to Division of Labor Statistics and Research, P.O. Box 420603, San Francisco, CA 94142-0603, and notify your local health officer by telephone within 24 hours.

	PLEASE DO NOT USE THIS COLUMN
1. INSURER NAME AND ADDRESS	
2. EMPLOYER NAME	Case No.
3. Address No. and Street City Zip	Industry
4. Nature of business (e.g., food manufacturing, building construction, retailer of women's clothes.)	County
5. PATIENT NAME (first name, middle initial, last name) 6. Sex ☐ Male ☐ Female 7. Date of Mo. Day Yr. Birth	Age
8. Address: No. and Street City Zip 9. Telephone number ( )	Hazard
10. Occupation (Specific job title) 11. Social Security Number - -	Disease
12. Injured at: No. and Street City County	Hospitalization
13. Date and hour of injury Mo. Day Yr. Hour or onset of illness _____ a.m. _____ p.m. 14. Date last worked Mo. Day Yr.	Occupation
15. Date and hour of first Mo. Day Yr. Hour examination or treatment _____ a.m. _____ p.m. 16. Have you (or your office) previously treated patient? ☐ Yes ☐ No	Return Date/Code

Patient please complete this portion, if able to do so. Otherwise, doctor please complete immediately, inability or failure of a patient to complete this portion shall not affect his/her rights to workers' compensation under the California Labor Code.

17. **DESCRIBE HOW THE ACCIDENT OR EXPOSURE HAPPENED.** (Give specific object, machinery or chemical. Use reverse side if more space is required.)

18. **SUBJECTIVE COMPLAINTS** (Describe fully. Use reverse side if more space is required.)

19. **OBJECTIVE FINDINGS** (Use reverse side if more space is required.)
   A. Physical examination

   B. X-ray and laboratory results (State if non or pending.)

20. **DIAGNOSIS** (if occupational illness specify etiologic agent and duration of exposure.) Chemical or toxic compounds involved?   ☐ Yes ☐ No
   ICD-9 Code ___ ___ ___ - ___ ___

21. Are your findings and diagnosis consistent with patient's account of injury or onset of illness? ☐ Yes ☐ No If "no", please explain.

22. Is there any other current condition that will impede or delay patient's recovery? ☐ Yes ☐ No If "yes", please explain.

23. **TREATMENT RENDERED** (Use reverse side if more space is required.)

24. If further treatment required, specify treatment plan/estimated duration.

25. If hospitalized as inpatient, give hospital name and location   Date admitted   Mo. Day Yr.   Estimated stay

26. WORK STATUS -- Is patient able to perform usual work?   ☐ Yes ☐ No
   If "no", date when patient can return to: Regular work ___/___/___
   Modified work ___/___/___   Specify restrictions _____

Doctor's Signature _____   CA License Number _____

Doctor Name and Degree (please type) _____   IRS Number _____

Address _____   Telephone Number (_____) _____

FORM 5021 (Rev. 4)
1992

Any person who makes or causes to be made any knowingly false or fraudulent material statement or material representation for the purpose of obtaining or denying workers' compensation benefits or payments is guilty of a felony.

Fig. 9.2

ASSIGNMENT 9.3 COMPLETE A DOCTOR'S FIRST REPORT OF OCCUPATIONAL INJURY OR ILLNESS FORM FOR A WORKERS' COMPENSATION CASE

Performance Objective

Task: Complete a Doctor's First Report of Occupational Injury or Illness form and define patient record abbreviations.

Conditions: Use the patient's record (Fig. 9.3a and 9.3b), a Doctor's First Report of Occupational Injury or Illness form (Fig. 9.4), and a computer.

Standards: Claim Productivity Measurement

              Time: _____ minutes

              Accuracy: _____

              (Note: The time element and accuracy criteria may be given by your instructor.)

Directions:

1. Complete the Doctor's First Report of Occupational Injury or Illness form for this temporary disability type of claim. Refer to Carlos A. Giovanni's patient record for November 11 through November 15.

2. Using a medical dictionary or an internet resource, define abbreviations found in the patient's medical record.

    After the instructor has returned your work to you, either make the necessary corrections and place your work in a three-ring notebook for future reference or, if you received a high score, place it in your portfolio for reference when applying for a job.

Abbreviations pertinent to this record:

pt	_____	H	_____
ER	_____	MDM	_____
C	_____	TD	_____
HX	_____	RTW	_____
PX	_____	approx	_____
CT	_____	HV	_____
R	_____	EPF	_____
tr	_____	M	_____
adm	_____	PO	_____
DC	_____	PF	_____
hosp	_____	SF	_____
OV	_____	X	_____
LC	_____	adv	_____
HA	_____	trt	_____
BP	_____	reg	_____
RTO	_____	W	_____
wks	_____	cons	_____

PATIENT RECORD NO. 15-4-5

Giovanni	Carlos	A.	10-24-55	M	555-677-3485
LAST NAME	FIRST NAME	MIDDLE NAME	BIRTH DATE	SEX	HOME PHONE

89 Beaumont Court	Woodland Hills	XY	12345
ADDRESS	CITY	STATE	ZIP CODE

	555-230-7788	555-677-3485		giovannic@wb.net
CELL PHONE	PAGER NO.	FAX NO.		E-MAIL ADDRESS

556-XX-9699	Y0394876
PATIENT'S SOC. SEC. NO.	DRIVER'S LICENSE

TV repairman	Giant Television Co. (TV repair company)
PATIENT'S OCCUPATION	NAME OF COMPANY

8764 Ocean Avenue, Woodland Hills, XY 12345	555-647-8851
ADDRESS OF EMPLOYER	PHONE

Maria B. Giovanni	homemaker
SPOUSE OR PARENT	OCCUPATION

EMPLOYER	ADDRESS	PHONE

State Compensation Insurance Fund, 600 S. Lafayette Park Place, Ehrlich, XY 12350
NAME OF INSURANCE

57780	
POLICY/CERTIFICATE NO.	GROUP NO.

REFERRED BY: Giant Television Company

Fig. 9.3a

DATE	PROGRESS NOTES
11-11-xx	Pt referred to College Hospital ER by employer for workers' compensation injury. I was called in as on-call
	neurosurgeon to evaluate the pt. Pt states that today at 2 PM he fell from the roof of a private home while
	installing an antenna at 2231 Duarte St., Woodland Hills, XY 12345 in Woodland Hills County. He describes the
	incident as follows: "When I was attaching the base of an antenna, the weight of the antenna shifted and knocked
	me off the roof." Pt complains of head pain and indicates brief loss of consciousness. I performed a C HX/PX.
	Complete skull x-rays showed fractured skull. CT of head/brain (without contrast) indicates well-defined R.
	subdural hematoma. Pt suffering from cerebral concussion; no open wound. Tr plan: Adm pt to College
	Hospital (5 PM) and schedule R infratentorial craniotomy to evacuate hematoma. (H/MDM). Obtained
	authorization and prepared Dr.'s First Report.
	AP/llf *Astro Parkinson, MD*
11-12-xx	Performed R infratentorial craniotomy and evacuated subdural hematoma. Pt stable and returned to room; will be
	seen daily. TD: Estimated RTW 1-15-xx. Possible cranial defect & head disfigurement resulting. Pt to be
	hospitalized for approx 2 weeks.
	AP/llf *Astro Parkinson, MD*
11-13-xx	HV (EPF HX/PX M/MDM). Pt improving; recommend consult with Dr. Graff for cranial defect. Authorization
	obtained from adjuster (Steve Burroughs) at State Comp.
	AP/llf *Astro Parkinson, MD*
11-14-xx	Pt seen in cons by Dr. Cosmo Graff who stated he does not recommend correcting PO cranial defect. Both
	Dr. Graff and I explained how the defect resulted from the injury; there may be some improvement over time.
	Pt states he is grateful to be alive (EPF HX/PX M/MDM).
	AP/llf *Astro Parkinson, MD*
11-15-xx	Daily HV (EPF HX/PX M/MDM). Pt progressing appropriately; no complications have occurred.
thru	
11-29-xx	AP/llf *Astro Parkinson, MD*
11-30-xx	DC from hosp. Permanent cranial defect resulting from fracture and surgery. RTO 1 wk.
	AP/llf *Astro Parkinson, MD*
12-7-xx	OV (EPF HX/PX LC/MDM) Pt doing very well. No HA or visual disturbances, BP 120/80, alert and oriented.
	He is anxious to return to work. Pt cautioned about maintaining low activity level until released. RTO 2 wks.
	AP/llf *Astro Parkinson, MD*
12-21-xx	OV (PF HX/PX SF/MDM). Pt continues to improve. Suggested he start a walking program 3 x wk and monitor
	symptoms. May do light activity and lifting (10 lbs). Adv to call if any symptoms return. RTO 10 days.
	AP/llf *Astro Parkinson, MD*
12-29-xx	OV (PF HX/PX SF/MDM). Pt did not experience any symptoms with increased activity. No further trt necessary.
	Pt will increase activity and call if any problems occur. Pt scheduled to resume reg W on 1-15-xx. Final report
	submitted to workers' compensation carrier.
	AP/llf *Astro Parkinson, MD*

Fig. 9.3b, cont'd

DOCTOR'S FIRST REPORT OF OCCUPATIONAL INJURY OR ILLNESS

Within 5 days of your initial examination, for every occupational injury or illness, send two copies of this report to the employer's workers' compensation insurance carrier or the insured employer. Failure to file a timely doctor's report may result in assessment of a civil penalty. In the case of diagnosed or suspected pesticide poisoning, send a copy of the report to Division of Labor Statistics and Research, P.O. Box 420603, San Francisco, CA 94142-0603, and notify your local health officer by telephone within 24 hours.

	PLEASE DO NOT USE THIS COLUMN
1. INSURER NAME AND ADDRESS	Case No.
2. EMPLOYER NAME	Industry
3. Address No. and Street City Zip	County
4. Nature of business (e.g., food manufacturing, building construction, retailer of women's clothes.)	County
5. PATIENT NAME (first name, middle initial, last name) 6. Sex ☐ Male ☐ Female 7. Date of Birth Mo. Day Yr.	Age
8. Address: No. and Street City Zip 9. Telephone number ( )	Hazard
10. Occupation (Specific job title) 11. Social Security Number - -	Disease
12. Injured at: No. and Street City County	Hospitalization
13. Date and hour of injury or onset of illness Mo. Day Yr. Hour ____ a.m. ____ p.m. 14. Date last worked Mo. Day Yr.	Occupation
15. Date and hour of first examination or treatment Mo. Day Yr. Hour ____ a.m. ____ p.m. 16. Have you (or your office) previously treated patient? ☐ Yes ☐ No	Return Date/Code

Patient please complete this portion, if able to do so. Otherwise, doctor please complete immediately, inability or failure of a patient to complete this portion shall not affect his/her rights to workers' compensation under the California Labor Code.

17. **DESCRIBE HOW THE ACCIDENT OR EXPOSURE HAPPENED.** (Give specific object, machinery or chemical. Use reverse side if more space is required.)

18. **SUBJECTIVE COMPLAINTS** (Describe fully. Use reverse side if more space is required.)

19. **OBJECTIVE FINDINGS** (Use reverse side if more space is required.)
   A. Physical examination

   B. X-ray and laboratory results (State if non or pending.)

20. **DIAGNOSIS** (if occupational illness specify etiologic agent and duration of exposure.) Chemical or toxic compounds involved?   ☐ Yes   ☐ No
   ICD-9 Code ___ ___ ___ - ___ ___

21. Are your findings and diagnosis consistent with patient's account of injury or onset of illness? ☐ Yes   ☐ No   If "no", please explain.

22. Is there any other current condition that will impede or delay patient's recovery? ☐ Yes   ☐ No   If "yes", please explain.

23. **TREATMENT RENDERED** (Use reverse side if more space is required.)

24. If further treatment required, specify treatment plan/estimated duration.

25. If hospitalized as inpatient, give hospital name and location   Date admitted   Mo. Day Yr.   Estimated stay

26. WORK STATUS -- Is patient able to perform usual work?   ☐ Yes   ☐ No
   If "no", date when patient can return to: Regular work ___/___/___
                                              Modified work ___/___/___   Specify restrictions _____

Doctor's Signature _____   CA License Number _____

Doctor Name and Degree (please type) _____   IRS Number _____

Address _____   Telephone Number (___)_____

FORM 5021 (Rev. 4)
1992

Any person who makes or causes to be made any knowingly false or fraudulent material statement or material representation for the purpose of obtaining or denying workers' compensation benefits or payments is guilty of a felony.

Fig. 9.4

105

10 Disability Income Insurance and Disability Benefits Programs

Linda M. Smith

KEY TERMS

Your instructor may wish to select some words pertinent to this chapter for a test. For definitions of the terms, further study, and/or reference, the words, phrases, and abbreviations may be found in the glossary at the end of the Textbook.

Some of the insurance terms presented in this chapter are shown marked with an asterisk (*) and may seem familiar from previous chapters. However, their meanings may or may not have a slightly different connotation when referring to disability income insurance. Key terms for this chapter follow.

accidental death and dismemberment
Armed Services Disability
benefit period*
Civil Service Retirement System
consultative examiner
cost-of-living adjustment
Disability Determination Services
disability income insurance
double indemnity
exclusions*
Federal Employees Retirement System
future purchase option
guaranteed renewable*
hearing
long-term disability insurance
noncancelable clause*
Non-VA Medical Care Program
partial disability*

reconsideration
residual benefits*
residual disability
short-term disability insurance
Social Security Administration
Social Security Disability Insurance program
State Disability Insurance
supplemental benefits
Supplemental Security Income
temporary disability*
temporary disability insurance
total disability*
unemployment compensation disability
Veterans Affairs disability program
Veterans Affairs outpatient clinic card
voluntary disability insurance
waiting period*
waiver of premium*

KEY ABBREVIATIONS

See how many abbreviations and acronyms you can translate and then use this as a handy reference list. Definitions for the key abbreviations are located near the back of the Textbook *in the glossary.*

AIDS _____

CE _____

COLA _____

CSRS _____

DDS _____

FERS _____

HIV _____

OASDI _____

SDI _____

SSA _____

SSDI program _____

SSI _____

TDI _____

UCD _____

VA _____

The student will be able to:

- Define and spell the key terms and key abbreviations for this chapter, given the information from the *Textbook* glossary, within a reasonable time period, and with enough accuracy to obtain a satisfactory evaluation.
- After reading the chapter, answer the fill in the blank, multiple choice, and true/false review questions with enough accuracy to obtain a satisfactory evaluation.

- Fill in the correct meaning of each abbreviation, given a list of common medical abbreviations and symbols that appear in chart notes, within a reasonable time period and with enough accuracy to obtain a satisfactory evaluation.
- Complete each state disability form, given the patients' medical chart notes and blank state disability forms, within a reasonable time period and with enough accuracy to obtain a satisfactory evaluation.

STUDY OUTLINE

Disability Claims
History
Disability Income Insurance
Individual
Group
Federal Disability Programs
Workers' Compensation
Disability Benefit Programs
State Disability Insurance
Background

Funding
Eligibility
Benefits
Time Limits
Medical Examinations
Restrictions
Voluntary Disability Insurance
Claims Submission Guidelines
Disability Income Claims
Conclusion

107

Part I Fill in the Blank

Review the objectives, key terms, glossary definitions of key terms, chapter information, and figures before completing the following review questions.

1. Insurance that provides monthly or weekly income when an individual is unable to work because of a nonindustrial illness or injury is called

   _____.

2. A _____ is the maximum amount of time that benefits will be paid to the injured or ill person for the disability.

3. When an individual who is insured under a disability income insurance policy cannot perform one or more of his or her regular job duties, this is known as

   _____ or _____ disability.

4. Ezra Jackson has disability income insurance under a group policy paid for by his employer. Ezra makes no contribution toward the policy premiums. One evening he goes inline skating and suffers a complex fracture of the patella, which necessitates several months off from work. Are his monthly disability benefits taxable?

   _____ Why or why not? _____

   _____

5. Some insurance contracts that pay twice the face amount of the policy if accidental death occurs may have a provision titled _____.

6. When an individual becomes permanently disabled and cannot pay the insurance premium, a desirable provision in an insurance contract is _____.

7. Give three examples of preexisting conditions that may be written into a disability contract as exclusions:

   a. _____

   b. _____

   c. _____

8. Two federal programs for individuals younger than 65 years of age who have a severe disability are:

   a. _____

   b. _____

9. The strict definition of *Disability* given by Social Security is _____

   _____.

10. When applying for SSDI benefits, there is a _____ waiting period during which time the individual will not receive SSA benefits.

11. The _____ program pays monthly income benefits to adults and children with limited income and resources who are disabled, blind, or age 65 or older.

12. The Social Security Administration may hire a physician to evaluate an applicant's disability. A physician's role may be any one of the following:

    a. _____

    b. _____

    c. _____

13. If Disability Determination Services determines that the claimant is not eligible for disability benefits, the first level of the appeals process is referred to as

    _____.

14. The two types of federal retirement which have provisions for those who become

    disabled are _____ and _____.

15. Jamie Woods, a Navy petty officer, suffered an accident aboard the USS *Denebola* three weeks after his honorable discharge. To receive veteran's benefits for this injury, the time

    limit in which a claim must be filed is _____.

16. Name the states and the territory that have nonindustrial state disability programs.

    a. _____

    b. _____

    c. _____

    d. _____

    e. _____

    f. _____

17. In your state, temporary disability insurance claims must be filed within _____ days.

18. How long can a person continue to draw state disability insurance benefits?

    _____

19. After a claim begins, when do basic state disability benefits become payable if the

    patient is confined to his or her home? _____ If the

    patient is hospitalized? _____

20. Nick Tyson has recovered since a previous illness ended and becomes ill again with the

    same ailment. Is he entitled to state disability benefits? _____

21. John S. Thatcher stubbed his toe as he was leaving work and going to his car parked on the street. Because the injury was only slightly uncomfortable, he thought no more about it. The next morning he found that his foot was too swollen to fit in his shoe, so he stayed home. When the swelling did not subside after three days, John went to the doctor. Radiographs showed a broken toe, which kept John home for two weeks. After one week he applied for temporary state disability benefits.

    Will he be paid? _____

    Why or why not? _____

22. Peggy Jonson has an ectopic pregnancy and is unable to work because of complications of this condition. Can she receive state temporary disability benefits?

    _____

23. Four states that allow for maternity benefits in normal pregnancy are:

    a. _____

    b. _____

    c. _____

    d. _____

24. Betty T. Kraft had to stay home from her job because her 10-year-old daughter had measles. She applied for temporary state disability benefits.

    Will she be paid? _____

    Why or why not? _____

25. Vincent P. Michael was ill with a bad cold for one week. Will he receive temporary state disability benefits? _____

    Why or why not? _____

26. Betsy C. Palm works in Hawaii and had an emergency appendectomy. She was hospitalized for three days. Will she receive state disability benefits?

    _____

    Why or why not? _____

27. Frank E. Thompson is a box boy at a supermarket on Saturdays and Sundays while a full-time student at college. He broke his leg while skiing and cannot work at the market, but he is able to attend classes with his leg in a cast. Can he collect state disability benefits for his part-time job? _____

    Why or why not? _____

28. Jerry L. Slate is out of a job and is receiving unemployment insurance benefits. He is now suffering from severe intestinal flu. The employment office calls him to interview for a job, but he is too ill to go. Can he collect temporary state disability benefits for this illness when he might have been given a job?

_____

Why or why not? _____

29. While walking the picket line with other employees on strike, Gene J. Berry came down with pneumonia and was ill for two weeks. Can he collect temporary state disability benefits?

Why or why not? _____

Gene went back to work for three weeks and then developed a slight cold and cough, which again was diagnosed as pneumonia. The doctor told him to stay home from work. Would he be able to collect temporary disability benefits?

_____

Why or why not? _____

30. A month after he retired, Roger Reagan had a gallbladder operation. Can he receive temporary state disability benefits?

Why or why not? _____

31. Jane M. Lambert fell in the back yard of her home and fractured her left ankle. She had a nonunion fracture and could not work for 28 weeks. For how long will she collect temporary state disability benefits? _____

32. Dr. Kay examines Ben Yates and completes a disability income claim form because of a prolonged illness. On receiving the information, the insurance adjuster notices some conflicting data. Name other documents that may be requested to justify payment of benefits.

a. _____

b. _____

c. _____

33. Trent Walters, a permanently disabled individual, applies for federal disability benefits. To establish eligibility for benefits under this program, data allowed must be _____ year/years old.

34. A Veterans Affairs patient is seen on an emergency basis by Dr. Onion. Name the two methods or options for billing this case.

a. _____

b. _____

Part II Multiple Choice

Choose the best answer.

35. Another disability income insurance term for benefits is:
    a. indemnity.
    b. supplemental benefits.
    c. guarantee.
    d. compensation.

36. When the purchase of insurance is investigated, the words to look for in the insurance contract that mean the premium cannot be increased at renewal time are:
    a. guaranteed renewable.
    b. conditional provision.
    c. noncancelable clause.
    d. optional provision.

37. Provisions that limit the scope of insurance coverage are known as:
    a. clauses.
    b. deductibles.
    c. conditions.
    d. exclusions.

38. A Social Security Administration division that determines an individual's eligibility to be placed under the federal disability program is called:
    a. Disability Determination Services.
    b. Social Security Disability.
    c. Supplemental Security Income.
    d. none of the above.

39. The time period from the beginning of disability to receiving the first payment of benefits is called a/an:
    a. exclusion period.
    b. waiting period.
    c. insurance period.
    d. elimination phase.

40. The entity responsible for notifying the insurance company of a disability income claim is:
    a. the insured.
    b. the claimant.
    c. the physician.
    d. both a and b.

Part III True/False

Write "T" or "F" in the blank to indicate whether you think the statement is true or false.

_____ 41. When a person insured under a disability income insurance policy cannot, for a limited period of time, perform all functions of his or her regular job duties, it is known as *permanent disability*.

_____ 42. Disability income policies provide medical expense benefits.

_____ 43. There is no standard definition for total disability.

_____ 44. Eligibility for the SSI program is based strictly on financial need.

_____ 45. To be eligible to apply for disability benefits under Social Security, an individual must be unable to perform any type of work for a period of not less than 12 months.

_____ 46. Hospital benefits may be paid for nonoccupational illness or injury under state temporary disability benefits.

_____ 47. If a woman has an abnormal condition that arises from her pregnancy (e.g., diabetes or varicose veins) and is unable to work because of the condition, she may not receive state disability benefits.

_____ 48. When a claim form is submitted for a patient applying for state disability benefits, the most important item required on the form is the claimant's Social Security number.

_____ 49. To justify payment of disability benefits, an insurance company may request an employee's wage statements.

_____ 50. A person receiving state disability benefits must report any income received to the state disability insurance office because it can affect benefits.

Performance Objective

Task: Complete two state disability insurance forms and define patient record abbreviations.

Conditions: Use the patient's record (Fig. 10.1), a New York State Notice and Proof of Claim for Disability Benefits (Fig. 10.2), and a computer.

Standards: Time: _____ minutes

              Accuracy: _____

              (Note: The time element and accuracy criteria may be given by your instructor.)

Directions:

1. To familiarize you with what information the employee must furnish, this assignment will encompass completing the New York State Notice and Proof of Claim for Disability Benefits.

2. Mr. Broussard (see Fig. 10.1) is applying for state disability benefits, and he does not receive sick leave pay from his employer. The language he prefers is English. He does not want any disclosure of benefit payment information to his employer. During his disability, he was not in the custody of law enforcement authorities for any violation and he has no alcoholic tendencies.

3. Date the Claimant's Information November 5 of the current year, and date the Health Care Provider's Statement November 10 of the current year.

4. Refer to Chapter 10 and Fig. 10.2 of the *Textbook* to assist you in completing this form.

After the instructor has returned your work to you, either make the necessary corrections and place your work in a three-ring notebook for future reference or, if you received a high score, place it in your portfolio for reference when applying for a job.

Abbreviations pertinent to this record:

NP	_____	c/o	_____
LBP	_____	pt	_____
lt	_____	wk	_____
reg	_____	exam	_____
SLR	_____	rt	_____
WNL	_____	STAT	_____
MRI	_____	RTO	_____
imp	_____	retn	_____

PATIENT RECORD

Broussard	Jeff	L.	03-09-52	M	555-466-2490
LAST NAME	FIRST NAME	MIDDLE NAME	BIRTH DATE	SEX	HOME PHONE

3577 Plain Street	Woodland Hills	XY	12345	
ADDRESS	CITY	STATE	ZIP CODE	

555-667-7654	555-399-5903	555-466-2490	broussard@wb.net
CELL PHONE	PAGER NO.	FAX NO.	E-MAIL ADDRESS

566-XX-0090	F0394588
PATIENT'S SOC. SEC. NO.	DRIVER'S LICENSE

carpenter Payroll #2156	Ace Construction Company
PATIENT'S OCCUPATION	NAME OF COMPANY

4556 West Eighth Street, Dorland, XY 12347	555-447-8900
ADDRESS OF EMPLOYER	PHONE

Harriet M. Broussard	secretary
SPOUSE OR PARENT	OCCUPATION

Merit Accounting Company, 6743 Main Street, Woodland Hills, XY 12345	555-478-0980
EMPLOYER ADDRESS	PHONE

Blue Cross	Jeff L. Broussard
NAME OF INSURANCE	INSURED OR SUBSCRIBER

466-XX-9979	6131
POLICY/CERTIFICATE NO.	GROUP NO.

REFERRED BY: Harold B. Hartburn (friend)

DATE	PROGRESS NOTES
10-21-xx	8:30 a.m. NP seen c/o ongoing LBP. On 9-12-xx after swinging a golf club, pt had sudden onset of severe
	pain in low back with radiation to lt side. Pt unable to work 9-13 but resumed wk on 8-17 and has been working
	full time but doing no lifting while working. Pain is exacerbating affecting his work and reg duties. Exam
	showed SLR strongly positive on lt, on rt causes pain into lt side. Neurological exam WNL. Ordered STAT
	MRI. Off work. RTO.
	RS/mtf *Raymond Skeleton, MD*
10-23-xx	Pt returns for test results. MRI showed huge defect of L4-5. Imp: acute herniated disc L4-5 with spinal stenosis.
	Recommended laminotomy, foraminotomy, and diskectomy L4-5.
	RS/mtf *Raymond Skeleton, MD*
11-1-xx	Admit to College Hospital. Operation: Lumbar laminotomy with exploration and decompression of spinal
	cord with diskectomy L4-5; lumbar anterior arthrodesis.
	RS/mtf *Raymond Skeleton, MD*
11-5-xx	Pt seen daily in hosp. At 3 p.m. pt discharged to home. Will retn to wk 12-15-XX.
	RS/mtf *Raymond Skeleton, MD*

Fig. 10.1

DB-450 9-17

New York State
NOTICE AND PROOF OF CLAIM FOR DISABILITY BENEFITS

Use this form if you became disabled **while employed** or if you became disabled **within four (4) weeks after termination of employment** OR if you became **disabled after having been unemployed for more than four (4) weeks**. Please answer all questions in Part A and questions 1 through 3 in Part B. Read all instructions on this form carefully. Health care providers must complete Part B on page 2.

PART A - CLAIMANT'S INFORMATION (Please Print or Type)

1. Last Name: _____ First Name: _____ MI: ___

2. Mailing Address (Street & Apt. #): _____
   City: _____ State: _____ Zip: _____ Country: _____

3. Daytime Phone #: _____ 4. Email Address: _____

5. Social Security #: ___ - ___ - _____ 6. Date of Birth: ___ - ___ - _____ 7. Gender: ☐ Male ☐ Female

8. My disability is (if injury, also state <u>how</u>, <u>when</u> and <u>where</u> it occurred): _____

9. I became disabled or became ineligible for Unemployment Insurance because of this disability on: ___ / ___ / _____
   I worked on that day: ☐ Yes ☐ No
   Have you recovered from this disability? ☐ Yes ☐ No   If Yes, what was the date you were able to work: ___ / ___ / _____
   Have you since worked for wages or profit? ☐ Yes ☐ No   If Yes, list dates: _____

10. Give name of last employer. If more than one employer during last eight (8) weeks, name all employers. Average Weekly Wage is based on all wages earned in last eight (8) weeks worked.

LAST EMPLOYER			PERIOD OF EMPLOYMENT		Average Weekly Wage (Include Bonuses, Tips, Commissions, Reasonable Value of Board, Rent, etc.)
Firm or Trade Name	Address	Phone Number	First Day	Last Day Worked	
			Mo. Day Yr.	Mo. Day Yr.	

OTHER EMPLOYER (during last eight (8) weeks)			PERIOD OF EMPLOYMENT		Average Weekly Wage (Include Bonuses, Tips, Commissions, Reasonable Value of Board, Rent, etc.)
Firm or Trade Name	Address	Phone Number	First Day	Last Day Worked	
			Mo. Day Yr.	Mo. Day Yr.	
			Mo. Day Yr.	Mo. Day Yr.	

11. My job is or was: _____ 12. Union Member: ☐ Yes ☐ No If "Yes": _____
    _{Occupation}   _{Name of Union or Local Number}

13. Were you claiming or receiving unemployment prior to this disability? ☐ Yes ☐ No
    If you did **not** claim or if you claimed but did **not** receive unemployment insurance benefits after LAST DAY WORKED, explain reasons fully: _____

14. For the period of disability covered by this claim:
    A. Are you <u>**receiving**</u> wages, salary or separation pay: ☐ Yes ☐ No
    B. Are you <u>**receiving**</u> or <u>**claiming**</u>:
       1. Workers' compensation for work-connected disability: ☐ Yes ☐ No
       2. Paid Family Leave: ☐ Yes ☐ No
       3. No-Fault motor vehicle accident (check box): ☐ Yes ☐ No or personal injury involving third party (check box): ☐ Yes ☐ No
       4. Long-term disability benefits under the Federal Social Security Act for this disability: ☐ Yes ☐ No

    IF "YES" IS CHECKED IN ANY OF THE ITEMS IN 14, COMPLETE THE FOLLOWING:
    I have: ☐ received ☐ claimed from: _____ for the period: ___ / ___ / _____ to: ___ / ___ / _____

15. In the year (52 weeks) **before** your disability began, have you received disability benefits for other periods of disability? ☐ Yes ☐ No
    If "Yes", fill in the following: Paid by: _____ from: ___ / ___ / _____ to: ___ / ___ / _____

16. In the year (52 weeks) **before** your disability began, have you received Paid Family Leave? ☐ Yes ☐ No
    If "Yes", fill in the following: Paid by: _____ from: ___ / ___ / _____ to: ___ / ___ / _____

I hereby claim Disability Benefits and certify that for the period covered by this claim I was disabled. If my disability began while I was unemployed, I certify that I had been unemployed for more than four (4) weeks. I have read the instructions on page 2 of this form and that the foregoing statements, including any accompanying statements are, to the best of my knowledge, true and complete.

_____   _____
Claimant's Signature   **Date**
An individual may sign on behalf of the claimant only if he or she is legally authorized to do so and the claimant is a minor, mentally incompetent or incapacitated. If signed by other than claimant, print information below and complete and submit Form OC-110A, Claimant's Authorization to Disclose Workers' Compensation Records.

_____   _____   _____
On behalf of Claimant   **Address**   **Relationship to Claimant**

DB-450 (9-17) Page 1 of 2

Fig. 10.2   (From New York State Workers' Compensation Board.)

Continued

PART B - HEALTH CARE PROVIDER'S STATEMENT (Please Print or Type)

THE HEALTH CARE PROVIDER'S STATEMENT MUST BE FILLED IN COMPLETELY. THE ATTENDING HEALTH CARE PROVIDER SHALL COMPLETE AND RETURN TO THE CLAIMANT WITHIN SEVEN (7) DAYS OF RECEIPT OF THIS FORM. For item 7-d, you must give estimated date. If disability is caused by or arising in connection with pregnancy, enter estimated delivery date in item 9. **INCOMPLETE ANSWERS MAY DELAY PAYMENT OF BENEFITS.**

1. Last Name: _____ First Name: _____ MI: ___

2. Gender: ☐ Male ☐ Female   3. Date of Birth: ___ / ___ / _____

4. Diagnosis/Analysis: _____ Diagnosis Code: _____

   a. Claimant's symptoms: _____

   b. Objective findings: _____

5. Claimant hospitalized?: ☐ Yes ☐ No   From: ___ / ___ / ___   To: ___ / ___ / ___

6. Operation indicated?: ☐ Yes ☐ No   a. Type _____   b. Date ___ / ___ / ___

7. ENTER DATES FOR THE FOLLOWING	MONTH	DAY	YEAR
a Date of your first treatment for this disability			
b. Date of your most recent treatment for this disability			
c. Date Claimant was unable to work because of this disability			
d. Date Claimant will again be able to perform work (Even if considerable question exists, estimate date. Avoid use of terms such as unknown or undetermined.)			
e. If pregnancy related, please check box and enter the date ☐ estimated delivery date OR ☐ actual delivery date			

8. In your opinion, is this disability the result of injury arising out of and in the course of employment or occupational disease?:
☐ Yes ☐ No   If "Yes", has Form C-4 been filed with the Board? ☐ Yes ☐ No

I certify that I am a:

_____
(Physician, Chiropractor, Dentist, Podiatrist, Psychologist, Nurse-Midwife)   Licensed or Certified in the State of _____   License Number _____

_____
Health Care Provider's Printed Name   Health Care Provider's Signature   Date

_____
Health Care Provider's Address   Phone #

CLAIMANT: READ THESE INSTRUCTIONS CAREFULLY

PLEASE NOTE: Do not date and file this form prior to your first date of disability. In order for your claim to be processed, Parts A and B must be completed.

1. If you are using this form because you became disabled **while employed** or you became disabled **within four (4) weeks after termination of employment**, your completed claim should be mailed **within thirty (30) days to your employer or your last employer's insurance carrier.** You may find your employer's disability insurance carrier on the Workers' Compensation Board's website using Employer Coverage Search.

2. If you are using this form because you became **disabled after having been unemployed for more than four (4) weeks**, your completed claim should be mailed to: **Workers' Compensation Board, Disability Benefits Bureau, 328 State Street, Schenectady, NY 12305.** If you answered "Yes" to question 14.B.3, please complete and attach Form DB-450.1.

If you have any questions about claiming disability benefits, you may contact the Board's Disability Benefits Bureau at (800) 353-3092. Additional information may be obtained at the Board's website: www.wcb.ny.gov, or you may write to the Disability Benefits Bureau at the address listed above.

Notification Pursuant to the New York Personal Privacy Protection Law (Public Officers Law Article 6-A) and the Federal Privacy Act of 1974 (5 U.S.C. § 552a). The Workers' Compensation Board's (Board's) authority to request that claimants provide personal information, including their social security number, is derived from the Board's investigatory authority under Workers' Compensation Law (WCL) § 20, and its administrative authority under WCL § 142. This information is collected to assist the Board in investigating and administering claims in the most expedient manner possible and to help it maintain accurate claim records. Providing your social security number to the Board is voluntary. There is no penalty for failure to provide your social security number on this form; it will not result in a denial of your claim or a reduction in benefits. The Board will protect the confidentiality of all personal information in its possession, disclosing it only in furtherance of its official duties and in accordance with applicable state and federal law

HIPAA NOTICE - In order to adjudicate a workers' compensation claim or disability benefits claim, WCL 13-a(4)(a) and 12 NYCRR 325-1.3 require health care providers to regularly file medical reports of treatment with the Board and the insurance carrier or employer. Pursuant to 45 CFR 164.512 these legally required medical reports are exempt from HIPAA's restrictions on disclosure of health information.

Disclosure of Information: The Board will not disclose any information about your case to any unauthorized party without your consent. If you choose to have such information disclosed to an unauthorized party, you must file with the Board an original signed Form OC-110A, Claimant's Authorization to Disclose Workers' Compensation Records, or an original signed, notarized authorization letter. You may telephone your local WCB office to have Form OC-110A sent to you, or you may download it from our website, www.wcb.ny.gov. It can be found under Forms on the 'List of All Common Workers' Compensation Board Forms' web page. Mail the completed authorization form to the address listed above.

An employer or insurer, or any employee, agent, or person acting on behalf of an employer or insurer, who KNOWINGLY MAKES A FALSE STATEMENT OR REPRESENTATION as to a material fact in the course of reporting, investigation of, or adjusting a claim for any benefit or payment under this chapter for the purpose of avoiding provision of such payment or benefit SHALL BE GUILTY OF A CRIME AND SUBJECT TO SUBSTANTIAL FINES AND IMPRISONMENT.

DB-450 (9-17) Page 2 of 2

Fig. 10.2, cont'd

ASSIGNMENT 10.3 COMPLETE TWO STATE DISABILITY INSURANCE FORMS

Performance Objective

Task: Complete two state disability insurance forms and define patient record abbreviations.

Conditions: Use the patient's record (Fig. 10.3), a New York State Notice and Proof of Claim for Disability Benefits (Fig. 10.4), and a computer.

Standards: Time: _____ minutes

Accuracy: _____

(Note: The time element and accuracy criteria may be given by your instructor.)

Directions:

1. Assume that the Claim Statement of Employee has been completed satisfactorily by Mr. Fred E. Thorndike (see Fig. 10.3). Complete the New York State Notice and Proof of Claim for Disability Benefits (Fig. 10.4) and date it December 2. In completing this portion of the assignment, look at the first entry made by Dr. Practon on November 25 only.

2. Mr. Thorndike returns to see Dr. Practon on December 7, at which time his disability leave needs to be extended. Complete the Health Care Provider's Statement (Fig. 10.4) by referring to the entry made during the second visit, and date the certificate December 7. Remember that this is not a claim for payment to the physician, so no ledger card has been furnished for this patient.

3. Refer to Chapter 10 and Fig. 10.2 of the *Textbook* to assist you in completing these forms.

After the instructor has returned your work to you, either make the necessary corrections and place your work in a three-ring notebook for future reference or, if you received a high score, place it in your portfolio for reference when applying for a job.

Abbreviations pertinent to this record:

pt   _____

PE   _____

dx   _____

RTO _____

est   _____

c̄   _____

reg   _____

SDI   _____

wks   _____

Cont _____

wk   _____

FU   _____

CXR _____

PATIENT RECORD

Thorndike	Fred	E.	02-17-54	M	555-465-7820
LAST NAME	FIRST NAME	MIDDLE NAME	BIRTH DATE	SEX	HOME PHONE

5784 Helen Street	Woodland Hills	XY	12345
ADDRESS	CITY	STATE	ZIP CODE

555-432-7744	555-320-5500	555-466-7820	thorndike@wb.net
CELL PHONE	PAGER NO.	FAX NO.	E-MAIL ADDRESS

549-XX-8721	M00430548
PATIENT'S SOC. SEC. NO.	DRIVER'S LICENSE

salesman Payoll No. 6852	Easy on Paint Company
PATIENT'S OCCUPATION	NAME OF COMPANY

4586 West 20th Street, Woodland Hills, XY 12345	555-467-8898
ADDRESS OF EMPLOYER	PHONE

Jennifer B. Thorndike	homemaker
SPOUSE OR PARENT	OCCUPATION

EMPLOYER	ADDRESS	PHONE

Pacific Mutual Insurance Company,120 South Main Street, Merck, XY 12346
NAME OF INSURANCE

	6709	Fred E. Thorndike
POLICY/CERTIFICATE NO.	GROUP NO.	INSURED OR SUBSCRIBER

REFERRED BY: John Diehl (Friend)

DATE	PROGRESS NOTES
11-25-xx	On or about 11-3-xx, pt began to have chest pain and much coughing. On 11-24-xx, pt too ill to work and
	decided to file for SDI benefits. Pt states illness is not work connected and he does not receive sick pay.
	PE: Pt examined and complained of productive cough of 3 wks duration and chest pain. Chest x-rays
	confirmed dx-mucopurulent chronic bronchitis. Cont home rest and prescribed antibiotic medication. RTO
	12-7-xx. Pt will be capable of returning to wk 12-8-xx.
	GP/mtf *Gerald Practon, MD*
12-07-xx	Est pt returns for F/U c bronchitis. Chest pain improved. Still running low grade temp $\bar{c}$ productive cough.
	F/U CXR shows clearing. Recommended bed rest x 7d. Will extend disability to 12-15-xx at which time pt
	can resume reg work. No complications anticipated.
	GP/mtf *Gerald Practon, MD*

Fig. 10.3

DB-450 9-17

Use this form if you became disabled **while employed** or if you became disabled **within four (4) weeks after termination of employment** OR if you became **disabled after having been unemployed for more than four (4) weeks**. Please answer all questions in Part A and questions 1 through 3 in Part B. Read all instructions on this form carefully. Health care providers must complete Part B on page 2.

PART A - CLAIMANT'S INFORMATION (Please Print or Type)

1. Last Name: _____ First Name: _____ MI: ____

2. Mailing Address (Street & Apt. #): _____

   City: _____ State: _____ Zip: _____ Country: _____

3. Daytime Phone #: _____ 4. Email Address: _____

5. Social Security #: _____ - ____ - _____ 6. Date of Birth: ____ - ____ - _____ 7. Gender: ☐ Male ☐ Female

8. My disability is (if injury, also state how, when and where it occurred): _____

_____

9. I became disabled or became ineligible for Unemployment Insurance because of this disability on: ____ / ____ / _____

   I worked on that day: ☐ Yes ☐ No

   Have you recovered from this disability? ☐ Yes ☐ No   If Yes, what was the date you were able to work: ____ / ____ / _____

   Have you since worked for wages or profit? ☐ Yes ☐ No   If Yes, list dates: _____

10. Give name of last employer. If more than one employer during last eight (8) weeks, name all employers. Average Weekly Wage is based on all wages earned in last eight (8) weeks worked.

LAST EMPLOYER			PERIOD OF EMPLOYMENT		Average Weekly Wage (Include Bonuses, Tips, Commissions, Reasonable Value of Board, Rent, etc.)
Firm or Trade Name	Address	Phone Number	First Day	Last Day Worked	
			Mo. Day Yr.	Mo. Day Yr.	

OTHER EMPLOYER (during last eight (8) weeks)			PERIOD OF EMPLOYMENT		Average Weekly Wage (Include Bonuses, Tips, Commissions, Reasonable Value of Board, Rent, etc.)
Firm or Trade Name	Address	Phone Number	First Day	Last Day Worked	
			Mo. Day Yr.	Mo. Day Yr.	
			Mo. Day Yr.	Mo. Day Yr.	

11. My job is or was: _____   12. Union Member: ☐ Yes ☐ No If "Yes": _____
                              Occupation   Name of Union or Local Number

13. Were you claiming or receiving unemployment prior to this disability? ☐ Yes ☐ No

    If you did **not** claim or if you claimed but did **not** receive unemployment insurance benefits after LAST DAY WORKED, explain reasons fully: _____

_____

14. For the period of disability covered by this claim:

    A. Are you **receiving** wages, salary or separation pay: ☐ Yes ☐ No

    B. Are you **receiving** or **claiming**:

        1. Workers' compensation for work-connected disability: ☐ Yes ☐ No

        2. Paid Family Leave: ☐ Yes ☐ No

        3. No-Fault motor vehicle accident (check box): ☐ Yes ☐ No or personal injury involving third party (check box): ☐ Yes ☐ No

        4. Long-term disability benefits under the Federal Social Security Act for this disability: ☐ Yes ☐ No

IF "YES" IS CHECKED IN ANY OF THE ITEMS IN 14, COMPLETE THE FOLLOWING:

I have: ☐ received ☐ claimed from: _____ for the period: ____ / ____ / _____ to: ____ / ____ / _____

15. In the year (52 weeks) **before** your disability began, have you received disability benefits for other periods of disability? ☐ Yes ☐ No

    If "Yes", fill in the following: Paid by: _____ from: ____ / ____ / _____ to: ____ / ____ / _____

16. In the year (52 weeks) **before** your disability began, have you received Paid Family Leave? ☐ Yes ☐ No

    If "Yes", fill in the following: Paid by: _____ from: ____ / ____ / _____ to: ____ / ____ / _____

I hereby claim Disability Benefits and certify that for the period covered by this claim I was disabled. If my disability began while I was unemployed, I certify that I had been unemployed for more than four (4) weeks. I have read the instructions on page 2 of this form and that the foregoing statements, including any accompanying statements are, to the best of my knowledge, true and complete.

_____   _____
Claimant's Signature   Date

An individual may sign on behalf of the claimant only if he or she is legally authorized to do so and the claimant is a minor, mentally incompetent or incapacitated. If signed by other than claimant, print information below and complete and submit Form OC-110A, Claimant's Authorization to Disclose Workers' Compensation Records.

_____   _____   _____
On behalf of Claimant   Address   Relationship to Claimant

DB-450 (9-17) Page 1 of 2

Fig. 10.4   (From Employment Development Department, State of California.)

Continued

119

PART B - HEALTH CARE PROVIDER'S STATEMENT (Please Print or Type)

THE HEALTH CARE PROVIDER'S STATEMENT MUST BE FILLED IN COMPLETELY. THE ATTENDING HEALTH CARE PROVIDER SHALL COMPLETE AND RETURN TO THE CLAIMANT WITHIN SEVEN (7) DAYS OF RECEIPT OF THIS FORM. For item 7-d, you must give estimated date. If disability is caused by or arising in connection with pregnancy, enter estimated delivery date in item 9. **INCOMPLETE ANSWERS MAY DELAY PAYMENT OF BENEFITS.**

1. Last Name: _____ First Name: _____ MI: ___

2. Gender: ☐ Male ☐ Female   3. Date of Birth: ___ / ___ / _____

4. Diagnosis/Analysis: _____ Diagnosis Code: _____

   a. Claimant's symptoms: _____

   b. Objective findings: _____

5. Claimant hospitalized?: ☐ Yes ☐ No   From: ___ / ___ / _____   To: ___ / ___ / _____

6. Operation indicated?: ☐ Yes ☐ No   a. Type _____   b. Date ___ / ___ / _____

7. ENTER DATES FOR THE FOLLOWING	MONTH	DAY	YEAR
a. Date of your first treatment for this disability			
b. Date of your most recent treatment for this disability			
c. Date Claimant was unable to work because of this disability			
d. Date Claimant will again be able to perform work (Even if considerable question exists, estimate date. Avoid use of terms such as unknown or undetermined.)			
e. If pregnancy related, please check box and enter the date ☐ estimated delivery date OR ☐ actual delivery date			

8. In your opinion, is this disability the result of injury arising out of and in the course of employment or occupational disease?:
☐ Yes ☐ No   If "Yes", has Form C-4 been filed with the Board? ☐ Yes ☐ No

I certify that I am a:

_____
(Physician, Chiropractor, Dentist, Podiatrist, Psychologist, Nurse-Midwife)   **Licensed or Certified in the State of**   **License Number**

_____
Health Care Provider's Printed Name   **Health Care Provider's Signature**   **Date**

_____
Health Care Provider's Address   **Phone #**

CLAIMANT: READ THESE INSTRUCTIONS CAREFULLY

PLEASE NOTE: Do not date and file this form prior to your first date of disability. In order for your claim to be processed, Parts A and B must be completed.

1. If you are using this form because you became disabled **while employed** or you became disabled **within four (4) weeks after termination of employment,** your completed claim should be mailed **within thirty (30) days to your employer or your last employer's insurance carrier.** You may find your employer's disability insurance carrier on the Workers' Compensation Board's website using Employer Coverage Search.

2. If you are using this form because you became **disabled after having been unemployed for more than four (4) weeks,** your completed claim should be mailed to: **Workers' Compensation Board, Disability Benefits Bureau, 328 State Street, Schenectady, NY 12305.** If you answered "Yes" to question 14.B.3, please complete and attach Form DB-450.1.

If you have any questions about claiming disability benefits, you may contact the Board's Disability Benefits Bureau at (800) 353-3092. Additional information may be obtained at the Board's website: www.wcb.ny.gov, or you may write to the Disability Benefits Bureau at the address listed above.

DB-450 (9-17) Page 2 of 2

Fig. 10.4, cont'd

ASSIGNMENT 10.4 COMPLETE A STATE DISABILITY INSURANCE FORM

Performance Objective

Task: Complete a state disability insurance form and define patient record abbreviations.

Conditions: Use the patient's record (Fig. 10.5), a New York State Notice and Proof of Claim for Disability Benefits (Fig. 10.6), and a computer.

Standards: Time: _____ minutes

                Accuracy: _____

                (Note: The time element and accuracy criteria may be given by your instructor.)

Directions:

1. Assume that the Claimant's Information has been completed satisfactorily by Mr. James T. Fujita (see Fig. 10.5). Complete the Health Care Provider's Statement (see Fig. 10.6) and date it December 15.

2. Refer to Chapter 10 of the *Textbook* to assist you in completing this form.

After the instructor has returned your work to you, either make the necessary corrections and place your work in a three-ring notebook for future reference or, if you received a high score, place it in your portfolio for reference when applying for a job.

Abbreviations pertinent to this record:

pt   _____   exam   _____

hx   _____   neg   _____

WBC _____   imp   _____

wk   _____   SDI   _____

PATIENT RECORD

Fujita	James	T.	03-27-54	M	555-677-2881
LAST NAME	FIRST NAME	MIDDLE NAME	BIRTH DATE	SEX	HOME PHONE

3538 South A Street	Woodland Hills	XY		12345
ADDRESS	CITY	STATE		ZIP CODE

555-499-6556	555-988-4100	555-677-2881	fujita@wb.net
CELL PHONE	PAGER NO.	FAX NO.	E-MAIL ADDRESS

567-XX-8898	M4387931
PATIENT'S SOC. SEC. NO.	DRIVER'S LICENSE

electrician Payoll No. 8834	Macy Electric Company
PATIENT'S OCCUPATION	NAME OF COMPANY

2671 North C Street, Woodland Hills, XY 12345	555-677-2346
ADDRESS OF EMPLOYER	PHONE

Mary J. Fujita	homemaker
SPOUSE OR PARENT	OCCUPATION

EMPLOYER	ADDRESS	PHONE

Atlantic Mutual Insurance Company, 111 South Main Street, Woodland Hills, XY 12345
NAME OF INSURANCE

F20015		James T. Fujita
POLICY/CERTIFICATE NO.	GROUP NO.	INSURED OR SUBSCRIBER

REFERRED BY: Cherry Hotta (aunt)

DATE	PROGRESS NOTES
12-07-XX	Today pt could not go to work and came for exam complaining of pain in abdomen, nausea, and no vomiting. Pt
	has hx of mesentery adenopathy. Exam neg except abdomen showed tenderness all over with voluntary guarding.
	WBC 10,000. Imp: Mesenteric adenitis. Advised strict bed rest at home and bland diet. To return in 1 wk. Will file
	for SDI benefits. Pt states illness is not work connected and he receives sick leave pay of $150/wk.
	GI/mtf *Gaston Input, MD*
12-15-xx	Exam showed normal nontender abdomen. No nausea. Pt tolerating food well. WBC 7,500. Pt will be capable of
	returning to work 12-22-xx.
	GI/mtf *Gaston Input, MD*

Fig. 10.5

DB-450 9-17

Use this form if you became disabled **while employed** or if you became disabled **within four (4) weeks after termination of employment** OR if you became **disabled after having been unemployed for more than four (4) weeks.** Please answer all questions in Part A and questions 1 through 3 in Part B. Read all instructions on this form carefully. Health care providers must complete Part B on page 2.

PART A - CLAIMANT'S INFORMATION (Please Print or Type)

1. Last Name: _____ First Name: _____ MI: ___

2. Mailing Address (Street & Apt. #): _____

   City: _____ State: _____ Zip: _____ Country: _____

3. Daytime Phone #: _____ 4. Email Address: _____

5. Social Security #: ____ - ____ - _____ 6. Date of Birth: ___ - ___ - _____ 7. Gender: ☐ Male ☐ Female

8. My disability is (if injury, also state <u>how</u>, <u>when</u> and <u>where</u> it occurred): _____
_____

9. I became disabled or became ineligible for Unemployment Insurance because of this disability on: ____ / ____ / _____

   I worked on that day: ☐ Yes ☐ No

   Have you recovered from this disability? ☐ Yes ☐ No   If Yes, what was the date you were able to work: ____ / ____ / _____

   Have you since worked for wages or profit? ☐ Yes ☐ No   If Yes, list dates: _____

10. Give name of last employer. If more than one employer during last eight (8) weeks, name all employers. Average Weekly Wage is based on all wages earned in last eight (8) weeks worked.

LAST EMPLOYER			PERIOD OF EMPLOYMENT		Average Weekly Wage (Include Bonuses, Tips, Commissions, Reasonable Value of Board, Rent, etc.)
Firm or Trade Name	Address	Phone Number	First Day	Last Day Worked	
			Mo. Day Yr.	Mo. Day Yr.	

OTHER EMPLOYER (during last eight (8) weeks)			PERIOD OF EMPLOYMENT		Average Weekly Wage (Include Bonuses, Tips, Commissions, Reasonable Value of Board, Rent, etc.)
Firm or Trade Name	Address	Phone Number	First Day	Last Day Worked	
			Mo. Day Yr.	Mo. Day Yr.	

11. My job is or was: _____
                        Occupation
12. Union Member: ☐ Yes ☐ No If "Yes": _____
                                           Name of Union or Local Number

13. Were you claiming or receiving unemployment prior to this disability? ☐ Yes ☐ No

   If you did **not** claim or if you claimed but did **not** receive unemployment insurance benefits after LAST DAY WORKED, explain reasons fully: _____
_____

14. For the period of disability covered by this claim:

   A. Are you <u>receiving</u> wages, salary or separation pay: ☐ Yes ☐ No

   B. Are you <u>receiving</u> or <u>claiming</u>:

      1. Workers' compensation for work-connected disability: ☐ Yes ☐ No

      2. Paid Family Leave: ☐ Yes ☐ No

      3. No-Fault motor vehicle accident (check box): ☐ Yes ☐ No or personal injury involving third party (check box): ☐ Yes ☐ No

      4. Long-term disability benefits under the Federal Social Security Act for this disability: ☐ Yes ☐ No

IF "YES" IS CHECKED IN ANY OF THE ITEMS IN 14, COMPLETE THE FOLLOWING:

I have: ☐ received ☐ claimed from: _____ for the period: ____ / ____ / _____ to: ____ / ____ / _____

15. In the year (52 weeks) **before** your disability began, have you received disability benefits for other periods of disability? ☐ Yes ☐ No

   If "Yes", fill in the following: Paid by: _____ from: ____ / ____ / _____ to: ____ / ____ / _____

16. In the year (52 weeks) **before** your disability began, have you received Paid Family Leave? ☐ Yes ☐ No

   If "Yes", fill in the following: Paid by: _____ from: ____ / ____ / _____ to: ____ / ____ / _____

I hereby claim Disability Benefits and certify that for the period covered by this claim I was disabled. If my disability began while I was unemployed, I certify that I had been unemployed for more than four (4) weeks. I have read the instructions on page 2 of this form and that the foregoing statements, including any accompanying statements are, to the best of my knowledge, true and complete.

_____   _____
Claimant's Signature   Date

An individual may sign on behalf of the claimant only if he or she is legally authorized to do so and the claimant is a minor, mentally incompetent or incapacitated. If signed by other than claimant, print information below and complete and submit Form OC-110A, Claimant's Authorization to Disclose Workers' Compensation Records.

_____   _____   _____
On behalf of Claimant   Address   Relationship to Claimant

DB-450 (9-17) Page 1 of 2

Fig. 10.6   (From Employment Development Department, State of California.)

Continued

Chapter **10** Disability Income Insurance and Disability Benefits Programs

PART B - HEALTH CARE PROVIDER'S STATEMENT (Please Print or Type)

THE HEALTH CARE PROVIDER'S STATEMENT MUST BE FILLED IN COMPLETELY. THE ATTENDING HEALTH CARE PROVIDER SHALL COMPLETE AND RETURN TO THE CLAIMANT WITHIN SEVEN (7) DAYS OF RECEIPT OF THIS FORM. For item 7-d, you must give estimated date. If disability is caused by or arising in connection with pregnancy, enter estimated delivery date in item 9. **INCOMPLETE ANSWERS MAY DELAY PAYMENT OF BENEFITS.**

1. Last Name: _____ First Name: _____ MI: ____

2. Gender: ☐ Male ☐ Female   3. Date of Birth: ____ / ____ / _____

4. Diagnosis/Analysis: _____ Diagnosis Code: _____

   a. Claimant's symptoms: _____

   b. Objective findings: _____

5. Claimant hospitalized?: ☐ Yes ☐ No   From: ____ / ____ / _____   To: ____ / ____ / _____

6. Operation indicated?: ☐ Yes ☐ No   a. Type _____   b. Date ____ / ____ / _____

7.	ENTER DATES FOR THE FOLLOWING	MONTH	DAY	YEAR
a	Date of your first treatment for this disability			
b.	Date of your most recent treatment for this disability			
c.	Date Claimant was unable to work because of this disability			
d.	Date Claimant will again be able to perform work (Even if considerable question exists, estimate date. Avoid use of terms such as unknown or undetermined.)			
e.	If pregnancy related, please check box and enter the date ☐ estimated delivery date OR ☐ actual delivery date			

8. In your opinion, is this disability the result of injury arising out of and in the course of employment or occupational disease?:
☐ Yes ☐ No   If "Yes", has Form C-4 been filed with the Board? ☐ Yes ☐ No

I certify that I am a:

_____   _____   _____
(Physician, Chiropractor, Dentist, Podiatrist, Psychologist, Nurse-Midwife)   Licensed or Certified in the State of   License Number

_____   _____   _____
Health Care Provider's Printed Name   Health Care Provider's Signature   Date

_____   _____
Health Care Provider's Address   Phone #

CLAIMANT: READ THESE INSTRUCTIONS CAREFULLY

PLEASE NOTE: Do not date and file this form prior to your first date of disability. In order for your claim to be processed, Parts A and B must be completed.

1. If you are using this form because you became disabled **while employed** or you became disabled **within four (4) weeks after termination of employment**, your completed claim should be mailed **within thirty (30) days to your employer or your last employer's insurance carrier.** You may find your employer's disability insurance carrier on the Workers' Compensation Board's website using Employer Coverage Search.

2. If you are using this form because you became **disabled after having been unemployed for more than four (4) weeks**, your completed claim should be mailed to: **Workers' Compensation Board, Disability Benefits Bureau, 328 State Street, Schenectady, NY 12305.** If you answered "Yes" to question 14.B.3, please complete and attach Form DB-450.1.

If you have any questions about claiming disability benefits, you may contact the Board's Disability Benefits Bureau at (800) 353-3092. Additional information may be obtained at the Board's website: www.wcb.ny.gov, or you may write to the Disability Benefits Bureau at the address listed above.

DB-450 (9-17) Page 2 of 2

Fig. 10.6, cont'd

ASSIGNMENT 10.5 COMPLETE A STATE DISABILITY INSURANCE FORM

Performance Objective

Task: Complete a state disability insurance form and define patient record abbreviations.

Conditions: Use the patient's record (Fig. 10.7), a New York State Notice and Proof of Claim for Disability Benefits (Fig. 10.8), and a computer.

Standards: Time: _____ minutes

Accuracy: _____

(Note: The time element and accuracy criteria may be given by your instructor.)

Directions:

1. Mr. Vincent P. Michael (see Fig. 10.7) is applying for state disability benefits. Complete the New York State Notice and Proof of Claim for Disability Benefits (Fig. 10.8) and date it September 22. Assume that the Claimant's Information has been completed satisfactorily by Mr. Michael. Remember that this is not a claim for payment to the physician, so no ledger card has been furnished for this patient.

2. Refer to Chapter 10 of the *Textbook* to assist you in completing this form.

After the instructor has returned your work to you, either make the necessary corrections and place your work in a three-ring notebook for future reference or, if you received a high score, place it in your portfolio for reference when applying for a job.

Abbreviations pertinent to this record:

Pt   _____   exam   _____

ESR   _____   mm   _____

hr   _____   imp   _____

CVA   _____   adv   _____

retn   _____   wk   _____

approx _____   L   _____

PATIENT RECORD

Michael	Vincent	P.	05-17-55	M		555-567-9001
LAST NAME	FIRST NAME	MIDDLE NAME	BIRTH DATE	SEX		HOME PHONE

1529 1/2 Thompson Boulevard	Woodland Hills	XY	12345
ADDRESS	CITY	STATE	ZIP CODE

555-398-5677	555-311-0098	555-567-9001	michael@wb.net
CELL PHONE	PAGER NO.	FAX NO.	E-MAIL ADDRESS

562-XX-8888	E0034578
PATIENT'S SOC. SEC. NO.	DRIVER'S LICENSE

assembler "A"	Burroughs Corporation
PATIENT'S OCCUPATION	NAME OF COMPANY

5411 North Lindero Canyon Road, Woodland Hills, XY 12345	555-560-9008
ADDRESS OF EMPLOYER	PHONE

Helen J. Michael	homemaker
SPOUSE OR PARENT	OCCUPATION

EMPLOYER	ADDRESS	PHONE

Blue Shield	Vincent P. Michael
NAME OF INSURANCE	INSURED OR SUBSCRIBER

T8411981A	677899AT
POLICY/CERTIFICATE NO.	GROUP NO.

REFERRED BY: Robert T. Smith (friend)

DATE	PROGRESS NOTES
9-20-xx	Patient calls the office complaining of having had the flu, headache, dizziness, and of being tired. Pt unable to go to work today. Exam shows weakness of L hand. Pt exhibits light dysphasia and confusion. Pt is referred to XYZ Radiology for chest x-ray, frontal and lateral, and to the lab at College Hospital for ESR. Pt to return tomorrow at 11 AM for results.
	BC/mtf *Brady Coccidioides, MD*
9-21-xx	Chest x-rays show cardiomegaly and slight pulmonary congestion. ESR 46 mm/hr. Imp. Post flu syndrome, transient ischemic attack, possible CVA. Prescribed medication for the congestion and adv. pt. to take aspirin 1/day. Pt to stay off work and retn in 1 week. Approx. date of retn to work 10-16-xx.
	BC/mtf *Brady Coccidioides, MD*

Fig. 10.7

DB-450 9-17

New York State
NOTICE AND PROOF OF CLAIM FOR DISABILITY BENEFITS

Use this form if you became disabled **while employed** or if you became disabled **within four (4) weeks after termination of employment** OR if you became **disabled after having been unemployed for more than four (4) weeks**. Please answer all questions in Part A and questions 1 through 3 in Part B. Read all instructions on this form carefully. Health care providers must complete Part B on page 2.

PART A - CLAIMANT'S INFORMATION (Please Print or Type)

1. Last Name: _____ First Name: _____ MI: ___

2. Mailing Address (Street & Apt. #): _____

    City: _____ State: _____ Zip: _____ Country: _____

3. Daytime Phone #: _____ 4. Email Address: _____

5. Social Security #: ____ - ___ - _____ 6. Date of Birth: ___ - ___ - ___ 7. Gender: ☐ Male ☐ Female

8. My disability is (if injury, also state <u>how</u>, <u>when</u> and <u>where</u> it occurred): _____

_____

9. I became disabled or became ineligible for Unemployment Insurance because of this disability on: ___ / ___ / _____

    I worked on that day: ☐ Yes ☐ No

    Have you recovered from this disability? ☐ Yes ☐ No   If Yes, what was the date you were able to work: ___ / ___ / _____

    Have you since worked for wages or profit? ☐ Yes ☐ No   If Yes, list dates: _____

10. Give name of last employer. If more than one employer during last eight (8) weeks, name all employers. Average Weekly Wage is based on all wages earned in last eight (8) weeks worked.

LAST EMPLOYER			PERIOD OF EMPLOYMENT		Average Weekly Wage (Include Bonuses, Tips, Commissions, Reasonable Value of Board, Rent, etc.)
Firm or Trade Name	Address	Phone Number	First Day	Last Day Worked	
			Mo. Day Yr.	Mo. Day Yr.	

OTHER EMPLOYER (during last eight (8) weeks)			PERIOD OF EMPLOYMENT		Average Weekly Wage (Include Bonuses, Tips, Commissions, Reasonable Value of Board, Rent, etc.)
Firm or Trade Name	Address	Phone Number	First Day	Last Day Worked	
			Mo. Day Yr.	Mo. Day Yr.	

11. My job is or was: _____ 12. Union Member: ☐ Yes ☐ No If "Yes": _____
                                Occupation   Name of Union or Local Number

13. Were you claiming or receiving unemployment prior to this disability? ☐ Yes ☐ No

    If you did **not** claim or if you claimed but did **not** receive unemployment insurance benefits after LAST DAY WORKED, explain reasons fully: _____

14. For the period of disability covered by this claim:

    A. Are you <u>**receiving**</u> wages, salary or separation pay: ☐ Yes ☐ No

    B. Are you <u>**receiving**</u> or <u>**claiming**</u>:

       1. Workers' compensation for work-connected disability: ☐ Yes ☐ No

       2. Paid Family Leave: ☐ Yes ☐ No

       3. No-Fault motor vehicle accident (check box): ☐ Yes ☐ No or personal injury involving third party (check box): ☐ Yes ☐ No

       4. Long-term disability benefits under the Federal Social Security Act for this disability: ☐ Yes ☐ No

IF "YES" IS CHECKED IN ANY OF THE ITEMS IN 14, COMPLETE THE FOLLOWING:

I have: ☐ received ☐ claimed from: _____ for the period: ___ / ___ / _____ to: ___ / ___ / _____

15. In the year (52 weeks) **before** your disability began, have you received disability benefits for other periods of disability? ☐ Yes ☐ No

    If "Yes", fill in the following: Paid by: _____ from: ___ / ___ / _____ to: ___ / ___ / _____

16. In the year (52 weeks) **before** your disability began, have you received Paid Family Leave? ☐ Yes ☐ No

    If "Yes", fill in the following: Paid by: _____ from: ___ / ___ / _____ to: ___ / ___ / _____

I hereby claim Disability Benefits and certify that for the period covered by this claim I was disabled. If my disability began while I was unemployed, I certify that I had been unemployed for more than four (4) weeks. I have read the instructions on page 2 of this form and that the foregoing statements, including any accompanying statements are, to the best of my knowledge, true and complete.

_____   _____
       Claimant's Signature   **Date**

An individual may sign on behalf of the claimant only if he or she is legally authorized to do so and the claimant is a minor, mentally incompetent or incapacitated. If signed by other than claimant, print information below and complete and submit Form OC-110A, Claimant's Authorization to Disclose Workers' Compensation Records.

_____   _____   _____
      On behalf of Claimant   **Address**   **Relationship to Claimant**

DB-450 (9-17) Page 1 of 2

Fig. 10.8   (From Employment Development Department, State of California.)

Continued

       Chapter **10** Disability Income Insurance and Disability Benefits Programs

PART B - HEALTH CARE PROVIDER'S STATEMENT (Please Print or Type)

THE HEALTH CARE PROVIDER'S STATEMENT MUST BE FILLED IN COMPLETELY. THE ATTENDING HEALTH CARE PROVIDER SHALL COMPLETE AND RETURN TO THE CLAIMANT WITHIN SEVEN (7) DAYS OF RECEIPT OF THIS FORM. For item 7-d, you must give estimated date. If disability is caused by or arising in connection with pregnancy, enter estimated delivery date in item 9. **INCOMPLETE ANSWERS MAY DELAY PAYMENT OF BENEFITS.**

1. Last Name: _____ First Name: _____ MI: ___

2. Gender: ☐ Male ☐ Female   3. Date of Birth: ___ / ___ / ____

4. Diagnosis/Analysis: _____ Diagnosis Code: _____

   a. Claimant's symptoms: _____

   _____

   b. Objective findings: _____

   _____

5. Claimant hospitalized?: ☐ Yes ☐ No   From: ___ / ___ / _____   To: ___ / ___ / _____

6. Operation indicated?: ☐ Yes ☐ No   a. Type _____   b. Date ___ / ___ / ___

7. ENTER DATES FOR THE FOLLOWING	MONTH	DAY	YEAR
a Date of your first treatment for this disability			
b. Date of your most recent treatment for this disability			
c. Date Claimant was unable to work because of this disability			
d. Date Claimant will again be able to perform work (Even if considerable question exists, estimate date. Avoid use of terms such as unknown or undetermined.)			
e. If pregnancy related, please check box and enter the date ☐ estimated delivery date OR ☐ actual delivery date			

8. In your opinion, is this disability the result of injury arising out of and in the course of employment or occupational disease?:
☐ Yes ☐ No   If "Yes", has Form C-4 been filed with the Board? ☐ Yes ☐ No

I certify that I am a:

_____   _____   _____
(Physician, Chiropractor, Dentist, Podiatrist, Psychologist, Nurse-Midwife)   Licensed or Certified in the State of   License Number

_____   _____   _____
Health Care Provider's Printed Name   Health Care Provider's Signature   Date

_____   _____
Health Care Provider's Address   Phone #

CLAIMANT: READ THESE INSTRUCTIONS CAREFULLY

PLEASE NOTE: Do not date and file this form prior to your first date of disability. In order for your claim to be processed, Parts A and B must be completed.

1. If you are using this form because you became disabled **while employed** or you became disabled **within four (4) weeks after termination of employment**, your completed claim should be mailed **within thirty (30) days to your employer or your last employer's insurance carrier.** You may find your employer's disability insurance carrier on the Workers' Compensation Board's website using Employer Coverage Search.

2. If you are using this form because you became **disabled after having been unemployed for more than four (4) weeks**, your completed claim should be mailed to: **Workers' Compensation Board, Disability Benefits Bureau, 328 State Street, Schenectady, NY 12305.** If you answered "Yes" to question 14.B.3, please complete and attach Form DB-450.1.

If you have any questions about claiming disability benefits, you may contact the Board's Disability Benefits Bureau at (800) 353-3092. Additional information may be obtained at the Board's website: www.wcb.ny.gov, or you may write to the Disability Benefits Bureau at the address listed above.

DB-450 (9-17) Page 2 of 2

Fig. 10.8, cont'd

11 Medical Documentation and the Electronic Health Record

Cheryl Fassett

KEY TERMS

Your instructor may wish to select some words pertinent to this chapter for a test. For definitions of the terms, further study, and/or reference, the words, phrases, and abbreviations may be found in the glossary at the end of the Textbook. *Key terms for this chapter follow.*

acute
attending physician
chief complaint
chronic
clinical documentation improvement
cloned note
comorbidity
comprehensive
concurrent care
consultation
consulting physician
continuity of care
counseling
critical care
degaussing
detailed
documentation
electronic health record
emergency care
eponym
established patient
expanded problem focused
external audit
family history
health record
high complexity
history of present illness
internal review
legible

low complexity
medical decision making
medical necessity
moderate complexity
morbidity
mortality
new patient
non-physician practitioner
ordering physician
past history
physical examination
prepayment audit
primary care physician
problem focused
prospective review
query
referral
referring physician
resident physician
retrospective review
review of systems
social history
straightforward
subacute
subpoena
subpoena duces tecum
teaching physician
treating or performing physician
zeroization

KEY ABBREVIATIONS

See how many abbreviations and acronyms you can translate and then use this as a handy reference list. Definitions for the key abbreviations are located near the back of the Textbook *in the glossary.*

ARRA _____

C level of history or examination _____

CC _____

CDI _____

CCU _____

D level of history or examination _____

129

dx or Dx _____   NPP _____

ED or ER _____   PCP _____

EHR _____   PE or PX _____

E/M service _____   PF level of history or examination _____

EMR _____   PFSH _____

EPF level of history or examination _____   PH _____

ESI _____   POMR system _____

FH _____   RCU _____

HC medical decision making _____   RLQ _____

HIM _____   R/O _____

HIV _____   ROS _____

HPI _____   RUQ _____

ICU _____   SF medical decision making _____

LC medical decision making _____   SH _____

LLQ _____   SOAP style _____

LUQ _____   SOR system _____

MC medical decision making _____   WNL _____

MDM _____

PERFORMANCE OBJECTIVES

The student will be able to:

- Define and spell the key terms and key abbreviations for this chapter, given the information from the *Textbook* glossary, within a reasonable time period and with enough accuracy to obtain a satisfactory evaluation.
- Answer the fill in the blank, mix and match, multiple choice, and true/false review questions after reading the chapter, with enough accuracy to obtain a satisfactory evaluation.
- Use critical thinking to solve an office problem about patients' medical records.
- Abstract subjective and objective data from patient records, within a reasonable time period and with enough accuracy to obtain a satisfactory evaluation.

- Review a patient record and obtain answers to questions about the documentation presented, within a reasonable time period and with enough accuracy to obtain a satisfactory evaluation.
- Select the correct medicolegal form, create a letter with appropriate content, prepare an envelope, and properly complete US Postal Service documents for the physician's signature, given the patients' chart notes and ledger cards, within a reasonable time period and with enough accuracy to obtain a satisfactory evaluation.

STUDY OUTLINE

The Documentation Process
    Health Record
    Electronic Health Records
Incentive Programs for Adoption of Electronic Health Records
General Principles of Health Record Documentation
    Documenters
    Clinical Documentation Improvement
    Legible Documentation
    Common Documentation Errors
    Medical Necessity
    Legalities of Health Record Billing Patterns
    Termination of a Case
Documentation Terminology
    Terminology for Evaluation and Management Services
    Diagnostic Terminology and Abbreviations
    Directional Terms
    Surgical Terminology
Abstracting From Medical Records
    Life or Health Insurance Applications

Review and Audit of Health Records
    Internal Reviews
    External Reviews
    Software Edit Checks
Release and Retention of Health Records
    Subpoena
    Retention of Records
    Data Storage
    Data Disposal
    Electronic Power Protection
    Prevention of Legal Problems
Documentation Guidelines for Evaluation and Management Services
    Audit Point System
    Documentation of History
    Documentation of Examination
    Documentation of Medical Decision Making

Part I Fill in the Blank

Review the objectives, key terms, glossary definitions to key terms, chapter information, and figures before completing the following review questions.

1. Written or graphic information about patient care is termed a/an _____.

2. List the two types of health record systems that can be used in a medical practice.

   a. _____

   b. _____

3. The difference between an EMR and an EHR is that the _____ is an individual physician's record of the patient's care, whereas the _____ is all of the patient's health records, from many different information systems and providers.

4. The greatest advantage of an EHR system is the improvement of quality of care and patient safety through the _____ of medical records between providers and other health care organizations.

5. What is the Centers for Medicare and Medicaid Services (CMS) definition of *legible documentation?*

   _____

   _____

6. _____ is the performance of services or procedures consistent with the diagnosis, done with standards of good medical practice and a proper level of care given in the appropriate setting.

7. Medicare administrative contractors have _____ to access a medical practice without an appointment or search warrant to conduct a review of documentation, audits, and evaluations.

8. If a medical practice is audited by Medicare officials and intentional miscoding is discovered, _____ may be levied and providers may be _____.

9. Define the following terms in relationship to billing.

   a. New patient _____

   _____

   b. Established patient _____

   _____

10. Explain the difference between a consultation and the referral of a patient.

    a. Consultation:

    _____

    _____

    b. Referral:

    _____

    _____

11. Medical care for a patient who has received treatment for an illness and is referred to a second physician for treatment of the same condition is a situation called

    _____.

12. An emergency medical condition, as defined by Medicare, is a medical condition

    manifesting itself by _____ of _____ such that the absence of immediate medical attention could reasonably be expected to result in placing the patient's health in serious jeopardy, serious impairment to body functions, or serious dysfunction of any body organ or part.

13. For EHRs, how should an insurance billing specialist correct an error on a patient's record?

    _____

14. For paper-based records, how should an error be corrected on a patient's record?

    _____

15. Name the six documentation components of a patient's history.

    a. _____

    b. _____

    c. _____

    d. _____

    e. _____

    f. _____

16. List the eight descriptive elements that can be documented in the HPI.

    a. _____

    b. _____

    c. _____

    d. _____

    e. _____

    f. _____

    g. _____

    h. _____

17. List four of the body systems that are recognized for the reporting of the review of systems (ROS).

    a. _____

    b. _____

    c. _____

    d. _____

18. A problem-focused examination is a/an _____ examination of the affected body area or organ system.

19. Medical decision making (MDM) is the process performed after taking the patient's history and performing the examination, which results in a/an

_____.

20. Any charts that are amended with additional notes must be labeled "_____" or "late entry," dated on the day of the amendment, and signed by the physician.

Part II Mix and Match

21. Match the following terms in the right column with their descriptions, and fill in the blank with the appropriate letter.

_____ Renders a service to a patient

_____ Directs selection, preparation, and administration of tests, medication, or treatment

_____ Legally responsible for the care and treatment given to a patient

_____ Gives an opinion regarding a specific problem that is requested by another doctor

_____ Sends the patient for tests or treatment or to another doctor for consultation

_____ Oversees care of patients in managed care plans and refers patients to see specialists when needed

_____ Responsible for training and supervising medical students

_____ Clinical nurse specialist or licensed social worker who treats a patient for a specific medical problem and uses the results of a diagnostic test in managing a patient's medical problem

_____ Performs one or more years of training in a specialty area while working at a hospital (medical center)

a. Attending physician

b. Consulting physician

c. Non-physician practitioner

d. Ordering physician

e. Primary care physician

f. Referring physician

g. Resident physician

h. Teaching physician

i. Treating or performing physician

Part III Multiple Choice
Choose the best answer.

22. Chart chasing is eliminated when using which type of record system?
    a. Paper-based
    b. EHR
    c. Problem-oriented
    d. Integrated record

23. Regarding the SOAP style of documentation that a physician uses to chart a patient's progress in the health record, SOAP stands for:
    a. signature, observation, assessment, and progress.
    b. subjective, objective, assessment, and plan.
    c. symptoms, objective findings, and professional services.
    d. subjective, opinions, assistance, and present illness.

24. During the performance of an external audit to review a medical practice's health records, the system used to show deficiencies in documentation is called a/an:
    a. SOAP system.
    b. electronic recording system.
    c. information record system.
    d. point system.

25. Which of these elements is a requirement for all levels of history?
    a. Chief complaint (CC)
    b. History of present illness (HPI)
    c. Review of systems (ROS)
    d. Past, family, or social history (PFSH)

26. When there is an underlying disease or other conditions are present at the time of the patient's office visit, this is termed:
    a. mortality.
    b. continuity.
    c. comorbidity.
    d. complexity.

27. Critical care is rendered in:
    a. the coronary care unit.
    b. the intensive care unit.
    c. the emergency room.
    d. all of the above.

28. Verification of successful backups by comparing original records with copied records should be performed:
    a. once a day.
    b. once a week.
    c. once a month.
    d. once a year.

29. An acceptable method for ensuring that electronic PHI (ePHI) cannot be recovered from a hard drive that is being disposed of is by:
    a. deletion of files.
    b. formatting drives.
    c. incineration.
    d. all of the above.

Part IV True/False

Write "T" or "F" in the blank line to indicate whether you think the statement is true or false.

_____ 30. A patient's hospital discharge summary contains the discharge diagnosis but not the admitting diagnosis.

_____ 31. An eponym should not be used when a comparable anatomic term can be used in its place.

_____ 32. If the phrase "rule out" appears in a patient's health record in connection with a disease, then code the condition as if it existed.

_____ 33. During a prospective review or prebilling audit, all procedures or services and diagnoses listed on the encounter form must match the data on the insurance claim form.

_____ 34. Willful disregard of a subpoena is punishable as contempt of court.

_____ 35. Based on Medicare Conditions of Participation, hospitals must retain medical records for a period of at least 4 years.

_____ 36. Assigned insurance claims for Medicaid and Medicare cases must be kept for a period of 7 years.

_____ 37. If a patient fails to make payment on an overdue account, the physician has the right to formally withdraw from providing care to the patient.

_____ 38. There are very few circumstances that insurance billers may be faced with when executing their job duties that may lead to a case of lawsuit.

_____ 39. Deleting files or formatting the hard drive is sufficient to keep electronic protected health information from being accessed.

ASSIGNMENT 11.2 REVIEW DIAGNOSTIC TERMINOLOGY AND ABBREVIATIONS

In the Textbook, review Fig. 11.6, and use a medical dictionary to complete the assignment.

1. Place the appropriate letter on a blank line before the phrase.

_____ Taking or letting out fluids from a body part   a. alteration

_____ Act of cutting out   b. bypass

_____ Modifying a body part without affecting function   c. control

_____ Taking out or off a device from a body part   d. drainage

_____ Stop or attempt to stop bleeding   e. excision

_____ Altering the route of passage with anastomoses   f. removal

2. Write in the meaning of these abbreviations and/or symbols commonly encountered in a patient's medical record:

RLQ _____

DC _____

WNL _____

R/O _____

URI _____

3. When documenting incisions, the unit of measure for length should be listed in _____.

Multiple Choice Questions

4. If a physician called and asked for a patient's medical record STAT, what does he or she mean?
   a. The physician wants a statistic from a patient's record.
   b. The physician wants the record delivered on Tuesday.
   c. The physician wants the record delivered immediately.

5. If a physician asks you to locate the results of the last UA, what would you be searching for?
   a. A urinalysis report
   b. An x-ray report of the ulna
   c. Uric acid test results

6. If a physician telephoned and asked for a copy of the last H&P to be emailed, what is being requested?
   a. Heart and pulmonary findings
   b. H2 antagonist test results
   c. A history and physical

7. If a hospital nurse telephoned and asked you to read the results of the patient's last CBC, what would you be searching for?
   a. Carcinoma basal cell report
   b. Complete blood count
   c. Congenital blindness, complete report

8. If you were asked to make a photocopy of the patient's last CT, what would you be searching for?
   a. Chemotherapy record
   b. Connective tissue report
   c. Computed tomography scan

ASSIGNMENT 11.3 CRITICAL THINKING: SOLVE AN OFFICE PROBLEM

Performance Objective

Task: Answer questions after reviewing the case study using critical thinking skills.

Conditions: Use a case study and a pen or pencil.

Standards: Time: _____ minutes

              Accuracy: _____

Directions: Answer questions after reviewing the case study using your critical thinking skills. Record your answer on the blank lines.

1. A patient comes into the office for treatment. He does not return, because he is dissatisfied with Dr. Practon's treatment. Is it necessary to keep his records when he

   obviously will not return? _____

   Why? _____

   _____

ASSIGNMENT 11.4 ABSTRACT SUBJECTIVE OBSERVATIONS AND OBJECTIVE FINDINGS FROM PATIENT RECORDS

Performance Objective

Task: List subjective observations and objective findings after reading each of the case studies.

Conditions: Use a pencil and four case studies.

Standards: Time: _____ minutes

                    Accuracy: _____

                    (Note: The time element and accuracy criteria may be given by your instructor.)

Case Study 1 Mrs. Smith is 25 years old and was brought into the emergency department of College Hospital with complaints of difficulty breathing and chest pain. Her vital signs show an elevated temperature of 101°F and pulse rate of 90. Respirations are labored at 30 per minute. Blood pressure is 140/80. Her skin is warm and diaphoretic (perspiring). She states, "This condition has been going on for the past three days."

Subjective observations: _____

Objective findings: _____

Case Study 2 Mr. Jones is 56 years old and was admitted to the hospital with chest pain and elevated pulse and blood pressure. His skin is cold and clammy.

Subjective observations: _____

Objective findings: _____

Case Study 3 You are assisting the radiology technician with Sally Salazar, a 6-year-old Hispanic girl who was brought into the pediatrician's office with a suspected fracture of the right arm. Sally states she was "running at school, tripped on my shoelace, and fell." She tells you her "arm hurts," points out how "funny my arm looks," and starts to cry. You notice her arm looks disfigured and is covered with dirt. Sally is cradling her arm against her body and is unwilling to let go because "it's going to fall off."

Subjective observations: _____

Objective findings: _____

Case Study 4 You are working in the business office of College Hospital. A former patient in your hospital comes in complaining of his billing. He states he was never catheterized, never had any of the medications listed on his itemized bill, and has "never been in this hospital for that length of time." His face is red, his voice is gradually getting louder, and you notice he is standing with the aid of crutches because his left leg is in a full cast.

Subjective observations: _____

Objective findings: _____

ASSIGNMENT 11.5 REVIEW OF A PATIENT RECORD

Performance Objective

Task: Answer questions after reviewing a patient's record.

Conditions: Use a pencil, internal record review sheet, medical dictionary, abbreviation reference list, drug reference book (e.g., *Mosby's MD Consult*), and laboratory reference book.

Standards: Time: _____ minutes

              Accuracy: _____

              (Note: The time element and accuracy criteria may be given by your instructor.)

Directions: In many instances, when developing the skill of reviewing a patient record, you may need critical thinking in addition to efficient use of reference books. Answer only those questions you think can be justified by the documentation presented in the patient's record. Because the content of each record is variable, you may or may not have answers to all eight questions.

Answer the questions by recording on the blank lines the documentation found identifying the components from the patient's record.

If your answers vary, perhaps you have a reason for them that may or may not be valid. List your reasons in the response section. Differences may be reviewed with your instructor privately or via class discussion.

Patient Record

10-21-20xx
HPI
This new pt is an 80-year-old white male who has had problems with voiding since 9-5-20xx.

During the night, the pt had only 50 mL output and was catheterized this morning because of his poor urinary output (200 mL). He was thought to have a distended bladder; he complains of pressure in the suprapubic region. He has not had any gross hematuria. He has difficulty voiding, especially lying down. His voiding pattern is improved while standing and sitting.

Gene Ulibarri, MD

1. Location: In what body system is the sign or symptom occurring?

    Response: _____

2. Quality: Is the symptom or pain burning, gnawing, stabbing, pressure-like, squeezing, fullness?

    Response: _____

3. Severity: In this case, how would you rank the symptom (how was distress relieved) or pain (slight, mild, severe, persistent)?

    Response: _____

4. Duration: How long has the symptom been present, or how long does it last?

    Response: _____

5. Timing: When does(do) a sign(s) or symptom(s) occur (AM, PM, after or before meals)?

    Response: _____

6. Context: Is the pain/symptom associated with big meals, dairy products, etc.?

   Response: _____

7. Modifying factors: What actions make symptoms worse or better?

   Response: _____

8. Associated signs and symptoms: What other system or body area produces complaints when the presenting problem occurs? (Example: Chest pain leads to shortness of breath.)

   Response: _____

12 Diagnostic Coding

Cheryl Fassett

KEY TERMS

Your instructor may wish to select some words pertinent to this chapter for a test. For definitions of the terms, further study, and/or reference, the words, phrases, and abbreviations may be found in the glossary at the end of the Textbook. *Key terms for this chapter follow.*

adverse effect
benign tumor
carcinoma in situ
chief complaint
combination code
complication
computer-assisted coding
conventions
eponym
essential modifiers
etiology
Excludes 1
Excludes 2
external causes of morbidity
International Classification of Diseases, Tenth Revision, Clinical Modification
International Classification of Diseases, Tenth Revision, Procedure Coding System
intoxication
late effect
laterality
malignant tumor
manifestation

medical necessity
metastasis
morbidity
mortality
neoplasm
nonessential modifiers
not elsewhere classifiable
not otherwise specified
Official Guidelines for Coding and Reporting
ordinality of encounter
placeholder
poisoning
primary diagnosis
principal diagnosis
prophylaxis
residual subcategories
rule out
secondary diagnosis
sequela
sequencing
syndrome
Uncertain Behavior
Z codes

KEY ABBREVIATIONS

AHA _____

AHIMA _____

CAC _____

CC _____

CM _____

CPT _____

DM _____

GEMS _____

HIV _____

ICD-10-CM _____

ICD-10-PCS _____

ICD-11 _____

MRI _____

NCHS _____

NEC _____

NOS _____

WHO _____

PERFORMANCE OBJECTIVES

The student will be able to:

- Define and spell the key terms and key abbreviations for this chapter, given the information from the textbook glossary, within a reasonable time period and with enough accuracy to obtain a satisfactory evaluation.
- Answer the fill-in-the-blank, multiple choice, and true/false review questions after reading the chapter, with enough accuracy to obtain a satisfactory evaluation.
- Indicate main terms, subterms, subterms to subterms, and carryover lines, given a section of a page from the ICD-10-CM code book, with enough accuracy to obtain a satisfactory evaluation.

- Answer questions, given a section of a page from the ICD-10-CM code book, with enough accuracy to obtain a satisfactory evaluation.
- Select the correct diagnostic code numbers and given diagnoses, and locate the conditions using Volumes 1 and 2 of the ICD-10-CM code book, with enough accuracy to obtain a satisfactory evaluation.
- Select the correct diagnostic code numbers, given a series of scenarios and diagnoses, using Volumes 1 and 2 of the ICD-10-CM code book, with enough accuracy to obtain a satisfactory evaluation.

STUDY OUTLINE

Diagnosis Coding Overview
   Assigning a Diagnosis Code
   Sequencing of Diagnostic Codes
   Admitting Diagnoses
   Medical Necessity
International Classification of Diseases
   History
   Transition From ICD-9-CM to ICD-10-CM
   ICD-10 Diagnosis and Procedure Codes
   ICD-10-CM
   ICD-10-PCS
   ICD-10-CM and Its Compliance With HIPAA
   Organization and Format of ICD-10-CM
   Alphabetic Index to Diseases and Injuries
   Special Points to Remember in the Alphabetic Index

   Tabular List of Diseases and Injuries
   Special Points to Remember in the Tabular List
Official Coding Guidelines for ICD-10-CM
   Selection of a Coding Manual
   Diagnostic Code Book Conventions
   General Coding Guidelines
   Chapter-Specific Coding Guidelines
   Diagnostic Coding and Reporting Guidelines for Outpatient Services
   Handy Hints for Diagnostic Coding
   Computer-Assisted Coding
The Future of Diagnosis Coding
Basic Steps in Selecting Diagnostic Codes from ICD-10-CM

Part I Fill in the Blank on ICD-10-CM

Review the objectives, key terms, and chapter information before completing the following review questions.

1. When submitting insurance claims for patients seen by a healthcare organization office or in an outpatient hospital setting, the _____ diagnosis is listed first, but in the inpatient hospital setting, the _____ diagnosis is used.

2. Claims to insurance carriers often are denied because of lack of _____, which indicates that the procedure provided was not payable for the diagnosis submitted.

3. Diagnosis coding for services provided by a healthcare organization are reported using ICD-10-CM effective with dates of service _____.

4. The abbreviation ICD-10-CM means _____.

5. The official version of the International Classification of Disease (ICD) was developed by the _____.

6. ICD-10-CM requires _____ documentation in the medical record than the previous coding system, ICD-9-CM.

7. ICD-10-PCS is the coding system for reporting inpatient services by hospitals and replaces _____ of the ICD-9-CM coding system.

8. ICD-10-CM is the standard code set required under _____ legislation and must be used by covered entities when assigning diagnostic codes.

9. Volume 2, Diseases, is a/an _____ index or listing of code numbers.

10. Volume 1, Diseases, is a/an _____ listing of code numbers.

11. When using the ICD-10-CM coding system, the _____ is used as a placeholder to save space for future code expansion.

12. Conventions are _____ used in the diagnostic code books to assist in the selection of correct codes for the diagnosis encountered.

13. The abbreviation NEC appearing in the ICD-10-CM code book means

_____.

14. _____ are used to enclose synonyms in the Tabular List.

15. If a condition is documented in the medical record, but it is not specified as to whether the condition is acute or chronic, then the _____ code should be assigned.

16. When selecting a code that corresponds with the condition stated in the medical record, the coder should first locate the term in the _____ and then confirm the code in the _____.

17. The instructional note _____ listed in the Tabular List assists the coder as to when it is appropriate to report a secondary code.

18. A condition that is produced after the acute phase of an illness is listed as the main term _____ in the Alphabetic Index.

19. When reporting a condition that affects the left side of the patient, the character _____ is reported to indicate laterality.

20. The Neoplasm Table has column headings for _____, _____, _____, and _____.

21. In juvenile diabetes, the patient's _____ does not function and produce enough insulin.

22. When coding for diabetes in pregnancy, a code from category _____ is assigned as the primary diagnosis.

23. _____ hypertension is indicative of a life-threatening condition.

24. Full-term uncomplicated _____ deliveries are always reported with the code O80.

25. When reporting accidents and injuries, a seventh character of "A" identifies that the encounter is _____.

26. Additional external cause codes are _____ when reporting poisonings using combination codes from T36 through T65.

27. If documentation states that the incident related to a poisoning was a suspected suicide attempt, the code would be reported from the column titled _____.

28. If a patient falls and fractures his or her wrist, the fracture code is the primary code, followed by a/an _____ code to explain how the accident occurred.

29. When a person encounters health services to receive a vaccination, the diagnosis is reported with a/an _____.

Part II Multiple Choice on ICD-10-CM

Choose the best answer.

30. The consequences of inaccurate assignment of diagnostic codes include:
    a. delay in payment of claim.
    b. denial of claim.
    c. change in level of reimbursement.
    d. all of the above.

31. Diagnosis codes should be reported to the highest level of:
    a. specificity.
    b. medical necessity.
    c. etiology.
    d. sequel.

32. When a provider makes a hospital visit, the encounter should be reported with a diagnosis code that represents:
    a. the reason the patient was admitted to the hospital.
    b. the condition the provider evaluated and treated during the encounter.
    c. the condition that was requested by the admitting physician.
    d. the final discharge diagnosis.

33. To determine the diagnosis codes that would support medical necessity of a specific procedure, such as magnetic resonance imaging (MRI), under Medicare guidelines, the coder should consult:
    a. *Current Procedural Terminology* (CPT) guidelines.
    b. local coverage determinations (LCDs) and national coverage determinations (NCDs).
    c. all of the above.
    d. none of the above.

34. Passage of which legislation, in 1988, placed requirements on physicians to report appropriate diagnosis codes on all claims to Medicare?
    a. Affordable Care Act
    b. Health Insurance Portability and Accountability Act (HIPAA)
    c. American Recovery and Reinvestment Act
    d. Medicare Catastrophic Coverage Act

35. ICD-10-PCS (Procedure Coding System) was developed by 3M Health Information Systems under contract with the:
    a. National Center for Health Statistics.
    b. World Health Organization.
    c. Centers for Disease Control.
    d. Centers for Medicare and Medicaid Services.

36. Annual updates to ICD-10-CM are published:
    a. by the AMA and AHA.
    b. by the AHA and AHIMA.
    c. by the AHA, AHIMA, and US Printing Office.
    d. by the AMA, AHA, AHIMA, and US Printing Office.

37. The Alphabetic Index to Diseases and Injuries is placed:
    a. after Volume 1, the Tabular Index.
    b. first in the coding manual.
    c. after the Table of Drugs and Chemicals.
    d. after the Index to External Causes.

38. How many chapters does the Tabular List contain?
    a. 17
    b. 17 with two supplementary classifications
    c. 19
    d. 21

39. When two diagnoses are classified with a single code, it is referred to as:
    a. a combination code.
    b. a manifestation.
    c. an external cause code.
    d. a Z code.

40. An essential modifier is also referred to as a:
    a. main term.
    b. nonessential modifier.
    c. subterm.
    d. convention.

41. The equivalent of unspecified is:
    a. NEC.
    b. NOS.
    c. nonessential.
    d. secondary.

42. When reporting outpatients' services, signs and symptoms are acceptable for reporting purposes:
    a. in all situations.
    b. in addition to the definitive diagnosis.
    c. when a definitive diagnosis has not been determined.
    d. under no circumstances.

43. When conditions documented as "threatened" are referenced in the Alphabetic Index and there is no entry for the threatened condition, report:
    a. with signs and symptoms.
    b. as if the patient has the condition.
    c. the existing underlying condition.
    d. all of the above.

44. When reporting laterality, the final character "3" is reported to indicate:
    a. right side.
    b. left side.
    c. bilateral.
    d. unspecified.

45. When reporting an encounter for testing of human immunodeficiency virus (HIV), the code should be assigned as:
    a. B20.
    b. R75.
    c. Z11.4.
    d. Z21.

46. When fractures are documented, but there is no indication of whether the fracture is open or closed,
    a. report as closed.
    b. report as open.
    c. it does not matter if it is reported as open or closed.
    d. report as unspecified.

47. When identifying the total body surface area of a burn, the front torso is considered as:
a. 1%.
b. 9%.
c. 18%.
d. 36%.

48. Why are external cause codes used?
a. To generate additional revenue
b. To establish injury prevention programs
c. All of the above
d. None of the above

Part III True/False

Write "T" or "F" in the blank to indicate whether you think the statement is true or false.

_____ 49. Diagnoses that relate to the patient's previous medical problem must always be reported.

_____ 50. The concept of "principal diagnosis" is applicable to outpatient and inpatient cases.

_____ 51. The diagnosis coding system is designed to provide statistical mortality rate data that include information about causes of diseases.

_____ 52. The process for looking up a diagnosis code in the ICD-9-CM coding system is the same as in the ICD-10-CM coding system.

_____ 53. ICD-10 was published by the World Health Organization (WHO) and clinically modified by the Centers for Medicare and Medicaid Services (CMS).

_____ 54. The Alphabetic Index contains the Table of Drugs and Chemicals.

_____ 55. ICD-10-CM codes can contain up to seven characters.

_____ 56. Signs and symptoms that are not typically associated with a disease process should be reported when documented.

_____ 57. When a person who is not currently sick encounters health services for some specific purpose, such as to receive a vaccination, a Z code is used.

_____ 58. _Code conventions_ are rules or principles for determining a diagnostic code when using a diagnostic code book.

_____ 59. Because there are annual ICD-10-CM code revisions, there is a three-month grace period to implement these changes and revisions.

_____ 60. An external cause code may never be sequenced as the primary diagnosis in the first position.

Performance Objective

Task: Answer questions pertaining to categories G00-G09 of ICD-10-CM, Volume 2.

Conditions: Use the abstracted section from ICD-10-CM, Volume 2, and pen or pencil.

Standards: Time: _____ minutes

              Accuracy: _____

              (Note: The time element and accuracy criteria may be given by your instructor.)

Directions: Refer to a section from a page of ICD-10-CM, Volume 2 (Fig. 12.1), and answer questions pertaining to categories G00 through G09.

1. Locate the section title. _____

2. Place an X in front of each of the following diagnostic statements included in category code G00 and its subcategories.

   _____ bacterial leptomeningitis

   _____ bacterial meningitis

   _____ bacterial meningomyelitis

   _____ leptospirosis

   _____ tuberculous meningitis

   _____ meningoencephalitis

   _____ bacterial arachnoiditis

3. Refer to the *Exclusion* 1 note located under category code G01, titled "Meningitis in bacterial diseases classified elsewhere." Place an X in front of the following code number(s) that are excluded.

   _____ gonococcal meningitis A54.81

   _____ meningitis as a result of measles (B05.1)

   _____ meningitis in neurosyphilis (A52.13)

   _____ *Hemophilus* meningitis (G00.0)

   _____ meningitis as a result of candidal meningitis (B37.5)

   _____ Lyme disease (A69.21)

4. Place an X in front of each of the following diagnostic statements included in category code G04 and its subcategories.

   _____ meningomyelitis

   _____ meningoencephalitis

   _____ pyogenic meningitis

   _____ epidemic meningitis

   _____ tuberculous meningitis

   _____ acute ascending myelitis

147

5. Write the code numbers for category G04.0 that require a fifth digit.

_____

INFLAMMATORY DISEASES OF THE CENTRAL NERVOUS SYSTEM (G00-G09)

● **G00 Bacterial meningitis, not elsewhere classified**
   An infection of the cerebrospinal fluid surrounding the spinal cord and brain.

   | **Includes** | bacterial arachnoiditis
   bacterial leptomeningitis
   bacterial meningitis
   bacterial pachymeningitis

   | **Excludes1** | bacterial:
   meningoencephalitis (G04.2)
   meningomyelitis (G04.2)

   G00.0 Hemophilus meningitis
      Meningitis due to Hemophilus influenzae

   G00.1 Pneumococcal meningitis

   G00.2 Streptococcal meningitis
      Use additional code to further identify organism (B95.0-B95.5)

   G00.3 Staphylococcal meningitis
      Use additional code to further identify organism (B95.61-B95.8)

   G00.8 Other bacterial meningitis
      Meningitis due to Escherichia coli
      Meningitis due to Friedländer bacillus
      Meningitis due to Klebsiella

      Use additional code to further identify organism (B96.-)

   ▪ **G00.9 Bacterial meningitis, unspecified**
      Meningitis due to gram-negative bacteria, unspecified
      Purulent meningitis NOS
      Pyogenic meningitis NOS
      Suppurative meningitis NOS

● ▶ _**G01 Meningitis in bacterial diseases classified elsewhere**_

   Code first underlying disease

   | **Excludes1** | meningitis (in):
   gonococcal (A54.81)
   leptospirosis (A27.81)
   listeriosis (A32.11)
   Lyme disease (A69.21)
   meningococcal (A39.0)
   neurosyphilis (A52.13)
   tuberculosis (A17.0)
   meningoencephalitis and meningomyelitis
      in bacterial diseases classified
      elsewhere (G05)

Fig. 12.1

G02 *Meningitis in other infectious and parasitic diseases classified elsewhere*
 Code first underlying disease, such as:
 African trypanosomiasis (B56.-)
 poliovirus infection (A80.-)

 Excludes1 candidal meningitis (B37.5)
 coccidioidomycosis meningitis (B38.4)
 cryptococcal meningitis (B45.1)
 herpesviral [herpes simplex] meningitis (B00.3)
 infectious mononucleosis complicated by meningitis (B27.- with fourth character 2)
 measles complicated by meningitis (B05.1)
 meningoencephalitis and meningomyelitis in other infectious and parasitic diseases classified elsewhere (G05)
 mumps meningitis (B26.1)
 rubella meningitis (B06.02)
 varicella [chickenpox] meningitis (B01.0)
 zoster meningitis (B02.1)

G03 **Meningitis due to other and unspecified causes**
 Includes arachnoiditis NOS
 leptomeningitis NOS
 meningitis NOS
 pachymeningitis NOS

 Excludes1 meningoencephalitis (G04.-)
 meningomyelitis (G04.-)

 G03.0 **Nonpyogenic meningitis**
 Aseptic meningitis
 Nonbacterial meningitis

 G03.1 **Chronic meningitis**

 G03.2 **Benign recurrent meningitis [Mollaret]**

 G03.8 **Meningitis due to other specified causes**

 G03.9 **Meningitis, unspecified**
 Arachnoiditis (spinal) NOS

G04 **Encephalitis, myelitis and encephalomyelitis**
 Includes acute ascending myelitis
 meningoencephalitis
 meningomyelitis

 Excludes1 encephalopathy NOS (G93.40)
 other noninfectious acute disseminated encephalomyelitis (noninfectious ADEM) (G04.81)

 Excludes2 acute transverse myelitis (G37.3-)
 alcoholic encephalopathy (G31.2)
 benign myalgic encephalomyelitis (G93.3)
 multiple sclerosis (G35)
 subacute necrotizing myelitis (G37.4)
 toxic encephalitis (G92)
 toxic encephalopathy (G92)

 G04.0 **Acute disseminated encephalitis and encephalomyelitis (ADEM)**

 Excludes1 acute necrotizing hemorrhagic encephalopathy (G04.3-)

 G04.00 **Acute disseminated encephalitis and encephalomyelitis, unspecified**

G04.01 **Postinfectious acute disseminated encephalitis and encephalomyelitis (postinfectious ADEM)**

 Excludes1 post chickenpox encephalitis (B01.1)
 post measles encephalitis (B05.0)
 post measles myelitis (B05.1)

G04.02 **Postimmunization acute disseminated encephalitis, myelitis and encephalomyelitis**
 Encephalitis, post immunization
 Encephalomyelitis, post immunization
 Use additional code to identify the vaccine (T50.A-, T50.B-, T50.Z-)

G04.1 **Tropical spastic paraplegia**

G04.2 **Bacterial meningoencephalitis and meningomyelitis, not elsewhere classified**

G04.3 **Acute necrotizing hemorrhagic encephalopathy**
 Sudden and severe CNS disease with pathology of hemorrhages and necrosis of white matter

 Excludes1 acute disseminated encephalitis and encephalomyelitis (G04.0-)

 G04.30 Acute necrotizing hemorrhagic encephalopathy, unspecified

 G04.31 Postinfectious acute necrotizing hemorrhagic encephalopathy

 G04.32 Postimmunization acute necrotizing hemorrhagic encephalopathy
 Use additional code to identify vaccine (T50.A-, T50.B-, T50.Z-)

 G04.39 Other acute necrotizing hemorrhagic encephalopathy
 Code also underlying etiology, if applicable

G04.8 **Other encephalitis, myelitis and encephalomyelitis**
 Code also any associated seizure (G40.-, R56.9)

 G04.81 Other encephalitis and encephalomyelitis
 Noninfectious acute disseminated encephalomyelitis (noninfectious ADEM)

 G04.89 Other myelitis

G04.9 **Encephalitis, myelitis and encephalomyelitis, unspecified**

 G04.90 Encephalitis and encephalomyelitis, unspecified
 Ventriculitis (cerebral) NOS

 G04.91 Myelitis, unspecified

Fig. 12.1, cont'd

DIAGNOSTIC CODING ASSIGNMENTS

In this chapter, the points awarded for assignments that require diagnostic codes are 1 point for each correct digit.

ASSIGNMENT 12.3 OBTAIN GENERAL DIAGNOSTIC CODES FOR CONDITIONS

Performance Objective

Task: Locate the correct diagnostic code for each diagnosis listed.

Conditions: Use pen or pencil and ICD-10-CM diagnostic code book.

Standards: Time: _____ minutes

            Accuracy: _____

            (Note: The time element and accuracy criteria may be given by your instructor.)

Directions: Using the ICD-10-CM code book, read each diagnosis and locate the condition in Volume 2, the Alphabetic Index. Then go to Volume 1, to the Tabular List of Diseases. Match the definition as closely as possible to the written description and assign the correct code, entering it on the blank line.

Problems	ICD-10-CM Codes
1. Breast mass	_____
2. *Klebsiella* pneumonia	_____
3. Acute lateral wall myocardial infarction; initial episode	_____
4. Acute cerebrovascular accident	_____
5. Atherosclerotic cardiovascular disease	_____
6. Dyspnea, rule out (R/O) cystic fibrosis	_____
7. Ileitis	_____
8. Osteoarthritis of elbow	_____
9. Tinnitus	_____
10. Acute exacerbation of chronic asthmatic bronchitis	_____

ASSIGNMENT 12.4 CODE DIAGNOSES FROM MEDICAL RECORDS

Performance Objective

Task: Locate the correct diagnostic code for each case scenario.

Conditions: Use pen or pencil and ICD-10-CM diagnostic code book.

Standards: Time: _____ minutes

             Accuracy: _____

             (Note: The time element and accuracy criteria may be given by your instructor.)

Directions: This exercise will give you experience in basic diagnostic coding for physicians' insurance claims. First list the ICD-10-CM code for the diagnosis, condition, problem, or other reason for the admission and/or encounter (visit) shown in the medical record to be chiefly responsible for the services provided. Then list additional diagnostic codes that describe any coexisting conditions that affect patient care. Always assign codes to their highest level of specificity—the more digits, the more specific. Do not code probable, R/O, suspected, or questionable conditions. Assign the correct code(s), entering it (them) on the blank line.

Problems   ICD-10-CM Codes

Problem 1. A patient, Mrs. Jennifer Hanson, calls Dr. Input's office stating she has blood in her stool. Dr. Input suspects a gastrointestinal bleed and tells Mrs. Hanson to come in immediately. It is discovered that the reason for the blood in the stool is a bleeding duodenal ulcer. Code the diagnosis to be listed on the insurance claim for the office visit.   _____

Problem 2. a. Jason Belmen comes in with a fractured humerus. He also has chronic obstructive pulmonary disease (COPD), which is not treated. Code the diagnosis.   _____

b. Assume Mr. Belmen needs general anesthesia for open reduction of the fractured humerus. The COPD could now be considered a risk factor. List the diagnostic code in the second part of this scenario.   _____

Problem 3. Margarita Sanchez came into the office for removal of sutures. Code the diagnosis.   _____

Problem 4. A patient, George Martin, has benign prostatic hypertrophy (BPH). He is seen for catheterization because of urinary retention. Code the primary and secondary diagnoses for the office visit. (Note: BPH is an enlargement of the prostate gland, caused by overgrowth of androgen-sensitive glandular elements, which occurs naturally with aging.)   _____

Problem 5. Mia Bartholomew is seen in the office complaining of a sore throat. A throat culture is done, and the specimen is sent to an outside laboratory for a culture and sensitivity study to determine the presence of *Streptococcus*. List the diagnostic code the physician would use if the insurance claim is submitted before the results are known. List the diagnostic code used if the physician submits the insurance claim after the laboratory report is received indicating *Streptococcus* is present.   _____

Chapter **12** Diagnostic Coding

ASSIGNMENT 12.5 CODE DIAGNOSES USING Z CODES

Performance Objective

Task: Locate the correct diagnostic code for each case scenario.

Conditions: Use pen or pencil and ICD-10-CM diagnostic code book.

Standards: Time: _____ minutes

Accuracy: _____

(Note: The time element and accuracy criteria may be given by your instructor.)

Directions: In this exercise, you will be reviewing Z codes in the ICD-10-CM code book. Assign the correct code, entering it on the blank line. These are some keywords under which Z codes may be located in Volume 2:

admission	checking/checkup	donor	insertion of	status post
aftercare	conflict	evaluation	maintenance	vaccination
attention to	contact	examination	observation	
border	contraception	fitting of	person with	
care of	counseling	follow-up	problem with	
carrier	dialysis	history of	screening	

Problems   ICD-10-CM Codes

1. Kathy Osborn, a patient, is seen in the office for an annual checkup.   _____

2. Daniel Matsui is seen in the office for adjustment of a lumbosacral corset.   _____

3. Philip O'Brien comes into the office to receive a prophylactic flu shot.   _____

4. Bernadette Murphy is seen in the office for a pregnancy test; the result is positive.   _____

5. Michiko Fujita is seen in the office for a fractured rib. No x-rays are taken because Mrs. Fujita thinks she is pregnant.   _____

6. Dr. Perry Cardi sees Kenneth Pickford in the office for a cardiac pacemaker adjustment. The pacemaker was implanted because of sick sinus syndrome.   _____

7. Frank Meadows returns for follow-up, postoperative transurethral prostatic resection (TURP) for prostate cancer after treatment has been completed.   _____

Performance Objective

Task: Locate the correct diagnostic code for each diagnosis listed.

Conditions: Use pen or pencil and ICD-10-CM diagnostic code book.

Standards: Time: _____ minutes

                      Accuracy: _____

                      (Note: The time element and accuracy criteria may be given by your instructor.)

Directions: In this exercise, you will be reviewing diagnostic codes in the ICD-10-CM code book involving neoplasms. Assign the correct code, entering it on the blank line.

Problems   ICD-10-CM Codes

1. Leiomyoma, uterus   _____

2. Ewing's sarcoma, forearm   _____

3. Adenocarcinoma, right breast, central portion, female   _____

4. Dyspnea resulting from carcinoma of the breast, female with metastasis to the upper lobe, right lung   _____

5. Patient is seen for a yearly examination 1 year after a mastectomy for breast cancer; she is disease-free at this time.   _____

ASSIGNMENT 12.7 CODE DIAGNOSES FOR PATIENTS WITH DIABETES

Performance Objective

Task: Locate the correct diagnostic code for each diagnosis listed.

Conditions: Use pen or pencil and ICD-10-CM diagnostic code book.

Standards: Time: _____ minutes

               Accuracy: _____

               (Note: The time element and accuracy criteria may be given by your instructor.)

Directions: In this exercise, you will review diagnostic codes in the ICD-10-CM code book involving cases of patients with diabetes. The diabetes codes are combination codes that include the type of diabetes, the body system affected, and the complications affecting that body system. Use as many codes as are necessary to describe all of the complications of the disease. Assign as many codes from categories E08 through E13 as needed to identify all of the associated conditions that the patient has.

Example: If a patient with type 2 uncontrolled diabetes is treated for a skin ulcer on the lower extremity, look up "diabetes" in Volume 2 and find the subterm "with skin ulcer." The diabetes code listed is E11.622. Go to Volume 1 and verify. Volume 1 instructs you to *"use additional code to identify site of ulcer"* (L97.-, L98.-). The additional code L97.809 is selected, as it describes "Nonpressure chronic ulcer of other part of unspecified lower leg with unspecified severity."

Always verify all codes in Volume 1 before assigning them. Assign the correct code(s) for each case involving diabetes, entering it (them) on the blank line.

Problems   ICD-10-CM Codes

1. Diabetes mellitus   _____

2. Type 2, non–insulin-dependent diabetes mellitus with neuropathy. _____

3. Diabetic gangrene (type 1 diabetes)   _____

4. Type 2 diabetes with cataract   _____

5. Type 1 diabetes with diabetic polyneuropathy and retinopathy   _____

ASSIGNMENT 12.8 CODE DIAGNOSES FOR PATIENTS WITH HYPERTENSION

Performance Objective

Task: Locate the correct diagnostic code for each diagnosis listed.

Conditions: Use pen or pencil and ICD-10-CM diagnostic code book.

Standards: Time: _____ minutes

              Accuracy: _____

              (Note: The time element and accuracy criteria may be given by your instructor.)

Directions: In this exercise, you will review diagnostic codes in the ICD-10-CM code book involving patients who have hypertension. To begin coding, look in Volume 2 under "hypertension."
    Assign the correct code(s) for each case, entering it (them) on the blank line.

Problems	ICD-10-CM Codes
1. High blood pressure reading	_____
2. Malignant hypertension	_____
3. Hypertension complicating pregnancy	_____
4. Hypertension with kidney disease	_____
5. Hypertension as a result of arteriosclerotic cardiovascular disease (ASCVD) and systolic congestive heart failure (CHF)	_____
6. Myocarditis and CHF as a result of malignant hypertension	_____

ASSIGNMENT 12.9 CODE DIAGNOSES FOR INJURIES, FRACTURES, BURNS, LATE EFFECTS, AND COMPLICATIONS

Performance Objective

Task: Locate the correct diagnostic code for each diagnosis listed.

Conditions: Use pen or pencil and ICD-10-CM diagnostic code book.

Standards: Time: _____ minutes

                   Accuracy: _____

                   (Note: The time element and accuracy criteria may be given by your instructor.)

Directions: In this exercise, you will review diagnostic codes from the ICD-10-CM code book involving patients who have suffered injuries, burns, fractures, and late effects. Here are some guidelines for coding injuries, fractures, burns, late effects, and complications.

Injuries

When coding injuries, assign separate codes for each injury unless a combination code is provided, in which case the combination code is assigned. The code for the most serious injury, as determined by the provider and the focus of treatment, is sequenced first.

Fractures

Fractures are presumed to be closed unless otherwise specified. Fracture not indicated, whether displaced or not displaced, should be coded as displaced.

Burns

Multiple burns at the same site, but of different degrees, are coded to the most severe degree.

Code the extent of body surface involved (percentage of body surface), when specified, as an additional code.

Late Effects

A residual, late effect is defined as the current condition resulting from a previous acute illness or injury that is no longer the current problem. Late effects are coded using the residual or late effect as the primary diagnosis. The cause of the residual or late effect is coded second.

Complications

For conditions resulting from the malfunction of internal devices, use the subterm "mechanical" found under the main term "complication."

Postoperative complications are sometimes found under the subterm "postoperative," which appears under the main term identifying the condition. If not found there, look for a subterm identifying the type of procedure, type of complication, or surgical procedure under the main term "complication."

Problems   ICD-10-CM Codes

1. Supracondylar fracture of right femur with intracondylar extension of lower end; initial encounter   _____

2. Fracture of left humerus and left foot; subsequent encounter   _____

3. Comminuted fracture of left radius and ulna, not displaced; initial encounter   _____

4. Pathologic fracture of right hip caused by drug-induced osteoporosis; initial encounter for fracture   _____

5. Lacerations of the upper arm with embedded glass; initial encounter   _____

6. Burns on the face and neck; sequela   _____

7. Second- and third-degree burns on chest wall; 20% of body involved, 10% third-degree; initial encounter   _____

8. Bursitis of the knee resulting from crushing injury to the knee 1 year ago   _____

Performance Objective

Task: Locate the correct diagnostic code for each case scenario.

Conditions: Use pen or pencil and ICD-10-CM diagnostic code book.

Standards: Time: _____ minutes

             Accuracy: _____

             (Note: The time element and accuracy criteria may be given by your instructor.)

Directions: In this exercise, you will review diagnostic codes from the ICD-10-CM code book involving patients who have conditions involving pregnancy and delivery, and newborn infants.

For the supervision of a normal pregnancy, turn to Volume 2 and look up "pregnancy." This is a long category. Look up the subterm "supervision" and find the sub-subterm "normal" (NEC Z34.8-) and "first" (Z34.0-). Check Volume 1 to verify these codes. Also see code Z33.1, "pregnancy state, incidental." This code is used in the second position to tell the insurance carrier that the patient is pregnant in addition to any other diagnosis.

If a patient has complications, turn to Volume 2 and look under the main term "pregnancy." Find the subterm "complicated by" and find the sub-subterm stating the complication. These are codes from ICD-10-CM Chapter 15: "Pregnancy, Childbirth, and Puerperium" (O00-O9a).

Delivery in a completely normal case is coded O80 and is listed under the main term "delivery, uncomplicated." *Normal* is described as "delivery requiring minimal or no assistance, with or without episiotomy, without fetal manipulation (e.g., rotation version) or instrumentation (forceps) of a spontaneous, cephalic, vaginal, full-term, single, live-born infant." This code is for use as a single diagnosis code and is not to be used with any other code from Chapter 15.

When coding deliveries, always include a code for the status of the infant. Look up "outcome of delivery" in Volume 2, and you will find various Z37 codes listing possible outcomes. These codes would be listed as secondary codes on the insurance claim form for the delivery.

On the insurance claim form for the newborn, turn to "newborn" in Volume 2. You will find codes from Z38.0 to Z38.8 describing the birth of the newborn. Use these codes in the first position when billing for services for the newborn infant.

Assign the correct code(s) for each case, entering it (them) on the blank line.

Problems   ICD-10-CM Codes

1. A pregnant patient who is due to deliver in 6 weeks presents in the office with preeclampsia. _____

2. A patient presents with a chief complaint of severe episodes of pain and vaginal hemorrhage. The physician determines that the patient has an incomplete spontaneous abortion complicated by excessive hemorrhage; she was 6 weeks pregnant. _____

3. A patient comes in who is diagnosed with a kidney stone; the patient is pregnant. _____

4. A patient is delivered of twins, both live born by cesarean section because of cephalopelvic disproportion, which caused an obstruction. Code the mother's chart. _____

Performance Objective

Task: Locate the correct diagnostic code for each diagnosis listed.

Conditions: Use pen or pencil and the ICD-10-CM diagnostic code book.

Standards: Time: _____ minutes

             Accuracy: _____

             (Note: The time element and accuracy criteria may be given by your instructor.)

Directions: In this exercise, you will be reviewing diagnostic codes from the ICD-10-CM code book involving patients who may have had an adverse effect from ingesting a toxic substance. Read the definitions for poisoning and drug intoxication in the *Textbook.*

Injury codes T36 through T65 are combination codes that include the substances related to adverse effects, poisonings, toxic effects, and underdosing, as well as the external cause. No additional external cause code is required to report poisonings, toxic effects, adverse effects, or underdosing codes.

A code from categories T36 through T65 is sequenced first, followed by the code or codes that specify the nature of the adverse effect, poisoning, or toxic effect.

Assign the correct code(s) for each case and enter it (them) on the blank line.

Problems	ICD-10-CM Codes
1. Light-headedness caused by digitalis intoxication; initial encounter	_____
2. Treatment of a rash after an initial dose of penicillin is given	_____
3. Initial encounter for accidental overdose of meperidine (Demerol)	_____
4. A 20-month-old baby accidentally ingests approximately 15 aspirin and is severely nauseated.	_____
5. A patient presents in the physician's office with a vague complaint of not feeling well. The physician notices that the patient has ataxia (a staggering gait). After reviewing the patient's history, the physician determines the ataxia is caused by the meprobamate the patient is taking.	_____
6. Initial visit for internal bleeding: abnormal reaction to a combination of chloramphenicol and warfarin (Coumadin)	_____

13 Procedural Coding

Cheryl Fassett

KEY TERMS

Your instructor may wish to select some words pertinent to this chapter for a test. For definitions of the terms, further study, and/or reference, the words, phrases, and abbreviations may be found in the glossary at the end of the textbook. *Key terms for this chapter follow.*

bilateral
bundled codes
comprehensive code
conversion factor
Current Procedural Terminology
customary fee
downcoding
durable medical equipment
emergency department
fee schedule
global surgery policy
Healthcare Common Procedure Coding System
modifiers
National Correct Coding Initiative
never event

physical status modifiers
procedure code numbers
professional component
qualifying circumstance modifiers
reasonable fee
relative value studies
relative value unit
resource-based relative value scale
surgical package
technical component
unbundling
upcoding
usual, customary, and reasonable

KEY ABBREVIATIONS

See how many abbreviations and acronyms you can translate and then use this as a handy reference list. Definitions for the key abbreviations are located near the back of the textbook in the glossary.

CF _____

CPT _____

DME _____

ECG _____

ED _____

E/M _____

EOB _____

FTC _____

GAF _____

GPCIs _____

HCPCS _____

NCCI edits _____

PC _____

PS _____

QC _____

RBRVS _____

RVS _____

RVU _____

TC _____

UCR _____

159

Copyright © 2020 Elsevier, Inc. All Rights Reserved.

Chapter **13** **Procedural Coding**

The student will be able to:

- Define and spell the key terms and key abbreviations for this chapter, given the information from the textbook glossary, within a reasonable time period and with enough accuracy to obtain a satisfactory evaluation.
- Answer the fill-in-the-blank, mix and match, multiple choice, and true/false review questions after reading the chapter, with enough accuracy to obtain a satisfactory evaluation.
- Select the five-digit procedure code numbers, modifiers, and/or descriptors of each service, given a series of problems relating to various medical procedures and services and using the *Current Procedural Terminology* (CPT) code book, with enough accuracy to obtain a satisfactory evaluation.
- Fill in the correct meaning of each abbreviation given in a list of common medical abbreviations and symbols that appear in chart notes, with enough accuracy to obtain a satisfactory evaluation.

STUDY OUTLINE

Understanding the Importance of Procedural Coding Skills
A Coding Specialist's Tools
Health Care Procedure Coding System
    Level I: CPT Codes
    Level II: HCPCS Codes
CPT Content and Format
    Category I: Codes
    Category II: Performance Measurement Codes
    Category III: New and Emerging Technology Codes
    Code Book Symbols
    Unlisted Procedures
    Evaluation and Management Services
    Anesthesia Services
    Surgery Guidelines
    Integumentary System
    Musculoskeletal System
    Respiratory System
    Cardiovascular System
    Urinary System
    Male Genital System
    Female Reproductive System
    Endocrine System
    Nervous System
    Eye and Auditory System

    Radiology
    Pathology and Laboratory
    Medicine Section
Code Modifiers
    Common CPT Modifiers
    HCPCS Modifiers
Correct Coding Edits and Practices
    National Correct Coding Initiative (NCCI)
    Bundling
    Unbundling
    Downcoding
    Upcoding
    Code Monitoring
Methods of Payment
    Fee Schedule
    Usual, Customary, and Reasonable
    Relative Value Studies
    Resource-Based Relative Value Scale
    Medicare Fee Schedule
    Developing a Fee Schedule Using RBRVS
Procedure 13.1: Choose Correct Procedural Codes for Professional Services
Procedure 13.2: Locate Correct Level II HCPCS Codes for Professional Services

ASSIGNMENT 13.1 REVIEW QUESTIONS

Part I Fill in the Blank

Review the objectives, key terms, and chapter information before completing the following review questions.

1. The coding system used for billing professional medical services and procedures is found in a book titled _____.

2. The Medicare program uses a system of coding composed of two levels, and this is called _____.

3. A medical service or procedure performed that differs in some way from the code description may be shown by using a CPT code with a/an _____.

4. A *relative value scale* or *schedule* is a listing of procedure codes indicating the relative value of services performed, which is shown by _____.

5. Name three methods for basing payments adopted by insurance companies and by state and federal programs.

   a. _____

   b. _____

   c. _____

6. List four of the situations that can occur in a medical practice when referring to charges and payments from a fee schedule.

   a. _____

   b. _____

   c. _____

   d. _____

7. Name the six sections of Category I in the CPT code book published by the American Medical Association.

   a. _____

   b. _____

   c. _____

   d. _____

   e. _____

   f. _____

8. Name five criteria for Medicare's definition of DME.

a. _____

b. _____

c. _____

d. _____

e. _____

9. A surgical package includes:

_____

_____

_____

_____

10. A function of computer software that performs online checking of codes on an insurance claim to detect improper code submission is called a/an _____.

11. A single code that describes two or more component codes bundled together as one unit is known as a/an _____.

12. Grouping related codes together is commonly referred to as _____.

13. Use of many procedural codes to identify procedures that may be described by one code is termed _____.

14. A code used on a claim that does not match the code system used by the third-party payer and is converted to the closest code rendering less payment is termed

_____.

15. Intentional manipulation of procedural codes to generate increased reimbursement is called _____.

16. Give eight reasons for using modifiers on insurance claims.

a. _____

b. _____

c. _____

d. _____

e. _____

f. _____

g. _____

h. _____

17. What modifier is usually used when billing for an assistant surgeon who is not in a teaching hospital?

_____

18. Explain when to use the -99 modifier code.

_____

_____

Part II Mix and Match

19. Match the symbols in the first column with the definitions in the second column. Write the correct letters on the blanks.

_____	▶◀	a. New code
_____	●	b. Modifier -51 exempt
_____	↗	c. Add-on code
_____	⊘	d. New or revised text
_____	+	e. Revised code
_____	▲	f. Reference material

20. Match the two-digit modifiers in the first column with the definitions in the second column. Write the correct letters on the blanks.

_____ -23		a. Increased procedural service
_____ -22		b. Multiple procedures
_____ -25		c. Staged or related procedure
_____ -26		d. Decision for surgery
_____ -51		e. Significant, separately identifiable evaluation and management (E/M) service by the same physician on the same day of the procedure or other service
_____ -52		f. Unusual anesthesia
_____ -57		g. Reduced services
_____ -58		h. Professional component

Part III Multiple Choice Questions

Choose the best answer.

21. The codes used to bill ambulance services, surgical supplies, and durable medical equipment are:
    a. CPT codes.
    b. CPT modifiers
    c. Level I HCPCS CPT codes.
    d. Level II HCPCS national codes.

22. A complex reimbursement system in which three fees are considered in calculating payment is known as:
    a. usual, customary, and reasonable (UCR).
    b. relative value studies (RVS).
    c. resource-based relative value scale (RBRVS).
    d. relative value unit (RVU).

23. Medicare defines the postoperative global periods as:
    a. 0, 25, 50, or 100 days.
    b. 0, 10, or 90 days.
    c. 0, 10, 20, or 50 days.
    d. 0, 20, 50, or 90 days.

24. To code numerous CPT codes to identify a procedure that can be described in a single comprehensive code is referred to as:
    a. unbundling.
    b. downcoding.
    c. bundling.
    d. upcoding.

25. When two surgeons work together as primary surgeons performing distinct parts of a procedure, and each doctor bills for performing his or her distinct part of the procedure, the CPT surgical code is listed with modifier:
    a. -62.
    b. -66.
    c. -80.
    d. -82.

Part IV True/False

Write "T" or "F" in the blank to indicate whether you think the statement is true or false.

_____ 26. Procedure coding is the transformation of written descriptions of procedures and professional services into numeric designations (code numbers).

_____ 27. Category II codes describe clinical components that may be typically included in evaluation and management services or clinical services and do not have a relative value associated with them.

_____ 28. When multiple lacerations have been repaired using the same technique and are in the same anatomic category, each repair should be assigned a separate code when billing an insurance claim.

_____ 29. When listing a sterile tray for an in-office surgical procedure, the tray is bundled with the procedure, unless other supplies are needed in addition to those usually used.

_____ 30. HCPCS Level II modifiers consist of only two numeric characters.

PROCEDURE CODING ASSIGNMENTS

In this chapter, the points awarded for assignments that require procedure codes are 1 point for each correct digit.

ASSIGNMENT 13.2 INTRODUCTION TO CPT AND CODING EVALUATION AND MANAGEMENT SERVICES

Performance Objective

Task: Locate the correct information and/or procedure code for each question and/or case scenario.

Conditions: Use pen or pencil and the CPT code book.

Standards: Time: _____ minutes

             Accuracy: _____

             (Note: The time element and accuracy criteria may be given by your instructor.)

1. To become acquainted with the sections of the CPT code book, match the code number in the left column with the appropriate description in the right column by writing the letters in the blanks. Locate each code number in the CPT code book. As you progress through the assignment, the problems get more difficult and complex.

   99231 _____ a.   Chest x-ray

   59400 _____ b.   Anesthesia for procedures on cervical spine and cord

   71045 _____ c.   Subsequent hospital care

   00600 _____ d.   Supplies and materials

   85025 _____ e.   Routine OB care, antepartum and postpartum

   99070 _____ f.   CBC

2. Name the section of the CPT where each of the following codes is located.

   a. 65091 _____

   b. 86038 _____

   c. 92596 _____

   d. 75984 _____

   e. 0042T _____

   f. 01320 _____

   g. 99324 _____

   h. 0503F _____

3. Evaluation and Management (E/M) codes are used by physicians to report a significant portion of their services. Remember, it is the physician's responsibility to assign E/M codes, and the exercises presented here are only for familiarization. The problems will acquaint you with terminology for this section of the CPT code book. Select the appropriate **new patient** office visit codes using the key components:

a. This is a Level 3 case: Detailed history

   Detailed examination

   Low-complexity decision making _____

b. This is a Level 1 case: Problem-focused history

   Problem-focused examination

   Straightforward decision making _____

c. This is a Level 5 case: Comprehensive history

   Comprehensive examination

   High-complexity decision making _____

4. Select the appropriate **established patient** office visit codes using the key components. Coding these cases illustrates consideration of two of three components.

a. This is a Level 4 case: Detailed history

   Detailed examination

   Low-complexity decision making _____

b. This is a Level 5 case: Comprehensive history

   Comprehensive examination

   Moderate-complexity decision making _____

c. This is a Level 5 case: Detailed history

   Comprehensive examination

   High-complexity decision making _____

5. Evaluation and Management (E/M) codes **99201** to **99239** are used for services provided in the physician's office or in a hospital facility. Read the brief statement and then locate the code number in the *Current Procedural Terminology* code book.

a. Office visit of a 20-year-old patient seen within the past 3 years for instruction in diabetes injection sites by RN (minimal problem). Patient not seen by physician at this brief visit. _____

b. Office visit of a 30-year-old new patient with allergic rhinitis. This case had an expanded problem-focused history & examination and straightforward decision making. _____

c. Discussion of medication with the son of an 80-year-old patient with dementia on discharge from the observation unit. _____

d. Admission to hospital of 60-year-old established patient in acute respiratory distress with bronchitis. Comprehensive history & examination and medical decision making of moderate complexity. _____

e. Hospital visit of a 4-year-old boy, now stable, who will be discharged the next day. This is a problem-focused interval history & examination and medical decision making of low complexity. _____

f. New patient seen in the office for chest pain, congestive heart failure, and hypertension. Comprehensive history & examination and highly complex decision making. _____

6. Evaluation and Management codes **99241** to **99255** are used for consultations provided in the physician's office or in an outpatient or inpatient hospital facility. A *consultation* is a service provided by a physician whose opinion about a case is requested by another physician. Read the brief statement and then locate the code number in the *Current Procedural Terminology* code book.

   a. Office consultation for a 30-year-old woman complaining of palpitations and chest pains. Her family physician described a mild systolic click. This is an expanded problem-focused history & examination and straightforward decision making.   _____

   b. Subsequent inpatient consultation for a 54-year-old woman, who is now stable, admitted 2 days ago for a bleeding ulcer. This case requires a detailed history & examination and low-complexity decision making.   _____

   c. Office consultation for a 14-year-old boy with poor grades in school and suspected alcohol abuse. This is a comprehensive history & examination and medical decision making of moderate complexity.   _____

   d. Subsequent inpatient consultation for a 50-year-old man who is diabetic and is suffering with fever, chills, gangrenous heel ulcer, rhonchi, and dyspnea (difficulty breathing), an unstable condition. The patient appears lethargic and tachypneic (rapid breathing). This case is a comprehensive history & examination with highly complex medical decision making.   _____

   e. Initial emergency department (ED) consultation for a senior who presents with thyrotoxicosis, exophthalmos, cardiac arrhythmia, and congestive heart failure. This case is a comprehensive history & examination with highly complex medical decision making.   _____

   f. Initial hospital consultation for a 30-year-old woman, post-abdominal surgery, who is exhibiting a fever. This case is an expanded problem-focused history & examination and straightforward medical decision making.   _____

7. Evaluation and Management codes **99281** to **99499** are used for emergency department, critical care, nursing facility, rest home, custodial care, home, prolonged, physician standby, and preventive medicine services. Read the brief statement and then locate the code number in the *Current Procedural Terminology* code book.

a. First hour of critical care of a senior who, after major surgery, suffers a cardiac arrest from a pulmonary embolus.   _____

b. A 40-year-old woman is admitted to the Obstetrical unit, and the primary care physician has requested the neonatologist to stand by for possible cesarean section and neonatal resuscitation. Code for a 1-hour standby.   _____

c. A child is seen in the ED with a fever, diarrhea, abdominal cramps, and vomiting. This case had an expanded problem-focused history & examination, and a moderately complex medical decision was made.   _____

d. A patient is seen for an annual visit at a nursing facility for detailed history & comprehensive examination and low-complexity medical decision making.   _____

e. An initial visit is made to a domiciliary care facility for a developmentally disabled individual with a mild rash on hands and face. This case had an expanded problem-focused history & examination and low-complexity medical decision making.   _____

f. A 50-year-old man with a history of asthma comes into the office with acute bronchospasm and moderate respiratory distress. Office treatment is initiated. The case requires intermittent physician face-to-face time with the patient for 2 hours and prolonged services. Assume the appropriate E/M code has been assigned for this case.   _____

Performance Objective

Task: Locate the correct procedure and modifier, if necessary, for each question and/or case scenario.

Conditions: Use pen or pencil and CPT code book.

Standards: Time: _____ minutes

                   Accuracy: _____

                   (Note: The time element and accuracy criteria may be given by your instructor.)

Directions: Anesthesia codes **00100** to **01999** may be used by anesthesiologists and physicians. Some plastic surgeons, other medical specialists, and large clinics may have a room set aside to perform surgical procedures that might be performed in a hospital outpatient surgical department. Read the brief statement and then locate the Anesthesia Code in the *Current Procedural Terminology* code book. Special modifiers **P1** through **P6** may be needed when coding for this section, as well as code numbers for cases that have difficult circumstances. Definitions for abbreviations may be found in Appendix A of this *Workbook.*

a. Cesarean delivery after neuraxial labor anesthesia, normal healthy
   patient   _____   _____

b. Reduction mammoplasty of a woman with mild systemic disease   _____

c. Total right hip replacement, 71-year-old patient, normal healthy patient   _____   _____

d. Repair of cleft palate, newborn infant, normal healthy patient   _____   _____

e. TURP, normal healthy male   _____

Performance Objective

Task: Locate the correct procedure code and modifier, if necessary, for each question and/or case scenario.

Conditions: Use pen or pencil and *Current Procedural Terminology* code book.

Standards: Time: _____ minutes

                Accuracy: _____

                (Note: The time element and accuracy criteria may be given by your instructor.)

Directions: Surgery codes **10040** to **69979** are used for each anatomic part of the body. Read over each case carefully. Use the *Current Procedural Terminology* code book to obtain the correct code number for each descriptor given. Full descriptors for services rendered have been omitted in some instances to give you practice in abstracting the correct descriptor from the available information. Indicate the correct two-digit modifier if necessary. The skill of critical thinking enters this section of the assignment, in that you may have to use your own judgment to code because the cases do not contain full details. Remember to use the index at the back of the CPT code book.

a. Suppose you work in an office that has an encounter form listing code 43228. Check your edition of CPT and see whether you can locate this code number. If the code does not appear, what code number are you directed to use? _____

Integumentary System 10040-19499

b. Removal of benign lesion from the back (1.0 cm) and left foot (0.5 cm) _____

c. Drainage of deep breast abscess _____

d. Laser destruction of two benign facial lesions _____

Musculoskeletal System 20000-29909

Reminder: Be sure to read the "Application of casts and strapping" guidelines in your CPT code book that appear before the 29000 codes.

e. Aspiration of fluid (arthrocentesis) from right knee joint; not infectious _____

f. Deep tissue biopsy of left upper arm _____

g. Fracture of the left tibia, closed treatment _____

   Does the procedural code include application and removal of the first cast? _____

   If done as an office procedure, may supplies be coded? _____

   Does the procedural code include subsequent replacement of a cast for follow-up care? _____

   If not, list the code number for application of a walking short leg cast. _____

Respiratory System 30000-32999

h. Parietal pleurectomy _____

i. Removal of two nasal polyps, simple _____

j. Diagnostic bronchoscopy with bronchial biopsy _____

Cardiovascular System 33010-37799

k. Pacemaker insertion with transvenous electrode, atrial _____

l. Thromboendarterectomy with patch graft _____

m. Introduction of intracatheter and injection procedure for contrast venography _____

Hemic/Lymphatic/Diaphragm 38100-39599

n. Repair, esophageal/diaphragmatic hernia, transthoracic _____

o. Partial splenectomy _____

p. Excision, two deep cervical nodes _____

Digestive System 40490-49999

q. T & A, 12-year-old boy _____

r. Endoscopic balloon dilation of esophagus _____

Urinary System/Male and Female Genital 50010-55980

s. Removal of urethral diverticulum from female patient _____

t. Anastomosis of single ureter to bladder _____

Laparoscopy/Peritoneoscopy/Hysteroscopy/Female Genital/ Maternity 56300-59899

u. Routine OB care, antepartum and postpartum care _____

v. Therapeutic D & C, nonobstetric _____

w. Enucleation of eye, with implant, muscles attached to implant _____

x. Strabismus surgery, superior oblique muscle _____

y. Cochlear device implantation _____

z. Bilateral, myringotomy including aspiration, requiring general anesthesia _____

Performance Objective

Task: Locate the correct procedure code and modifier, if necessary, for each question and/or case scenario.

Conditions: Use pen or pencil and *Current Procedural Terminology* code book.

Standards: Time: _____ minutes

               Accuracy: _____

               (Note: The time element and accuracy criteria may be given by your instructor.)

Radiologists, as well as other physicians in many specialties, perform these studies. A physician who interprets, dictates, and signs a report may not bill for the report separately because it is considered part of the radiology procedure.

   Some medical practices perform basic laboratory tests under a waived test certificate that complies with the rules of the Clinical Laboratory Improvement Amendments (CLIA) of 1988, implemented in September 1992.

a. Upper GI x-ray study with films and KUB   _____

b. Ultrasound, pregnant uterus after first trimester, two gestations   _____ and _____

c. Routine urinalysis with microscopy, nonautomated   _____

d. Hemoglobin (Hgb), electrophoretic method   _____

Performance Objective

Task: Locate the correct procedure code and modifiers, if necessary, for each case scenario.

Conditions: Use pen or pencil and *Current Procedural Terminology* code book.

Standards: Time: _____ minutes

             Accuracy: _____

             (Note: The time element and accuracy criteria may be given by your instructor.)

Directions: Find the correct procedure codes and modifiers, if necessary. This assignment will reinforce what you have already learned about procedural coding because code numbers for the case scenarios presented are located in all the sections of the CPT code book. Also search for codes in the Medicine section, if necessary.

1. A new patient had five benign skin lesions on the right arm destroyed with surgical curettement. Complete the coding for the surgery.

Code Number	*Description*
a. _____	Level 3, detailed history and examination with low-complexity decision making, initial new patient office visit
b. _____	Destruction of five benign skin lesions rt arm

2. Mrs. Stayman had four moles on her back. Dr. Davis excised the multiple nevi in one new-patient office visit after an expanded problem-focused history & examination and straightforward medical decision making. The information on the pathology report stated nonmalignant lesions measuring 2.2 cm, 1.5 cm, 1 cm, and 0.75 cm.

Code Number		*Description*
a. _____	_____	Initial OV
b. _____		Excision, benign lesion 2.2 cm
c. _____	_____	Excision, benign lesion 1.5 cm
d. _____	_____	Excision, benign lesion 1 cm
e. _____	_____	Excision, benign lesion 0.75 cm

   In another case, if a patient required removal of a 1-cm lesion on the back and a 0.5-cm

   lesion on the neck, the procedural codes would be _____ for the back lesion

   and _____ for the neck lesion.

3. Dr. Davis stated on his operative report that Mr. Allen was suffering from a complex, complicated nasal fracture. Dr. Davis debrided the wound because it was contaminated and performed an open reduction with internal fixation in a complex and complicated procedure.

Code Number   *Description*

a. _____   _____   Initial OV, complex history & examination, moderate-complexity decision making

b. _____   Open tx nasal fracture, complicated

c. _____   _____   Debridement, skin, subcutaneous tissue, muscle, and bone

4. A registered nurse (RN), an established patient, age 40 years, sees the doctor for an annual physical. A Pap (Papanicolaou) smear is obtained and sent to an outside laboratory. The patient also has a furuncle on the right axilla at the time of the visit, which the doctor incises and drains (I & D).

Code Number   *Description*

a. _____   _____   Periodic physical examination

b. _____   Handling of specimen

c. _____   I & D, furuncle, right axilla

d. _____   5-mL penicillin IM injection

5. While making his rounds in the hospital during the noon hour, Dr. James sees a new patient in the ED for a laceration of the forehead, 5-cm long. The doctor does a workup for a possible concussion.

Code Number   *Description*

a. _____   _____   ED care, expanded problem-focused history, expanded problem-focused examination, low-complexity decision making

b. _____   Repair of laceration, simple, face

6. The physician sees a new patient in the office with the same condition as the patient in Problem 5; however, an infection has developed, and the patient is seen for daily dressing changes. On day 11, the sutures are removed, and on day 12, a final dressing change is made, and the patient is discharged.

Code Number   *Description*

a. _____   _____   Level 3, detailed history & examination with low-complexity decision making, initial new patient office visit

b. _____   Repair of laceration

c. _____   Tet tox (tetanus toxoid) 0.5 mL

d. _____   Administration intramuscular injection

e. _____   Minimal service, OV (suture removal)

f. _____   Minimal service, OV (dressing change)

Note: Some fee schedules allow no follow-up days; Medicare fee schedule allows 10 follow-up days for the procedural code number for repair of laceration.

     Chapter **13** **Procedural Coding**

7. The physician sees 13-year-old Bobby Jones (established patient) for a Boy Scout physical. Bobby is in good health and well groomed. His troop is going for a 1-week camping trip in 12 days. The physician reviewed safety issues with Bobby, talked to him about school, and counseled him about not getting into drugs or alcohol. Bobby denied any problems with that or of being sexually active. He said that he plays baseball. He has no allergies. The physician performed a detailed examination. The physician completed information for scouting papers and cleared him for camping activity.

Code Number	Description
a. _____	Periodic preventive evaluation and management

8. A new patient, David Ramsey, age 15 years, was seen by Dr. Menter for lapses of memory and frequent headaches. The doctor performed an electroencephalogram (EEG) and some psychological tests (including a psychodiagnostic assessment using personality and psychopathology tests [Rorschach and MMPI]). Dr. Astro Parkinson was called in as a consultant. All the test results were negative, and the patient was advised to come in for weekly psychotherapy.

Code Number	Description

Dr. Menter's bill:

a. _____	OV, comprehensive history & examination, moderate-complexity decision making
b. _____	EEG, extended monitoring (1 hour)
c. _____	Psychological tests (Rorschach and MMPI)
d. _____	Psychotherapy (60 minutes—done on a different day)

Dr. Parkinson's bill:

e. _____	Consultation, expanded problem-focused history & examination, straightforward decision making

9. An established patient, age 70 years, requires repair of a bilateral initial inguinal hernia (reducible). The code for this initial procedure is

a. _____ _____

ASSIGNMENT 13.7 HCPCS/MODIFIER CODE MATCH

Performance Objective

Task: Locate the correct HCPCS code and modifier, if necessary, for each medical drug, supply item, or service presented.

Conditions: Use pen or pencil and HCPCS code reference list in Appendix B of this *Workbook*.

Standards: Time: _____ minutes

Accuracy: _____

(Note: The time element and accuracy criteria may be given by your instructor.)

Directions: Match the HCPCS code in the first or second column with the description of the drug, supply item, or service presented in the third or fourth column. Write the correct letters on the blanks.

Code		Code		Description		Description
E1280	_____	J0760	_____	a. Vitamin B_{12}, 1000 mg		k. Blood (whole) for transfusion/unit
E0141	_____	A9150	_____	b. Injection, insulin per 5 units		l. Heavy-duty wheel-chair with detachable arms
J0290	_____	J2001	_____	c. Rigid walker, wheeled, without seat		m. Ampicillin inj, up to 500 mg
J3420	_____	L0160	_____	d. Waiver of liability statement on file		n. Dimethyl sulfoxide (DMSO) inj
J1815	_____	L3100-RT	_____	e. Nonemergency transportation, taxi		o. Urine strips
P9010	_____	A4250	_____	f. Inj of colchicine		p. Vancomycin (Vancocin) inj
J1212	_____	J2590	_____	g. Cervical occipital/mandibular support		q. Oxytocin (Pitocin) inj
J3370	_____	A4927	_____	h. Inj of lidocaine (Xylocaine)		r. Wide, heavy-duty wheelchair with detachable arms and leg rests
E1092	_____	A0100	_____	i. Gloves, nonsterile		s. Rt hallux valgus night splint
A4211	_____	-GA	_____	j. Supplies for self-administered drug injections		t. nonprescription drug

Chapter **13** Procedural Coding

Performance Objective

Task: Locate the correct procedure code and modifier, if necessary, for each case scenario.

Conditions: Use pen or pencil and *Current Procedural Terminology* code book.

Standards: Time: _____ minutes

             Accuracy: _____

             (Note: The time element and accuracy criteria may be given by your instructor.)

Directions: Find the correct procedure codes and modifiers, if necessary, for each case scenario.

1. The physician sees Horace Hart, a 60-year-old new patient, in the office for bronchial asthma, arteriosclerotic heart disease (ASHD), and hypertension. He performs an electrocardiogram (ECG) and urinalysis (UA) without microscopy and obtains x-rays. Comprehensive metabolic and lipid panels and a complete blood count (CBC) are done by an outside laboratory.

   Code Number   *Description*

   Physician's bill:

   a. _____   Initial OV, comprehensive history & examination, high-complexity decision making

   b. _____   ECG with interpret and report

   c. _____   UA, routine, nonautomated

   d. _____   Chest x-ray, two views

   e. _____   Routine venipuncture for handling of specimen

   f. _____   Handling of specimen

   Laboratory's bill:

   g. _____   Comprehensive metabolic panel: albumin, bilirubin, calcium, carbon dioxide, chloride, creatinine, glucose, phosphatase (alkaline), potassium, protein, sodium, ALT, AST, and urea nitrogen

   h. _____   Lipid panel

   i. _____   CBC, completely automated with complete automated differential

   If the doctor decides to have the chest x-rays interpreted by a radiologist, the procedural code billed by the radiologist would be _____.

2. Mr. Hart is seen again in the office on May 12. On May 25, he is seen at home at 2 AM with asthma exacerbation, possible myocardial infarct, and congestive heart failure. The doctor consulted with a thoracic cardiovascular surgeon by telephone. He also called to make arrangements for hospitalization. To complete the patient care, these services required 2 hours and 40 minutes of non–face-to-face time in addition to the time spent examining the patient during the house call.

Code Number   *Description*

a. _____   OV, problem-focused history & examination, straightforward decision making

b. _____   Home visit, detailed interval history & examination, high- complexity decision making

c. _____   Detention time, prolonged (list time required)

3. On June 9, Horace Hart is seen again in the hospital. The thoracic cardiovascular surgeon who was telephoned the previous day was called in for consultation to formally examine the patient and says that surgery is necessary, which is scheduled the following day. The patient's physician sees the patient for his asthmatic condition and acts as assistant surgeon. The surgeon does the follow-up care and assumes care in the case.

Code Number   *Description*

Primary care physician/assistant surgeon's bill:

a. _____   Hospital visit, problem-focused history & examination, low-complexity decision making

b. _____   Pericardiotomy

Thoracic cardiovascular surgeon's bill:

c. _____   Consultation, comprehensive history & examination, moderate-complexity decision making

d. _____   Pericardiotomy

Performance Objective

Task: Locate the correct procedure code and modifier, if necessary, for each case scenario.

Conditions: Use pen or pencil and *Current Procedural Terminology* code book.

Standards: Time: _____ minutes

Accuracy: _____

(Note: The time element and accuracy criteria may be given by your instructor.)

Directions: Read through this progress note on Roy A. Takashima. Abstract information from the note about the subjective symptoms, objective findings, and diagnoses. List the diagnostic and procedure codes you think this case would warrant.

Takashima, Roy A.
October 5, 20xx

Patient presents with many things going on. First, he's had no difficulties after the feral cat bite, and the cat was normal on quarantine.

He seemed to be recovering from the flu but is plagued with a persistent cough and pain down the center of his chest attributed to bronchitis without fever or grossly discolored phlegm.

Physical examination shows expiratory rhonchi and gross exacerbation of his cough on forced expiration. Spirometry before and after bronchodilator was remarkably good; he is symptomatically improved with a Proventil inhaler, which he is given as a sample. I don't think other antibiotics would help.

His reflux is under good control with proprietary antacids with a clear examination.

He has several areas of seborrheic keratoses on his face and head that need attention.

Finally, in follow-up, he needs a complete physical examination.

Ting Cho, MD

Diagnosis: Influenza and acute bronchitis

Subjective symptoms _____

_____

Objective findings _____

_____

_____

Diagnosis code _____ _____

_____ _____

E/M code _____

Spirometry code _____ _____

Performance Objective

Task: Calculate and insert the correct amounts for the Medicare scenario.

Conditions: Use a pen or pencil, the description of the problem and the reference material listed in the problem.

Standards: Time: _____ minutes

              Accuracy: _____

              (Note: The time element and accuracy criteria may be given by your instructor.)

Problem: In the late 1980s, Medicare's Resource-Based Relative Value System (RBRVS) became the way payment was determined each year. However, since the early 1990s, annual fee schedules have been supplied by local fiscal intermediaries, so the RBRVS has become more useful in determining practice cost to convert patients to capitation in negotiations of managed care contracts. Because physicians may request determination of fees for certain procedures to discover actual cost and what compensation ratios should be, it is important to know how Medicare fees are determined. Each year, the *Federal Register* publishes geographic practice cost indices (GPCIs) by Medicare carrier and locality, as well as relative value units (RVUs) and related information. This assignment will give you some mathematical practice in using figures for annual conversion factors to determine fees for given procedures in various regions of the United States. Refer to Figs 13.1 and 13.2, which are pages of the *Federal Register*.

a. HCPCS Code 47600: Removal of gallbladder. The medical practice is located in Phoenix, Arizona.

	Work	*Overhead*	*Malpractice*
RVUs	_____	_____	_____
GPCI	× _____	× _____	× _____

+ _____ + _____ + _____ = Total adjusted RVUs

2018 conversion factor $35.99 Total adjusted RVUs _____ = allowed

amount $ _____ .

b. HCPCS Code 47715: Excision of bile duct cyst. The medical practice is located in Arkansas.

	Work	*Overhead*	*Malpractice*
RVUs	_____	_____	_____
GPCI	× _____	× _____	× _____

+ _____ + _____ + _____ = Total adjusted RVUs

2018 conversion factor $35.99 Total adjusted RVUs _____ = allowed

amount $ _____ .

c. HCPCS Code 48146: Pancreatectomy. The medical practice is located in Fresno, California.

	Work	*Overhead*	*Malpractice*
RVUs	_____	_____	_____
GPCI	× _____	× _____	× _____

+ _____ + _____ + _____ = Total adjusted RVUs

2018 conversion factor $35.99 Total adjusted RVUs 3 = allowed

amount $ _____ .

Carrier number	Locality number	Locality name	Work	Practice expense	Mal-practice	
510	5	Birmingham, AL	0.981	0.913	0.824	
510	4	Mobile, AL	0.964	0.911	0.824	
510	2	North Central AL	0.970	0.867	0.824	
510	1	Northwest AL	0.985	0.869	0.824	
510	6	Rest of AL	0.975	0.851	0.824	
510	3	Southeast AL	0.972	0.869	0.824	
1020	1	Alaska	1.106	1.255	1.042	
1030	5	Flagstaff (city), AZ	0.983	0.911	1.255	
1030	1	Phoenix, AZ	1.003	1.016	1.255	
1030	7	Prescott (city), AZ	0.983	0.911	1.255	
1030	99	Rest of Arizona	0.987	0.943	1.255	
1030	2	Tucson (city), AZ	0.987	0.989	1.255	
1030	8	Yuma (city), AZ	0.983	0.911	1.255	
520	13	Arkansas	0.960	0.856	0.302	
2050	26	Anaheim-Santa Ana, CA	1.046	1.220	1.370	
542	14	Bakersfield, CA	1.028	1.050	1.370	
542	11	Fresno/Madera, CA	1.006	1.009	1.370	
542	13	Kings/Tulare, CA	0.999	1.001	1.370	
2050	18	Los Angeles, CA (1st of 8)	1.060	1.196	1.370	
2050	19	Los Angeles, CA (2nd of 8)	1.060	1.196	1.370	

Fig. 13.1

HCPCS[1]	MOD	Status	Description	Work RVUs	Practice expense RVUs[2]	Malpractice RVUs	Total	Global period	Update
47399	....	C	Liver surgery procedure	0.00	0.00	0.00	0.00	YYY	S
47400	....	A	Incision of liver duct	19.11	8.62	1.38	29.11	090	S
47420	....	A	Incision of bile duct	15.48	9.59	2.01	27.08	090	S
47425	....	A	Incision of bile duct	14.95	11.84	2.48	29.27	090	S
47440	....	A	Incision of bile duct	18.51	10.61	2.23	31.35	090	S
47460	....	A	Incision of bile duct sphincter	14.57	15.71	1.84	32.12	090	N
47480	....	A	Incision of gallbladder	8.14	7.68	1.61	17.43	090	S
47490	....	A	Incision of gallbladder	6.11	3.61	0.38	10.10	090	N
47500	....	A	Injection for liver x-rays	1.98	1.53	0.14	3.65	000	N
47505	....	A	Injection for liver x-rays	0.77	1.34	0.14	2.25	000	N
47510	....	A	Insert catheter, bile duct	7.47	2.90	0.25	10.62	090	N
47511	....	A	Insert bile duct drain	10.02	2.90	0.25	13.17	090	N
47525	....	A	Change bile duct catheter	5.47	1.61	0.16	7.24	010	N
47530	....	A	Revise, reinsert bile tube	5.47	1.53	0.19	7.19	090	N
47550	....	A	Bile duct endoscopy	3.05	1.58	0.35	4.98	000	S
47552	....	A	Biliary endoscopy, thru skin	6.11	1.38	0.21	7.70	000	S
47553	....	A	Biliary endoscopy, thru skin	6.42	3.84	0.63	10.89	000	N
47554	....	A	Biliary endoscopy, thru skin	9.16	3.97	0.68	13.81	000	S
47555	....	A	Biliary endoscopy, thru skin	7.64	2.66	0.30	10.60	000	N
47556	....	A	Biliary endoscopy, thru skin	8.66	2.66	0.30	11.62	000	N
47600	....	A	Removal of gallbladder	10.80	7.61	1.60	20.01	090	S
47605	....	A	Removal of gallbladder	11.66	8.23	1.77	21.66	090	S
47610	....	A	Removal of gallbladder	14.01	9.47	2.02	25.50	090	S
47612	....	A	Removal of gallbladder	14.91	14.39	3.08	32.38	090	S
47620	....	A	Removal of gallbladder	15.97	11.35	2.39	29.71	090	S
47630	....	A	Removal of bile duct stone	8.40	3.79	0.40	12.59	090	N
47700	....	A	Exploration of bile ducts	13.90	7.71	1.60	23.21	090	S
47701	....	A	Bile duct revision	26.87	8.30	1.92	37.09	090	S
47710	....	A	Excision of bile duct tumor	18.64	12.19	2.49	33.32	090	S
47715	....	A	Excision of bile duct cyst	14.66	8.31	1.73	24.70	090	S
47716	....	A	Fusion of bile duct cyst	12.67	6.63	1.55	20.85	090	S
47720	....	A	Fuse gallbladder and bowel	12.03	9.26	1.95	23.34	090	S
47721	....	A	Fuse upper gi structures	14.57	11.55	2.50	28.62	090	S
47740	....	A	Fuse gallbladder and bowel	14.08	10.32	2.16	26.56	090	S
47760	....	A	Fuse bile ducts and bowel	20.15	11.74	2.56	34.45	090	S
47765	....	A	Fuse liver ducts and bowel	19.25	14.77	3.00	37.02	090	S
47780	....	A	Fuse bile ducts and bowel	20.63	13.22	2.76	36.61	090	S
47800	....	A	Reconstruction of bile ducts	17.91	13.37	2.46	33.74	090	S
47801	....	A	Placement, bile duct support	11.41	5.54	0.82	17.77	090	S
47802	....	A	Fuse liver duct and intestine	16.19	10.38	1.77	28.34	090	S
47999	....	C	Bile tract surgery procedure	0.00	0.00	0.00	0.00	YYY	S
48000	....	A	Drainage of abdomen	13.25	7.13	1.42	21.80	090	S
48001	....	A	Placement of drain, pancreas	15.71	8.22	1.91	25.84	090	S
48005	....	A	Resect/debride pancreas	17.77	9.29	2.16	29.22	090	S
48020	....	A	Removal of pancreatic stone	13.12	6.86	1.59	21.57	090	S
48100	....	A	Biopsy of pancreas	10.30	4.26	0.80	15.36	090	S
48102	....	A	Needle biopsy, pancreas	4.48	2.44	0.25	7.17	010	N
48120	....	A	Removal of pancreas lesion	12.93	9.83	2.09	24.85	090	S
48140	....	A	Partial removal of pancreas	18.47	13.44	2.86	34.77	090	S
48145	....	A	Partial removal of pancreas	19.30	15.88	3.20	38.38	090	S
48146	....	A	Pancreatectomy	21.97	16.67	1.94	40.58	090	S
48148	....	A	Removal of pancreatic duct	14.57	8.32	1.70	24.59	090	S
48150	....	A	Partial removal of pancreas	34.55	22.79	4.80	62.14	090	S
48151	....	D	Partial removal of pancreas	0.00	0.00	0.00	0.00	090	0
48152	....	A	Pancreatectomy	31.33	22.79	4.80	58.92	090	S
48153	....	A	Pancreatectomy	34.55	22.79	4.80	62.14	090	S
48154	....	A	Pancreatectomy	31.33	22.79	4.80	58.92	090	S
48155	....	A	Removal of pancreas	19.65	20.63	4.31	44.59	090	S
48160	....	N	Pancreas removal, transplant	0.00	0.00	0.00	0.00	XXX	0
48180	....	A	Fuse pancreas and bowel	21.11	12.74	2.66	36.51	090	S
48400	....	A	Injection, intraoperative	1.97	1.04	0.24	3.25	ZZZ	S
48500	....	A	Surgery of pancreas cyst	12.17	8.62	1.68	22.47	090	S
48510	....	A	Drain pancreatic pseudocyst	11.34	7.62	1.46	20.42	090	S
48520	....	A	Fuse pancreas cyst and bowel	13.11	11.43	2.46	27.00	090	S
48540	....	A	Fuse pancreas cyst and bowel	15.95	12.80	2.68	31.43	090	S
48545	....	A	Pancreatorrhaphy	14.81	7.75	1.81	24.37	090	S
48547	....	A	Duodenal exclusion	21.42	11.20	2.61	35.23	090	S

ADDENDUM B—RELATIVE VALUE UNITS (RVUs) AND RELATED INFORMATION

[1] All numeric CPT HCPCS Copyright 1993 American Medical Association.
[2] *Indicates reduction of Practice Expense RVUs as a result of OBRA 1993.

Fig. 13.2

14 The Paper Claim: CMS-1500

Cheryl Fassett

KEY TERMS

Your instructor may wish to select some words pertinent to this chapter for a test. For definitions of the terms, further study, and/or reference, the words, phrases, and abbreviations may be found in the glossary at the end of the Textbook. *Key terms for this chapter follow.*

Administrative Simplification Compliance Act
clean claim
deleted claim
dirty claim
durable medical equipment number
electronic claim
employer identification number
facility provider number
group National Provider Identifier (group NPI)
Health Insurance Claim Form (CMS-1500)
incomplete claim
intelligent character recognition

invalid claim
National Provider Identifier
National Uniform Claim Committee
optical character recognition
paper claim
pending claim
physically clean claim
rejected claim
Social Security number
state license number
suspended claim
taxonomy code

KEY ABBREVIATIONS

See how many abbreviations and acronyms you can translate and then use this as a handy reference list. Definitions for the key abbreviations are located near the back of the Text-book *in the glossary.*

ASCA _____

CMS-1500 _____

DME _____

DNA _____

EIN _____

EMG _____

EPSDT _____

ICR _____

LMP _____

MSP _____

NA, N/A _____

NPI _____

NUCC _____

OCR _____

SOF _____

SSN _____

PERFORMANCE OBJECTIVES

The student will be able to:

- Define and spell the key terms and key abbreviations for this chapter, given the information from the *Textbook* glossary, within a reasonable time period and with enough accuracy to obtain a satisfactory evaluation.
- After reading the chapter, answer the fill-in-the-blank, mix and match, multiple choice, and true/false review questions, with enough accuracy to obtain a satisfactory evaluation.
- Given a handwritten CMS-1500 form, type a CMS-1500 Health Insurance Claim Form and list the reasons

why the claim was either rejected or delayed, within a reasonable time period and with enough accuracy to obtain a satisfactory evaluation.
- Given the patients' medical chart notes and blank insurance claim forms, complete each CMS-1500 Health Insurance Claim Form for billing, within a reasonable time period and with enough accuracy to obtain a satisfactory evaluation.

STUDY OUTLINE

The Paper Claim CMS-1500
National Uniform Claim Committee
History of the Paper Claim CMS-1500
Types of Submitted Claims
Claim Status
Abstracting From Medical Records
Cover Letter Accompanying Insurance Claims
Health Insurance Claim Form (CMS-1500)
Basic Guidelines for Submitting a Claim
Completion of Insurance Claim Forms

Common Reasons Why Claim Forms Are Delayed or Rejected
Claim Completion Guidelines
Optical Character Recognition
Do's and Don'ts for Claim Completion
Instructions for the Health Insurance Claim Form (CMS-1500)
Block-by-Block Instructions for Completion of the CMS-1500
Insurance Program Templates

186

Part I Fill in the Blank

Review the objectives, key terms, chapter information, glossary definitions of key terms, and figures before completing the following review questions.

1. What legislation required all claims sent to the Medicare program be submitted electronically, effective October 16, 2003?

   _____

2. State the name of the health insurance claim form that was required for use effective

   April 1, 2014. _____

3. Does Medicare accept the CMS-1500 claim form?

   _____

4. What is a pended claim?

   _____

5. How many days will it take to process a Medicare claim that is submitted electronically?

   _____

6. If a claim is submitted on behalf of the patient, and coverage of the services is denied, what is the most effective way to present the situation to the patient?

   _____

7. What is *dual coverage*?

   _____

8. The insurance company with the first responsibility for payment of a bill for medical services is known as the

   _____

9. The CMS-1500 claim form allows for reporting of a maximum of _____ diagnosis codes per claim form.

10. What internet resource can be used to find physician provider numbers?

    _____

11. For electronic submission of claims, what allows the physician's name to be printed in the signature block where it would normally be signed?

    _____

12. When preparing a claim that is to be optically scanned, birth dates are keyed in with how many digits?

    _____

13. If circumstances make it impossible to obtain a signature each time a paper claim is submitted, the patient's signature may be obtained and maintained in the patient's medical record. The claim block should be completed with

_____ or _____, thus indicating the signature is on file.

Part II Mix and Match

14. Match the types of claims listed in the right column with their descriptions and fill in the blanks with the appropriate letters.

_____ Claim missing required information

_____ Phrase used when a claim is held back from payment

_____ Claim that is submitted and then optically scanned by the insurance carrier and converted to electronic form

_____ Claim that needs manual processing because of errors or to solve a problem

_____ Claim that needs clarification and answers to some questions

_____ Claim that is canceled or voided if the incorrect claim form is used or itemized charges are not provided

_____ Claim that is paperless

_____ Claim that is submitted within the time limit and correctly completed

_____ Medicare claim that contains information that is complete and necessary but is illogical or incorrect

a. Clean claim

b. Paper claim

c. Invalid claim

d. Dirty claim

e. Electronic claim

f. Pending claim

g. Rejected claim

h. Incomplete claim

i. Deleted claim

15. Match the types of numbers listed in the right column with their descriptions and fill in the blanks with the appropriate letters.

_____ A number issued by the federal government to each individual for personal use

_____ A Medicare lifetime provider number

_____ A number listed on a claim when submitting insurance claims to insurance companies under a group name

_____ A number that a health care provider must obtain to practice in a state

_____ A number used when billing for supplies and equipment

_____ A number issued to a hospital

_____ An individual health care provider's federal tax identification number issued by the Internal Revenue Service

a. State license number

b. Employer identification number

c. Social Security number

d. Group national provider number

e. National Provider Identifier

f. Durable medical equipment number

g. Facility provider number

PART III MULTIPLE CHOICE

Choose the best answer.

16. The basic paper claim form currently used by health care professionals and suppliers to bill insurance carriers for services provided to patients is the:
   a. UB-04 claim form.
   b. CMS-1500 claim form.
   c. Attending physician's statement.
   d. COMB-1.

17. What is the exception to the Administrative Simplification Compliance Act's (ASCA's) requirement for providers to send claims to Medicare electronically?
   a. Chiropractors
   b. Providers who have more than 25 full-time employees
   c. Providers with fewer than 10 full-time employees
   d. Any provider who requests a financial hardship

18. Under ASCA, plans other than Medicare:
    a. may allow submission of claims on paper.
    b. will never allow submission of claims on paper.
    c. only allow submission of claims on paper.
    d. must follow the claims submission guidance of the American Medical Association (AMA).

19. The National Uniform Claim Committee (NUCC) is made up of which of the following?
    a. AMA representatives
    b. Centers for Medicare and Medicaid Services (CMS) representatives
    c. Providers
    d. All of the above

20. The most recently revised version of the 1500 Health Insurance Claim Form developed in 2012 accommodates:
    a. the change in the names of the government agency from Health Care Finance Administration to Centers for Medicare and Medicaid Services (CMS).
    b. requirements for allowing optical scanning of the claim.
    c. changes in the Electronic Claims Submission Version 5010 837P.
    d. changes to the *Current Procedural Terminology* (CPT) coding system.

21. If a patient has dual coverage:
    a. insurance information for the primary carrier should be obtained.
    b. insurance information for both the primary and the secondary carrier should be obtained.
    c. insurance information for the secondary carrier can be obtained after the primary insurance carrier processes the claim.
    d. the primary carrier has insurance information for the secondary carrier and will automatically forward the claim to the secondary carrier if necessary.

22. Health Insurance Portability and Accountability Act (HIPAA) laws require that the provider rendering the service be identified on the claim form by:
    a. reporting of the correct provider number.
    b. reporting of the correct International Classification of Diseases (ICD)-10 code.
    c. reporting of the correct CPT code.
    d. reporting of the correct facility code.

23. The Omnibus Budget Reconciliation Act (OBRA) requires Medicare administrative contractors to:
    a. deny all claims received after 1 year from date of service.
    b. pay all clean claims that are submitted within 1 year from date of service.
    c. investigate all clean claims not paid on time.
    d. pay interest on all clean claims not paid on time.

24. A claim that is investigated on a postpayment basis that is found to be "not due" will require:
    a. resubmission of a claim.
    b. manual review of the claim.
    c. refund of the monies paid.
    d. additional medical records.

25. If there is a balance remaining on a patient's account after the patient's primary insurance has paid, and the patient has secondary coverage, the billing specialist should:
    a. send a bill to the patient for the remaining balance.
    b. send a claim form to the secondary insurance for the remaining balance.
    c. send a claim form to the secondary insurance with a copy of the explanation of benefits from the primary carrier.
    d. monitor the claim to determine whether the patient has sent a claim to the secondary carrier.

26. The maximum number of diagnostic codes that can be submitted on the CMS-1500 claim form is:
    a. four.
    b. six.
    c. eight.
    d. twelve.

27. National Provider Identifier (NPI) numbers are used to report:
    a. referring physicians.
    b. ordering physicians.
    c. performing physicians.
    d. all of the above.

28. NPI numbers are assigned:
    a. each time a health care provider contracts with a new payer.
    b. annually, per health care provider.
    c. once in a lifetime, per health care provider.
    d. each time the provider moves to another state.

29. To correct a claim that has been denied because of an invalid procedure code, the billing specialist should:
   a. check the patient registration form to ensure all data were reported accurately.
   b. confirm the code in the CPT manual to ensure it is valid for the date of service.
   c. confirm the code in the ICD-10 manual to ensure it is valid for the date of service.
   d. confirm the provider's NPI number to make sure it was reported accurately.

30. To correct a claim that was denied because more than six lines were entered on the claim, the billing specialist should:
   a. readjust the printer, so all claim lines fit on the form, reprint, and send.
   b. reenter data with the appropriate code range for the dates of service and bill on one line.
   c. bill six claim lines on one claim and complete an additional paper claim for the additional claim lines.
   d. write off the additional claim lines that have been denied.

PART IV TRUE/FALSE

Write "T" or "F" in the blank to indicate whether you think the statement is true or false.

_____ 31. The insurance billing specialist does not need to know how to complete a paper claim because most claims are submitted electronically.

_____ 32. Physicians who experience downtimes of internet services that are out of their control for more than two days may submit claims to Medicare on paper.

_____ 33. The goal of the NUCC is to provide a warehouse for providers to purchase CMS-1500 claim forms.

_____ 34. Effective June 1, 2013, providers were required to use only the CMS-1500 claim form.

_____ 35. Use of the standardized CMS-1500 claim form has simplified processing of paper claims.

_____ 36. Quantities of the CMS-1500 claim form can be purchased through CMS or downloaded from the CMS website and used for submission.

_____ 37. Interest rates that apply to the Prompt Payment Interest Rate can be located on the Treasury's Financial Fiscal Service page.

_____ 38. Medicare claims that require further investigation before being processed are referred to as "other" claims.

_____ 39. A diagnosis should never be submitted without supporting documentation in the medical record.

_____ 40. Claims for dates of services in two different years may be submitted on the same claim form.

_____ 41. Services that are inclusive in the global surgical package that have no charge associated with them should not be submitted on the CMS-1500 claim form.

_____ 42. Proofreading claims before submission can prevent denials and delay of claim processing.

_____ 43. When submitting supplemental documentation for processing of a claim, the patient's name and date of service need only be on the front of a two-sided document.

_____ 44. Handwriting is permitted on optically scanned paper claims.

_____ 45. Use the abbreviation "DNA" when information is not applicable.

ASSIGNMENT 14.2 COMPLETE A HEALTH INSURANCE CLAIM FORM FOR A PRIVATE CASE

Performance Objective

Task: Complete a health insurance claim form

Conditions: Use Merry M. McLean's patient record, one health insurance claim form, a computer or pen.

Standards: Claim Productivity Measurement

Time: _____ minutes

Accuracy: _____

(Note: The time element and accuracy criteria may be given by your instructor.)

Directions:

1. Complete the Health Insurance Claim Form, using NUCC guidelines, and send the form to the Prudential Insurance Company for Mrs. Merry M. McLean by referring to the patient record. Date the claim June 15 of the current year. Record on the financial account record/statement when you have billed the insurance company.

2. A Performance Evaluation Checklist may be reproduced from the "Instruction Guide to the Workbook" in a section before Chapter 1 if your instructor wishes you to submit it to assist with scoring and comments.

After the instructor has returned your work to you, either make the necessary corrections and place your work in a three-ring notebook for future reference, or, if you received a high score, place it in your portfolio for reference when applying for a job.

| COLLEGE CLINIC |
| 4567 Broad Avenue, Woodland Hills, XY 12345-0001 |
| (555)-486-9002 |
| Fax: (555) 487-8976 |
| NPI: 3664021CC |

PATIENT INFORMATION:

Name:	Merry M. McLean
Address:	4919 Dolphin Way
	Woodland Hills, XY 12345
Telephone:	(555) 486-1859
Date of Birth:	02/02/1948
Social Security:	459-XX-9989
Occupation:	SECRETARY
Employer:	Porter Company
	5490 Wilshire Blvd.
	Merck, XY 12346
Status:	Married
Spouse:	Harry L. McLean

INSURANCE INFORMATION:

Primary:	Prudential Insurance
	5621 Wilshire Blvd.
	Merck, XY 12346
	(555) 664-9023
Policy Number:	459-XX-9989
Group Number:	8832
Subscriber:	Harry L. McLean
Secondary:	None

DIAGNOSIS INFORMATION

1. N32.0   Vesicle fistula, not otherwise specified   5.

2. R32   Urinary incontinence, unspecified   6.

3.   7.

4.   8.

PROCEDURE INFORMATION

Description	Date	Code	Charge
1. Office visit, new patient	05/06/20XX	99203	70.92
2. Urinalysis	05/06/20XX	81000	8.00
3. Cystoscopy	05/10/20XX	52000	167.05
4. Initial hospital care	05/16/20XX	99221	73.00
5. Repair vesicovaginal fistula	05/17/20XX	51900	1196.82
6. Hospital visit	05/18/20XX	99024	N/C
7. Hospital visit	05/19/20XX	99024	N/C
8. Hospital visit	05/20/20XX	99024	N/C
9. Hospital visit	05/21/20XX	99024	N/C
10. Discharge	05/22/20XX	99024	N/C
11. Follow-up office visit	06/05/20XX	99024	N/C

NOTES: Referred by: Emdee Fine, MD, 5000 Wilshire Blvd., Merck, XY 12346
                                NPI: 73027175XX
                 Treating MD: Gene Ulibarri, MD
                                NPI: 25678831XX
        Place of service: College Clinic for 5/6–5/10, 6/5
                                College Hospital for 5/16–5/22
                                4500 Broad Avenue, Woodland Hills, XY 12345
                                NPI: X950731067

ASSIGNMENT 14.3 COMPLETE ONE HEALTH INSURANCE CLAIM FORM FOR A PRIVATE CASE

Performance Objective

Task: Complete one health insurance claim form.

Conditions: Use Walter J. Stone's E/M patient record, one health insurance claim form, a computer or pen.

Standards: Claim Productivity Measurement

Time: _____ minutes

Accuracy: _____

(Note: The time element and accuracy criteria may be given by your instructor.)

Directions: You will be billing for all services listed on the patient's progress notes for Dr. Clarence Cutler.

1. Complete one Health Insurance Claim Form, addressing it to Travelers Insurance Company for Mr. Walter J. Stone by referring to patient record. Date the claim May 5 of the current year. Use NUCC guidelines.

2. A Performance Evaluation Checklist may be reproduced from the "Instruction Guide to the Workbook" that appears in a section before Chapter 1 if your instructor wishes you to submit it to assist with scoring and comments.

After the instructor has returned your work to you, either make the necessary corrections and place your work in a three-ring notebook for future reference or, if you received a high score, place it in your portfolio for reference when applying for a job.

193

| COLLEGE CLINIC |
| 4567 Broad Avenue, Woodland Hills, XY 12345-0001 |
| (555)-486-9002 |
| Fax: (555) 487-8976 |
| NPI: 3664021CC |

PATIENT INFORMATION:		INSURANCE INFORMATION:	
Name:	Walter J. Stone	Primary:	Travelers Insurance
Address:	2008 Converse Street		5460 Olympic Blvd.
	Woodland Hills, XY 12345		Woodland Hills, XY 12345
Telephone:	(555) 345-0776	Policy Number:	456-XX-9989
Date of Birth:	03/14/1949	Group Number:	6754
Social Security:	456-XX-9989	Subscriber:	Walter J. Stone
Occupation:	ADVERTISING AGENT	Secondary:	None
Employer:	RV Black and Associates		
	1267 Broad Street		
	Woodland Hills, XY 12345		
Status:	Widowed		
Spouse:			

DIAGNOSIS INFORMATION

1. K25.0   Acute gastric ulcer with hemorrhage

2. K80.18   Calculus of gallbladder and bile duct with cholecystitis, unspecified, without obstruction

3. K92.2   Gastrointestinal hemorrhage, unspecified

4. I10   Essential hypertension, benign

PROCEDURE INFORMATION

Description	Date	Code	Charge
1. Initial hospital care	05/03/20XX	99222	120.80
2. Cholecystectomy	05/04/20XX	43255	741.99
3. Endoscopy	05/04/20XX	43255-51-59-99	281.51

NOTES: Referred by: Gaston Input, MD, College Hospital
           NPI: 32783127XX
       Treating MD: Clarence Cutler, MD
           NPI: 43050047XX
    Place of service: College Hospital
           4500 Broad Avenue, Woodland Hills, XY 12345
           NPI: X950731067

ASSIGNMENT 14.4 LOCATE ERRORS ON A COMPLETED HEALTH INSURANCE CLAIM FORM

Performance Objective

Task: Locate errors on a completed health insurance claim form and post the information to the patient's ledger card.

Conditions: Use Tom N. Parkinson's completed insurance claim (Fig. 14.1), one health insurance claim form, a computer or pen.

Standards: Time: _____ minutes

              Accuracy: _____

              (Note: The time element and accuracy criteria may be given by your instructor.)

Guidance: To alleviate frustration and ease the process of completing a claim form for the first time, you will be editing a claim and then taking the correct information and inserting it on a blank CMS-1500 form. Refer to Chapter 14 in the Textbook for block-by-block private payer instructions for completing the CMS-1500 insurance claim form. Refer to Fig. 14.3 in the Textbook for visual placement of data.

Directions: Study the completed claim form (Fig. 14.1) and search for missing or incorrect information. If possible, verify all information. Highlight or circle in red all incorrect or missing information. Insert the correct information on the claim form. Now transfer all the data to a blank CMS-1500 claim form. If mandatory information is missing, insert the word "NEED" in the corresponding block of the claim form.

A Performance Evaluation Checklist may be reproduced from the "Instruction Guide to the Workbook" that appears in a section before Chapter 1 if your instructor wishes you to submit it to assist with scoring and comments.

Optional: List, in block-by-block order, the reasons why the claim may either be rejected or delayed according to the errors found.

General Directions for Claim Form Completion

Assume that the Health Insurance Claim Form CMS-1500 is printed in red ink for processing by optical character recognition (OCR) or intelligent character recognition (ICR). Complete the form using NUCC guidelines and send it to the proper insurance carrier. Refer to Chapter 14 in the Textbook for block instructions. Claim form templates have been completed to use as visual examples for placement of data; they may be found at the end of Chapter 14 in the Textbook. Screened areas on each form do not apply to the insurance program example shown and should be left blank.

All physicians in College Clinic accept assignment of benefits for all types of insurance that you will be billing for; indicate this by checking "yes" in Block 27. For each claim completed, be sure to insert your initials at the lower left corner of the claim form.

DRAFT - NOT FOR OFFICIAL USE

HEALTH INSURANCE CLAIM FORM

APPROVED BY NATIONAL UNIFOR MCLAIM COMMITTEE (NUCC) 02/12

	PICA								PICA	

1. MEDICARE ☐ (Medicare#) MEDICAID ☐ (Medicaid#) TRICARE ☐ (ID#DoD#) CHAMPVA ☐ (Member ID#) GROUP HEALTH PLAN ☒ (ID#) FECA BLK LUNG ☐ (ID#) OTHER ☐ (ID#)

1a. INSURED'S I.D. NUMBER (For Program in Item 1)
PX4278A

2. PATIENT'S NAME (Last Name, First Name, Middle Initial)
Parkinson, Tom, N

3. PATIENT'S BIRTH DATE   SEX
MM 04 | DD 06 | YY 1993   M ☒ F ☐

4. INSURED'S NAME (Last Name, First Name, Middle Initial)
Parkinson, Jamie, B

5. PATIENT'S ADDRESS (No., Street)
4510 South A Street

6. PATIENT RELATIONSHIP TO INSURED
Self ☐ Spouse ☐ Child ☒ Other ☐

7. INSURED'S ADDRESS (No., Street)
4510 South A Street

CITY
Woodland Hills   STATE XY

8. RESERVED FOR NUCC USE

CITY
Woodland Hills   STATE XY

ZIP CODE
12345-0000

TELEPHONE (Include Area Code)
(555) 7421560

ZIP CODE
12345-0000

TELEPHONE (Include Area Code)
(555) 7421560

9. OTHER INSURED'S NAME (Last Name, First Name, Middle Initial)

10. IS PATIENT'S CONDITION RELATED TO:

11. INSURED'S POLICY GROUP OR FECA NUMBER

a. OTHER INSURED'S POLICY OR GROUP NUMBER

a. EMPLOYMENT? (Current or Previous)
☐ YES ☒ NO

a. INSURED'S DATE OF BIRTH
MM | DD | YY   SEX M ☐ F ☐

b. RESERVED FOR NUCC USE

b. AUTO ACCIDENT?
☐ YES ☒ NO   PLACE (State)

b. OTHER CLAIM ID (Designated by NUCC)

c. RESERVED FOR NUCC USE

c. OTHER ACCIDENT?
☐ YES ☒ NO

c. INSURANCE PLAN NAME OR PROGRAM NAME

d. INSURANCE PLAN NAME OR PROGRAM NAME

10d. CLAIM CODES (Designated by NUCC)

d. IS THERE ANOTHER HEALTH BENEFIT PLAN?
☐ YES ☒ NO   If yes, complete items 9, 9a, and 9d.

READ BACK OF FORM BEFORE COMPLETING & SIGNING THIS FORM.
12. PATIENT'S OR AUTHORIZED PERSON'S SIGNATUREI authorize the release of any medical or other information necessary to process this claim. I also request payment of government benefits either to myself or to the party who accepts assignment below.

SIGNED _____   DATE _____

13. INSURED'S OR AUTHORIZED PERSON'S SIGNATURE I authorize payment of medical benefits to the undersigned physician or supplier for services described below.

SIGNED _____

14. DATE OF CURRENT: ILLNESS, INJURY, or PREGNANCY(LMP)
MM | DD | YY   QUAL.

15. OTHER DATE
QUAL.   MM | DD | YY

16. DATES PATIENT UNABLE TO WORK IN CURRENT OCCUPATION
FROM MM | DD | YY   TO MM | DD | YY

17. NAME OF REFERRING PROVIDER OR OTHER SOURCE

17a.
17b. NPI

18. HOSPITALIZATION DATES RELATED TO CURRENT SERVICES
FROM MM | DD | YY   TO MM | DD | YY

19. ADDITIONAL CLAIM INFORMATION (Designated by NUCC)

20. OUTSIDE LAB? $ CHARGES
☐ YES ☒ NO

21. DIAGNOSIS OR NATURE OF ILLNESS OR INJURY Relate A-L to service line below (24E)   ICD Ind. 0

A. _____ B. _____ C. _____ D. _____
E. _____ F. _____ G. _____ H. _____
I. _____ J. _____ K. _____ L. _____

22. RESUBMISSION CODE   ORIGINAL REF. NO.

23. PRIOR AUTHORIZATION NUMBER

24. A. DATE(S) OF SERVICE						B. PLACE OF SERVICE	C. EMG	D. PROCEDURES, SERVICES, OR SUPPLIES (Explain Unusual Circumstances)		E. DIAGNOSIS POINTER	F. $ CHARGES		G. DAYS OR UNITS	H. EPSDT Family Plan	I. ID. QUAL.	J. RENDERING PROVIDER ID. #
From MM	DD	YY	To MM	DD	YY			CPT/HCPCS	MODIFIER							
07	14	20XX						99242			80	24	1		NPI	
07	14	20XX						71020		A	38	96	1		NPI	4627889700
															NPI	
															NPI	
															NPI	
															NPI	

25. FEDERAL TAX I.D. NUMBER   SSN ☐ EIN ☐
7034597

26. PATIENT'S ACCOUNT NO.

27. ACCEPT ASSIGNMENT? (For govt. claims, see back)
☒ YES ☐ NO

28. TOTAL CHARGE
$ 119 | 20

29. AMOUNT PAID
$

30. Rsvd for NUCC Use
$

31. SIGNATURE OF PHYSICIAN OR SUPPLIER INCLUDING DEGREES OR CREDENTIALS
(I certify that the statements on the reverse apply to this bill and are made a part thereof.)
Gerald Practon   071420XX
SIGNED *Gerald Practon*   DATE

32. SERVICE FACILITY LOCATION INFORMATION

a. NPI   b.

33. BILLING PROVIDER INFO & PH #   (555) 4869002
College Clinic
4567 Broad Avenue
Woodland Hills XY 12345-0001

a. 3664021CC   b.

NUCC Instruction Manual available at: www.nucc.org   *PLEASE PRINT OR TYPE*   OMB APPROVAL PENDING

196

ASSIGNMENT 14.5 COMPLETE A CLAIM FORM FOR A MEDICARE/MEDICAID CASE

Performance Objective

Task: Complete a CMS-1500 claim form for a Medicare/Medicaid case.

Conditions: Use Helen P. Nolan's patient record, one health insurance claim form, a pen or pencil.

Standards: Claim Productivity Measurement

Time: _____ minutes

Accuracy: _____

(Note: The time element and accuracy criteria may be given by your instructor.)

Directions:

1. Complete the CMS-1500 claim form, using NUCC guidelines for a Medicare/Medicaid case. If your instructor wants you to direct it to your local Medicare fiscal intermediary, obtain the name and address by going to the internet. Refer to Mrs. Helen P. Nolan's patient record for information. Date the claim May 31 of the current year.

2. Refer to Chapter 14 and Fig. 14.5 of the textbook for instructions on how to complete the CMS-1500 claim form.

3. A Performance Evaluation Checklist may be reproduced from the "Instruction Guide to the Workbook" that appears in a section before Chapter 1 if your instructor wishes you to submit it to assist with scoring and comments.

After the instructor has returned your work to you, either make the necessary corrections and place your work in a three-ring notebook for future reference or, if you received a high score, place it in your portfolio for reference when applying for a job.

COLLEGE CLINIC
4567 Broad Avenue, Woodland Hills, XY 12345-0001
(555)-486-9002
Fax: (555) 487-8976
NPI: 3664021CC

PATIENT INFORMATION:		INSURANCE INFORMATION:	
Name:	Helen P. Nolan	Primary:	Medicare
Address:	2588 Cedar Street		
	Woodland Hills, XY 12345	Policy Number:	632XX3209D
Telephone:	(555) 660-9878	Group Number:	
Date of Birth:	05/10/37	Subscriber:	
Social Security:	732-XX-1573	Secondary:	Medicaid
Occupation:	HOMEMAKER	Policy Number:	1960235894901XX
Employer:		Group Number:	
Status:	Widowed		
Spouse:			

DIAGNOSIS INFORMATION

1. I84.131   Internal and external bleeding hemorrhoids

2. K60.5   Anorectal fistula

3.

4.

PROCEDURE INFORMATION

Description	Date	Code	Charge
1. Office visit, new patient	05/01/20XX	99203-25	64.92
2. Diagnostic proctoscopy	05/01/20XX	46614	166.68
3. Hemorrhoidectomy with fistulectomy	05/08/20XX	46258	582.17

NOTES: Referred by: James B. Jeffers, MD, 100 S. Broadway, Woodland Hills, XY 12345
NPI: 12345069XX
Treating MD: Rex Rumsey, MD
NPI: 19999047XX
Place of service: 5/1 College Clinic
5/8 College Hospital
4500 Broad Avenue, Woodland Hills, XY 12345
NPI: X950731067

ASSIGNMENT 14.6 COMPLETE A CLAIM FORM FOR A MEDICARE CASE

Performance Objective

Task: Complete a CMS-1500 claim form for a Medicare case.

Conditions: Use Elsa M. Mooney's patient record, one health insurance claim form, a pen or pencil.

Standards: Claim Productivity Measurement

Time: _____ minutes

Accuracy: _____

(Note: The time element and accuracy criteria may be given by your instructor.)

Directions:

1. Complete the CMS-1500 claim form, using National Uniform Claim Committee (NUCC) guidelines for a Medicare case. If your instructor wants you to direct it to your local fiscal intermediary, obtain the name and address by going to the internet. Refer to Mrs. Elsa M. Mooney's patient record for information. Date the claim December 21 of the current year. Dr. Cardi is a participating physician who is accepting assignment.

2. Refer to Chapter 14 (Fig. 14.4) of the textbook for instructions on how to complete this claim form and a Medicare template.

3. A Performance Evaluation Checklist may be reproduced from the "Instruction Guide to the Workbook" that appears in a section before Chapter 1 if your instructor wishes you to submit it to assist with scoring and comments.

After the instructor has returned your work to you, either make the necessary corrections and place your work in a three-ring notebook for future reference or, if you received a high score, place it in your portfolio for reference when applying for a job.

COLLEGE CLINIC

COLLEGE CLINIC
4567 Broad Avenue, Woodland Hills, XY 12345-0001
(555)-486-9002
Fax: (555) 487-8976
NPI: 3664021CC

PATIENT INFORMATION:		INSURANCE INFORMATION:	
Name:	Elsa M. Mooney	Primary:	Medicare
Address:	5750 Canyon Road		
	Woodland Hills, XY 12345	Policy Number:	321XX2653A
Telephone:	(555) 452-4968	Group Number:	
Date of Birth:	02/06/1930	Subscriber:	
Social Security:	321-XX-2653	Secondary:	none
Occupation:	RETIRED SECRETARY	Policy Number:	
Employer:		Group Number:	
		Subscriber:	
Status:	Widowed		
Spouse:			

DIAGNOSIS INFORMATION

1. I25.119   Atherosclerotic heart disease of native coronary artery with unspecified angina pectoris
2.
3.
4.

PROCEDURE INFORMATION

Description	Date	Code	Charge
1. Initial office visit, new pt	12/15/20XX	99203	64.92
2. ECG with interpret & report	12/15/20XX	93000	31.36

NOTES: Referred by: George Gentle, MD, 1000 N. Main St., Woodland Hills, XY 12345
NPI: 40213102XX
Treating MD: Perry Cardi, MD
NPI: 67805027XX
Place of service: College Clinic
4500 Broad Avenue, Woodland Hills, XY 12345
NPI: X950731067

ASSIGNMENT 14.7 COMPLETE A CLAIM FORM FOR A MEDICAID CASE

Performance Objective

Task: Complete a CMS-1500 claim form.

Conditions: Use Rose Clarkson's patient record, one health insurance claim form, a pen or pencil.

Standards: Claim Productivity Measurement

Time: _____ minutes

Accuracy: _____

(Note: The time element and accuracy criteria may be given by your instructor.)

Directions:

1. Using National Uniform Claim Committee (NUCC) guidelines, complete the Health Insurance Claim Form and direct it to Medicaid for Rose Clarkson by referring to her patient record. Date the claim September 6 of the current year. If your instructor wants you to insert the name and address of your Medicaid fiscal agent on the claim, obtain the address by going to the internet.

2. Refer to Chapter 14 (Fig. 14.3) in the *Textbook* for instructions on how to complete this claim form and a Medicaid template.

3. A Performance Evaluation Checklist may be reproduced from the "Instruction Guide to the Workbook" in the section before Chapter 1 if your instructor wishes you to submit it to assist with scoring and comments.

After the instructor has returned your work to you, either make the necessary corrections and place your work in a three-ring notebook for future reference or, if you received a high score, place it in your portfolio for reference when applying for a job.

| COLLEGE CLINIC |
| 4567 Broad Avenue, Woodland Hills, XY 12345-0001 |
| (555)-486-9002 |
| Fax: (555) 487-8976 |
| NPI: 3664021CC |

PATIENT INFORMATION:		INSURANCE INFORMATION:	
Name:	Rose Clarkson	Primary:	Medicaid
Address:	3408 Jackson Street		
	Hempstead, XY 11551-0300	Policy Number:	CC99756329346X
Telephone:	(555) 487-2209	Group Number:	
Date of Birth:	03/09/1954	Subscriber:	
Social Security:	030-XX-9543	Secondary:	none
Occupation:	UNEMPLOYED	Policy Number:	
Employer:		Group Number:	
		Subscriber:	
Status:			
Spouse:			

DIAGNOSIS INFORMATION

1. I50.9   Congestive heart failure

2. I34.1   Nonrheumatic mitral valve prolapse

3.

4.

PROCEDURE INFORMATION

Description	Date	Code	Charge
1. Initial office visit, new pt	09/04/20XX	99203	70.92
2. 12 lead ECG	09/04/20XX	93000	34.26
3. Echocardiogram with Doppler	09/04/20XX	99306	250.73
4. Chest x-ray	09/04/20XX	71010	31.95

NOTES: Referred by: James Jackson, MD, 100 N. Main St., Hempstead, XY 11551
                        NPI: 72011337XX
            Treating MD: Perry Cardi, MD
                        NPI: 67805027XX
        Place of service: College Clinic
                        4500 Broad Avenue, Woodland Hills, XY 12345
                        NPI: X950731067

ASSIGNMENT 14.8 COMPLETE A CLAIM FORM FOR A MEDICAID CASE

Performance Objective

Task: Complete a CMS-1500 claim form for a Medicaid case

Conditions: Use Stephen M. Drake's patient record, one health insurance claim form, a pen or pencil.

Standards: Claim Productivity Measurement

Time: _____ minutes

Accuracy: _____

(Note: The time element and accuracy criteria may be given by your instructor.)

Directions:

1. Using NUCC guidelines, complete the Health Insurance Claim Form and direct it to Medicaid for Stephen M. Drake by referring to his patient record. Date the claim May 26 of the current year. If your instructor wants you to insert the name and address of your Medicaid fiscal agent on the claim, obtain it by going to the internet. Do not list services not charged for (N/C) on the claim form. Remember that the physician must always sign all forms on Medicaid cases; stamped signatures are not allowed.

2. Refer to Chapter 14 (Fig. 14.3) in the Textbook for instructions on how to complete this claim form and a Medicaid template.

3. A Performance Evaluation Checklist may be reproduced from the "Instruction Guide to the Workbook" that appears in the section before Chapter 1 if your instructor wishes you to submit it to assist with scoring and comments.

After the instructor has returned your work to you, either make the necessary corrections and place your work in a three-ring notebook for future reference or, if you received a high score, place it in your portfolio for reference when applying for a job.

COLLEGE CLINIC
4567 Broad Avenue, Woodland Hills, XY 12345-0001
(555)-486-9002
Fax: (555) 487-8976
NPI: 3664021CC

PATIENT INFORMATION:		INSURANCE INFORMATION:	
Name:	Stephen M. Drake	Primary:	Medicaid
Address:	2317 Charnwood Avenue		
	Woodland Hills, XY 12345	Policy Number:	197152403316X
Telephone:	(555) 277-5831	Group Number:	
Date of Birth:	04/03/1991	Subscriber:	
Social Security:	566-XX-0081	Secondary:	none
Occupation:	STUDENT	Policy Number:	
Employer:		Group Number:	
		Subscriber:	
Status:			
Spouse:			

DIAGNOSIS INFORMATION

1. J03.90   Acute tonsillitis, unspecified

2. J35.03   Chronic tonsillitis and adenoiditis

3. J02.0   Streptococcal sore throat

4.

PROCEDURE INFORMATION

Description	Date	Code	Charge
1. Initial office visit, new pt	05/01/20XX	99203	70.92
2. Strep culture	05/01/20XX	87081	25.00
3. Injection, antibiotic	05/01/20XX	90772	5.22
4. Bicillin	05/01/20XX	J0540	10.00
5. Follow-up office visit	05/08/20XX	99212-57	28.55
6. Remove tonsils and adenoids	05/09/20XX	42821	410.73
7. Post-op office visit	05/17/20XX	99024	N/C

NOTES: Referred by: James Jeffers, MD, 100 S. Broadway, Hempstead, XY 12345
NPI: 12345069XX
Treating MD: Gerald Practon, MD
NPI: 46278897XX
Place of service: College Clinic for 5/1–5/8, 5/17
College Hospital for 5/9
4500 Broad Avenue, Woodland Hills, XY 12345
NPI: X950731067

ASSIGNMENT 14.9 COMPLETE A CLAIM FORM FOR A TRICARE STANDARD CASE

Performance Objective

Task: Complete a CMS-1500 claim form for a TRICARE Standard case.

Conditions: Use Rosa M. Sandoval's patient record, one health insurance claim form, a pen or pencil.

Standards: Claim Productivity Measurement

Time: _____ minutes

Accuracy: _____

(Note: The time element and accuracy criteria may be given by your instructor.)

Directions:

1. Using National Uniform Claim Committee (NUCC) guidelines, complete the CMS-1500 claim form. Refer to Miss Rosa M. Sandoval's patient record for information. Date the claim May 31 of the current year. Dr. Atrics is not accepting assignment on this TRICARE Standard case but is completing the claim for the patient's convenience.

2. Refer to Chapter 14 (Fig. 14.8) of the Textbook for instructions on how to complete this claim form and to view a TRICARE template.

3. A Performance Evaluation Checklist may be reproduced from the "Instruction Guide to the Workbook" chapter if your instructor wishes you to submit it to assist with scoring and comments.

After the instructor has returned your work to you, either make the necessary corrections and place your work in a three-ring notebook for future reference or, if you received a high score, place it in your portfolio for reference when applying for a job.

COLLEGE CLINIC
4567 Broad Avenue, Woodland Hills, XY 12345-0001
(555)-486-9002
Fax: (555) 487-8976
NPI: 3664021CC

PATIENT INFORMATION:		INSURANCE INFORMATION:	
Name:	Rosa Sandoval	Primary:	Tricare Standard
Address:	209 West Maple St		PO Box 1234
	Woodland Hills, XY 12345		West End, YZ 01222
Telephone:	(555) 456-3322	Policy Number:	886-XX-0999
Date of Birth:	11/01/1991	Group Number:	
Social Security:	994-XX-1164	Subscriber:	Herman J. Sandoval
Guarantor:	Herman J. Sandoval (Father)		(DOB 2/10/70)
		Secondary:	none
		Policy Number:	
		Group Number:	
		Subscriber:	

DIAGNOSIS INFORMATION

1. H66.001   Acute suppurative otitis media without spontaneous rupture of ear drum, right ear

2. H66.3x1   Chronic suppurative otitis media, NOS, right ear

3.

4.

PROCEDURE INFORMATION

Description	Date	Code	Charge
1. Initial office visit, new pt	05/01/20XX	99202-25	51.91
2. Myringotomy	05/01/20XX	69420-RT	97.76
3. Post-op visit	05/03/20XX	99024	N/C
4. Post-op visit	05/08/20XX	99024	N/C

NOTES: Referred by: mother
        Treating MD: Pedro Atrics, MD
              NPI: 137640017XX
       Place of service: College Clinic
              4500 Broad Avenue, Woodland Hills, XY 12345
              NPI: X950731067

ASSIGNMENT 14.10 COMPLETE A CLAIM FORM FOR A TRICARE EXTRA CASE

Performance Objective

Task: Complete a CMS-1500 claim form for a TRICARE Extra case.

Conditions: Use Darlene B. Drew's patient record, one health insurance claim form, a pen or pencil.

Standards: Claim Productivity Measurement

Time: _____ minutes

Accuracy: _____

(Note: The time element and accuracy criteria may be given by your instructor.)

Directions:

1. Using NUCC guidelines, complete the CMS-1500 claim form. Refer to Mrs. Darlene B. Drew's patient record for information and post to the financial statement. Date the claim February 3 of the current year. Assume that the No Availability Statement (NAS) has been transmitted electronically so that the physician can treat the patient at College Hospital. Dr. Ulibarri is accepting assignment on this TRICARE Extra case.

2. Refer to Chapter 14 (Fig. 14.8) of the Textbook for instructions on how to complete this claim form and to view a TRICARE template.

3. A Performance Evaluation Checklist may be reproduced from the "Instruction Guide to the Workbook" shown in the section before Chapter 1 if your instructor wishes you to submit it to assist with scoring and comments.

After the instructor has returned your work to you, either make the necessary corrections and place your work in a three-ring notebook for future reference or, if you received a high score, place it in your portfolio for reference when applying for a job.

COLLEGE CLINIC
4567 Broad Avenue, Woodland Hills, XY 12345-0001
(555)-486-9002
Fax: (555) 487-8976
NPI: 3664021CC

PATIENT INFORMATION:		INSURANCE INFORMATION:	
Name:	Darlene Drew	Primary:	Tricare Extra
Address:	720 Ganley Street		PO Box 1234
	Woodland Hills, XY 12345		West End, YZ 01222
Telephone:	(555) 466-1002	Policy Number:	67531
Date of Birth:	12/22/1951	Effective date:	1/1/1980
Social Security:	450-XX-3762	Subscriber:	Harry M. Drew
Occupation:	SEAMSTRESS		Service# 221XX0711
Employer:	J. B. Talon Company		DOB 4/15/1937
	2111 Ventura Blvd.	Secondary:	none
	Merck, XY 12346		
Status:	Married		
Spouse:	Harry M. Drew		

DIAGNOSIS INFORMATION

1. N34.0   Abscess of urethral gland

2. B96.5   Pseudomonas (aeruginosa)

3.

4.

PROCEDURE INFORMATION

Description	Date	Code	Charge
1. Initial office visit, new pt	01/13/20XX	99203-25	70.92
2. Urinalysis	01/13/20XX	81000	8.00
3. Drainage of Skene's gland abscess	01/13/20XX	53060	147.95
4. Handling/transport culture specimen	01/13/20XX	99000	5.00
5. Office visit	01/18/20XX	99212	28.55
6. Excision of Skene's gland	01/24/20XX	53270-58	184.39
7. Post-op visit	01/27/20XX	99024	n/c

NOTES: Referred by: James B. Jeffers, MD, 100 S. Broadway, Woodland Hills, XY 12345
                  NPI: 12345069XX
            Treating MD: Gene Ulibarri, MD
                  NPI: 25678831XX
      Place of service: College Clinic for 1/13–18, 1/27
                  College Hospital for 1/24
                  4500 Broad Avenue, Woodland Hills, XY 12345
                  NPI: X950731067

ASSIGNMENT 14.11 COMPLETE A CLAIM FORM FOR A WORKERS' COMPENSATION CASE

Performance Objectives

Task: Complete a CMS-1500 claim form for a workers' compensation case.

Conditions: Use Glen M. Hiranuma's patient record, a CMS-1500 claim form, a pen or pencil.

Standards: Claim Productivity Measurement

          Time: _____ minutes

          Accuracy: _____

          (Note: The time element and accuracy criteria may be given by your instructor.)

Directions:

1. Using National Uniform Claim Committee (NUCC) guidelines, complete a CMS-1500 claim form and direct it to the proper workers' compensation carrier. Refer to Mr. Glen M. Hiranuma's patient record for information. As a result of this work-related injury, the patient was unable to work on 5/22 through the returning date of 6/5. Date the claim May 24 of the current year.

2. Refer to Chapter 14 (Fig. 14.10) of the Textbook for instructions on how to complete this claim form and to view a workers' compensation template.

3. A Performance Evaluation Checklist may be reproduced from the "Instruction Guide to the Workbook" that appears in the section before Chapter 1 if your instructor wishes you to submit it to assist with scoring and comments.

After the instructor has returned your work to you, either make the necessary corrections and place your work in a three-ring notebook for future reference or, if you received a high score, place it in your portfolio for reference when applying for a job.

COLLEGE CLINIC
4567 Broad Avenue, Woodland Hills, XY 12345-0001
(555)-486-9002
Fax: (555) 487-8976
NPI: 3664021CC

PATIENT INFORMATION:

		INSURANCE INFORMATION:	
Name:	Glen Hiranuma	Primary:	State Insurance Fund
Address:	4372 Hanley Avenue		14156 Magnolia Blvd.
	Woodland Hills, XY 12345		Torres, XY 12349
Telephone:	(555) 467-3383	Policy Number:	016-2432-211
Date of Birth:	12/24/1955	Date of Injury:	05/22/20XX
Social Security:	558-XX-9960	Subscriber:	
Occupation:	HOUSE PAINTER	Secondary:	none
Employer:	Pittsburgh Paint Company	Policy Number:	
	3725 Bonfield Avenue	Group Number:	
	Woodland Hills, XY 12345	Subscriber:	
Status:	Married		
Spouse:	Esme M. Hiranuma		

DIAGNOSIS INFORMATION

1. S06.0x1   Concussion with loss of consciousness of 30 minutes or less

2. S43.92   Unspecified sprain of left shoulder girdle

3. S70.212   Abrasion of left hip

4. S80.812   Abrasion left lower leg

5. W11.xxxA   Fall on and from ladder, initial encounter

PROCEDURE INFORMATION

Description	Date	Code	Charge
1. Hospital admit	05/22/20XX	99222	120.80
2. WC Report	05/22/20XX	99080	50.00
3. Discharge	05/23/20XX	99238	65.26

NOTES: Referred by: Pittsburgh Pain Company
          Treating MD: Gerald Practon, MD
                NPI: 46278897XX
          Place of service: College Hospital
                4500 Broad Avenue, Woodland Hills, XY 12345
                NPI: X950731067
                Patient unable to work from 5/23/20xx to 06/05/20xx

ASSIGNMENT 14.12 COMPLETE A CLAIM FORM FOR A WORKERS' COMPENSATION CASE

Performance Objective

Task: Complete a CMS-1500 claim form for a workers' compensation case.

Conditions: Use Carlos A. Giovanni's patient record, a CMS-1500 claim form, a pen or pencil.

Standards: Claim Productivity Measurement

Time: _____ minutes

Accuracy: _____

(Note: The time element and accuracy criteria may be given by your instructor.)

Directions:

1. Using NUCC guidelines, complete a CMS-1500 claim form for November dates of service and direct it to the correct workers' compensation carrier for this workers' compensation claim. Refer to Mr. Carlos A. Giovanni's patient record for information to record on the claim. Date the claim November 30 of the current year. Note: A progress report is being submitted with this claim; complete a separate CMS-1500 for services for December.

2. Refer to Chapter 14 (Fig. 14.10) of the textbook for instructions on how to complete this claim form and to view a workers' compensation template.

3. A Performance Evaluation Checklist may be reproduced from the "Instruction Guide to the Workbook" that appears in a section before Chapter 1 if your instructor wishes you to submit it to assist with scoring and comments.

After the instructor has returned your work to you, either make the necessary corrections and place your work in a three-ring notebook for future reference or, if you received a high score, place it in your portfolio for reference when applying for a job.

<table>
<tr><td colspan="2" align="center">COLLEGE CLINIC
4567 Broad Avenue, Woodland Hills, XY 12345-0001
(555)-486-9002
Fax: (555) 487-8976
NPI: 3664021CC</td></tr>
</table>

PATIENT INFORMATION:		INSURANCE INFORMATION:	
Name:	Carlos A. Giovanni	Primary:	State Compensation Ins Fund
Address:	89 Beaumont Court		600 S. Lafayette Park Place
	Woodland Hills, XY 12345		Ehrlich, XY 12350
Telephone:	(555) 677-3485		
Date of Birth:	10/24/1955	Policy Number:	57780
Social Security:	556-XX-9699	Date of Injury:	11/11/20XX
Occupation:	TV REPAIRMAN	Subscriber:	
Employer:	Giant Television Company	Secondary:	none
	8764 Ocean Avenue	Policy Number:	
	Woodland Hills, XY 12345	Group Number:	
Status:	Married	Subscriber:	
Spouse:	Maria Giovanni		

DIAGNOSIS INFORMATION

1.	S02.91xA	Fracture of skull and facial bones, initial encounter for closed fracture
2.	S06.0x1	Concussion with loss of consciousness of 30 minutes or less
3.	W13.xxxA	Fall from, out of or through building or structure

PROCEDURE INFORMATION

Description	Date	Code	Charge
1. Hospital admit	11/11/20XX	99223-57	152.98
2. WC Report	11/11/20XX	99080	50.00
3. Craniotomy	11/12/20XX	61314	2548.09
4. Hospital visits	11/13-29/20XX	99024	N/C
5. Discharge	11/30/20XX	99024	N/C
6. Office visit	12/07/20XX	99024	N/C
7. Office visit	12/21/20XX	99024	N/C
8. Office visit	12/29/20XX	99024	N/C
9. Medical report	12/29/20XX	99080	50.00

NOTES: Referred by: Giant Television Company
Treating MD: Astro Parkinson, MD
NPI: 46789377XX
Place of service: College Clinic for 12/7–12/29
College Hospital for 11/11–11/30
4500 Broad Avenue, Woodland Hills, XY 12345
NPI: X950731067
Patient unable to work from 11/12/20xx–01/14/20xx

15 The Electronic Claim

Cheryl Fassett

KEY TERMS

Your instructor may wish to select some words pertinent to this chapter for a test. For definitions of the terms, further study, and/or reference, the words, phrases, and abbreviations may be found in the glossary at the end of the Textbook. *Key terms for this chapter follow.*

Accredited Standards Committee X12
Accredited Standards Committee X12 Version 5010
Administrative Simplification Enforcement Tool
American National Standards Institute
application service provider
audit trail
batch
business associate agreement
cable modem
claim attachments
clearinghouse
code sets
covered entity
data elements
digital subscriber line

direct data entry
electronic data interchange
electronic funds transfer
electronic remittance advice
encoder
encryption
HIPAA Transaction and Code Set Rule
National Standard Format
real time
standard transactions
T-1
taxonomy codes
trading partner
trading partner agreement

KEY ABBREVIATIONS

See how many abbreviations and acronyms you can translate, and then use this as a handy reference list. Definitions for the key abbreviations are located near the back of the Textbook *in the glossary.*

ANSI _____

ASC X12 _____

ASET _____

ASP _____

ATM _____

DDE _____

DHHS _____

DSL _____

EDI _____

EFT _____

EHR _____

EMC _____

EOMB _____

ERA _____

HPID _____

IRS _____

MAC _____

NDC _____

NSF _____

PMS _____

TCS rule _____

PERFORMANCE OBJECTIVES

The student will be able to:

- Define and spell the key terms and key abbreviations for this chapter, given the information from the textbook glossary, within a reasonable time period and with enough accuracy to obtain a satisfactory evaluation.
- After reading the chapter, answer the fill-in-the-blank, multiple choice, and true/false review questions with enough accuracy to obtain a satisfactory evaluation.
- Decide whether keyed medical and nonmedical data elements are required, situational, or not used when electronically submitting the 837P health care claim.
- State which medical and nonmedical code sets for 837P electronic claims are required, situational, or not used.

- Input data into the element for place of service codes for 837P electronic claims submission.
- Indicate the patient's relationship to the insured by using the individual relationship code numbers for 837P electronic claims submission.
- Select the correct taxonomy codes for the specialists for submission of 837P electronic claims submission.
- Locate errors, given computer-generated insurance forms, within a reasonable time period and with enough accuracy to obtain a satisfactory evaluation.
- Fill in the correct meaning of each abbreviation, given a list of common medical abbreviations and symbols that appear in chart notes, with enough accuracy to obtain a satisfactory evaluation.

STUDY OUTLINE

Electronic Data Interchange
Electronic Claims
Advantages of Electronic Claim Submission
Clearinghouses
Transaction and Code Set Regulations: Streamlining Electronic Data Interchange
  Transaction and Code Set Standards
Electronic Standard HIPAA 837P
  Levels of Information for 837P Standard Transaction Format
  Accredited Standards Committee X12 Version 5010
Claims Attachments Standards
Standard Unique Identifiers
  Standard Unique Employer Identifier
  Standard Unique Health Care Provider Identifier
  Standard Unique Health Plan Identifier
  Standard Unique Patient Identifier
Practice Management System

Building the Claim
  Encounter or Multipurpose Billing Forms
  Keying Insurance Data for Claim Transmission
  Encoder
  Clean Electronic Claims Submission
Putting HIPAA Standard Transactions to Work
  Interactive Transactions
  Electronic Funds Transfer
  Electronic Remittance Advice
Methods for Sending Claims
Computer Claims Systems
  Carrier-Direct
  Clearinghouses
Transmission Reports
  Electronic Processing Problems
  Solutions to Electronic Processing Problems
  Billing and Account Management Schedule
  Administrative Simplification Enforcement Tool

Part I Fill in the Blank

Review the objectives, key terms, glossary definitions of key terms, chapter information, and figures before completing the following review questions.

1. Exchange of data in a standardized format through computer systems is a technology

   known as _____.

2. The act of converting computerized data into a code so that unauthorized users are

   unable to read it is a security system known as _____.

3. Payment to the provider of service of an electronically submitted insurance claim may

   be received in approximately _____.

4. Medical practices that do not use the services of clearinghouses submit claims through

   a _____ to the insurance company.

5. Refer to Table 15.1 in the *textbook* to list benefits of using Health Insurance Portability and Accountability Act (HIPAA) standard transactions and code sets.

   a. _____

   b. _____

   c. _____

   d. _____

   e. _____

   f. _____

6. Dr. Morgan has 10 or more full-time employees and submits insurance claims for his Medicare patients. Is his medical practice subject to the HIPAA transaction rules?

   _____

7. Dr. Maria Montez does not submit insurance claims electronically and has five full-time employees. Is she required to abide by HIPAA transaction rules?

   _____

8. Refer to Table 15.2 in the *textbook* to name the standard code sets used for the following:

   a. Physician services _____

   b. Diseases and injuries _____

   c. Pharmaceuticals and biologics _____

9. Refer to Table 15.3 in the *textbook* to complete these statements.

   a. The staff at College Clinic submit professional health care claims for each of their providers and must use the industry

      standard electronic format called _____ to transmit them electronically.

   b. The billing department at College Hospital must use the industry standard electronic format called

      _____ to transmit health care claims electronically.

215

c. The Medicare fiscal intermediary (insurance carrier) uses the industry standard electronic format called _____ to transmit payment information to the College Clinic and College Hospital.

d. It has been three weeks since Gordon Marshall's health care claim was transmitted to the XYZ insurance company, and you wish to inquire about the status of the claim. The industry standard electronic format that must be used to transmit this inquiry is called _____.

e. Dr. Practon's insurance billing specialist must use the industry standard electronic format called _____ to obtain information about Beatrice Garcia's health policy benefits and coverage from the insurance plan.

10. The family practice taxonomy code is _____.

11. The American National Standards Institute formed the _____, which developed the electronic data exchange standards.

12. Refer to Table 15.4 in the textbook to name the levels for data collected to construct and submit an electronic claim.

    a. _____

    b. _____

    c. _____

    d. _____

    e. _____

    f. _____

13. HIPAA electronic standards for claim submission were upgraded to Version _____, and all providers, payers, and clearinghouses were required to use it effective January 1, 2012.

14. The Claims Attachments Standards have not yet been adopted; however, it was mandated for compliance as of _____, as required under the Affordable Care Act.

15. The _____ is an all numeric 10-character number assigned to each provider and required for all transactions with health plans effective May 23, 2007.

16. The most important function of a practice management system is _____.

17. To look for and correct all errors before the health claim is transmitted to the insurance carrier, you _____ or _____.

18. Much of the patient and insurance information required to complete the CMS-1500 form can be found on the _____ that is used to post charges.

19. Add-on software to a practice management system that can reduce the time it takes to build or review a claim before batching is known as a/an _____.

20. Many insurance companies, such as Medicare, provide instant access to information about pending claims through online _____.

21. An electronic funds transfer (EFT) agreement may allow for health plans to _____ overpayments from a provider's bank account.

22. The Medicare electronic remittance advice was previously referred to as a/an

_____.

23. On completion of a signed agreement and approval of enrollment with a third-party payer for electronic claims submission, the provider will be assigned a/an _____ number.

24. When computer software is upgraded, the health care organization must submit a batch of _____ to the insurance carrier to determine whether claims can be transmitted successfully.

25. Under HIPAA transaction standard Accredited Standards Committee (ASC) X12 Version 5010, a _____ digit ZIP code is required to report service facility locations.

26. The _____ is an electronic tool that enables organizations to file a complaint against a noncompliant covered entity that is negatively affecting the efficient processing of claims.

Part II Multiple Choice
Choose the best answer.

27. Electronic claims are submitted by means of:
    a. the US Postal Service.
    b. fax transmission.
    c. phone transmission.
    d. electronic data interchange (EDI).

28. Today, most claims are submitted by means of:
    a. the US Postal Service.
    b. fax transmission.
    c. phone transmission.
    d. EDI.

29. The online error-edit process allows providers to:
    a. correct claim errors before transmission of the claim.
    b. decrease labor costs by freeing staff to do other duties.
    c. reduce postage fees and trips to the post office.
    d. reduce storage of claims.

30. Under HIPAA, data elements that are used uniformly to document why patients are seen (diagnosis) and what is done to them during their encounter (procedure) are known as:
    a. medical code sets.
    b. information elements.
    c. transaction and code set (TCS) standards.
    d. National Standard Format (NSF).

31. The standard transaction that replaces the paper CMS-1500 claim form and more than 400 versions of the electronic NSF is called the:
    a. 270.
    b. 837I.
    c. 837P.
    d. 837D.

32. The next version of the electronic claims submission that will be proposed for consideration once lessons are learned from implementation of Version 5010 will be:
   a. Version 5011.
   b. Version 5012.
   c. Version 6001.
   d. Version 7030.

33. A standard unique number that will be assigned to identify individual health plans under the Affordable Care Act is referred to as a/an:
   a. employer identification number (EIN).
   b. electronic remittance advice (ERA).
   c. health plan identifier (HPID).
   d. National Provider Identifier (NPI).

34. Uniform patient identifiers:
   a. were required on all claims effective May 23, 2007.
   b. were required on all claims effective October 1, 2012.
   c. were required on all claims effective October 1, 2014.
   d. are not yet required, and the proposal is on hold for implementation of the standard.

35. An authorization and assignment of benefits signature for a patient who was treated in the hospital but has never been to the provider's office:
   a. should be obtained by the provider when he or she sees the patient in the hospital.
   b. must be mailed to the patient for signature before submission of a claim.
   c. can be obtained from the patient at his or her first office visit.
   d. is not required; the authorization obtained by the hospital applies to that provider's claim filing.

36. A paperless computerized system that enables payments to be transferred automatically to a physician's bank account by a third-party payer may be done via:
   a. electronic savings account.
   b. ERA.
   c. EFT.
   d. EDI.

37. An electronic Medicare remittance advice that takes the place of a paper Medicare explanation of benefits (EOB) is referred to as:
   a. American National Standards Institute (ANSI) 277.
   b. ANSI 820.
   c. ANSI 830.
   d. ANSI 835.

38. A method for submitting claims electronically by keying information into the payer system for processing is accomplished through use of:
   a. a clearinghouse.
   b. carrier direct entry.
   c. an application service provider.
   d. digital subscriber line (DSL).

39. A report that is generated by a payer and sent to the provider to show how many claims were received as electronic claims and how many of the claims were automatically rejected and will not be processed is called a:
   a. send-and-receive file report.
   b. scrubber report.
   c. transaction transmission summary.
   d. rejection analysis report.

40. The HIPAA transaction standard ASC X12 Version 5010 requires that anesthesia services be reported:
   a. per day.
   b. per unit.
   c. per second.
   d. per minute.

Part III True/False

Write "T" or "F" in the blank to indicate whether you think the statement is true or false.

_____ 41. Like paper claims, electronic claims require the performing physician's signature.

_____ 42. Claims can be submitted to various insurance payers in a single-batch electronic transmission.

_____ 43. Under HIPAA, insurance payers can require health care providers to use the payer's own version of local code sets.

_____ 44. As *International Classification of Diseases* (ICD) and *Current Procedural Terminology* (CPT) codes are deleted and become obsolete, they should immediately be removed from the practice's computer system.

_____ 45. HIPAA has brought forth electronic formats for determination of eligibility for a health insurance plan.

_____ 46. HIPAA's electronic standard transactions are identified by a four-digit number that precedes "ASC X12N."

_____ 47. Implementation of ICD-10 resulted in the upgrade to HIPAA transaction standard ASC X12 Version 6020.

_____ 48. HIPAA requires that the NPI number be used to identify employers rather than inputting the actual name of the company when submitting claims.

_____ 49. HIPAA limits how computer systems may transmit data and formats for storage of data.

_____ 50. A paper remittance advice is generated by Medicare when using ANSI 835 Version 5010.

_____ 51. HIPAA transaction standard ASC X12 Version 5010 allows employer identification numbers to be used to report as a primary identifier.

_____ 52. When transmitting electronic claims, inaccuracies that violate the HIPAA standard transaction format are known as *syntax errors*.

_____ 53. An organization may file a complaint online against someone whose actions affect the ability of a transaction to be accepted or efficiently processed by using the Administration Simplification Enforcement Tool (ASET).

ASSIGNMENT 15.2 CRITICAL THINKING FOR MEDICAL AND NONMEDICAL CODE SETS FOR 837P ELECTRONIC CLAIMS SUBMISSION

Performance Objective

Task: Decide whether keyed medical and nonmedical data elements are required, situational, or not used when electronically submitting the 837P health care claim.

Conditions: List of keyed data elements (Table 15.5 in Textbook) and pen or pencil.

Standards: Time: _____ minutes

            Accuracy: _____

            (Note: The time element and accuracy criteria may be given by your instructor.)

Directions: When submitting the 837P health care claim, supporting code sets of medical and nonmedical data are composed of "Required" and "Situational" data elements. Read each keyed data element and answer whether you think it is **R** for required, **S** for situational, or **N** for not used.

a. Patient's type of insurance _____

b. Patient's ZIP code _____

c. Insured's name _____

d. Principal diagnosis code _____

e. Referring provider's NPI _____

f. Procedure code _____

g. Provider's signature _____

h. Date of service _____

i. Place of service _____

j. Procedure modifier _____

ASSIGNMENT 15.3 INPUT DATA INTO ELEMENT FOR PLACE OF SERVICE CODES FOR 837P ELECTRONIC CLAIMS SUBMISSIONS

Performance Objective

Task: Insert the correct place of service code for each location description where the medical professional service was rendered.

Conditions: Place of service codes reference (Fig. 15.1), list of places where medical care was rendered, and pen or pencil.

Standards: Time: _____ minutes

                Accuracy: _____

                (Note: The time element and accuracy criteria may be given by your instructor.)

Directions: When submitting the 837P electronic claim, place of service codes must be entered in data element 1331. Refer to the place of service codes reference list and insert the correct code for each place of service for the following locations.

    a. Inpatient psychiatric facility   _____

    b. Physician's office   _____

    c. Outpatient hospital   _____

    d. Intermediate nursing facility   _____

    e. Independent clinic   _____

    f. Independent laboratory   _____

    g. Birthing center   _____

    h. End-stage renal disease treatment facility   _____

    i. Inpatient hospital   _____

    j. Hospice   _____

PLACE OF SERVICE CODES	
Codes	**Place of Service**
01	Pharmacy
00-02	Unassigned
03	School
04	Homeless shelter
05	Indian health service free-standing facility
06	Indian health service provider-based facility
07	Tribal 638 free-standing facility
08	Tribal 638 provider-based facility
09	Prison/correctional facility
10	Unassigned
11	Doctor's office
12	Patient's home
13	Assisted living facility
14	Group home
15	Mobile unit
16	Temporary lodging
17-19	Unassigned
20	Urgent care facility
21	Inpatient hospital
22	Outpatient hospital or urgent care center
23	Emergency department—hospital
24	Ambulatory surgical center
25	Birthing center
26	Military treatment facility/uniformed service treatment facility
27-30	Unassigned
31	Skilled nursing facility (swing bed visits)
32	Nursing facility (intermediate/long-term care facilities)
33	Custodial care facility (domiciliary or rest home services)
34	Hospice (domiciliary or rest home services)
35-40	Unassigned
41	Ambulance—land
42	Ambulance—air or water
43-48	Unassigned
49	Independent clinic
50	Federally qualified health center
51	Inpatient psychiatric facility
52	Psychiatric facility—partial hospitalization
53	Community mental health care (outpatient, twenty-four-hours-a-day services, admission screening, consultation, and educational services)
54	Intermediate care facility/mentally retarded
55	Residential substance abuse treatment facility
56	Psychiatric residential treatment center
57	Nonresidential substance abuse treatment facility
58-59	Unassigned
60	Mass immunization center
61	Comprehensive inpatient rehabilitation facility
62	Comprehensive outpatient rehabilitation facility
63-64	Unassigned
65	End-stage renal disease treatment facility
66-70	Unassigned
71	State or local public health clinic
72	Rural health clinic
73-80	Unassigned
81	Independent laboratory
82-98	Unassigned
99	Other unlisted facility

Fig. 15.1

ASSIGNMENT 15.4 SELECT THE CORRECT INDIVIDUAL RELATIONSHIP CODE NUMBER FOR 837P ELECTRONIC CLAIMS SUBMISSION

Performance Objective

Task: Insert the correct individual relationship code for the patient's relationship to the insured.

Conditions: Individual relationship code number reference (Fig. 15.2), list of individuals or entities, and pen or pencil.

Standards: Time: _____ minutes

              Accuracy: _____

              (Note: The time element and accuracy criteria may be given by your instructor.)

Directions: Refer to the individual relationship code number list, choose the correct code for the patient's relationship to the insured for the following persons, and insert it on the lines.

a. Mother   _____

b. Spouse   _____

c. Child   _____

d. Father   _____

e. Stepdaughter   _____

f. Emancipated minor   _____

g. Adopted child   _____

h. Handicapped dependent _____

i. Stepson   _____

j. Sponsored dependent _____

Individual Relationship Code	
Code	**Relationship**
01	Spouse
04	Grandfather or grandmother
05	Grandson or granddaughter
07	Nephew or niece
09	Adopted child
10	Foster child
15	Ward
17	Stepson or stepdaughter
19	Child
20	Employee
21	Unknown
22	Handicapped dependent
23	Sponsored dependent
24	Dependent of a minor dependent
29	Significant other
32	Mother
33	Father
34	Other adult
36	Emancipated minor
39	Organ donor
40	Cadaver donor
41	Injured plaintiff
43	Child where insured has no financial responsibility
53	Life partner
G8	Other relationship

Fig. 15.2

ASSIGNMENT 15.5 SELECT THE CORRECT TAXONOMY CODES FOR MEDICAL SPECIALISTS FOR 837P ELECTRONIC CLAIMS SUBMISSION

Performance Objective

Task: Choose the correct taxonomy code for each specialist for submission of 837P electronic claims by referring to the Health Care Provider Taxonomy code list.

Conditions: Health Care Provider Taxonomy code list (Fig. 15.3), list of providers of service, and pen or pencil.

Standards: Time: _____ minutes

             Accuracy: _____

             (Note: The time element and accuracy criteria may be given by your instructor.)

Directions: Refer to the Health Care Provider Taxonomy code list, choose the correct code for each of the following specialists, and insert the code numbers on the lines.

a. Raymond Skeleton, MD, orthopedist   _____

b. Gaston Input, MD, gastroenterologist   _____

c. Vera Cutis, MD, dermatologist   _____

d. Gene Ulibarri, MD, urologist   _____

e. Bertha Caesar, MD, obstetrician/gynecologist   _____

f. Gerald Practon, MD, general practitioner   _____

g. Pedro Atrics, MD, pediatrician   _____

h. Astro Parkinson, MD, neurosurgeon   _____

i. Brady Coccidioides, MD, pulmonary disease   _____

j. Max Gluteus, RPT, physical therapist   _____

College Clinic Staff		
Health Care Provider Taxonomy Codes		
Name	**Specialty**	**Taxonomy Code**
Concha Antrum, MD	Otolaryngologist	207Y00000X
Pedro Atrics, MD	Pediatrician	208000000X
Bertha Caesar, MD	Obstetrician/Gynecologist	207V00000X
Perry Cardi, MD	Cardiologist	207RC0000X
Brady Coccidioides, MD	Pulmonary disease	207RP1001X
Vera Cutis, MD	Dermatologist	207N00000X
Clarence Cutler, MD	General surgeon	208600000X
Dennis Drill, DDS	Dentist	122300000X
Max Gluteus, RPT	Physical therapist	208100000X
Cosmo Graff, MD	Plastic surgeon	208200000X
Malvern Grumose, MD	Pathologist	207ZP0105X
Gaston Input, MD	Gastroenterologist	207RG0100X
Adam Langerhans, MD	Endocrinologist	207RE0101X
Cornell Lenser, MD	Ophthalmologist	207W00000X
Michael Menter, MD	Psychiatrist	2084P0800X
Arthur O. Dont, DDS	Orthodontist	1223X0400X
Astro Parkinson, MD	Neurosurgeon	207T00000X
Nick Pedro, MD	Podiatrist	213E00000X
Gerald Practon, MD	General practitioner	208D00000X
Walter Radon, MD	Radiologist	2085R0202X
Rex Rumsey, MD	Proctologist	208C00000X
Sensitive E. Scott, MD	Anesthesiologist	207L00000X
Raymond Skeleton, MD	Orthopedist	207X00000X
Gene Ulibarri, MD	Urologist	208800000X

Fig. 15.3

ASSIGNMENT 15.6 PROOFREAD A COMPUTER-GENERATED HEALTH INSURANCE CLAIM FORM AND LOCATE INCORRECT AND MISSING DATA

Performance Objective

Task: Locate and designate blocks on the computer-generated insurance claim form that have incorrect or missing information; correct or add data before submission to the insurance company.

Conditions: Use Brad E. Diehl's patient record (Fig. 15.4), completed insurance claim (Fig. 15.5), a highlighter, and a red-ink pen.

Standards: Time: _____ minutes

Accuracy: _____

(Note: The time element and accuracy criteria may be given by your instructor.)

Directions: Proofread the insurance claim form (see Fig. 15.5) and locate blocks that need correction or completion before submission to the insurance company. Highlight all errors you discover. Refer to the patient's record (see Fig. 15.4) to verify pertinent demographic and insurance information. Refer to the progress notes to verify procedures and determine diagnoses. Verify all entries on the claim form, including dates, codes, rounded-out fees, and physician identification numbers. Insert all corrections and missing information in red. If you cannot locate the necessary information but know it is mandatory, write "NEED" in the corresponding block.

Optional: Retype a blank CMS-1500 claim form with all corrections and changes.

Additional Coding

1. Assume that Mr. Diehl followed Dr. Input's treatment plan. Refer to his record, abstract information, and locate procedure codes that would be billed by providers outside of the office.

Site	Description of Service	Code
a. ABC Radiology	_____	_____
b. College Hospital	_____	_____
c. Surgeon	_____	_____

2. Code the symptoms Mr. Diehl was complaining about when he presented for the January 6, 20xx, office visit.

Symptom	ICD-10-CM Code
a. _____	_____
b. _____	_____
c. _____	_____
d. _____	_____
e. _____	_____

PATIENT RECORD NO. 8-6

Diehl	Brad	E.	09-21-46	M	555-222-0123
LAST NAME	FIRST NAME	MIDDLE NAME	BIRTH DATE	SEX	HOME PHONE

3975 Hills Road	Woodland Hills	XY	12345	
ADDRESS	CITY	STATE	ZIP CODE	

555-703-6600	555-321-0988	555-222-0123	Diehl@WB.net
CELL PHONE	PAGER NO.	FAX NO.	E-MAIL ADDRESS

561-XX-1501	M0983457
PATIENT'S SOC. SEC. NO.	DRIVER'S LICENSE

radio advertising salesman	KACY Radio
PATIENT'S OCCUPATION	NAME OF COMPANY

4071 Mills Road, Woodland Hills, XY 12335	555-201-6666
ADDRESS OF EMPLOYER	PHONE

Tak E. Diehl (birthdate 4-7-45)	legal secretary
SPOUSE OR PARENT	OCCUPATION

Attys. Dilman, Forewise & Gilson,	12 West Dix Street, Woodland Hills, XY 12345	555-222-6432
EMPLOYER	ADDRESS	PHONE

Aetna Insurance Co., 2412 Main Street, Woodland Hills, XY 12345	Brad E. Diehl
NAME OF INSURANCE	INSURED OR SUBSCRIBER

403119	
POLICY/CERTIFICATE NO.	GROUP NO.

REFERRED BY: Raymond Skeleton, MD

DATE	PROGRESS NOTES No. 8-7
1-6-20xx	NP pt comes in complaining of coughing and sneezing; some difficulty breathing.
	Occasional dizziness and epigastric abdominal pain with cramping. Symptoms started in
	July of last year. Performed a detailed history and physical examination with low
	complexity medical decision making. AP & lat chest x-rays taken; neg findings. BP 178/98.
	Pt to have cholecystography with oral contrast at ABC Radiology. Diagnostic colonoscopy
	(flexible) to be scheduled at College Hospital. Dx: hypertension and respiratory distress;
	R/O irritable colon. No disability at this time.
	GI/llf *Gaston Input, MD*
1-20-xx	Pt retns for a EPF hx/exam LC MDM. Oral cholecystography reveals a single 1.5 cm
	radiolucent calculus within the cholecyst. Colonoscopy confirmed irritable bowel
	syndrome. Blood drawn and CBC (auto with diff) performed in office indicates
	WBC 10,000. DX: cholecystitis with cholelithiasis. Adv. cholecystectomy
	(abdominal approach) as soon as possible; to be scheduled at College Hospital.
	GI/llf *Gaston Input, MD*

Fig. 15.4

HEALTH INSURANCE CLAIM FORM

APPROVED BY NATIONAL UNIFOR MCLAIM COMMITTEE (NUCC) 02/12

☐☐ PICA   PICA ☐☐

1. MEDICARE (Medicare#)	MEDICAID (Medicaid#)	TRICARE (ID#DoD#)	CHAMPVA (Member ID#)	GROUP HEALTH PLAN ☒ (ID#)	FECA BLK LUNG (ID#)	OTHER (ID#)	1a. INSURED'S I.D. NUMBER (For Program in Item 1) 403119

2. PATIENT'S NAME (Last Name, First Name, Middle Initial)	3. PATIENT'S BIRTH DATE / SEX	4. INSURED'S NAME (Last Name, First Name, Middle Initial)
Diehl, Brad, E	09 21 1946 M☐ F☐	Same

5. PATIENT'S ADDRESS (No., Street) — 3975 Hills Road

6. PATIENT RELATIONSHIP TO INSURED — Self ☒ Spouse ☐ Child ☐ Other ☐

7. INSURED'S ADDRESS (No., Street)

CITY — Woodland Hills   STATE XY

8. RESERVED FOR NUCC USE

CITY   STATE

ZIP CODE 12345-0000   TELEPHONE (Include Area Code) (555) 2220123

ZIP CODE   TELEPHONE (Include Area Code) ( )

9. OTHER INSURED'S NAME (Last Name, First Name, Middle Initial)

10. IS PATIENT'S CONDITION RELATED TO:

11. INSURED'S POLICY GROUP OR FECA NUMBER

a. OTHER INSURED'S POLICY OR GROUP NUMBER

a. EMPLOYMENT? (Current or Previous) ☐ YES ☒ NO

a. INSURED'S DATE OF BIRTH MM DD YY / SEX M☐ F☐

b. RESERVED FOR NUCC USE

b. AUTO ACCIDENT? ☐ YES ☒ NO   PLACE (State)

b. OTHER CLAIM ID (Designated by NUCC)

c. RESERVED FOR NUCC USE

c. OTHER ACCIDENT? ☐ YES ☒ NO

c. INSURANCE PLAN NAME OR PROGRAM NAME

d. INSURANCE PLAN NAME OR PROGRAM NAME

10d. CLAIM CODES (Designated by NUCC)

d. IS THERE ANOTHER HEALTH BENEFIT PLAN? ☐ YES ☒ NO — If yes, complete items 9, 9a, and 9d.

READ BACK OF FORM BEFORE COMPLETING & SIGNING THIS FORM.

12. PATIENT'S OR AUTHORIZED PERSON'S SIGNATURE I authorize the release of any medical or other information necessary to process this claim. I also request payment of government benefits either to myself or to the party who accepts assignment below.

SIGNED _Signature on file_   DATE _____

13. INSURED'S OR AUTHORIZED PERSON'S SIGNATURE I authorize payment of medical benefits to the undersigned physician or supplier for services described below.

SIGNED _Signature on file_

14. DATE OF CURRENT: ILLNESS, INJURY, or PREGNANCY(LMP) MM DD YY QUAL.	15. OTHER DATE QUAL. MM DD YY	16. DATES PATIENT UNABLE TO WORK IN CURRENT OCCUPATION FROM MM DD YY TO MM DD YY

17. NAME OF REFERRING PROVIDER OR OTHER SOURCE — DN Raymond Skeleton MD

17a.

17b. NPI 12678547XX

18. HOSPITALIZATION DATES RELATED TO CURRENT SERVICES FROM MM DD YY TO MM DD YY

19. ADDITIONAL CLAIM INFORMATION (Designated by NUCC)

20. OUTSIDE LAB? ☐ YES ☐ NO $ CHARGES

21. DIAGNOSIS OR NATURE OF ILLNESS OR INJURY Relate A-L to service line below (24E)   ICD Ind. 0

A. R06.00   B. I10   C. K80.60   D.
E.   F.   G.   H.
I.   J.   K.   L.

22. RESUBMISSION CODE   ORIGINAL REF. NO.

23. PRIOR AUTHORIZATION NUMBER

24. A. DATE(S) OF SERVICE From MM DD YY	To MM DD YY	B. PLACE OF SERVICE	C. EMG	D. PROCEDURES, SERVICES, OR SUPPLIES (Explain Unusual Circumstances) CPT/HCPCS	MODIFIER	E. DIAGNOSIS POINTER	F. $ CHARGES	G. DAYS OR UNITS	H. EPSDT Family Plan	I. ID. QUAL.	J. RENDERING PROVIDER ID. #
1	01 06 20XX		11		99203		A,B	70 92	1		NPI	32783127XX
2	01 06 20XX		11		71020		A	40 97	1		NPI	32783127XX
3	01 20 20XX		11		99213		C	40 20	1		NPI	32783127XX
4	01 20 20XX		11		85025		C	25 00	1		NPI	32783127XX
5	01 20 20XX		11				C		1		NPI	32783127XX
6											NPI	

25. FEDERAL TAX I.D. NUMBER   SSN ☐ EIN ☐

26. PATIENT'S ACCOUNT NO. — 8

27. ACCEPT ASSIGNMENT? (For govt. claims, see back) ☒ YES ☐ NO

28. TOTAL CHARGE $

29. AMOUNT PAID $

30. Rsvd for NUCC Use

31. SIGNATURE OF PHYSICIAN OR SUPPLIER INCLUDING DEGREES OR CREDENTIALS (I certify that the statements on the reverse apply to this bill and are made a part thereof.) — 012520XX

SIGNED   DATE

32. SERVICE FACILITY LOCATION INFORMATION — Same

a. NPI   b.

33. BILLING PROVIDER INFO & PH # (555) 4869002
College Clinic
4567 Broad Avenue
Woodland Hills XY 12345-0001

a. 3664021CC   b.

NUCC Instruction Manual available at: www.nucc.org   PLEASE PRINT OR TYPE   OMB APPROVAL PENDING

Fig. 15.5

229

  Chapter **15**   The Electronic Claim

ASSIGNMENT 15.7 PROOFREAD A COMPUTER-GENERATED HEALTH INSURANCE CLAIM FORM AND LOCATE INCORRECT AND MISSING DATA

Performance Objective

Task: Locate and designate blocks on the computer-generated insurance claim form that have incorrect information or need completion; correct or add data before submission to the insurance company.

Conditions: Use Evert I. Strain's patient record (Fig. 15.6), completed insurance claim (Fig. 15.7), a highlighter, and a red-ink pen.

Standards: Time: _____ minutes

             Accuracy: _____

             (Note: The time element and accuracy criteria may be given by your instructor.)

Directions: Proofread the insurance claim form (see Fig. 15.7) and locate blocks that need correction or completion before submission to the insurance company. Highlight all errors you discover. Refer to the patient's record (see Fig. 15.6) to verify pertinent demographic and insurance information. Refer to the progress notes to verify procedures and determine diagnoses. Verify all entries on the claim form, including dates, codes, rounded-out fees, and physician identification numbers. Insert all corrections and missing information in red. If you cannot locate the necessary information but know it is mandatory, write "NEED" in the corresponding block.

Optional: Retype a blank CMS-1500 claim form with all corrections and changes.

Additional Coding

1. Refer to Mr. Strain's medical record, abstract information, and code procedures that would be billed by outside providers.

Site	Description of Service	Code
a. ABC Laboratory	_____	_____
b. ABC Radiology	_____	_____

PATIENT RECORD NO. 8-7

Strain	Evert	I	09-11-46	M	555-678-0211
LAST NAME	FIRST NAME	MIDDLE NAME	BIRTH DATE	SEX	HOME PHONE

7650 None Such Road	Woodland Hills	XY	12345
ADDRESS	CITY	STATE	ZIP CODE

555-430-2101	555-320-9980	555-678-0211	Strain@WB.net
CELL PHONE	PAGER NO.	FAX NO.	E-MAIL ADDRESS

453-XX-4739	Y0923658
PATIENT'S SOC. SEC. NO.	DRIVER'S LICENSE

mechanical engineer	R & R Company
PATIENT'S OCCUPATION	NAME OF COMPANY

2400 Davon Road, Woodland Hills, XY 12345	555-520-8977
ADDRESS OF EMPLOYER	PHONE

Ester I. Strain (wife)	administrative assistant
SPOUSE OR PARENT	OCCUPATION

University College, 4021 Book Road, Woodland Hills, XY 12345	555-450-9908
EMPLOYER ADDRESS	PHONE

ABC Insurance Co., P.O. Box 130, Woodland Hills, XY 12345	Evert I. Strain
NAME OF INSURANCE	INSURED OR SUBSCRIBER

453-XX-4739	96476A
POLICY/CERTIFICATE NO.	GROUP NO.

REFERRED BY: Gerald C. Jones, MD, 1403 Haven Street, Woodland Hills, XY 12345   NPI # 54754966XX

DATE	PROGRESS NOTES	No. 8-8
1-8-20xx	Est pt comes in complaining of frequent urination, headaches, polyphagia; unable to	
	remember current events. These problems have been present for almost a year.	
	A comprehensive history is taken and compared to his last H & P 2 years ago.	
	A com PX is performed. BP 160/110; pt was prescribed antihypertensive medication but	
	discontinued it when the prescription ran out. Lab report, hand carried by pt from an	
	urgent care center, indicates SGOT in normal range and cholesterol elevated. Fasting blood	
	sugar extremely high. Dx: diabetes mellitus, malignant hypertensive, and ASCVD.	
	Pt to have 3 hour GTT tomorrow a.m. at ABC laboratory. STAT CT scan of head s̄ contrast	
	ordered at ABC radiology to follow lab work. Arrangement will be made for pt to be	
	admitted to College Hospital. Disability 1/9 through 1/31.	
	GI/llf *Gerald Practon, MD*	
1-9-xx	Admit to College Hospital (C hx/exam MC MDM).	
	GI/llf *Gerald Practon, MD*	
1-10-xx	Hosp visit (PF hx/exam SF MDM). CT scan of head reviewed, neg. findings. Pt alert and	
	comfortable. If blood sugar and BP remain stable, discharge planned for tomorrow.	
	BP 130/85.	
	GI/llf *Gerald Practon, MD*	
1-11-xx	DC from hosp. Pt to be seen in one week in ofc.	
	GI/llf *Gerald Practon, MD*	

Fig. 15.6

HEALTH INSURANCE CLAIM FORM

APPROVED BY NATIONAL UNIFOR MCLAIM COMMITTEE (NUCC) 02/12

| | PICA | | | | | | | | PICA | |

1. MEDICARE	MEDICAID	TRICARE	CHAMPVA	GROUP HEALTH PLAN	FECA BLK LUNG	OTHER	1a. INSURED'S I.D. NUMBER	(For Program in Item 1)
☐ (Medicare#)	☐ (Medicaid#)	☐ (ID#DoD#)	☐ (Member ID#)	☒ (ID#)	☐ (ID#)	☐ (ID#)	453 XX 4739	96476A

2. PATIENT'S NAME (Last Name, First Name, Middle Initial)
Strain, Evert, I

3. PATIENT'S BIRTH DATE MM 09 DD 21 YY 1946 **SEX** M ☒ F ☐

4. INSURED'S NAME (Last Name, First Name, Middle Initial)
Same

5. PATIENT'S ADDRESS (No., Street)
7650 None Such Road

6. PATIENT RELATIONSHIP TO INSURED
Self ☒ Spouse ☐ Child ☐ Other ☐

7. INSURED'S ADDRESS (No., Street)

CITY Woodland Hills **STATE** XY

8. RESERVED FOR NUCC USE

CITY **STATE**

ZIP CODE **TELEPHONE (Include Area Code)** ( )

ZIP CODE **TELEPHONE (Include Area Code)** ( )

9. OTHER INSURED'S NAME (Last Name, First Name, Middle Initial)

10. IS PATIENT'S CONDITION RELATED TO:

11. INSURED'S POLICY GROUP OR FECA NUMBER

a. OTHER INSURED'S POLICY OR GROUP NUMBER

a. EMPLOYMENT? (Current or Previous) ☐ YES ☒ NO

a. INSURED'S DATE OF BIRTH MM DD YY **SEX** M ☐ F ☐

b. RESERVED FOR NUCC USE

b. AUTO ACCIDENT? ☐ YES ☒ NO **PLACE (State)**

b. OTHER CLAIM ID (Designated by NUCC)

c. RESERVED FOR NUCC USE

c. OTHER ACCIDENT? ☐ YES ☒ NO

c. INSURANCE PLAN NAME OR PROGRAM NAME

d. INSURANCE PLAN NAME OR PROGRAM NAME

10d. CLAIM CODES (Designated by NUCC)

d. IS THERE ANOTHER HEALTH BENEFIT PLAN? ☐ YES ☐ NO **If yes**, complete items 9, 9a, and 9d.

READ BACK OF FORM BEFORE COMPLETING & SIGNING THIS FORM.

12. PATIENT'S OR AUTHORIZED PERSON'S SIGNATURE I authorize the release of any medical or other information necessary to process this claim. I also request payment of government benefits either to myself or to the party who accepts assignment below.

SIGNED _Signature on file_ DATE _____

13. INSURED'S OR AUTHORIZED PERSON'S SIGNATURE I authorize payment of medical benefits to the undersigned physician or supplier for services described below.

SIGNED _Signature on file_

14. DATE OF CURRENT: ILLNESS, INJURY, or PREGNANCY(LMP) MM DD YY QUAL.

15. OTHER DATE QUAL. MM DD YY

16. DATES PATIENT UNABLE TO WORK IN CURRENT OCCUPATION FROM MM DD YY TO MM DD YY

17. NAME OF REFERRING PROVIDER OR OTHER SOURCE DN Gerald C Jones
17a.
17b. NPI 54754966XX

18. HOSPITALIZATION DATES RELATED TO CURRENT SERVICES FROM 01 09 20XX TO 01 11 20XX

19. ADDITIONAL CLAIM INFORMATION (Designated by NUCC)

20. OUTSIDE LAB? ☐ YES ☒ NO **$ CHARGES**

21. DIAGNOSIS OR NATURE OF ILLNESS OR INJURY Relate A-L to service line below (24E) **ICD Ind.** 0

A. E11.9   B. I10   C. I25.10   D.
E.   F.   G.   H.
I.   J.   K.   L.

22. RESUBMISSION CODE ORIGINAL REF. NO.

23. PRIOR AUTHORIZATION NUMBER

24. A. DATE(S) OF SERVICE From MM DD YY	To MM DD YY	B. PLACE OF SERVICE	C. EMG	D. PROCEDURES, SERVICES, OR SUPPLIES (Explain Unusual Circumstances) CPT/HCPCS | MODIFIER	E. DIAGNOSIS POINTER	F. $ CHARGES	G. DAYS OR UNITS	H. EPSDT Family Plan	I. ID. QUAL.	J. RENDERING PROVIDER ID. #
1	01 08 20XX		11		99215		96 97	1		NPI	46278897XX
2	01 09 20XX		21		99222		120 80	1		NPI	46278897XX
3	1 10 20XX		21		99231		37 74	1		NPI	46278897XX
4	01 11 20XX		21		99231		65 26	1		NPI	46278897XX
5										NPI	
6										NPI	

25. FEDERAL TAX I.D. NUMBER 7034597 SSN ☐ EIN ☒

26. PATIENT'S ACCOUNT NO. 8-7

27. ACCEPT ASSIGNMENT? (For govt. claims, see back) ☒ YES ☐ NO

28. TOTAL CHARGE $ 320 77

29. AMOUNT PAID $

30. Rsvd for NUCC Use $

31. SIGNATURE OF PHYSICIAN OR SUPPLIER INCLUDING DEGREES OR CREDENTIALS (I certify that the statements on the reverse apply to this bill and are made a part thereof.)
Gerald Practon MD 012520XX
SIGNED _Gerald Practon MD_ DATE

32. SERVICE FACILITY LOCATION INFORMATION
Same
a. NPI b.

33. BILLING PROVIDER INFO & PH # (555) 4869002
College Clinic
4567 Broad Avenue
Woodland Hills XY 12345-0001
a. 3664021CC b.

NUCC Instruction Manual available at: www.nucc.org   *PLEASE PRINT OR TYPE*   OMB APPROVAL PENDING

Fig. 15.7

ASSIGNMENT 15.8 DEFINE PATIENT RECORD ABBREVIATIONS

Performance Objective

Task: Insert definitions of abbreviations.

Conditions: Use pencil or pen.

Standards: Time: _____ minutes

              Accuracy: _____

              (Note: The time element and accuracy criteria may be given by your instructor.)

Directions: After completing the assignments in this chapter, you will be able to define the abbreviations shown here.

Abbreviations pertinent to the record of Brad E. Diehl:

NP _____   R/O _____

LC _____   auto _____

pt _____   retn _____

MDM _____   diff _____

AP _____   EPF _____

cm _____   WBC _____

lat _____   hx _____

neg _____   DX _____

BP _____   exam _____

CBC _____   adv _____

Abbreviations pertinent to the record of Evert I. Strain:

est _____   lab _____

CT _____   hosp _____

pt _____   SGOT _____

C _____   PF _____

H & P _____   Dx _____

hx _____   SF _____

comp _____   ASCVD _____

exam _____   neg _____

PX _____   GTT _____

MC _____   DC _____

BP _____   STAT _____

MDM _____   ofc _____

16 Receiving Payments and Insurance Problem Solving

Linda M. Smith

KEY TERMS

Your instructor may wish to select some words pertinent to this chapter for a test. For definitions of the terms, further study, and/or reference, the words, phrases, and abbreviations may be found in the glossary at the end of the textbook. *Key terms for this chapter follow.*

Administrative Law Judge hearing	overpayment
aging report	peer review
appeal	Qualified Independent Contractor
claim denial management	rebill (resubmit)
delinquent claim	rejected claim
denied claim	reimbursement
explanation of benefits	remittance advice
inquiry	revenue cycle management
insurance payment poster	review
insurance payment posting	suspended claim
lost claim	suspense
medical necessity	tracer

KEY ABBREVIATIONS

See how many abbreviations and acronyms you can translate, and then use this as a handy reference list. Definitions for the key abbreviations are located near the back of the textbook *in the glossary.*

ALJ _____

CMS _____

DAB _____

EOB _____

HIPAA _____

NPI _____

QIC _____

RA _____

RCM _____

PERFORMANCE OBJECTIVES

The student will be able to:

- Define and spell the key terms and key abbreviations for this chapter, given the information from the *textbook* glossary, within a reasonable time period and with enough accuracy to obtain a satisfactory evaluation.

- After reading the chapter, answer the fill-in-the-blank, multiple choice, and true/false review questions with enough accuracy to obtain a satisfactory evaluation.

- Review an aging report to determine the method of follow-up needed to zero out all patient accounts.
- Locate the errors on each claim, given three returned insurance claims, within a reasonable time period and with enough accuracy to obtain a satisfactory evaluation.

- Complete form CMS-1965, Request for Medicare Hearing by an Administrative Law Judge, Part B, Medicare Claim, within a reasonable time period and with enough accuracy to obtain a satisfactory evaluation.
- File an appeal by composing and printing a letter with envelope, within a reasonable time period and with enough accuracy to obtain a satisfactory evaluation.

STUDY OUTLINE

Part I Fill in the Blank

Review the objectives, key terms, and chapter information before completing the following review questions.

1. The process in the health care organization uses to track services provided from registration and appointment scheduling to the final payment for services is referred to as

   _____.

2. Once a claim has been successfully submitted to the insurance carrier, the next step in

   the revenue cycle is for the insurance billing specialist to _____ the claim until a response is received from the responsible party and the service has been paid in full.

3. Who dictates the guidelines for claims submission, such as which services are covered, the reimbursement rates, and time limits for claim submission and payment?

   _____

4. Time limits for filing claims promptly can be found in the _____ or

   the _____.

5. What is the purpose of prompt payment laws?

   _____

6. After an insurance claim is processed by the insurance carrier (paid, suspended, rejected, or denied), a document known as a/an _____ is sent to the patient and to the provider of professional medical services.

7. A claim that is processed by a third-party payer but is held in an indeterminate state

   is referred to as a _____ claim.

8. Claims paid with no errors are designated as _____.

9. Claims that are not paid within 30 to 45 days of the service date are referred to as

   _____ claims.

10. A _____ claim is a submitted claim that does not follow specific third-party payer instructions or contains technical errors.

11. A service is considered _____ if it is provided in accordance with the generally accepted standards of medical practice and is clinically appropriate.

12. State the solution if a claim for routine foot care has been denied as a noncovered service.

    _____

    _____

    _____

13. State the solution if a claim has been denied because the professional service rendered was for an injury that is being considered as compensable under workers' compensation.

_____

_____

_____

14. When an insurance carrier changes the code submitted to one of lesser value and it reduces the reimbursement amount, it is referred to as _____.

15. When an insurance carrier reimburses a service at an amount over and above the amount due, it is referred to as an _____.

16. Patient accounts with a balance should be billed on a _____ basis.

17. A/an _____ is a request for a review and reconsideration of a claim that has been underpaid, incorrectly paid, or denied by an insurance company.

18. A/an _____ is an evaluation of a denied claim performed by a group of unbiased practicing physicians or other health care professionals to judge the effectiveness and efficiency of professional care rendered and to determine if payment can be made.

19. Name the five levels for appealing a Medicare claim.

    a. _____

    b. _____

    c. _____

    d. _____

    e. _____

20. A/an _____ is an independent contractor who conducts reconsiderations for Medicare claims going through the appeals process.

21. To pursue judicial review of a Medicare claim in federal district court, the amount of the case must meet the minimum dollar amount of _____ in 2018.

22. A TRICARE expedited appeal must be filed within _____ of the receipt of the initial denial.

23. A TRICARE nonexpedited appeal must be filed within _____ of the receipt of the initial denial.

24. _____ are public officials who regulate the Insurance Industry in their state.

25. Effective claim denial management starts with _____ the reason for denials.

Part II Multiple Choice

Choose the best answer.

26. A written request made to an insurance company to locate the status of an insurance claim is often referred to as:
    a. an inquiry.
    b. a follow-up.
    c. a tracer.
    d. all of the above.

27. When an electronic claim is transmitted for several services and one service is rejected for incomplete information, the solution is to:
    a. resubmit a paper claim with the needed data for the rejected services only.
    b. add the required information in field 19 that it is a retransmission
    c. add the required information and retransmit the rejected claim.
    d. not transmit a rejected claim.

28. A request for payment to a third-party payer asking for a review of an insurance claim that has been denied is referred to as a/an:
    a. review.
    b. appeal.
    c. request.
    d. demand.

29. When overpayments are identified, the Office of Inspector General (OIG) strongly advises that:
    a. service providers hold it for 30 days to make sure it was not due them.
    b. service providers place in a hold account until the insurance carrier requests it.
    c. service providers return the overpayment within 180 days of receipt of payment.
    d. service providers return the overpayment promptly when the insurance poster identifies it.

30. The steps in claim denial management are:
    a. Identify, Appeal, Categorize, Measure, Strategize.
    b. Appeal, Identify, Categorize, Strategize, Measure.
    c. Strategize, Categorize, Measure, Identify, Appeal.
    d. Identify, Measure, Categorize, Appeal, Strategize.

Part III True/False

Write "T" or "F" in the blank to indicate whether you think the statement is true or false.

_____ 31. An insurance billing specialist's primary goal is to assist in management of the revenue cycle.

_____ 32. A patient's insurance card specifies the detailed benefits and coverages.

_____ 33. All health insurance companies are obligated to reimburse health care organizations promptly for services rendered.

_____ 34. The elements within a remittance advice (RA) document and an explanation of benefits (EOB) document are different.

_____ 35. There is a standard format for EOB forms that all carriers are expected to follow.

_____ 36. Due to issues concerning timely filing, it is wise to be aggressive on claims that are outstanding for more than 30 to 45 days.

_____ 37. Information collected at the front desk does not impact denials.

_____ 38. Services are considered medically necessary if they are in accordance with the generally accepted standards of medical practice.

_____ 39. If any insurance carrier has downcoded a claim, thereby reducing reimbursement, there is no other recourse than to write off the balance.

_____ 40. If a claim has not been paid within a reasonable amount of time, the most effective follow-up method is to simply rebill the claim.

Performance Objective

Task: Use the aging report in Fig. 16.1 to complete follow-up.

Conditions: Refer to the aging report (see Fig. 16.1) and use a pen or computer.

Standards: Time: _____ minutes

Accuracy: _____

(Note: The time element and accuracy criteria may be given by your instructor.)

Directions: Review the aging report in Fig. 16.1 and consider the following scenario:

The Happy Day Primary Care Office is reviewing their aging report to follow up on outstanding payments. The office charges Aetna $260 for initial office visits and $145 for established patient office visits. Electronic claims that are filed to Aetna are reimbursed within to the office within 30 days of initial electronic claim submission. Answer the following questions.

1. Who were the three patients who were most recently billed?

_____

_____

_____

2. Do phone calls to Aetna need to be made for patients that are in the 0 to 30 days categories? Why or why not?

_____

_____

3. Which two patients have balances that are different from typical office visit charges submitted to Aetna?

_____

_____

4. What would account for the difference in the balance from the original total charges submitted to Aetna?

_____

_____

5. Would it be appropriate to send the patients in categories beyond 60 days to a collection agency? Why or why not?

_____

_____

AETNA

Patient Name	Acct #	Primary Insurance	Secondary Insurance	0–30 days	31–60 days	61–90 days	91–120 days	Over 120 days	Total Balance
Bassett, Eleanor	75846	AETNA		$145.00	$0.00	$0.00	$0.00	$0.00	$145.00
Herron, John	83029	AETNA		$0.00	$42.41	$0.00	$0.00	$0.00	$42.41
Holt, Maxine	64739	AETNA	BLUE SHIELD	$145.00	$0.00	$0.00	$0.00	$0.00	$145.00
Kellog, Keenan	24537	AETNA		$0.00	$0.00	$145.00	$0.00	$0.00	$145.00
Lincoln, Frank	85940	AETNA		$0.00	$15.00	$0.00	$0.00	$0.00	$15.00
Markham, Melanie	14263	AETNA	MEDICARE	$0.00	$0.00	$0.00	$260.00	$0.00	$260.00
McDonald, Lydia	56374	AETNA		$260.00	$0.00	$0.00	$0.00	$0.00	$260.00
McLean, Mary	24395	AETNA		$0.00	$0.00	$0.00	$0.00	$260.00	$260.00
				$550.00	$57.41	$145.00	$260.00	$260.00	$1,272.41

Fig. 16.1

Chapter **16** **Receiving Payments and Insurance Problem Solving**

ASSIGNMENT 16.3 POST TO A FINANCIAL ACCOUNTING RECORD (LEDGER) FROM AN EXPLANATION OF BENEFITS (EOB) DOCUMENT

Performance Objective

Task: Post data from an EOB document to a patient's financial accounting record (ledger).

Conditions: Use a blank financial accounting record (ledger) (Fig. 16.2), an EOB document (Fig. 16.3), and a pen or computer.

Standards: Time: _____ minutes

             Accuracy: _____

             (Note: The time element and accuracy criteria may be given by your instructor.)

Background: Most payments in the medical office are posted in the same practice management billing software that the electronic claims are submitted from. However, to develop the skills and understanding for payment posting, a paper financial accounting ledger has been provided.

Directions: Post in ink the payment received and preferred provider organization (PPO) adjustment to a patient's financial accounting record (ledger) (see Fig. 16.2) by referring to an EOB document (see Fig. 16.3). An EOB document is defined in Fig. 16.2 in the textbook.

After the instructor has returned your work to you, either make the necessary corrections and place your work in a three-ring notebook for future reference or, if you received a high score, place it in your portfolio for reference when applying for a job.

1. Locate patient's financial accounting record (ledger) and EOB.

2. Ledger lines 6 and 7: Insert date of service (DOS), reference (CPT code number, check number, or dates of service for posting adjustments or when insurance was billed), description of the transaction, charge amounts, payments, adjustments, and running current balance. The posting date is the actual date the transaction is recorded. If the DOS differs from the posting date, list the DOS in the reference or description column.

STATEMENT
Financial Account
COLLEGE CLINIC
4567 Broad Avenue
Woodland Hills, XY 12345-0001
Tel. 555-486-9002
Fax No. 555-487-8976

Mr. Jabe Bortolussi
989 Moorpark Road
Woodland Hills, XY 12345

Phone No. (H) __(555) 230-8870__   (W) __(555) 349-6689__   Birth date __04-07-71__

Primary Insurance Co. _____ABC Insurance Company_____   Policy/Group No. __4206/010__

DATE	REFERENCE	DESCRIPTION	CHARGES		CREDITS PYMNTS.	ADJ.	BALANCE	
			BALANCE FORWARD ⟶					
6-3-xx	99204	E/M NP Level 4	250	00			250	00
6-3-xx	94375	Respiratory flow vol loop	40	00			290	00
6-3-xx	94060	Spirometry	75	00			365	00
6-3-xx	94664	Aerosol inhalation	50	00			415	00
6-3-xx	94760	Pulse oximetry	50	00			465	00

PLEASE PAY LAST AMOUNT IN BALANCE COLUMN ⬆

THIS IS A COPY OF YOUR FINANCIAL ACCOUNT AS IT APPEARS ON OUR RECORDS

Fig. 16.2

ABC Insurance Company
P.O. Box 4300
Woodland Hills, XY 12345-0001

Claim No.:	1-00-16987087-00-zmm
Group Name:	COLLEGE CLINIC
Group No.:	010
Employee:	JABE V. BORTOLUSSI
Patient:	JABE V. BORTOLUSSI
SSN:	554-XX-8876
Plan No.:	4206
Prepared by:	M. SMITH
Prepared on:	07/04/20XX

GERALD PRACTON MD
4567 BROAD AVENUE
WOODLAND HILLS XY 12345

Patient Responsibility

Amount not covered:	00
Co-pay amount:	00
Deductible:	00
Co-insurance:	64.61
Patient's total responsibility:	64.61
Other insurance payment:	00

EXPLANATION OF BENEFITS

Treatment Dates	Service Code	CPT Code	Charge Amount	Not Covered	Reason Code	PPO Discount	Covered Amount	Deductible Amount	Co-pay Amount	Paid At	Payment Amount
06/03/xx	200	99204	250.00	00	48	136.00	114.00	00	00	80%	91.20
06/03/xx	540	94375	40.00	00	48	00	40.00	00	00	80%	32.00
06/03/xx	540	94060	75.00	00	48	00	75.00	00	00	80%	60.00
06/03/xx	200	94664	50.00	00	48	1.55	48.45	00	00	80%	38.76
06/03/xx	540	94760	50.00	00	48	4.40	45.60	00	00	80%	36.48
		TOTAL	465.00	00		141.95	323.05	00	00		258.44

Other Insurance Credits or Adjustments   00

CPT Code
99204 OFFICE/OUTPT VISIT E&M NEW MOD-HI SEVERIT
94375 RESPIRATORY FLOW VOLUM LOOP
94060 BRONCHOSPSM EVAL SPIROM PRE & POST BRON
94664 AEROSOL/VAPOR INHALA; INIT DEMO & EVAL
94760 NONINVASIVE EAR/PULSE OXIMETRY-02 SAT

Total Payment Amount   258.44

Reason Code
48 CON DISCOUNT/PT NOT RESPONSIBLE

Participant	Date	
GERALD PRACTON MD	07-04-xx	
Patient	ID Number	
JABE V. BORTOLUSSI	554-XX-8876	
Plan Number	Patient Number	Office No.
4206		010

GC 1234567890

258.44

PAY
TO THE
ORDER
OF

COLLEGE CLINIC
4567 BROAD AVENUE
WOODLAND HILLS XY 12345

J M Smith
_____
ABC Insurance Company

Fig. 16.3

ASSIGNMENT 16.4 LOCATE ERRORS ON A RETURNED INSURANCE CLAIM

Performance Objective

Task: Highlight the blocks on the insurance claim form where errors are discovered.

Conditions: Use an insurance claim form (Fig. 16.4) and a highlighter or red pen.

Standards: Time: _____ minutes

               Accuracy: _____

               (Note: The time element and accuracy criteria may be given by your instructor.)

Directions: An insurance claim (see Fig. 16.4) was returned by the Prudential Insurance Company. Highlight or circle in red all blocks on the claim form where errors are discovered.

Option 1: Retype the claim and either insert the correction, if data are available to fix the error, or insert the word "NEED" in the block of the claim form.

Option 2: On a separate sheet of paper, list the blocks from 1 to 33 and state where errors occur. A Performance Evaluation Checklist may be reproduced from the "Instruction Guide to the Workbook" chapter if your instructor wishes you to submit it to assist with scoring and comments.

After the instructor has returned your work to you, either make the necessary corrections and place your work in a three-ring notebook for future reference or, if you received a high score, place it in your portfolio for reference when applying for a job.

HEALTH INSURANCE CLAIM FORM

APPROVED BY NATIONAL UNIFOR MCLAIM COMMITTEE (NUCC) 02/12

Prudential Insurance Company
500 South Bend Street
Woodland Hills XY 12345-0001

CARRIER →

| | | PICA | | | | | | | | PICA | | |

1. MEDICARE	MEDICAID	TRICARE	CHAMPVA	GROUP HEALTH PLAN	FECA BLK LUNG	OTHER	1a. INSURED'S I.D. NUMBER	(For Program in Item 1)
☐ (Medicare#)	☐ (Medicaid#)	☐ (ID#DoD#)	☐ (Member ID#)	☐ (ID#)	☐ (ID#)	☒ (ID#)		

2. PATIENT'S NAME (Last Name, First Name, Middle Initial)	3. PATIENT'S BIRTH DATE / SEX	4. INSURED'S NAME (Last Name, First Name, Middle Initial)
Johnson, Emily B.	MM 02 DD 12 YY 1963 M ☐ F ☐	Johnson, Erron T.

5. PATIENT'S ADDRESS (No., Street)
4391 Everett Street

6. PATIENT RELATIONSHIP TO INSURED
Self ☐ Spouse ☒ Child ☐ Other ☐

7. INSURED'S ADDRESS (No., Street)
Same

CITY: Woodland Hills STATE: XY

8. RESERVED FOR NUCC USE

CITY STATE

ZIP CODE: 12345-0001 TELEPHONE (Include Area Code) (   )

ZIP CODE TELEPHONE (Include Area Code) (   )

9. OTHER INSURED'S NAME (Last Name, First Name, Middle Initial)

10. IS PATIENT'S CONDITION RELATED TO:

11. INSURED'S POLICY GROUP OR FECA NUMBER

a. OTHER INSURED'S POLICY OR GROUP NUMBER

a. EMPLOYMENT? (Current or Previous) ☐ YES ☐ NO

a. INSURED'S DATE OF BIRTH MM DD YY SEX M ☐ F ☐

b. RESERVED FOR NUCC USE

b. AUTO ACCIDENT? ☐ YES ☐ NO PLACE (State)

b. OTHER CLAIM ID (Designated by NUCC)

c. RESERVED FOR NUCC USE

c. OTHER ACCIDENT? ☐ YES ☐ NO

c. INSURANCE PLAN NAME OR PROGRAM NAME

d. INSURANCE PLAN NAME OR PROGRAM NAME

10d. CLAIM CODES (Designated by NUCC)

d. IS THERE ANOTHER HEALTH BENEFIT PLAN?
☐ YES ☒ NO *If yes,* complete items 9, 9a, and 9d.

READ BACK OF FORM BEFORE COMPLETING & SIGNING THIS FORM.
12. PATIENT'S OR AUTHORIZED PERSON'S SIGNATUREI authorize the release of any medical or other information necessary to process this claim. I also request payment of government benefits either to myself or to the party who accepts assignment below.

SIGNED *Emily B. Johnson* DATE 1/4/2020

13. INSURED'S OR AUTHORIZED PERSON'S SIGNATURE I authorize payment of medical benefits to the undersigned physician or supplier for services described below.

SIGNED *Emily B. Johnson*

14. DATE OF CURRENT: ILLNESS, INJURY, or PREGNANCY(LMP) MM DD YY QUAL.

15. OTHER DATE QUAL. MM DD YY

16. DATES PATIENT UNABLE TO WORK IN CURRENT OCCUPATION FROM MM DD YY TO MM DD YY

17. NAME OF REFERRING PROVIDER OR OTHER SOURCE

17a.
17b. NPI 67805027XX

18. HOSPITALIZATION DATES RELATED TO CURRENT SERVICES FROM MM DD YY TO MM DD YY

19. ADDITIONAL CLAIM INFORMATION (Designated by NUCC)

20. OUTSIDE LAB? ☐ YES ☒ NO $ CHARGES

21. DIAGNOSIS OR NATURE OF ILLNESS OR INJURY Relate A-L to service line below (24E) ICD Ind. 0

A. ___ B. ___ C. ___ D. ___
E. ___ F. ___ G. ___ H. ___
I. ___ J. ___ K. ___ L. ___

22. RESUBMISSION CODE ORIGINAL REF. NO.

23. PRIOR AUTHORIZATION NUMBER

24. A. DATE(S) OF SERVICE From MM DD YY To MM DD YY	B. PLACE OF SERVICE	C. EMG	D. PROCEDURES, SERVICES, OR SUPPLIES (Explain Unusual Circumstances) CPT/HCPCS MODIFIER	E. DIAGNOSIS POINTER	F. $ CHARGES	G. DAYS OR UNITS	H. EPSDT Family Plan	I. ID. QUAL.	J. RENDERING PROVIDER ID. #
1 01 04 20XX	11		99213	A	125 00	1		NPI	705687717XX
2 01 04 20XX	11		99213	A	125 00			NPI	
3								NPI	
4								NPI	
5								NPI	
6								NPI	

25. FEDERAL TAX I.D. NUMBER SSN EIN
7180561XX ☐ ☐

26. PATIENT'S ACCOUNT NO.
237819

27. ACCEPT ASSIGNMENT? (For govt. claims, see back)
☒ YES ☐ NO

28. TOTAL CHARGE $ 250 00

29. AMOUNT PAID $ 0 00

30. Rsvd for NUCC Use $

31. SIGNATURE OF PHYSICIAN OR SUPPLIER INCLUDING DEGREES OR CREDENTIALS (I certify that the statements on the reverse apply to this bill and are made a part thereof.)

SIGNED *Vera Cutis, MD* DATE 01/06/20XX

32. SERVICE FACILITY LOCATION INFORMATION

a. NPI b.

33. BILLING PROVIDER INFO & PH # (555) 4869002
College Clinic
4567 Broad Avenue
Woodland Hills XY 12345-0001

a. 3664021CC b.

NUCC Instruction Manual available at: www.nucc.org

PLEASE PRINT OR TYPE

OMB APPROVAL PENDING

Fig. 16.4

250

Performance Objective

Task: Highlight the blocks on the insurance claim form where errors are discovered.

Conditions: Use an insurance claim form (Fig. 16.5) and a highlighter or red pen.

Standards: Time: _____ minutes

               Accuracy: _____

               (Note: The time element and accuracy criteria may be given by your instructor.)

Directions: An insurance claim was returned by the Healthtech Insurance Company. Highlight or circle in red all blocks on the claim form where errors are discovered.

   Option 1: Retype the claim and either insert the correction if data are available to fix the error or insert the word "NEED" in the block of the claim form.

   Option 2: On a separate sheet of paper, list the blocks from 1 to 33 and state where errors occur. A Performance Evaluation Checklist may be reproduced from the "Instruction Guide to the Workbook" that appears in the section before Chapter 1 if your instructor wishes you to submit it to assist with scoring and comments.

   After the instructor has returned your work to you, either make the necessary corrections and place your work in a three-ring notebook for future reference or, if you received a high score, place it in your portfolio for reference when applying for a job.

HEALTH INSURANCE CLAIM FORM

APPROVED BY NATIONAL UNIFOR MCLAIM COMMITTEE (NUCC) 02/12

DRAFT - NOT FOR OFFICIAL USE

Healthtech Insurance Company
4821 West Lake Avenue
Woodland Hills XY 12345-0001

| | PICA | | | | | | | | PICA | | |

| 1. MEDICARE (Medicare#) | MEDICAID [X] (Medicaid#) | TRICARE [X] (ID#DoD#) | CHAMPVA (Member ID#) | GROUP HEALTH PLAN (ID#) | FECA BLK LUNG (ID#) | OTHER [X] (ID#) | 1a. INSURED'S I.D. NUMBER (For Program in Item 1) 433129870ANC |

2. PATIENT'S NAME (Last Name, First Name, Middle Initial)
Dugan, Charles C

3. PATIENT'S BIRTH DATE
MM 12 DD 24 YY 1968 SEX M [X] F [ ]

4. INSURED'S NAME (Last Name, First Name, Middle Initial)
Same

5. PATIENT'S ADDRESS (No., Street)
5900 Elm Street

6. PATIENT RELATIONSHIP TO INSURED
Self [X] Spouse [ ] Child [ ] Other [ ]

7. INSURED'S ADDRESS (No., Street)
Same

CITY Woodland Hills   STATE XY

8. RESERVED FOR NUCC USE

CITY   STATE

ZIP CODE 12345-0001
TELEPHONE (Include Area Code) (555) 5593300

ZIP CODE
TELEPHONE (Include Area Code) ( )

9. OTHER INSURED'S NAME (Last Name, First Name, Middle Initial)

10. IS PATIENT'S CONDITION RELATED TO:

11. INSURED'S POLICY GROUP OR FECA NUMBER

a. OTHER INSURED'S POLICY OR GROUP NUMBER

a. EMPLOYMENT? (Current or Previous) YES [ ] NO [X]

a. INSURED'S DATE OF BIRTH MM DD YY SEX M [ ] F [ ]

b. RESERVED FOR NUCC USE

b. AUTO ACCIDENT? YES [ ] NO [X] PLACE (State)

b. OTHER CLAIM ID (Designated by NUCC)

c. RESERVED FOR NUCC USE

c. OTHER ACCIDENT? YES [ ] NO [X]

c. INSURANCE PLAN NAME OR PROGRAM NAME

d. INSURANCE PLAN NAME OR PROGRAM NAME

10d. CLAIM CODES (Designated by NUCC)

d. IS THERE ANOTHER HEALTH BENEFIT PLAN? YES [ ] NO [ ] If yes, complete items 9, 9a, and 9d.

READ BACK OF FORM BEFORE COMPLETING & SIGNING THIS FORM.
12. PATIENT'S OR AUTHORIZED PERSON'S SIGNATURE I authorize the release of any medical or other information necessary to process this claim. I also request payment of government benefits either to myself or to the party who accepts assignment below.

SIGNED _____ DATE _____

13. INSURED'S OR AUTHORIZED PERSON'S SIGNATURE I authorize payment of medical benefits to the undersigned physician or supplier for services described below.

SIGNED _____

14. DATE OF CURRENT: ILLNESS, INJURY, or PREGNANCY(LMP) MM DD YY QUAL.

15. OTHER DATE QUAL. MM DD YY

16. DATES PATIENT UNABLE TO WORK IN CURRENT OCCUPATION FROM MM DD YY TO MM DD YY

17. NAME OF REFERRING PROVIDER OR OTHER SOURCE
17a.
17b. NPI 67805027XX

18. HOSPITALIZATION DATES RELATED TO CURRENT SERVICES FROM MM DD YY TO MM DD YY

19. ADDITIONAL CLAIM INFORMATION (Designated by NUCC)

20. OUTSIDE LAB? YES [ ] NO [X] $ CHARGES

21. DIAGNOSIS OR NATURE OF ILLNESS OR INJURY Relate A-L to service line below (24E)   ICD Ind. 0

A. S51.801   B. ____   C. ____   D. ____
E. ____   F. ____   G. ____   H. ____
I. ____   J. ____   K. ____   L. ____

22. RESUBMISSION CODE   ORIGINAL REF. NO.

23. PRIOR AUTHORIZATION NUMBER

24. A. DATE(S) OF SERVICE From MM DD YY	To MM DD YY	B. PLACE OF SERVICE	C. EMG	D. PROCEDURES, SERVICES, OR SUPPLIES (Explain Unusual Circumstances) CPT/HCPCS MODIFIER	E. DIAGNOSIS POINTER	F. $ CHARGES	G. DAYS OR UNITS	H. EPSDT Family Plan	I. ID. QUAL.	J. RENDERING PROVIDER ID. #
1	09 55 20XX		11		99203	A	70 92	1		NPI	46278897XX
2	09 55 20XX		11		12001	A				NPI	46278897XX
3										NPI	
4										NPI	
5										NPI	
6										NPI	

25. FEDERAL TAX I.D. NUMBER 7034597XX SSN [ ] EIN [X]

26. PATIENT'S ACCOUNT NO. 238293

27. ACCEPT ASSIGNMENT? (For govt. claims, see back) YES [X] NO [ ]

28. TOTAL CHARGE $

29. AMOUNT PAID $

30. Rsvd for NUCC Use $

31. SIGNATURE OF PHYSICIAN OR SUPPLIER INCLUDING DEGREES OR CREDENTIALS (I certify that the statements on the reverse apply to this bill and are made a part thereof.)
SIGNED Gerald Practon, MD DATE 09/30/20XX

32. SERVICE FACILITY LOCATION INFORMATION
College Hospital
4500 Broad Avenue
Woodland Hills XY 12345-0001
a. 937310XX b.

33. BILLING PROVIDER INFO & PH # (555) 4869002
College Clinic
4567 Broad Avenue
Woodland Hills XY 12345-0001
a. 3664021CC b.

NUCC Instruction Manual available at: www.nucc.org   *PLEASE PRINT OR TYPE*   OMB APPROVAL PENDING

Fig. 16.5

ASSIGNMENT 16.6 LOCATE ERRORS ON A RETURNED INSURANCE CLAIM

Performance Objective

Task: Highlight the blocks on the insurance claim form where errors are discovered.

Conditions: Use an insurance claim form (Fig. 16.6) and a highlighter or red pen.

Standards: Time: _____ minutes

              Accuracy: _____

              (Note: The time element and accuracy criteria may be given by your instructor.)

Directions: An insurance claim (see Fig. 16.6) was returned by an insurance plan. Highlight or circle in red all blocks on the claim form where errors are discovered.

    Option 1: Retype the claim and either insert the correction if data are available to fix the error or insert the word "NEED" in the block of the claim form.

    Option 2: On a separate sheet of paper, list the blocks from 1 to 33 and state where errors occur. A Performance Evaluation Checklist may be reproduced from the "Instruction Guide to the Workbook" that appears in the section before Chapter 1 if your instructor wishes you to submit it to assist with scoring and comments.

    After the instructor has returned your work to you, either make the necessary corrections and place your work in a three-ring notebook for future reference or, if you received a high score, place it in your portfolio for reference when applying for a job.

HEALTH INSURANCE CLAIM FORM

APPROVED BY NATIONAL UNIFOR MCLAIM COMMITTEE (NUCC) 02/12

American Insurance Company
509 Main Street
Woodland Hills XY 12345-0001

CARRIER →

| | | PICA | | | | | | | | | PICA | | |

1. MEDICARE	MEDICAID	TRICARE	CHAMPVA	GROUP HEALTH PLAN	FECA BLK LUNG	OTHER	1a. INSURED'S I.D. NUMBER	(For Program in Item 1)
☐ (Medicare#)	☐ (Medicaid#)	☐ (ID#DoD#)	☐ (Member ID#)	☐ (ID#)	☐ (ID#)	☒ (ID#)		

2. PATIENT'S NAME (Last Name, First Name, Middle Initial)	3. PATIENT'S BIRTH DATE	SEX	4. INSURED'S NAME (Last Name, First Name, Middle Initial)
Mary T Avery	MM 05 DD 07 YY 1980	M ☐ F ☐	Same

5. PATIENT'S ADDRESS (No., Street)	6. PATIENT RELATIONSHIP TO INSURED	7. INSURED'S ADDRESS (No., Street)
4309 Main Street	Self ☒ Spouse ☐ Child ☐ Other ☐	

CITY	STATE	8. RESERVED FOR NUCC USE	CITY	STATE
Woodland Hills	XY			

ZIP CODE	TELEPHONE (Include Area Code)	ZIP CODE	TELEPHONE (Include Area Code)
12345-0001	(555) 4509899		( )

9. OTHER INSURED'S NAME (Last Name, First Name, Middle Initial)	10. IS PATIENT'S CONDITION RELATED TO:	11. INSURED'S POLICY GROUP OR FECA NUMBER
a. OTHER INSURED'S POLICY OR GROUP NUMBER	a. EMPLOYMENT? (Current or Previous) ☐ YES ☒ NO	a. INSURED'S DATE OF BIRTH MM DD YY SEX M ☐ F ☐
b. RESERVED FOR NUCC USE	b. AUTO ACCIDENT? ☐ YES ☒ NO PLACE (State)	b. OTHER CLAIM ID (Designated by NUCC)
c. RESERVED FOR NUCC USE	c. OTHER ACCIDENT? ☐ YES ☒ NO	c. INSURANCE PLAN NAME OR PROGRAM NAME
d. INSURANCE PLAN NAME OR PROGRAM NAME	10d. CLAIM CODES (Designated by NUCC)	d. IS THERE ANOTHER HEALTH BENEFIT PLAN? ☐ YES ☐ NO If yes, complete items 9, 9a, and 9d.

READ BACK OF FORM BEFORE COMPLETING & SIGNING THIS FORM.

12. PATIENT'S OR AUTHORIZED PERSON'S SIGNATURE I authorize the release of any medical or other information necessary to process this claim. I also request payment of government benefits either to myself or to the party who accepts assignment below.

SIGNED *Mary T. Avery*   DATE 11/20/2007

13. INSURED'S OR AUTHORIZED PERSON'S SIGNATURE I authorize payment of medical benefits to the undersigned physician or supplier for services described below.

SIGNED *Mary T. Avery*

PATIENT AND INSURED INFORMATION →

14. DATE OF CURRENT: ILLNESS, INJURY, or PREGNANCY(LMP) MM DD YY QUAL.	15. OTHER DATE QUAL. MM DD YY	16. DATES PATIENT UNABLE TO WORK IN CURRENT OCCUPATION MM DD YY MM DD YY FROM 11 09 20XX TO 11 30 20XX

17. NAME OF REFERRING PROVIDER OR OTHER SOURCE	17a.	18. HOSPITALIZATION DATES RELATED TO CURRENT SERVICES
Gerald Practon MD	17b. NPI	MM DD YY MM DD YY FROM 11 11 20XX TO 11 12 20XX

19. ADDITIONAL CLAIM INFORMATION (Designated by NUCC)	20. OUTSIDE LAB? ☐ YES ☒ NO	$ CHARGES

21. DIAGNOSIS OR NATURE OF ILLNESS OR INJURY Relate A-L to service line below (24E)   ICD Ind. 0

A. J03.90   B.   C.   D.
E.   F.   G.   H.
I.   J.   K.   L.

22. RESUBMISSION CODE _____ ORIGINAL REF. NO. _____

23. PRIOR AUTHORIZATION NUMBER

24. A. DATE(S) OF SERVICE			B. PLACE OF SERVICE	C. EMG	D. PROCEDURES, SERVICES, OR SUPPLIES (Explain Unusual Circumstances)		E. DIAGNOSIS POINTER	F. $ CHARGES	G. DAYS OR UNITS	H. EPSDT Family Plan	I. ID. QUAL.	J. RENDERING PROVIDER ID. #
From MM DD YY	To MM DD YY				CPT/HCPCS	MODIFIER						
11 10 20XX			11		99203		A	50 00	1		NPI	43050047XX
11 11 20XX			21		99222		A	120 80			NPI	43050047XX
11 11 20XX			21		42821		A	410 73			NPI	43050047XX
11 22 20XX			21		99231		A	20 00			NPI	43050047XX
											NPI	
											NPI	

25. FEDERAL TAX I.D. NUMBER	SSN EIN	26. PATIENT'S ACCOUNT NO.	27. ACCEPT ASSIGNMENT? (For govt. claims, see back)	28. TOTAL CHARGE	29. AMOUNT PAID	30. Rsvd for NUCC Use
715737291XX	☐ ☒	456273	☐ YES ☐ NO	$	$	

31. SIGNATURE OF PHYSICIAN OR SUPPLIER INCLUDING DEGREES OR CREDENTIALS (I certify that the statements on the reverse apply to this bill and are made a part thereof.)	32. SERVICE FACILITY LOCATION INFORMATION	33. BILLING PROVIDER INFO & PH # (555) 4869002
	College Hospital 4500 Broad Avenue Woodland Hills XY 12345-0001	College Clinic 4567 Broad Avenue Woodland Hills XY 12345-0001
SIGNED _____ DATE 11/15/20XX	a. X950731067 b.	a. 3664021CC b.

PHYSICIAN OR SUPPLIER INFORMATION →

NUCC Instruction Manual available at: www.nucc.org   *PLEASE PRINT OR TYPE*   OMB APPROVAL PENDING

Fig. 16.6

254

ASSIGNMENT 16.7 REQUEST FOR MEDICARE HEARING BY AN ADMINISTRATIVE LAW JUDGE

Performance Objective

Task: Insert information on a Request for Medicare Hearing by an Administrative Law Judge (Form OMHA-100)

Conditions: Request for Medicare Hearing by an Administrative Law Judge (Form OMHA-100) (Fig. 16.7), and a computer with printer.

Standards: Time: _____ minutes

             Accuracy: _____

             (Note: The time element and accuracy criteria may be given by your instructor.)

Directions: You receive a Medicare EOB and payment check for the patient Bill Hutch, but the amount is incorrect because of an excessive reduction in the allowed payment. An appeal was made in September and denied; the document control number assigned by Medicare Blue Shield is 240-577-9008. Dr. Brady Coccidioides believes that a mistake has been made and wishes to request a hearing.

Complete the Request for Medicare Hearing by an Administrative Law Judge (Form OMHA-100) for this case (see Fig. 16.7 in the textbook). Mr. Hutch's e-mail address is bhutch@gmail.net. Complete the form as the appellant and do not fill in the representative's portion. The Health Insurance Claim Number is the patient's Medicare identification number, Block 1a. No additional evidence is to be presented; the doctor does not wish to appear for the hearing. Date the form December 5, 20xx. The beneficiary has assigned his appeal rights to the provider.

After the instructor has returned your work to you, either make the necessary corrections and place your work in a three-ring notebook for future reference or, if you received a high score, place it in your portfolio for reference when applying for a job.

DEPARTMENT OF HEALTH AND HUMAN SERVICES
Office of Medicare Hearings and Appeals
REQUEST FOR ADMINISTRATIVE LAW JUDGE (ALJ)
HEARING OR REVIEW OF DISMISSAL

Section 1: Which Medicare Part are you appealing (if known)? (*Check one*)

☐ Part A ☐ Part B ☐ Part C (*Medicare Advantage*) or Medicare Cost Plan ☐ Part D (*Prescription Drug Plan*)

Section 2: Which party are you, or which party are you representing? (*Check one*)

☐ The Medicare beneficiary or enrollee, or a successor (such as an estate), who received or requested the items or services being appealed, or is appealing a Medicare Secondary Payer issue.

☐ The provider or supplier that furnished the items or services to the Medicare beneficiary or enrollee, a Medicaid State agency, or an applicable plan appealing a Medicare Secondary Payer issue.

☐ Other. *Please explain:*

Section 3: What is your (the appealing party's) information? (*Representative information in next section*)

Name (*First, Middle Initial, Last*)	Firm or Organization (*if applicable*)		

Address where appeals correspondence should be sent	City	State	ZIP Code

Telephone Number	Fax Number	E-Mail

Section 4: What is the representative's information? (*Skip if you do not have a representative*)

Name	Firm or Organization (*if applicable*)		

Mailing Address	City	State	ZIP Code

Telephone Number	Fax Number	E-Mail

Did you file an appointment of representation (form CMS-1696) or other documents authorizing your representation at a prior level of appeal?

☐ No. *Please file the document(s) with this request.*
☐ Yes

Section 5: What is being appealed? *Submit a separate request for each Reconsideration or Dismissal that you wish to appeal. If the appeal involves multiple beneficiaries or enrollees, use the multiple claim attachment (OMHA-100A).*

Name of entity that issued the Reconsideration or Dismissal (*or attach a copy of the Reconsideration or Dismissal*)	Reconsideration (Medicare Appeal or Case) Number (*or attach a copy of the Reconsideration or Dismissal*)		

Beneficiary or Enrollee Name	Health Insurance Claim Number		

Beneficiary or Enrollee Mailing Address	City	State	ZIP Code

What item(s) or service(s) are you appealing? (*N/A if appealing a Dismissal*)	Date(s) of service being appealed (*if applicable*)

Supplier or Provider Name (*N/A for Part D appeals*)	Supplier or Provider Telephone Number (*N/A for Part D appeals*)

Supplier or Provider Mailing Address (*N/A for Part D appeals*)	City	State	ZIP Code

Section 6: For appeals of prescription drugs ONLY (*Skip for all other appeals*)

Part D Prescription Drug Plan Name	What drug(s) are you appealing?

Are you requesting an expedited hearing?
(*An expedited hearing is only available if your appeal is not solely related to payment (for example, you do not have the drug) and applying the standard time frame for a decision (90 days) may jeopardize your health, life, or ability to regain maximum function*)

☐ No. ☐ Yes. *On a separate sheet, please explain or have your prescriber explain why applying the standard time frame for a decision (90 days) may jeopardize your health, life, or ability to regain maximum function.*

OMHA-100 (03/17)   **PAGE 1 OF 2**   PSC Publishing Services (301) 443-6740. EF

Fig. 16.7   (From Department of Health and Human Services, Office of Medicare Hearings and Appeals.)

Section 7: Why do you disagree with the Reconsideration or Dismissal being appealed? (*Attach a continuation sheet if necessary*)

Section 8: Are you submitting evidence with this request, or do you plan to submit evidence?

☐ I am not planning to submit evidence at this time. (*Skip to Section 9, below*)

☐ I am submitting evidence with this request.

☐ I plan to submit evidence. Indicate what you plan to submit and when you plan to submit it:

Was the evidence already submitted for the matter that you are appealing?	☐ No. *Part A and Part B appeals only. If you are a provider or supplier, or a provider or supplier that is representing a beneficiary, you must include a statement explaining why the evidence is being submitted for the first time and was not submitted previously.* ☐ Yes.

Section 9: Is there other information about your appeal that we should know?

Are you aggregating claims to meet the amount in controversy requirement? (*If yes, attach your aggregation request. See 42 C.F.R. § 405.1006(e) and (f), and 423.1979(c) for request requirements.*)	☐ No	☐ Yes
Are you waiving the oral hearing before an ALJ and requesting a decision based on the record? (*If yes, attach a completed form OMHA-104 or other explanation. N/A if requesting review of a dismissal.*)	☐ No	☐ Yes
Does the request involve claims that were part of a statistical sample? (*If yes, please explain the status of any appeals for claims in the sample that are not included in this request.*)	☐ No	☐ Yes

Section 10: Certification of copies sent to other parties (*Part A and Part B appeals only*)

If another party to the claim or issue that you are appealing was sent a copy of the Reconsideration or Dismissal, you must send a copy of your request for an ALJ hearing or review of dismissal to that party. Indicate the party (or their representative) to whom and address where you are sending a copy of the request, and when the copy will be sent (*attach a continuation sheet if there are multiple parties*).	Name of Recipient
	Mailing Address

City	State	ZIP Code
Date of Mailing		

☐ Check here if no other parties were sent a copy of the Reconsideration or Dismissal.

Section 11: Filing instructions

Your appealed claim must meet the current amount in controversy requirement to file an appeal. See the Reconsideration or Dismissal or visit www.hhs.gov/omha for information on the current amount in controversy. Send this request form to the entity in the appeal instructions that came with your reconsideration (for example, requests for hearing following a Part C reconsideration are generally sent to the entity that conducted the reconsideration). If instructed to send to OMHA, use the addresses below.

Beneficiaries and enrollees, send your request to:	For expedited Part D appeals, send your request to:	All other appellants, send your request to:
OMHA Centralized Docketing Attn: Beneficiary Mail Stop 200 Public Square, Suite 1260 Cleveland, Ohio 44114-2316	OMHA Centralized Docketing Attn: Expedited Part D Mail Stop 200 Public Square, Suite 1260 Cleveland, Ohio 44114-2316	OMHA Centralized Docketing 200 Public Square, Suite 1260 Cleveland, Ohio 44114-2316

We must receive this request within 60 calendar days after you received the Reconsideration or Dismissal that you are appealing. We will assume that you received the Reconsideration or Dismissal 5 calendar days after the date of the Reconsideration or Dismissal, unless you provide evidence to the contrary. *If you are filing this request late, attach a completed form OMHA-103 or other explanation for the late filing.*

PRIVACY ACT STATEMENT

The legal authority for the collection of information on this form is authorized by the Social Security Act (section 1155 of Title XI and sections 1852(g)(5), 1860D-4(h)(1), 1869(b)(1), and 1876 of Title XVIII). The information provided will be used to further document your appeal. Submission of the information requested on this form is voluntary, but failure to provide all or any part of the requested information may affect the determination of your appeal. Information you furnish on this form may be disclosed by the Office of Medicare Hearings and Appeals to another person or governmental agency only with respect to the Medicare Program and to comply with Federal laws requiring the disclosure of information or the exchange of information between the Department of Health and Human Services and other agencies.

If you need large print or assistance, please call 1-855-556-8475

OMHA-100 (03/17) **PAGE 2 OF 2**

Fig. 16.7, cont'd

257

ASSIGNMENT 16.8 FILE AN APPEAL

Performance Objective

Task: Compose, format, key, proofread, and print a letter of appeal, and attach to this document photocopies of information to substantiate reimbursement requested.

Conditions: Computer, printer, letterhead paper, envelope, attachments, thesaurus, English dictionary, medical dictionary, and pen or pencil.

Standards: Time: _____ minutes

               Accuracy: _____

               (Note: The time element and accuracy criteria may be given by your instructor.)

Scenario: After retyping and resubmitting Mary T. Avery's insurance claim in Assignment 16.7 (see Fig. 16.6), the insurance company sends an EOB/RA (health insurance claim number 123098) with a check in the amount of $300 to the College Clinic for payment of the claim. Dr. Cutler wishes an appeal to be made for an increase of the payment of an additional $100. (Note: This patient's marital status is single, and the insured's identification number is T45098.)

    Directions: Use the retyped claim to Assignment 16.7 for Mary T. Avery. Follow these basic step-by-step procedures.

1. Compose, format, key, proofread, and print a letter.

2. Include the beneficiary's name, health insurance claim number, dates of service in question, and items or services in question with name, address, and signature of the provider.

3. Compose a letter with an introduction that stresses the medical practice's qualifications, the physician's commitment to complying with regulations and providing appropriate services, and the importance of the practice to the payer's panel of physicians or specialists.

4. Provide a detailed account of the necessity of the treatment given and its relationship to the patient's problems and chief complaint. You might cross-reference the medical record and emphasize parts of it that the reviewer may have missed.

5. Explain the reason why the provider does not agree with the payment. Use a blank sheet, labeling it "Explanation of Benefits," because you do not have this printed document to attach.

6. Abstract excerpts from the coding resource book if necessary.

7. Direct the correspondence to Mr. Donald Pearson, a claims adjuster at the American Insurance Company, 509 Main Street, Woodland Hills, XY 12345.

8. Address an envelope for the letter.

9. Retain copies of all data sent for the physician's files.

17 Collection Strategies

Linda M. Smith

KEY TERMS

Your instructor may wish to select some words pertinent to this chapter for a test. For definitions of the terms, further study, and/or reference, the words, phrases, and abbreviations may be found in the glossary at the end of the textbook. *Key terms for this chapter follow.*

accounts receivable
age analysis
automatic stay
balance
bankruptcy
bonding
cash flow
collateral
collection ratio
credit
credit card
creditor
cycle billing
debit card
debt
debtor
discount
dun messages

embezzlement
estate administrator
estate executor
fee schedule
financial accounting record
garnishment
itemized statement
lien
netback
no charge
nonexempt assets
professional courtesy
secured debt
skip
statute of limitations
unsecured debt
write-off

KEY ABBREVIATIONS

See how many abbreviations and acronyms you can translate and then use this as a handy reference list. Definitions for the key abbreviations are located near the back of the text-book *in the glossary.*

A/R _____

ATM _____

e-check _____

ERISA _____

FACT _____

FCBA _____

FCRA _____

FDCPA _____

FEHBA _____

FTC _____

N/A _____

NC _____

NSF _____

TILA _____

W2 _____

PERFORMANCE OBJECTIVES

The student will be able to:

- Define and spell the key terms and key abbreviations for this chapter, given the information from the *textbook* glossary, within a reasonable time period and with enough accuracy to obtain a satisfactory evaluation.
- After reading the chapter, answer the fill-in-the-blank, mix and match, multiple choice, and true/false review questions with enough accuracy to obtain a satisfactory evaluation.
- Select an appropriate dun message for a patient's bill, given a patient's ledger/statement, within a reasonable time period and with enough accuracy to obtain a satisfactory evaluation.
- Post a courtesy adjustment, given a patient's ledger/statement, within a reasonable time period and with enough accuracy to obtain a satisfactory evaluation.

- Post a patient's charges and payment to the patient's financial accounting record, within a reasonable time period and with enough accuracy to obtain a satisfactory evaluation.
- Compose a collection letter for a delinquent account, given letterhead stationery, within a reasonable time period and with enough accuracy to obtain a satisfactory evaluation.
- Complete a financial agreement, given a patient's ledger/statement, within a reasonable time period and with enough accuracy to obtain a satisfactory evaluation.

STUDY OUTLINE

Collection Strategies
Accounts Receivable
Patient Education
　Patient Registration Form
Fees
　Fee Schedule
　Missed Appointments
　Fee Adjustments
　Discussing Fees
　Collecting Fees

Credit and Collection Laws
　Statute of Limitations
The Collection Process
　Telephone Collection Procedures
　Collection Letters
　Insurance Collection
　Collection Agencies
　Small Claims Court
　Tracing a Skip
　Special Collection Issues

Part I Fill in the Blank

Review the objectives, key terms, chapter information, glossary definitions of key terms, and figures before completing the following review questions.

1. Third-party payers who generate a large percentage of reimbursement to health care organizations are composed of

   a. _____

   b. _____

   c. _____

   d. _____.

2. The unpaid balance due from patients for professional services rendered is known as a/an

   _____.

3. An important document that provides demographic and identifying data for each patient and assists in billing and collection is called a/an

   _____.

4. A term preferable to "write-off" when used in a medical practice is _____.

5. To verify a check, ask the patient for a/an _____

   and _____.

6. The procedure of systematically arranging the accounts receivable, by age, from the

   date of service is called _____.

7. Write the formula for calculating the office accounts receivable (A/R) ratio.

   _____

   _____

   _____

8. What is the collection rate if a total of $40,300 was collected for the month and the

   total of the accounts receivable is $50,670? _____

9. Patient accounts that are open to charges made from time to time are referred to as

   _____

10. A court order attaching a debtor's property or wages to pay off a debt is known as

    _____.

11. An individual who owes on an account and moves, leaving no forwarding address, is

    called a/an _____.

12. Translate these credit and collection abbreviations.

NSF _____   T _____

WCO _____   SK _____

PIF _____   FN _____

NLE _____   UE _____

13. A straight petition in bankruptcy or absolute bankruptcy is also known as a/an _____.

14. A wage earner's bankruptcy is sometimes referred to as a/an _____.

15. State three bonding methods.

a. _____

b. _____

c. _____

16. A system of billing accounts at spaced intervals during the month on the basis of a breakdown of accounts by alphabet, account number, insurance type, or date of service

is known as _____.

Part II Mix and Match

17. Match the credit and collection terms in the right column with the descriptions, and fill in the blank with the appropriate letter.

_____ Reductions of the normal fee based on a specific amount of money or a percentage of the charge	a. debtor
_____ Phrase to remind a patient about a delinquent account	b. itemized statement
_____ Item that permits bank customers to withdraw cash at any hour from an automated teller machine	c. fee schedule
_____ Individual owing money	d. discounts
_____ Claim on the property of another as security for a debt	e. financial account record (ledger)
_____ Individual record indicating charges, payments, adjustments, and balances owed for services rendered	f. creditor
_____ Detailed summary of all transactions of a creditor's account	g. dun message
_____ Person to whom money is owed	h. debit card
_____ Listing of accepted charges or established allowances for specific medical procedures	i. lien

18. Match the following federal acts with their descriptions, and fill in the blank with the appropriate letter.

_____ Law stating that a person has 60 days to complain about an error from the date that a statement is mailed

_____ Consumer protection act that applies to anyone who charges interest or agrees on payment of a bill in more than four installments, excluding a down payment

_____ Regulates collection practices of third-party debt collectors and attorneys who collect debts for others

_____ Federal law prohibiting discrimination in all areas of granting credit

_____ Regulates agencies that issue or use credit reports on consumers

a. Equal Credit Opportunity Act

b. Fair Credit Reporting Act

c. Fair Credit Billing Act

d. Truth in Lending Act

e. Fair Debt Collection Practices Act

Part III Multiple Choice

Choose the best answer.

19. Signing another person's name on a check to obtain money or pay off a debt without permission is called:
    a. embezzlement.
    b. stealing.
    c. garnishing.
    d. forgery.

20. When sending monthly statements to patients for balances due, the postal service can forward mail if the addressed envelopes contain the statement:
    a. "Please Forward."
    b. "Forwarding Service Requested."
    c. "Forwarding and Return Receipt Requested."
    d. "Send Forward."

21. When accepting a credit card as payment on an account, the proper guideline(s) to follow is/are to:
    a. ask for photo identification.
    b. accept a card only from the person whose name is on the card.
    c. get approval from the credit card company.
    d. all of the above.

22. A service offered by a nonprofit agency assisting people in paying off their debts is known as:
    a. credit counseling.
    b. debt solutions.
    c. grant-in-aid under the Hill-Burton Act.
    d. small claims court.

23. Insurance payment checks should be stamped in the endorsement area on the back "For Deposit Only," which is called a/an:
    a. conditional endorsement.
    b. qualified endorsement.
    c. special endorsement.
    d. restrictive endorsement.

Part IV True/False

Write "T" or "F" in the blank to indicate whether you think the statement is true or false.

_____ 24. Insurance companies and the federal government do not recommend waiving copayments to patients.

_____ 25. Regulation Z of the Truth in Lending Consumer Credit Cost Disclosure law applies if the patient is making three payments.

_____ 26. Most state collection laws allow telephone calls to the debtor between 8 AM and 9 PM.

_____ 27. When a patient has declared bankruptcy, it is permissible to continue to send monthly statements for a balance due.

_____ 28. A collection agency must follow all the laws stated in the Fair Debt Collection Practices Act.

Performance Objective

Task: Select an appropriate dun message and insert it on a patient's financial accounting record (ledger card).

Conditions: Use the patient's financial accounting record (Fig. 17.1), computer, and a printer.

Standards: Time: _____ minutes

Accuracy:_____

(Note: The time element and accuracy criteria may be given by your instructor.)

Background: Most patient account activities are recorded in the medical billing software. However, to develop the skills and understanding for payment posting, a paper financial accounting statement has been provided.

Directions: Read the scenario and refer to the patient's financial accounting record (see Fig. 17.1). Select appropriate dun messages for each month the patient has been billed. You may wish to refer to Fig. 17.5 in the textbook.

Scenario: Carrie Jones was on vacation in June and July and did not pay on her account. It is August (current year).

June 1, 20XX, dun message _____

July 1, 20XX, dun message _____

August 1, 20XX, dun message _____

After the instructor has returned your work to you, either make the necessary corrections and place your work in a three-ring notebook for future reference or, if you received a high score, place it in your portfolio for reference when applying for a job.

STATEMENT
Financial Account
COLLEGE CLINIC
4567 Broad Avenue
Woodland Hills, XY 12345-0001
Tel. 555-486-9002
Fax No. 555-487-8976

Carrie Jones
15543 Dean Street
Woodland Hills, XY 12345

Phone No. (H) ___(555) 439-8800___ (W) ___(555) 550-8706___   Birth date ___05-14-72___

Primary Insurance Co. ___Prudential Insurance Company___   Policy/Group No. ___450998___

	REFERENCE	DESCRIPTION	CHARGES	CREDITS PYMNTS.	ADJ.	BALANCE	
				BALANCE FORWARD ➔		20	00
4-16--xx	99215	C hx/exam HC DM DX 582				154	99
4-17--xx		Prudential billed (4-16-xx)				154	99
5-27--xx		Rec'd insurance ck #435		30	00	124	99
6-1-xx		Billed pt				124	99
7-1-xx		Billed pt				124	99
8-1-xx		Billed pt				124	99

PLEASE PAY LAST AMOUNT IN BALANCE COLUMN

THIS IS A COPY OF YOUR FINANCIAL ACCOUNT AS IT APPEARS ON OUR RECORDS

Fig. 17.1

ASSIGNMENT 17.3 MANUALLY POST A COURTESY ADJUSTMENT

Performance Objective

Task: Post a courtesy adjustment to a patient's financial accounting record (ledger card).

Conditions: Use the patient's financial accounting record (Fig. 17.2) and a pen.

Standards: Time: _____ minutes

               Accuracy: _____

               (Note: The time element and accuracy criteria may be given by your instructor.)

Background: Most patient account activities are recorded in the medical billing software. However, to develop the skills and understanding for payment posting, a paper financial accounting statement has been provided.

Directions: Read the case scenario and refer to the patient's financial accounting record (see Fig. 17.2). You may wish to refer to Fig. 17.5 in the textbook. Post a courtesy adjustment to her financial accounting record.

Scenario: Maria Smith recently lost her job and is raising two children as a single parent. It is September 1 (current year). A discussion with Dr. Gerald Practon leads to a decision to write off the balance of the current charges on the account but not the balance forward.

   After the instructor has returned your work to you, either make the necessary corrections and place your work in a three-ring notebook for future reference or, if you received a high score, place it in your portfolio for reference when applying for a job.

Acct No. 10-3

STATEMENT
Financial Account
COLLEGE CLINIC
4567 Broad Avenue
Woodland Hills, XY 12345-0001
Tel. 555-486-9002
Fax No. 555-487-8976

Ms. Maria Smith
3737 Unser Road
Woodland Hills, XY 12345

Phone No. (H) (555) 430-8877   (W)   (555) 908-1233   Birth date 06-11-80

Primary Insurance Co.   Metropolitan Insurance Company   Policy/Group No.   4320870

	REFERENCE	DESCRIPTION	CHARGES		CREDITS PYMNTS.	ADJ.	BALANCE	
						BALANCE FORWARD ⟶	20	00
5-19-xx	99214	OV DX 582	61	51			81	51
5-20-xx		Metropolitan billed (5-19-xx)					81	51
6-20-xx		Rec'd ins ck #6778			25	00	56	51
7-1-xx		Pt billed					56	51
8-1-xx		Pt billed					56	51

PLEASE PAY LAST AMOUNT IN BALANCE COLUMN ⇧

THIS IS A COPY OF YOUR FINANCIAL ACCOUNT AS IT APPEARS ON OUR RECORDS

Fig. 17.2

ASSIGNMENT 17.4 MANUALLY POST A PATIENT'S CHARGES AND PAYMENT

Performance Objective

Task: Post a payment to a patient's financial accounting record (ledger card).

Conditions: Use the patient's financial accounting record (Fig. 17.3), and a pen.

Standards: Time: _____ minutes

            Accuracy: _____

            (Note: The time element and accuracy criteria may be given by your instructor.)

Background: Most patient account activities are recorded in the medical billing software. However, to develop the skills and understanding for payment posting, a paper financial accounting statement has been provided.

Directions: Read the case scenario; refer to the patient's financial accounting record (see Fig. 17.3). You may wish to refer to Fig. 17.5 in the textbook. Post the charges for the services rendered and payment to the patient's financial accounting record.

Scenario:

Date of service: October 12 (current year)
Patient: Kenneth Brown; 8896 Aster Drive; Woodland Hills, XY, 12345
Patient Phone: 555-760-5211 (home) 555-987-3855 (work)
Date of birth: 1/15/82
Insurance: None
Service Provided: EKG (CPT 93000) fee = $34.26
Service Provided: New patient visit level III (CPT 99203) fee = $70.92
Patient paid by personal check: $50.00 (check #3421)

After the instructor has returned your work to you, either make the necessary corrections and place your work in a three-ring notebook for future reference or, if you received a high score, place it in your portfolio for reference when applying for a job.

STATEMENT
Financial Account
COLLEGE CLINIC
4567 Broad Avenue
Woodland Hills, XY 12345-0001
Tel. 555-486-9002
Fax No. 555-487-8976

Mr. Kenneth Brown
8896 Aster Drive
Woodland Hills, XY 12345

Phone No. (H) __(555) 760-5211__   (W) __(555) 987-3355__   Birth date __01-15-82__

Primary Insurance Co. __none__   Policy/Group No. _____

| | REFERENCE | DESCRIPTION | CHARGES | CREDITS | | BALANCE |
				PYMNTS.	ADJ.	
			BALANCE FORWARD ⟶			

PLEASE PAY LAST AMOUNT IN BALANCE COLUMN ⟱

THIS IS A COPY OF YOUR FINANCIAL ACCOUNT AS IT APPEARS ON OUR RECORDS

Fig. 17.3

ASSIGNMENT 17.5 COMPOSE A COLLECTION LETTER

Performance Objective

Task: Compose a letter for the physician's signature and post the entry on the patient's financial accounting record (ledger card).

Conditions: Use the patient's financial accounting record (Fig. 17.4), one sheet of letterhead paper (Fig. 17.5), a number 10 envelope, English dictionary, thesaurus, medical dictionary, computer, printer, and pen.

Standards: Time: _____ minutes

                Accuracy: _____

                (Note: The time element and accuracy criteria may be given by your instructor.)

Background: Most patient account activities are recorded in the medical billing software. However, to develop the skills and understanding for payment posting, a paper financial accounting statement has been provided.

Directions: Read the case scenario, refer to the patient's financial accounting record (see Fig. 17.4), and compose a collection letter, using your signature and requesting payment. Print on letterhead stationery in full block format (paragraphs to left margin). Include a paragraph stating that a copy of the delinquent statement is enclosed. You may wish to refer to Fig. 17.16 in the textbook. Post an entry on the patient's financial accounting record.

Scenario: It is December 1 (current year), and you have sent Mr. Ron Kelsey two statements with no response. You have tried to reach him by telephone without success and have decided to send him a collection letter (see Fig. 17.5).

After the instructor has returned your work to you, either make the necessary corrections and place your work in a three-ring notebook for future reference or, if you received a high score, place it in your portfolio for reference when applying for a job.

Acct No. 10-5

STATEMENT
Financial Account
COLLEGE CLINIC
4567 Broad Avenue
Woodland Hills, XY 12345-0001
Tel. 555-486-9002
Fax No. 555-487-8976

Mr. Ron Kelsey
6321 Ocean Street
Woodland Hills, XY 12345

Phone No. (H) (555) 540-9800   (W) (555) 890-7766   Birth date 03-25-75

Primary Insurance Co. XYZ Insurance Company   Policy/Group No. 8503Y

	REFERENCE	DESCRIPTION	CHARGES		CREDITS PYMNTS.	ADJ.	BALANCE	
			BALANCE FORWARD →					
07-09-xx	99283	ER new pt EPF hx/exam MC DM	66	23			66	23
07-10-xx		XYZ Insurance billed (3-9-xx)					66	23
09-20-xx		EOB rec'd pt has not met deductible					66	23
10-01-xx		Billed pt					66	23
11-01-xx		Billed pt					66	23

PLEASE PAY LAST AMOUNT IN BALANCE COLUMN ⇧

THIS IS A COPY OF YOUR FINANCIAL ACCOUNT AS IT APPEARS ON OUR RECORDS

Fig. 17.4

COLLEGE CLINIC
4567 Broad Avenue
Woodland Hills, XY 12345-0001
Tel. (555) 486-9002
FAX (555) 487-8976

Fig. 17.5

ASSIGNMENT 17.6 ACCEPTING CREDIT CARD PAYMENTS

Performance Objective

Task: Accept a credit card payment through various tools and post the credit entry on the patient's ledger.

Conditions: Use a credit card terminal, credit card reader attachment, or secured online web portal for credit card payments and credit card receipts, and pen or pencil.

Standards: Time: _____ minutes

            Accuracy: _____

            (Note: The time element and accuracy criteria may be given by your instructor.)

Background: The medical office has many different tools to accept credit card payments, such as:

- *Credit card terminal payment:* These lightweight devices use an internet connection to complete the payment transaction. The terminal can scan the credit card data including the cardholder's name, credit card number, and expiration date, through a swipe. The terminal also can process credit card transactions in which the user manually enters credit card information; in this scenario, the transaction requires the credit card number, the expiration date, the card security code (CVV), and the patient's billing ZIP code. Both transactions, the swipe method and the manual method, cause the terminal to typically print out two receipts per transaction, one for the medical office and one for the patient. If the credit card is swiped, the patient signs the medical office receipt because it states their name in the transaction. When manually entering the credit card data, the receipt will not print the patient's name, so the medical assistant must document the patient name, date of service, and/or medical record number on the receipt. Renting a credit card terminal can be costly, so smaller medical offices prefer to use other credit card accepting options.

- *Credit card reader payment:* A smaller medical office might choose a pay-for-use credit card that accepts software packages. The package includes a tablet or smartphone attachment device for scanning credit cards and a downloadable application (Fig. 17.11 in the textbook). The application is user friendly and is able to send the patient a receipt via email or by text message. There is a minimal fee per transaction ($0.25 to $0.30) and a percent charged based on the total amount.

- *Online credit card payment:* Some medical offices use an online merchant service to accept patient credit card payments. Through a secure web portal, patients can view their medical bills online and make payments by credit card or through a service such as PayPal. The transaction receipt is emailed to the patient and to the medical office. When the medical assistant receives the transaction via email, he or she updates the patient's account to reflect the current balance. There is a per transaction cost for this service similar to other credit card acceptance applications.

Directions: Read each case scenario, review the accompanying figures, and answer the following questions:

A. Kevin Long is attending the College Clinic on May 26 (current year) for an office visit and needs to pay for his $30 copay. He presents a credit card for payment (Fig. 17.6A).

   1. What should the medical assistant do to verify Kevin Long's identity before accepting the credit card for payment?

     _____

   2. Which tool can be used to accept Kevin Long's payment?

     _____

   3. Will the credit card receipt have Kevin's name printed? Why or why not?

     _____

   4. Does the medical office credit card receipt require the patient's signature? Why or why not?

     _____

   5. Was the expiration date or CVV needed for this transaction? Why or why not?

     _____

B. It is November 6 (current year), and you receive a phone call at the College Clinic. It is Kevin Long, who has an unpaid balance of $24.32, and it is up to you to discuss this delinquency with Mr. Long and come to an agreement on how the account can be paid. After discussion, Mr. Long decides to pay the total balance due by credit card, giving you his authorization (Fig. 17.6B).

1. Which tool can be used to accept Kevin Long's payment?

_____

2. Will the credit card receipts have Kevin's name printed? Why or why not?

_____

3. What must a medical assistant do to the receipt if the patient's name is not printed?

_____

4. Was the CVV needed for this transaction?

_____

5. How can a credit card receipt be sent to the patient?

_____

C. Kevin Long received a statement from the College Clinic for an outstanding balance of $63.52 from a date of service December 12 (current year). He notices that the clinic allows him to log in to pay online. He visits the medical office's website and clicks the "Pay Your Bill" feature. The secure online web portal asks Kevin to complete a form requests his name, billing address, an email address, the credit card number, expiration date, and CVV (Fig. 17.6C). Prior to submitting the online form, Kevin notices the following statement: "By clicking this box, the user agrees to the terms of this transaction." Kevin checks the box and clicks submit to send his credit card payment electronically. A receipt for the transaction is emailed to Kevin.

1. Which tool can be used to accept Kevin Long's payment?

_____

2. Will the credit card receipt have Kevin's name printed? Why or why not?

_____

3. Was the CVV needed for this transaction?

_____

4. How is the credit card receipt sent to the patient?

_____

5. What should the medical assistant do with the transaction email received?

_____

After the instructor has returned your work to you, either make the necessary corrections and place your work in a three-ring notebook for future reference or, if you received a high score, place it in your portfolio for reference when applying for a job.

COLLEGE CLINIC
4567 Broad Avenue
Woodland Hills, XY 12345-0001

05/26/20XX   09:39:14
Merchant ID: 00000000262026XX
Terminal ID: 038802XX
0150302859XX

CREDIT CARD

MC SALE

Name	Kevin Long
CARD#	XXXXXXXXXX4021
INVOICE	009
Batch #:	00716
Approval Code:	4123P
Entry Method:	Swiped

SALE AMOUNT   **$30.00**

Kevin Long

_____
Customer Signature

MERCHANT COPY

Fig. 17.6

Continued

COLLEGE CLINIC
4567 Broad Avenue
Woodland Hills, XY 12345-0001

11/6 /20XX	09:39:14
Merchant ID:	0000000262026XX
Terminal ID:	038802XX
0150302859XX	

CREDIT CARD

MC SALE

CARD#	XXXXXXXXXX4021
INVOICE	009
Batch#:	00716
Approval Code:	4123P
Entry Method:	Manual Entry
Mode:	Online

SALE AMOUNT	**$24.32**

Approved by patient over the phone.

_____
Customer Signature

MERCHANT COPY

11/6/20XX: Spoke with Kevin Long (MR 354689); he agreed to pay balance in full with a credit card over the phone. Payment for date of service 7/3/20XX. Balance paid in full.

Fig. 17.6, cont'd

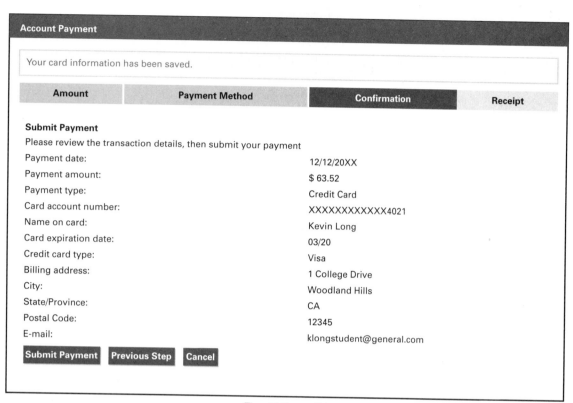

Account Payment

Your card information has been saved.

| Amount | Payment Method | **Confirmation** | Receipt |

Submit Payment

Please review the transaction details, then submit your payment

Payment date:	12/12/20XX
Payment amount:	$ 63.52
Payment type:	Credit Card
Card account number:	XXXXXXXXXXXX4021
Name on card:	Kevin Long
Card expiration date:	03/20
Credit card type:	Visa
Billing address:	1 College Drive
City:	Woodland Hills
State/Province:	CA
Postal Code:	12345
E-mail:	klongstudent@general.com

Submit Payment **Previous Step** **Cancel**

Fig. 17.6, cont'd

STATEMENT
Financial Account
COLLEGE CLINIC
4567 Broad Avenue
Woodland Hills, XY 12345-0001
Tel. 555-486-9002
Fax No. 555-487-8976

Mr. Kevin O. Long
2443 Davis Street
Woodland Hills, XY 12345

Phone No. (H) (555) 244-5600   (W)   (555) 970-4466   Birth date 08-15-76

Primary Insurance Co. Blue Cross   Policy/Group No. 130-XX-0987

	REFERENCE	DESCRIPTION	CHARGES		CREDITS PYMNTS.	ADJ.	BALANCE	
			BALANCE FORWARD ➡					
09-08-xx	99205	OV Level V DX 582	132	28			132	28
09-09-xx		Blue Cross billed (9-8-xx)					132	28
10-12-xx		BC EOB rec'd pt has not met deductible					132	28
10-23-xx		Not covered by insurance. Balance due					132	28

PLEASE PAY LAST AMOUNT IN BALANCE COLUMN ⬆

THIS IS A COPY OF YOUR FINANCIAL ACCOUNT AS IT APPEARS ON OUR RECORDS

Fig. 17.7

ASSIGNMENT 17.7 COMPLETE A FINANCIAL AGREEMENT

Performance Objective

Task: Complete a financial agreement and post an entry on the patient's ledger.

Conditions: Patient's ledger card is Fig. 17.8 and the financial agreement form is Fig. 17.9.

Standards: Time: _____ minutes

_____ Accuracy: _____

(Note: The time element and accuracy criteria may be given by your instructor.)

Background: Most patient account activities are recorded in the medical billing software. However, to develop the skills and understanding for payment posting, a paper financial accounting statement has been provided.

Directions: Read the case scenario. Complete a financial agreement (see Fig. 17.9 by subtracting the down payment from the total debt. Refer to the patient's ledger/statement (see Fig. 17.8) and post an appropriate entry to the ledger/statement using a pen. Review the completed financial agreement with the patient (role played by another student). Ask the patient to sign the financial agreement.

Scenario: Mr. Joseph Small has a large balance due. Create a payment plan for this case. You have discussed the installment plan concerning the amount of the total debt, the down payment, amount and date of each installment, and the date of final payment. On June 1 (current year), Mr. Small is paying $500 cash as a down payment, and the balance is to be divided into five equal payments, due on the first of each month. There will be no monthly finance charge. Mr. Small's daytime telephone number is 555-760-5502. He is a patient of Dr. Brady Coccidioides.

After the instructor has returned your work to you, either make the necessary corrections and place your work in a three-ring notebook for future reference or, if you received a high score, place it in your portfolio for reference when applying for a job.

STATEMENT
Financial Account
COLLEGE CLINIC
4567 Broad Avenue
Woodland Hills, XY 12345-0001
Tel. 555-486-9002
Fax No. 555-487-8976

Mr. Joseph Small
655 Sherry Street
Woodland Hills, XY 12345

Phone No. (H) (555) 320-8801   (W) (555) 760-5502   Birth date 11-04-77

Primary Insurance Co. Blue Shield   Policy/Group No. 870-XX-4398

	REFERENCE	DESCRIPTION	CHARGES		CREDITS PYMNTS.		ADJ.		BALANCE	
				BALANCE FORWARD ➡					20	00
04-19-xx	99215	OV Level	96	97					116	97
04-30-xx	99218	Adm hosp	74	22					191	19
04-30-xx	32440	Pneumonectomy, total	1972	10					2163	29
05-20-xx		Blue Shield billed (1-19 to 30-xx)							2163	29
05-15-xx		BS EOB Pt deductible $2000 rec'd ck #544			163	29			2000	00

PLEASE PAY LAST AMOUNT IN BALANCE COLUMN ⬆

THIS IS A COPY OF YOUR FINANCIAL ACCOUNT AS IT APPEARS ON OUR RECORDS

Fig. 17.8

College Clinic
4567 Broad Avenue
Woodland Hills, XY 12345-0001
Phone: 555/486-9002
Fax: 555/487-8976

FINANCIAL PAYMENT PLAN AGREEMENT

For medical professional services rendered to:

Patient Name _____ Account No. _____

Responsible Party _____

Address _____

_____

Telephones: Home_____

Mobile _____

Business _____

1. Cash price of total medical treatment	$	_____
2. Down payment (partial payment)	$	_____
3. Amount covered by insurance plan	$	_____
4. Unpaid balance due	$	_____
5. **ANNUAL PERCENTAGE RATE** (interest rate)	_____ %	
6. **FINANCE CHARGE** ($ amt of cost to patient)	$	_____
7. Total amount of unpaid balance due	_____	
8. Monthly payment amount	$	_____

TERMS:
1. ALL PAYMENTS ARE DUE ON OR BEFORE YOUR DUE DATE EACH MONTH.

2. The patient agrees to be fully responsible for the total payment of medical services performed in this office including any amounts not covered by any health insurance plan.

3. The patient has the right at any time to pay the unpaid balance due without penalty.

4. First payment due _____/_____/_____ and subsequent payments on the same day of each consecutive month until paid in full.

_____

Signature of Patient/Responsible Party   Date

_____

Physician's signature or Authorized representative   Date

Fig. 17.9

18 Ambulatory Surgery Centers

Rachael D'Andrea

KEY TERMS

Your instructor may wish to select some words pertinent to this chapter for a test. For definitions of the terms, further study, and/or reference, the words, phrases, and abbreviations may be found in the glossary at the end of the Textbook. *Key terms for this chapter follow.*

Accreditation Association for Ambulatory
   Health Care (AAAHC)
Ambulatory Payment Classification (APC) System
Ambulatory Surgery Center (ASC)
Ambulatory Surgical Unit (ASU)
Ambulatory Quality Reporting (ASCQR)
clearinghouse
CMS-1500
Current Procedural Terminology (CPT)
conversion factor (CF)
discounted fee-for-service
discounting
first listed diagnosis
geographic practice cost index (GPCI)
Health care Common Procedure Coding
   System (HCPCS)
International Classification of Diseases, Tenth Revision,
   Clinical Modification (ICD-10-CM)
local coverage determinations (LCDs)

medical necessity
Medicare Physician Provider Fee Schedule (MPFS)
modifiers
National Coverage Determinations (NCDs)
National Correct Coding Initiative (NCCI)
National Uniform Billing Committee (NUBC)
national unadjusted payment
Outpatient Prospective Payment System (OPPS)
packaged pass throughs
preadmission
preauthorization
Prospective Payment System (PPS)
Relative Value Unit (RVU)
Resource-Based Relative Value Scale (RBRVS)
revenue code
revenue cycle
Revenue Cycle Management (RCM)
status (payment) indicator
Uniform Bill 04 (UB-04)

KEY ABBREVIATIONS

AMA _____

APC_____

ASC_____

ASCQR _____

ASU_____

CF _____

CMS _____

CPT_____

ECS _____

EMR _____

GCPI _____

HCPCS _____

LCDs_____

MPFS _____

NCDs_____

NCCI_____

OPPS _____

PPS _____

RBRVS _____

RCM _____

RVU _____

UB-04 _____

PERFORMANCE OBJECTIVES

The student will be able to:

- Define and spell the key terms and key abbreviations for this chapter, given the information from the textbook glossary, within a reasonable time period and with enough accuracy to obtain a satisfactory evaluation.

- After reading the chapter, answer the multiple choice and essay questions with enough accuracy to obtain a satisfactory evaluation.

Part I Multiple Choice

Choose the best answer.

1. Linking refers to which of the following?
   a. Pairing professional charges to technical charges on the claim.
   b. Substituting a HCPCS code for the appropriate CPT code
   c. Assigning a diagnosis code to a CPT code on the claim
   d. Appending modifiers to CPT/HCPCS codes

2. The function of a clearinghouse is to:
   a. transfer electronic claims to specific insurers in a secure way.
   b. confirm that the data entry is correct.
   c. manage the claims appeal process.
   d. enter and validate charges on the claims.

3. Which reimbursement methodology uses work, practice cost and malpractice cost as its variables?
   a. Capitation
   b. Standard charges
   c. Resource-Based Relative Value System
   d. Fee-for-service

4. When multiple surgical procedures are listed on the CMS-1500 claim form, the fees are listed as:
   a. a percentage of the full fee.
   b. discounted charges.
   c. sequenced by the surgeon.
   d. in numerical order.

5. The component of the RBRVS that depicts the health care professional's labor value is the:
   a. conversion factor.
   b. practice expense relative value unit.
   c. work relative value unit.
   d. work GPCI.

6. Medicare global periods define:
   a. the postoperative period for procedures.
   b. bundling.
   c. diagnosis distribution.
   d. CPT and HCPCS services.

7. Components of the Medicare global period include:
   a. preoperative visits after the decision is made to operate.
   b. intraoperative services that are part of the surgical procedure.
   c. additional surgical services required of the surgeon during the postoperative period of surgery.
   d. all of the above.

8. Level II modifiers, or HCPCS modifiers, consist of two alpha or alphanumeric characters in the sequence:
   a. –21 through –59.
   b. –01 through –99.
   c. AA through VP.
   d. A1 through XX.

9. What should be entered in field 24e of the CMS-1500 claim form to properly link the diagnosis to the service?
   a. The CPT code
   b. The ICD-10-CM code
   c. The place of service
   d. One linking reference letter from box 21

10. The fee schedule database is used to:
    a. identify the amount of revenue from each CPT code.
    b. record the transfer of claims.
    c. provide a list of all of the services performed.
    d. maintain charge information about CPT/HCPCS codes.

11. Which of the following data elements are required to calculate the Medicare approved amount? Check all that apply.
    a. RVU total value
    b. GPCI values
    c. RVU component values
    d. Conversion factor

12. The type of payment used by insurance carriers to control costs that are considered risky for the health care professional is:
    a. reimbursement.
    b. coinsurance.
    c. fee-for-service.
    d. capitation.

13. The _____ is the process of patient health and financial information moving into, through and out of the Ambulatory Surgery Center.
    a. revenue stream
    b. revenue cycle
    c. audit procedure
    d. managed care method

14. The term that is used to describe an insurance company that pays for the health care of the covered individual is:
    a. first party payer.
    b. second party payer.
    c. third party payer.
    d. beneficiary.

15. The specified amount of money paid to the ASC or physician, which covers the cost of the health plan member's health care services for a specific length of time is:
    a. global payment.
    b. capitation.
    c. fee-for-service.
    d. self-pay.

16. The prospective review which involves the obtaining of approval from a health insurance company prior to the health care service being rendered is the:
    a. post review audit.
    b. medical evaluation.
    c. preauthorization.
    d. precertification.

17. The payment methodology that combines the professional and technical components of a procedure is:
    a. global payment.
    b. prospective payment.
    c. retrospective payment.
    d. managed care reimbursement.

18. The verification that the patient is currently covered by the insurance plan on the date of service for the procedure is:
    a. medical necessity.
    b. medical evaluation.
    c. eligibility.
    d. predetermined rate setting.

19. The professional component of a service is the part of the service provided by:
    a. the ACS.
    b. the surgeon or physician.
    c. the hospital.
    d. none of the above.

20. The technical component of a service is the part of the service provided by (Check all that apply):
    a. the ACS.
    b. the surgeon or physician.
    c. the hospital.
    d. none of the above.

21. The _____ gained approval from CMS in 2018 to accredit ASCs.
    a. JCAHO
    b. AAAHC
    c. Medicare Advisory Committee
    d. AMA

22. When a hospital-based surgery center is not certified as an ASC, the _____ reimbursement rules apply.
    a. third party payer
    b. beneficiary
    c. HOPPS
    d. organization-specific

23. Which law was enacted by Congress to establish the outpatient use of the HCPCS code set?
    a. OBRA
    b. PPS
    c. HIPAA
    d. ACA

24. The HCPCS Level II codes are maintained by:
    a. AMA.
    b. CMS.
    c. Medicaid.
    d. AHIMA.

25. Medicare payment for ambulatory surgical center (ASC) services is based on rates set under:
    a. Part A.
    b. Part B.
    c. Part A and Part B.
    d. State authority.

Part II True/False

Write "T" or "F" in the blank to indicate whether you think the statement is true or false.

_____ 26. Health insurance payers have a variety of reimbursement plans and contracts with individual providers for payment. This means that the same type of service to two different patients may be paid differently depending on the type of contract or insurance that each patient has.

_____ 27. A prospective payment system is a method of reimbursement in which Medicare payment is based on a predetermined fixed amount.

_____ 28. An appeal must be filed within 6 months of a claim determination.

_____ 29. Column 1/Column 2 edits are part of the NCCI.

_____ 30. The electronic version of the CMS-1500 claim form is called the 837E.

_____ 31. A free source of information about the number of global surgical days assigned to a code is the Medicare Fee Schedule Lookup Tool.

_____ 32. The Administrative Simplification Compliance Act (ASCA) requires that claims be sent electronically to Medicare as a condition for payment.

_____ 33. The Place of Service Codes Set is required for use in the implementation guide adopted as the national standard for electronic transmission of professional health care claims under the provisions of the Health Insurance Portability and Accountability Act of 1996 (HIPAA).

_____ 34. CMS will continue to look at ASC payment reform, specifically site neutrality and efficiency of care.

_____ 35. Coverage and subsequent payment of a Medicare service depends on that service being medically necessary and medically reasonable.

_____ 36. According to Medicare, ASCs are permitted to share space with Critical Access Hospital outpatient surgery departments and with Medicare participating Independent Diagnostic Testing Facilities (IDTF).

_____ 37. The Medicare rules state that non-ASC facility services that are separately reimbursable include the physician's professional services; sale, lease, or rental of durable medical equipment for ASC patients to use at home; services performed by an independent laboratory; and hospital-based ambulance services.

_____ 38. Because an ASC bills to Part B of Medicare, the physician NCCI edits are the ones that apply.

_____ 39. The NCCI contains one table of PTP edits for physicians/practitioners and one table of PTP edits for outpatient hospital services.

_____ 40. All payers use the same modifiers.

Part III Essays

41. Discuss how correctly linking diagnoses to procedures on the CMS-1500 form can corroborate the medical necessity for a procedure that has been performed.

42. Describe how to locate the local coverage determination (LCD) for the local Medicare administrative contractor (MAC).

43. Explain the reason for assigning CPT/HCPCS modifiers.

44. If an improper payment has been paid by a third-party payer, what are the steps that should be performed prior to the appeal?

45. Define the two types of ASCs and the main differences between the billing procedures.

289

46. Explain three reasons for the increase in ASCs since 1970.

47. Medicare and other payers may consider a procedure to be a noncovered service when performed in an ASC for several reasons. List two.

48. For a procedure or service to be considered medically necessary, the following criteria must be met:
    ■ The procedure or service matches the diagnosis
    ■ The procedure or service is not experimental or investigational
    ■ The procedure or service is necessary
    ■ The procedure or service is provided at the most appropriate level that is safe and effective
    ■ The procedure or service is not elective.
    Discuss these five criteria.

49. What is the reason for the NCCI?

50. Identify two reasons for the use of the status indicator.

19 Hospital Outpatient and Inpatient Billing

Nanette Sayles

KEY TERMS

Your instructor may wish to select some words pertinent to this chapter for a test. For definitions of the terms, further study, and/or reference, the words, phrases, and abbreviations may be found in the glossary at the end of the Textbook. *Key terms for this chapter follow.*

72-hour rule
admission
admission review
against medical advice
ambulatory payment classifications
capitation
Case Mix Groups
chargemaster
concurrent review
complication
comorbidity
continued stay review
cost outlier
covered entity
diagnosis-related groups
discharge disposition
Discharge Not Final Billed
discounting
discussion
downcoding
DRG creep
gatekeeper
grouper
Health Insurance Portability and Accountability Act
hospital acquired condition
inpatient
Inpatient Prospective Payment System
Inpatient Psychiatric Facility Prospective Payment System
Inpatient Rehabilitation Facility Patient Assessment
    Instrument
Inpatient Rehabilitation Facility Prospective Payment System
inpatient only
International Classification of Diseases, Tenth Revision,
    Clinical Modification

International Classification of Diseases, Tenth Revision,
    Procedure Coding System
Long-Term Acute Care Hospital Prospective Payment System
major complication/comorbidity
major diagnostic categories
Medicare Administrative Contractor
observation
Outpatient Prospective Payment System
per diem
preadmission
preadmission testing
preauthorization
present on admission
principal diagnosis
prospective review
prospective payment system
Quality Improvement Organization
reason for encounter
relative weight
Resource-Based Relative Value Scale
retrospective review
revenue code
revenue cycle
Rehabilitation Impairment Category
self-pay
status indicator
swing bed
Tax Equity and Fiscal Responsibility Act of 1982
transaction set
upcoding
utilization management

KEY ABBREVIATIONS

See how many abbreviations and acronyms you can translate, and then use this as a handy reference list. Definitions for the key abbreviations are located near the back of the Text-book *in the glossary.*

ABN _____

AMA _____

ANSI _____

APC _____

ASC _____

CC _____

CE _____

CMG _____

CPT _____

DNFB _____

DRG _____

EMTALA _____

HAC _____

HIPAA _____

ICD-10-CM _____

ICD-10-PCS _____

IPO _____

IPF PPS _____

IPPS _____

IRF PAI _____

IRF PPS _____

LTCH _____

LTCH PPS _____

MAC _____

MCC _____

MDC _____

MS-DRG _____

OPPS _____

PA _____

PAT _____

POA _____

PPS _____

QIO _____

RBRVS _____

RICs _____

TEFRA _____

UB-04 _____

UM _____

PERFORMANCE OBJECTIVES

The student will be able to:

- Define and spell the key terms and key abbreviations for this chapter, given the information from the *Textbook* glossary, within a reasonable time period and with enough accuracy to obtain a satisfactory evaluation.
- After reading the chapter, answer the fill-in-the-blank, mix and match, multiple choice, and true/false review questions, with enough accuracy to obtain a satisfactory evaluation.
- Answer questions about the insurance verification process by reviewing a couple of health insurance cards within a reasonable time period and with enough accuracy to obtain a satisfactory evaluation.
- Explain the revenue cycle of hospital claims.
- Manage the Discharge Not Final Billed Report.
- Discuss the 72-hour rule.

- Explain utilization management and its role in the hospital reimbursement system.
- Explain the chargemaster.
- Explain the *International Classification of Diseases, Tenth Revision, Procedure Coding System* (ICD-10-PCS).
- Explain the role of *International Classification of Diseases,* Tenth Revision, Procedure Coding System (ICD-10-PCS) in hospital billing.
- Explain the role of Current Procedural Terminology in hospital billing.
- Explain the role of Health care Coding Procedural Coding System.
- Assign the present on admission indicator.
- Explain the reimbursement methods used when receiving reimbursement for Medicare hospital services.

STUDY OUTLINE

Revenue Cycle
Preadmission
   Preauthorization
   Inpatient Only List
Patient Care
   Utilization Management
   Posting Charges
   Chargemaster
   Discharge
Postadmission
   Coding
   Health Care Claim
   Receipt of Reimbursement
   Hospital Acquired Conditions
   Discharge Not Final Billed Report

Types of Reimbursement Methodologies
Medicare
   Medicare Administrative Contractor
   Quality Improvement Organizations
   Medicare Reimbursement Methodologies
   Acute Inpatient Prospective Payment System
   Hospital Outpatient Prospective Payment System
   Resource-Based Relative Value Scale
   Long Term Care Hospital Prospective Payment System
   Inpatient Rehabilitation Facility Prospective Payment System
   Psychiatric Prospective Payment System
   Ambulance Fee Schedule

293

Part I Fill in the Blank

Review the objectives, key terms, glossary definitions of key terms, chapter information, and figures before completing the following review questions.

1. _____ is the term used when the second procedure is paid at 50% of the APC rate.

2. In packaging, all of the supplies, medications and other services are _____ in the APC.

3. _____ is coding to a lower level than deserved.

4. _____ is the reimbursement that Medicare uses for observation services.

5. Additional reimbursement for the MS-DRG for teaching medical residents is known as a/an _____.

6. The diagnosis established after examination and listed for admission to the hospital for an illness or injury is called a/an _____ diagnosis.

7. A _____ is a diagnosis or condition that arises after admission that increases the patient's length of stay 75% of the time.

8. _____ are the basis of the IPPS.

9. _____ allows the hospital to bill for each service provided.

10. _____ is important when assigning the present on admission indicator.

PART II MIX AND MATCH

1. Match the words or phrases used for managed care reimbursement methods in the left column with the definitions in the right column. Write the correct letters in the blanks.

_____ Discharge disposition

_____ Revenue cycle

_____ Admission review

_____ TEFRA

_____ Admission

_____ Ambulatory payment classifications

_____ Observation patient

_____ 72-hour rule

_____ Preauthorization

_____ Upcoding

_____ Revenue code

_____ IPF PPS

_____ Capitation

_____ Interrupted stay

_____ Inpatient Rehabilitation Facility Patient Assessment Instrument

a. The basis for the OPPS

b. Location where patient is going after leaving the hospital

c. When patient is formally admitted for care

d. Timeframe when outpatient services are folded into inpatient claim

e. Flat rate provided to care for patient

f. Receiving reimbursement is the end result of this

g. Code used to group charges on health care claim

h. Reviews admission for appropriateness

i. Outpatient who stays overnight

j. Obtaining permission from insurer before service

k. The federal law that mandated the use of prospective payment systems for Medicare

l. Recertification is required at day 12 and at least every 30 days

m. Period where patient leaves hospital

n. Tool used in the IRF PPS

o. Coding to increase reimbursement over what is deserved.

Part III Multiple Choice

Choose the best answer.

1. The result of upcoding is:
   a. downcoding.
   b. DRG creep.
   c. bundling.
   d. packaging.

2. Identify the true statement about APCS.
   a. APCs are used for inpatient claims.
   b. The hospital can receive multiple APCs for a patient visit.
   c. APCs use the fee-for-service methodology
   d. APCs use a per diem reimbursement strategy.

3. The average relative weight is:
   a. 1.
   b. 1.0000.
   c. 1.5.
   d. 1.0.

4. A preexisting condition that will, because of its effect on the specific principal diagnosis, require more intensive therapy or cause an increase in length of stay (LOS) by at least 1 day in approximately 75% of cases is called a:
   a. chronic condition.
   b. coexisting condition.
   c. comorbidity.
   d. complication.

5. A chargemaster contains:
   a. a grouper.
   b. the IRF PAI.
   c. a revenue code.
   d. the DNFB report.

Part IV True/False

Write "T" or "F" in the blank to indicate whether you think the statement is true or false.

_____ 1. A short stay outliner in the LTCH PPS is 4/5 of the length of stay.

_____ 2. 75% of the patients at an inpatient rehabilitation facility must fall into specific conditions.

_____ 3. MS-DRGs are a three-tiered system.

Research the internet and identify 10 procedures that frequently require preauthorization from the insurer before completion.

ASSIGNMENT 19.3 CALCULATING MS-DRG

For each of the MS-DRGs identified, complete the table. Use the most current MS-DRG tables from the Centers for Medicare and Medicaid Services website and the information therein to calculate the MS-DRG reimbursement if the facility base rate is $4,022.00 and the add-on is $340.

MS-DRG	Relative Weight	Calculations
10		
61		
101		
206		
329		

ASSIGNMENT 19.4 APC DISCOUNTING

Determine which of the following is subject to discounting.

The status indicator legend can be found at: https://med.noridianmedicare.com/web/jea/provider-types/opps/opps-payment-status-indicators

SCENARIO 1

APC	Status Indicator	Subject to Discounting Yes/No
1	C	
2	S	
3	J1	
4	T	

ASSIGNMENT 19.5 CRITIQUE OF THE INPATIENT REHABILITATION FACILITY-PATIENT ASSESSMENT INSTRUMENT (IRF-PAI)

Review the IRF-PAI document found at: https://www.cms.gov/Medicare/Medicare-Fee-for-Service-Payment/InpatientRehabFacPPS/IRFPAI.html.

Critique the assessment instrument. What do you like about it? What do you dislike? What, if anything, on the assessment instrument surprised you? Use content from the book and the IRF-PAI to support your opinions.

20 Seeking a Job and Attaining Professional Advancement

Linda M. Smith

KEY TERMS

Your instructor may wish to select some words pertinent to this chapter for a test. For definitions of the terms, further study, and/or reference, the words, phrases, and abbreviations may be found in the glossary at the end of the textbook. *Key terms for this chapter follow.*

application form
auditor
blind mailing
business associate agreement
certification
Certified Coding Specialist
Certified Coding Specialist-Physician
Certified Medical Assistant
Certified Medical Billing Specialist
Certified Professional Coder
Chargemaster Coordinator
chronologic résumé
Clinical Documentation Improvement Specialist
claims assistance professional
coding specialist
combination résumé
compliance specialist

continuing education
cover letter
employment agencies
functional résumé
immigrant
interview
mentor
National Certified Insurance and Coding Specialist
networking
portfolio
Registered Medical Assistant
Registered Medical Coder
résumé
Revenue Cycle Manager
self-employment
service contract

KEY ABBREVIATIONS

See how many abbreviations and acronyms you can translate, and then use this as a handy reference list. Definitions for the key abbreviations are located near the back of the textbook *in the glossary.*

AAPC _____

AHIMA _____

CAP _____

CCAP _____

CCS _____

CCS-P _____

CECP _____

CMA _____

CMBS _____

CMRS _____

CPC _____

CPC-A _____

CPC-H _____

ECP _____

EEOC _____

HRS _____

NCICS _____

PAHCOM _____

RMA _____

RMC _____

USCIS _____

301

PERFORMANCE OBJECTIVES

The student will be able to:

- Define and spell the key terms and key abbreviations for this chapter, given the information from the *textbook* glossary, within a reasonable time period and with enough accuracy to obtain a satisfactory evaluation.
- After reading the chapter, answer the fill-in-the-blank, multiple choice, and true/false review questions with enough accuracy to obtain a satisfactory evaluation.
- Research information in preparation for creating a résumé, given a worksheet to complete, within a reasonable time period and with enough accuracy to obtain a satisfactory evaluation.
- Create an accurate résumé in a suitable font and print onto plain paper, within a reasonable time period, to obtain a satisfactory evaluation.

- Compose and print on plain paper a letter of introduction to go with the résumé and place it in a typed envelope, using one sheet of plain typing paper and a number 10 envelope, within a reasonable time period, to obtain a satisfactory evaluation.
- Complete an application form for a job, given an application for position form, within a reasonable time period and with enough accuracy to obtain a satisfactory evaluation.
- Compose and print a follow-up thank-you letter onto one sheet of plain paper. Print the address on a number 10 envelope, within a reasonable time period, to obtain a satisfactory evaluation.
- Access the internet and visit websites to research and/or obtain data, within a reasonable time period and with enough accuracy to obtain a satisfactory evaluation.

STUDY OUTLINE

Employment Opportunities
    Insurance Billing Specialist
    Advanced Job Opportunities
Professional Organizations
    Certification
Job Search
    Online Job Search
    Job Fairs
    Application
    Letter of Introduction
    Résumé
    Interview
    Follow-Up Letter

Self-Employment
    Setting Up an Office
    Finances to Consider
    Business Associate Under the Health Insurance Portability and Accountability Act
    Security and Equipment
    Marketing, Advertising, Promotion, and Public Relations
    Business Incubator
    Reassess and Continue With Success
Attaining Professional Advancement
    Networking
    Find a Mentor
Procedure 20.1: Creating an Electronic Résumé

ASSIGNMENT 20.1 REVIEW QUESTIONS

Part I Fill in the Blank

Review the objectives, key terms, glossary definitions of key terms, chapter information, and figures before completing the following review questions.

1. Name three job titles that the insurance billing specialist may find advertised.

   a. _____

   b. _____

   c. _____

2. A _____ specialist works with physicians and other health care professionals to ensure that the documentation in the health record is complete and granular.

3. The process of earning a credential through a professional organization by gaining advanced education and experience is known as _____.

4. You have just completed a 1-year medical insurance billing course at a college. Name some preliminary job search contacts to make on campus.

   a. _____

   b. _____

   c. _____

   d. _____

5. When completing a job application form, the first step should be _____.
   Why? _____

6. Name skills that may be listed on an application form or in a résumé when a person is seeking a position as an insurance billing specialist.

   a. _____

   b. _____

   c. _____

   d. _____

   e. _____

   f. _____

7. A question appears on a job application form about salary. Two ways in which to handle this question are:

   a. _____

   b. _____

8. State the chief purpose of a cover letter when a résumé is sent to a prospective employer.

   _____

9. What information may be omitted from a résumé, under the Civil Rights Act of 1964, informed by the EEOC?

   _____

10. A/an _____ is a formal consultation with an employer to evaluate the qualifications of a prospective job applicant.

11. List the items to be compiled in a portfolio.

    a. _____

    b. _____

    c. _____

    d. _____

    e. _____

    f. _____

    g. _____

    h. _____

    i. _____

12. You are being interviewed for a job and the interviewer asks this question: "What is your religious preference?" How would you respond?

    _____

    _____

13. If a short period of time elapses after an interview and the applicant has received no word from the prospective employer, what follow-up steps may be taken?

    a. _____

    b. _____

14. If an individual creates a billing company and coding services are to be part of the offerings, the coding professional should have what type of professional status?

    _____

15. When considering self-employment, remember that the key to a successful business is to begin with a _____.

16. Hugh Beason was the owner of XYZ Medical Reimbursement Service. A fire occurred, damaging some of the equipment and part of the office premises requiring him to stop working for a month so that repairs could be made. What type/types of insurance would be helpful for this kind of problem?

    _____

17. A document that outlines the obligations of a billing service and a health care organization stating the responsible party for each specific duty and task is a/an

    _____.

18. List three methods a self-employed insurance billing specialist may use to price their services.

a. _____

b. _____

c. _____

19. A business _____ is an environment that grows and nurtures small businesses in their early years of existence by offering a wide range of business assistance and shared resources.

20. Gwendolyn Stevens has an insurance billing company and is attending a professional meeting where she has given business cards to a few attendees. Give two reasons for using this business marketing strategy.

a. _____

b. _____

21. Give the names of at least two national organizations that certify billers and coders.

a. _____

b. _____

Part II Multiple Choice

Choose the best answer.

22. A résumé format that emphasizes work experience dates is known as:
    a. functional.
    b. combination.
    c. business.
    d. chronologic.

23. When an individual plans to start an insurance billing company, he or she should have enough funds to operate the business for a period of:
    a. 6 months or more.
    b. 18 months or more.
    c. 1 year or more.
    d. 2 years.

24. Under Health Insurance Portability and Accountability Act (HIPAA) regulations, if a physician's insurance billing is outsourced to a person, this individual

    is known as a/an _____ because he or she uses and discloses individuals' identifiable health information.
    a. billing specialist
    b. business associate
    c. outside contractor
    d. outside vendor

25. When insurance billing is outsourced to a company, a document should be created, signed, and notarized by both parties; it is known as a:
    a. contract agreement.
    b. business agreement.
    c. service contract.
    d. legal contract.

26. A guide who offers advice, criticism, and guidance to an inexperienced person to help him or her reach a goal is known as a/an:
    a. mentor.
    b. counselor.
    c. associate.
    d. instructor.

Part III True/False

Write "T" or "F" in the blank to indicate whether you think the statement is true or false.

_____ 27. A résumé format that stresses job skills is known as functional.

_____ 28. When job applicants have similar skills and education, surveys have shown that hiring by employers has been based on bilingual skills.

_____ 29. Enhancing knowledge and keeping up-to-date are responsibilities of an insurance billing specialist.

_____ 30. Professional status of an insurance billing specialist may be obtained by passing a national examination for a Certified Medical Reimbursement Specialist (CMRS).

_____ 31. To earn the status of a claims assistance professional, this may be obtained by passing a national examination as a certified coding specialist (CCS).

Performance Objective

Task: Read these job advertisements. Then read the interests and abilities of the applicants to decide which job title belongs to each job hunter.

Conditions: Use the job advertisements and pen or pencil.

Standards: Time: _____ minutes

Accuracy: _____

(Note: The time element and accuracy criteria may be given by your instructor.)

Directions: These advertisements appeared in your local newspaper. Read the ads and then read the interests and abilities of each job applicant. Insert the job title for each applicant.

Job Titles

Insurance Biller	Insurance Coder	Bilingual Collections Manager
HS grad, computer exp, typing 40 wpm needed for busy output clinic, insurance claims knowledge	Detail-oriented individual, Dx and proc coder. 2 years exp preferred	Self-motivated individual with good communications skills. Bilingual. Enjoys working in health care.

Trudy

Trudy is bilingual in English and Spanish and enjoys working with people. She is especially good with the telephone and likes communications.

Job Title: _____

Walter

Walter wants to work in the health care field. He has taken diagnostic and procedure coding classes and enjoys problem solving.

Job Title: _____

Ilona

Ilona has experience with inputting patient data and transmitting insurance claims. She says she is honest and dependable.

Job Title: _____

Performance Objective

Task: Respond to a job advertisement by completing a worksheet and typing a résumé by abstracting data from your worksheet.

Conditions: Use two sheets of plain typing paper, a newspaper advertisement (Fig. 20.1), and a computer.

Standards: Time: _____ minutes

Accuracy: _____

(Note: The time element and accuracy criteria may be given by your instructor.)

Directions: An advertisement appeared in your local newspaper (see Fig. 20.1). You decide to apply for the position. Complete a worksheet in preparation for typing your résumé. Some of the information requested on the worksheet should not appear on the résumé but should be available if you are asked to provide it. Ask a classmate to review and comment about the information in your worksheet. Extract data that you think are relevant from the worksheet, and type a rough draft of your résumé. Ask the instructor for suggestions to improve the rough draft. Refer to Chapter 20 and Fig. 20.6 in the textbook to help organize your résumé into an attractive format before you type the final copy.

1. Insert title of personal data sheet from worksheet.

2. Insert heading: name, address, telephone number, and so on.

3. Select one of three formats for data.

4. Insert heading and data for education information.

5. Insert heading and data for skill information.

6. Insert heading and data for employment information.

7. Insert reference information.

8. Proofread résumé.

9. Print résumé.

MEDICAL INSURANCE CODING/REIMBURSEMENT SPECIALIST

Mid-Atlantic Clinic, a 20-physician, multi-specialty group practice in Chicago, Illinois, has a need for a coding and reimbursement specialist. Knowledge of medical terminology, CPT and ICD-9-CM coding systems, Medicare regulations, third-party insurance reimbursement, and physician billing procedures required. Proficiency in the interpretation and coding of procedural and diagnostic codes is strongly preferred. Successful candidates must have excellent communication and problem-solving skills. This position offers a competitive salary and superior benefits. Please send resume to:

George B. Pason, Personnel Director
Mid-Atlantic Clinic
1230 South Main Street
Chicago, IL 60611

Fig. 20.1

ASSIGNMENT 20.4 COMPLETE A COVER LETTER

Performance Objective

Task: Compose a cover letter to accompany your résumé.

Conditions: Use one sheet of plain typing paper, a number 10 envelope, computer, printer, thesaurus, and English dictionary.

Standards: Time: _____ minutes

               Accuracy: _____

               (Note: The time element and accuracy criteria may be given by your instructor.)

Directions: Compose a cover letter introducing yourself, and create a rough draft. Consult the instructor for suggestions. Print the cover letter on plain bond paper in a form that can be mailed. Refer to the sample letter in Chapter 20 and Fig. 20.5 in the textbook as a guide to help organize your thoughts. Type the name and address of the employer on a number 10 envelope, and insert the letter with the résumé from Assignment 20.3.

ASSIGNMENT 20.5 COMPLETE A JOB APPLICATION FORM

Performance Objective

Task: Complete a job application form by using data from your résumé.

Conditions: Use an application form (Fig. 20.2), your résumé, and a computer.

Standards: Time: _____ minutes

               Accuracy: _____

               (Note: The time element and accuracy criteria may be given by your instructor.)

Directions: Assume that the employer asked you to come to his or her place of business to complete an application form and make an appointment for an interview. Using your data and résumé, complete an application form (see Fig. 20.2).

APPLICATION FOR POSITION/ Medical or Dental Office
AN EQUAL OPPORTUNITY EMPLOYER

(In answering questions, use extra blank sheet if necessary)

No employee, applicant, or candidate for promotion training or other advantage shall be discriminated against (or given preference) because of race, color, religion, sex, age, physical handicap, veteran status, or national origin.
PLEASE READ CAREFULLY AND WRITE OR PRINT ANSWERS TO ALL QUESTIONS. DO NOT TYPE.

Date of application

A. PERSONAL INFORMATION

Name- Last	First	Middle	Social Security No.	Area Code/Phone No. ( )

Present Address: -Street	(Apt. #)	City	State	Zip	How long at this address?

Previous Address: -Street	CIty	State	Zip	Person to notify in case of Emergency or Accident - Name:
From:	To:			Address:	Telephone:

B. EMPLOYMENT INFORMATION

For what position are you applying?	☐ Full-time ☐ Part-time ☐ Either	Date available for employment?:	Wage/Salary Expectations:

List hrs./days you prefer to work:	List any hrs./days you are not available: (Except for times required for religious practices or observances)	Can you work overtime, if necessary? ☐ Yes ☐ No

Are you employed now? ☐ Yes ☐ No

If so, may we inquire of your present employer? ☐ No ☐ Yes, If yes:

Name of employer:

Phone number: ( )

Have you ever been bonded? ☐ Yes ☐ No

If required for position, are you bondable? ☐ Yes ☐ No ☐ Uncertain

Have you applied for a position with this office before? ☐ No ☐ Yes, If yes, when?:

Referred by/ or where did you hear of this job?:

Can you, upon employment, submit verification of your legal right to work in the United States? ☐ Yes ☐ No
Submit proof that you meet legal age requirement for employment? ☐ Yes ☐ No

Language(s) applicant speaks or writes (if use of a language other than English is relevant to the job for which applicant is applying):

C. EDUCATIONAL HISTORY

Name and address of schools attended (Include current)	Dates From	Thru	Highest grade/level completed	Diploma/degree(s) obtained/areas of study:
High school				
College				Degree/Major
Post graduate				Degree/Major
Other				Course/Diploma/License Certificate

Specific training, education, or experiences which will assist you in the job for which you have applied:

Future educational plans:

D. SPECIAL SKILLS

CHECK BELOW THE KINDS OF WORK YOU HAVE DONE:

☐ BLOOD COUNTS	☐ DENTAL ASSISTANT	☐ MEDICAL INSURANCE FORMS	☐ RECEPTIONIST
☐ BOOKKEEPING	☐ DENTAL HYGIENIST	☐ MEDICAL TERMINOLOGY	☐ TELEPHONES
☐ COLLECTIONS	☐ FILING	☐ MEDICAL TRANSCRIPTION	☐ TYPING
☐ COMPOSING LETTERS	☐ INJECTIONS	☐ NURSING	☐ STENOGRAPHY
☐ COMPUTER INPUT	☐ INSTRUMENT STERILIZATION	☐ PHLEBOTOMY (Draw Blood)	☐ URINALYSIS
OFFICE EQUIPMENT USED: ☐ COMPUTER	☐ DICTATING EQUIPMENT	☐ POSTING	☐ X-RAY
		☐ WORD PROCESSOR	☐ OTHER:

Other kinds of tasks performed or skills that may be applicable to position:

Typing speed:

Shorthand speed:

(PLEASE COMPLETE OTHER SIDE)

Fig. 20.2

E. EMPLOYMENT RECORD

LIST MOST RECENT EMPLOYMENT FIRST   May we contact your previous Employer(s) for a reference? ☐ yes ☐ no

1) Employer	Work performed. Be specific.
Address Street City State Zip code	
Phone number ( )	
Type of business / Dates Mo. Yr. Mo. Yr. From To	
Your position / Hourly rate/Salary Starting Final	
Supervisor's name	
Reason for leaving	

2) Employer	Work performed. Be specific.
Address Street City State Zip code	
Phone number ( )	
Type of business / Dates Mo. Yr. Mo. Yr. From To	
Your position / Hourly rate/Salary Starting Final	
Supervisor's name	
Reason for leaving	

3) Employer	Work performed. Be specific.
Address Street City State Zip code	
Phone number ( )	
Type of business / Dates Mo. Yr. Mo. Yr. From To	
Your position / Hourly rate/Salary Starting Final	
Supervisor's name	
Reason for leaving	

F. REFERENCES: FRIENDS/ACQUAINTANCES NON-RELATED

1) _____
   Name   Address   Telephone Number (☐ Work ☐ Home)   Occupation   Years acquainted
2) _____
   Name   Address   Telephone Number (☐ Work ☐ Home)   Occupation   Years acquainted

Please feel free to add any information which you feel will help us consider you for employment.

READ THE FOLLOWING CAREFULLY, THEN SIGN AND DATE THE APPLICATION

I certify that all answers given by me on this application are true, correct and complete to the best of my knowledge. I acknowledge notice that the information contained in this application is subject to check. I agree that, if hired, my continued employment may be contingent upon the accuracy of that information. If employed, I further agree to comply with company/office rules and regulations.

Signature _____ Date: _____

RM NO. 72-110   ©1976 BIBBERO SYSTEMS INC.   PETALUMA, CA (MB-CO) # 6-7 (REV. 4/92)   TO REORDER CALL 800-BIBBERO (800) 242-2376

Fig. 20.2, cont'd

ASSIGNMENT 20.6 PREPARE A FOLLOW-UP THANK-YOU LETTER

Performance Objective

Task: Prepare a follow-up thank-you letter after the interview, sending it to the interviewer.

Conditions: Use one sheet of plain typing paper, a number 10 envelope, computer, printer, thesaurus, and English dictionary.

Standards: Time: _____ minutes

              Accuracy: _____

              (Note: The time element and accuracy criteria may be given by your instructor.)

Directions: After the interview, you decide to send a follow-up thank-you letter to the person who interviewed you. Compose a letter and address a number 10 envelope. Refer to Chapter 20 and Fig. 20.11 in the handook to help organize your thoughts.

ASSIGNMENT 20.7 VISIT WEBSITES FOR JOB OPPORTUNITIES

Performance Objective

Task: Access the internet and visit several websites.

Conditions: Use a computer with a printer and/or a pen or pencil to make notes.

Standards: Time: _____ minutes

             Accuracy: _____

             (Note: The time element and accuracy criteria may be given by your instructor.)

Directions: Visit at least five websites by using either a search engine (Yahoo, Google, Bing) or a job-search website. Some suggestions are:

www.healthcarejobs.org
www.indeed.com
www.juju.com
www.topusajobs.com
www.monster.com

Enter a keyword or job title, such as "medical billing specialist" or "medical coder." Enter your city and state to locate listings near you. Click on the search button. If you get some results, print the listings that appeal to you for sharing and discussing in class.

Performance Objective

Task: Write a paragraph describing the benefits of becoming certified in this field.

Conditions: Use a computer with printer and/or a pen or pencil.

Standards: Time: _____ minutes

Accuracy: _____

(Note: The time element and accuracy criteria may be given by your instructor.)

Directions: Write a paragraph or two describing why you would like to become certified in this field, and incorporate a numbered list of benefits. Make sure grammar, punctuation, and spelling are correct.

Tests

TEST 1: PROCEDURE (E/M AND MEDICINE SECTIONS) AND DIAGNOSTIC PROCEDURE CODE TEST

Directions: Using a *Current Procedural Terminology* (CPT) code book insert the correct code numbers and modifiers for each service rendered. Give a brief description for each professional service rendered. An optional exercise is to abstract the pertinent data from each case, then use the *International Classification of Diseases*, Tenth Revision, Clinical Modifications (ICD-10-CM) code book to insert the diagnosis code.

Insert year of the CPT code book used:

_____

Insert year of the ICD-10-CM code book used:

_____

1. Dr. Input sees a new patient, Mrs. Post, in the office for acute abdominal distress. The physician spends approximately 1 hour obtaining a comprehensive history and physical examination with high-complexity decision making. Several diagnostic studies are ordered, and Mrs. Post is given an appointment to return in 1 week.

Description

_____ CPT # _____

_____ ICD-10-CM # _____

2. Mr. Nakahara, an established patient, sees Dr. Practon in the office on January 11 for a reevaluation of his type 2 diabetic condition. Dr. Practon takes a detailed history and performs a detailed examination. Decision making is moderately complex.

Description

_____ CPT # _____

_____ ICD-10-CM # _____

3. Dr. Cardi sees Mrs. Franklin for a follow-up office visit for her hypertension. A problem-focused history and examination of her cardiovascular system are obtained and reveal a blood pressure of 140/100. Decision making is straightforward, with medication being prescribed. The patient is advised to return in 2 weeks to have her blood pressure checked by the nurse. Mrs. Franklin returns 2 weeks later, and the nurse checks her blood pressure.

Description

_____	CPT # _____
_____	ICD-10-CM # _____
_____	CPT # _____
_____	ICD-10-CM # _____

4. Dr. Skeleton receives a call at 7 PM from Mrs. Snyder. Her husband, a patient of Dr. Skeleton's, has been very ill for 2 hours with profuse vomiting. Dr. Skeleton goes to their home to see Mr. Snyder and spends considerable time obtaining a detailed history and examination. The medical decision making is of a highly complex nature. The physician administers an injection of prochlorperazine (Compazine).

Description

_____	CPT # _____
_____	CPT # _____
_____	ICD-10-CM # _____

5. Dr. Cutis sees an established patient, a registered nurse, for determination of pregnancy. A detailed history and examination are obtained, with moderate-complexity medical decision making. A Papanicolaou smear is taken, a blood sample is drawn, and the specimens are sent to an independent laboratory for a qualitative human chorionic gonadotropin (hCG) test. The patient also complains of something she has discovered under her armpit. On examination, there is a furuncle of the left axilla, which is incised and drained during this visit. The laboratory requires CPT coding on the laboratory requisition. List how these laboratory procedures would appear on the requisition sheet. The Papanicolaou smear is processed according to the Bethesda System and under physician supervision.

Professional Service Rendered by Dr. Cutis

_____	CPT # _____
_____	CPT # _____
_____	CPT # _____
_____	CPT # _____
_____	ICD-10-CM # _____
_____	ICD-10-CM # _____

Laboratory Service on Requisition Sheet

_____	CPT # _____
_____	CPT # _____

6. Dr. Antrum makes a house call on Betty Mason, an established patient, for a problem-focused history of acute otitis media. A problem-focused examination is performed, with straightforward medical decision making. While there, Dr. Antrum also sees Betty's younger sister, Sandra, whom she has seen previously in the office, for acute tonsillitis. A problem-focused history and examination are performed with low-complexity decision making. In addition to the examinations, Dr. Antrum gives both children injections of penicillin.

Professional Service Rendered to Betty

_____ CPT # _____

_____ CPT # _____

_____ ICD-10-CM # _____

Professional Service Rendered to Sandra

_____ CPT # _____

_____ CPT # _____

_____ ICD-10-CM # _____

7. Two weeks later, Dr. Antrum is called to the emergency department at College Hospital at 2 AM on Sunday to see Betty Mason for recurrent chronic otitis media with suppuration. A problem-focused history and examination are performed with straightforward decision making. Dr. Antrum administers a second injection of penicillin.

Description

_____ CPT # _____

_____ CPT # _____

_____ CPT # _____

_____ ICD-10-CM # _____

8. While at the hospital, Dr. Antrum is asked to see another patient in the emergency department, who is new to her. A problem-focused history is taken. She performs a problem-focused examination and straightforward decision making for an intermediate 3.5 cm laceration of the scalp. The laceration is sutured, and the patient is advised to come to the office in 4 days for a dressing change. Four days later, the patient comes into the office for a dressing change by the nurse.

Description

_____ CPT # _____

_____ CPT # _____

_____ ICD-10-CM # _____

9. Dr. Menter, a psychiatrist, sees the following patients in the hospital. Code each procedure.

Ms. Blake: consultation, expanded problem-focused history and examination and straightforward decision making; referred by Dr. Practon

CPT # _____

Mrs. Clark: group psychotherapy (50 min)

CPT # _____

Mrs. Samson: group psychotherapy (50 min)

CPT # _____

Mr. Shoemaker: group psychotherapy (50 min)

CPT # _____

Miss James: individual psychotherapy (25 min)

CPT # _____

10. Dr. Input, a gastroenterologist, sees Mrs. Chan in the hospital at the request of Dr. Practon for an esophageal ulcer. In addition to the detailed history and examination and the low-complexity decision making, Dr. Input performs a flexible, transoral esophagogastroduodenoscopy with washings. Two days later, he sees Mrs. Chan in a follow-up hospital visit and obtains a problem-focused interval history and examination with low-complexity decision making.

Description

_____ CPT # _____

_____ CPT # _____

_____ ICD-10-CM # _____

_____

_____ CPT # _____

_____ ICD-10-CM # _____

11. Mrs. Galati, a new patient, goes to Dr. Cardi because of chest pain (moderate to severe), weakness, fatigue, and dizziness. Dr. Cardi takes a comprehensive history and performs a comprehensive examination, followed by a treadmill ECG with interpretation and report. He also performs a vital capacity test and dipstick urinalysis, and draws blood for triiodothyronine (T_3) testing and for analysis by sequential multiple analyzer computer (SMAC) (16 panel tests, including complete blood cell count [CBC]), which are sent to and billed by a laboratory. Medical decision making is of high complexity.

Description

_____ CPT # _____

_____ CPT # _____

_____ CPT # _____

_____ CPT # _____

_____ CPT # _____

_____ CPT # _____

_____ ICD-10-CM # _____

_____ ICD-10-CM # _____

_____ ICD-10-CM # _____

12. Jake Wonderhill has not had his eyes examined by Dr. Lenser for about 5 years. He is seen by Dr. Lenser, who performs the following ophthalmologic procedures in addition to a comprehensive eye examination: fluorescein angioscopy and electroretinography. Mr. Wonderhill receives a diagnosis of retinitis pigmentosa.

Description

_____ CPT # _____

_____ CPT # _____

_____ CPT # _____

_____ ICD-10-CM # _____

13. Dr. Practon is making rounds at the College Hospital and answers an urgent call on Third Floor East. He performs cardiopulmonary resuscitation on Mr. Sanchez for cardiac arrest and orders the patient taken to the critical care unit. Chest radiographs, laboratory work, blood gas measurements, and ECG are performed. The physician is detained 2 hours in constant attendance on the patient.

Description

_____ CPT # _____

_____ CPT # _____

_____ CPT # _____

_____ ICD-10-CM # _____

14. Mrs. Powers, a new patient, sees Dr. Skeleton for low sciatica. Dr. Skeleton takes a detailed history and performs a detailed examination of the patient's lower back and extremities. Medical decision making is of low complexity. Diathermy (30 minutes) is given. The next day the patient comes in for therapeutic exercises in the Hubbard tank (30 minutes).

Description

_____ CPT # _____

_____ CPT # _____

_____ ICD-10-CM # _____

_____ CPT # _____

_____ ICD-10-CM # _____

15. a. Mrs. Garcia, a new patient, is seen by Dr. Caesar for occasional vaginal spotting (detailed history/examination and low-complexity decision making). The doctor determines that the bleeding is coming from the cervix and asks her to return in 3 days for cryocauterization of the cervix. During the initial examination, Mrs. Garcia asks for an evaluation for possible infertility. Dr. Caesar advises her to wait 2 to 3 weeks and make an appointment for two infertility tests.

   b. When the patient returns in 3 days for cryocauterization, the doctor also takes a wet mount for bacteria/fungi, which is sent to and billed by a laboratory.

   c. Three weeks later, an injection procedure for hysterosalpingography and endometrial biopsy are performed.

Description

a. _____   CPT # _____

   _____   ICD-10-CM # _____

b. _____   CPT # _____

   _____   CPT # _____

   _____   ICD-10-CM # _____

c. _____   CPT # _____

   _____   CPT # _____

   _____   ICD-10-CM # _____

Multiple Choice

After reading the boxed codes with descriptions, select the answer/answers that is/are best in each case.

59120	surgical treatment of ectopic pregnancy; tubal or ovarian, requiring salpingectomy and/or oophorectomy, abdominal or vaginal approach
59121	tubal or ovarian, without salpingectomy and/or oophorectomy
59130	abdominal pregnancy
59135	interstitial, uterine pregnancy requiring total hysterectomy
59136	interstitial, uterine pregnancy with partial resection of uterus
59140	cervical, with evacuation

16. In regard to this section of CPT codes, which of the following statements is true about codes 59120 through 59140? Mark all that apply.
    a. They refer to abdominal hysterotomy.
    b. They involve laparoscopic treatment of ectopic pregnancy.
    c. They refer to treatment of ectopic pregnancy by surgery.
    d. They involve tubal ligation.

17. In regard to this section of CPT codes, for treatment of a tubal ectopic pregnancy, necessitating oophorectomy, the code to select is
    a. 59121.
    b. 59120.
    c. 59135.
    d. 59136.
    e. 59130.

18. In regard to this section of CPT codes, for treatment of an ectopic pregnancy (interstitial, uterine) requiring a total hysterectomy, the code/codes to select is/are
    a. 59135.
    b. 59135 and 59120.
    c. 59120.
    d. 59130 and 59120.
    e. 59121.

Directions: Match the description given in the right column with the procedure code/modifier combination in the left column. Write the letter in the blank.

Procedure With Modifier

1. 99214-25   _____

2. 99204-57   _____

3. 58150-80   _____

4. 32440-55   _____

5. 72080-26   _____

6. 29425-58   _____

7. 54640-50   _____

8. 99253-24   _____

Description

a. Dr. Practon assisted Dr. Caesar with a total abdominal hysterectomy and bilateral salpingo-oophorectomy.

b. Dr. Skeleton interprets a thoracolumbar x-ray film that was taken at College Hospital.

c. Mrs. Ulwelling saw Dr. Antrum for an office visit as a new patient, and she recommended that the patient undergo a laryngoscopy, with stripping of vocal cords to be done the following day.

d. Mrs. Gillenbach walked through a plate glass window and underwent a rhinoplasty, performed by Dr. Graff on February 16, 20xx. On February 26, 20xx, she came to see Dr. Graff for a consultation regarding reconstructive surgery on her right leg.

e. An established patient, Mrs. Mercado, is seen in a follow-up exam for type 2 diabetes. The patient asks Dr. Langerhans to look at some skin tags. The doctor examines them and says they need to be removed (11200). The evaluation and management service was detailed and of a moderate complexity.

f. Dr. Cutler performed a bilateral orchiopexy (inguinal approach) on baby Kozak.

g. Dr. Skeleton applied a short leg-walking cast to Mrs. Belchere's right leg 4 weeks after his initial treatment of her fractured tibia.

h. Dr. Cutler went on vacation, and Dr. Coccidioides took care of Mrs. Ash during the postoperative period after her total pneumonectomy.

Directions: Using a CPT code book, insert the correct code numbers and modifiers for each service rendered. Give a brief description for each professional service rendered.

9. Dr. Input performs a gastrojejunostomy for carcinoma in situ of the duodenum and calls in Dr. Scott to administer the anesthesia and Dr. Cutler to assist. This intraperitoneal surgery takes 2 hours, 30 minutes. The patient is otherwise normal and healthy. List the procedure and diagnostic code numbers with appropriate modifiers for each physician.

Professional Service Rendered by Dr. Input

_____   CPT # _____

_____   ICD-10-CM # _____

Professional Service Rendered by Dr. Scott

_____   CPT # _____

_____   ICD-10-CM # _____

Professional Service Rendered by Dr. Cutler

_____ CPT # _____

_____ ICD-10-CM # _____

10. Dr. Rumsey assists Dr. Cutler with a total colectomy (intraperitoneal procedure) with ileostomy. Dr. Scott is the anesthesiologist. Surgery takes 2 hours, 55 minutes. The patient has a secondary malignant neoplasm of the colon (severe systemic disease). List the procedure code numbers with appropriate modifiers and diagnostic code numbers for each physician.

Professional Service Rendered by Dr. Rumsey

_____ CPT # _____

_____ ICD-10-CM # _____

Professional Service Rendered by Dr. Scott

_____ CPT # _____

_____ ICD-10-CM # _____

Professional Service Rendered by Dr. Cutler

_____ CPT # _____

_____ ICD-10-CM # _____

11. Dr. Cutis removes a malignant tumor from a patient's back (1.5 cm) and does the local anesthesia herself.

Description

_____ CPT # _____

_____ ICD-10-CM # _____

12. Dr. Skeleton sees Mr. Richmond, a new patient worked into the office schedule on an emergency basis after a motor vehicle traffic accident with another car. Mr. Richmond has multiple lacerations of the face, arm, and chest and a fracture of the left tibia. The physician takes a comprehensive history and performs a comprehensive examination. Decision making is moderately complex. Dr. Skeleton orders bilateral radiographs of the tibia and fibula and two views of the chest and left wrist to be taken in his office. Then he closes the following lacerations: 2.6 cm, simple, face; 2.0 cm, intermediate, face; 7.5 cm, intermediate, right arm; 4.5 cm, intermediate, chest. All radiographs are negative except that of the left tibia. Dr. Skeleton performs a manipulative reduction of the left tibial shaft and applies a cast. Code this case as if you were actually listing the codes on the CMS-1500 claim form.

Description

_____ CPT # _____ and _____

_____ CPT # _____

_____ CPT # _____

_____ CPT # _____

_____ CPT # _____

_____ CPT # _____

_____ CPT # _____

_____ CPT # _____

_____ CPT # _____

_____ CPT # _____

_____ ICD-10-CM # _____

_____ ICD-10-CM # _____

_____ ICD-10-CM # _____

_____ ICD-10-CM # _____

_____ ICD-10-CM # _____

Six weeks later, Dr. Skeleton sees the same patient for an office visit and obtains radiographs (two views) of the left tibia and fibula. Treatment involves application of a cast below the patient's left knee to the toes, including a walking heel.

Description

_____ CPT # _____

_____ CPT # _____

_____ CPT # _____

_____ ICD-10-CM # _____

13. Dr. Cutler performs an incisional biopsy of a patient's breast for a breast lump, which requires 40 minutes of anesthesia. Dr. Scott is the anesthesiologist. The patient is otherwise normal and healthy. List the procedure and diagnostic code numbers for each physician.

Professional Service Rendered by Dr. Cutler

_____ CPT # _____

_____ ICD-10-CM # _____

Professional Service Rendered by Dr. Scott

_____ CPT # _____

_____ ICD-10-CM # _____

14. Mrs. DeBeau is aware that Dr. Input will be out of town for 6 weeks; however, she decides to have him perform the recommended combined anterior-posterior colporrhaphy with enterocele repair for vaginal enterocele. Dr. Practon agrees to perform the follow-up care and assist. Dr. Scott is the anesthesiologist. The anesthesia time is 2 hours, 15 minutes. The patient is normal and healthy. List the procedure and diagnostic code numbers for each physician. Note: Emphasis for this problem should be placed on the choice of CPT modifiers.

Professional Service Rendered by Dr. Input

_____ CPT # _____

_____ ICD-10-CM # _____

Professional Service Rendered by Dr. Practon

_____ CPT # _____

_____ CPT modifier _____

_____ CPT modifier _____

_____ ICD-10-CM # _____

Professional Service Rendered by Dr. Scott

_____ CPT # _____

_____ ICD-10-CM # _____

15. Mr. Wong, a new patient, is seen in the College Hospital and undergoes a comprehensive history and physical examination (H&P) with moderately complex decision making. Dr. Coccidioides performs a bronchoscopy with biopsy. Results of the biopsy confirm the diagnosis: malignant neoplasm of upper left lobe of lung. The following day the physician performs a total pneumonectomy. Dr. Cutler assists on the total pneumonectomy (pulmonary resection), and Dr. Scott is the anesthesiologist. Surgery takes 3 hours, 45 minutes. The patient has mild systemic disease. List the procedure and diagnostic code numbers for each physician.

Professional Service Rendered by Dr. Coccidioides

_____ CPT # _____

_____ CPT # _____

_____ CPT # _____

_____ ICD-10-CM # _____

Professional Service Rendered by Dr. Cutler

_____ CPT # _____

_____ ICD-10-CM # _____

Professional Service Rendered by Dr. Scott

_____ CPT # _____

_____ ICD-10-CM # _____

When completing the CMS-1500 claim form for Dr. Scott, in which block would you list anesthesia minutes? _____

327

Directions: Using a CPT code book, insert the correct procedure code numbers and modifiers and diagnostic codes for each service rendered. Give a brief description for each professional service rendered.

1. Mrs. Cahn sees Dr. Skeleton because of severe pain in her right shoulder. She is a new patient. Dr. Skeleton takes a detailed history and performs a detailed examination. A complete x-ray study of the right shoulder is done. Decision making is of low complexity. A diagnosis of bursitis is made, and an injection into the bursa is administered.

Description

_____ CPT # _____

_____ CPT # _____

_____ CPT # _____

_____ ICD-10-CM # _____

2. John Murphy comes into the Broxton Radiologic Group, Inc., for an extended radiation therapy consultation for prostatic cancer. The radiologist takes a detailed history and does a detailed examination. Decision making is of low complexity. The physician determines a simple treatment plan involving simple simulation-aided field settings. Basic dosimetry calculations are done, and the patient returns the following day and receives radiation therapy to a single treatment area (6 to 10 MeV).

Description

_____ CPT # _____

_____ CPT # _____

_____ CPT # _____

_____ CPT # _____

_____ CPT # _____

Diagnosis:

_____ ICD-10-CM # _____

3. Dr. Input refers Mrs. Horner to the Nuclear Medicine Department of the Broxton Radiologic Group, Inc., for a bone marrow imaging of the whole body, and imaging of the liver and spleen. List the procedure code numbers after each radiologic procedure to show how the radiology group would bill. Also, list the diagnosis of malignant neoplasm of the bone marrow.

Description

Total body bone marrow, imaging   CPT # _____

Radiopharmaceuticals, diagnostic (iodine I-123)   HCPCS # _____

Liver and spleen imaging   CPT # _____

Radiopharmaceuticals, diagnostic (iodine I-123)   HCPCS # _____

Diagnosis:

_____   ICD-10-CM # _____

4. Dr. Input also refers Mrs. Horner to XYZ Laboratory for the following tests. List the procedure code numbers to indicate how the laboratory would bill.

Description

CBC, automated, and automated differential   CPT # _____

Urinalysis, automated with microscopy   CPT # _____

Urine culture (quantitative, colony count)   CPT # _____

Urine antibiotic sensitivity (microtiter)   CPT # _____

5. The general laboratory at College Hospital receives a surgical tissue specimen (ovarian biopsy) for gross and microscopic examination from a patient with Stein-Leventhal syndrome. List the procedure and diagnostic code numbers to indicate what the hospital pathology department would bill.

Description

_____   CPT # _____

Diagnosis:

_____   ICD-10-CM # _____

6. Dr. Langerhans refers Jerry Cramer to XYZ Laboratory for a lipid panel. He has a family history of cardiovascular disease. List the procedure and diagnostic code number or numbers to indicate how the laboratory would bill.

Description

_____   CPT # _____

Diagnosis:

_____   ICD-10-CM # _____

7. Dr. Caesar is an OB/GYN specialist who has her own ultrasound machine. Carmen Cardoza, age 45, is referred to Dr. Caesar for an obstetric consultation and an amniocentesis with ultrasonic guidance. The diagnosis is Rh incompatibility. The doctor performs a detailed history and physical examination, and decision making is of low complexity.

Description

_____ CPT # _____

_____ CPT # _____

Diagnosis:

_____ ICD-10-CM # _____

8. Mr. Marcos's medical record indicates that a retrograde pyelogram followed by a percutaneous nephrostolithotomy, with basket extraction of a 1 cm stone, was performed by Dr. Ulibarri for nephrolithiasis.

Description

_____ CPT # _____

_____ CPT # _____

Diagnosis:

_____ ICD-10-CM # _____

9. Broxton Radiologic Group, Inc., performs the following procedures on Mrs. Stephens at the request of Dr. Input. List the procedure code numbers after each radiologic procedure. On the laboratory slip, the following congenital diagnoses are listed: diverticulum of the stomach and colon; cystic lung. Locate the corresponding diagnostic codes.

Barium enema   CPT # _____

Evaluation of upper gastrointestinal tract with small bowel   CPT # _____

Complete chest x-ray   CPT # _____

Diagnosis:

_____ ICD # _____

Diagnosis:

_____ ICD # _____

Diagnosis:

_____ ICD # _____

10. Two weeks later, Mrs. Stephens is referred again for further radiologic studies for flank pain. List the procedure and diagnostic code numbers after each radiologic procedure.

Intravenous pyelogram (IVP) with drip infusion   CPT # _____

Oral cholecystography   CPT # _____

Diagnosis:

_____   ICD # _____

TEST 4: COMPLETE A CMS-1500 CLAIM FORM

Performance Objective

Task: Complete a CMS-1500 claim form for a private case and post transactions to the patient's financial accounting record.

Conditions: Use the patient's record (Fig. 1) and financial statement (Fig. 2); one health insurance claim form; a computer or pen; procedural and diagnostic code books; and Appendix A in this *Workbook*.

Standards: Claim Productivity Management

Time: _____ minutes

Accuracy: _____

(Note: The time element and accuracy criteria may be given by your instructor.)

Directions:

1. Using NUCC guidelines, complete a CMS-1500 claim form and direct it to the private carrier. Refer to Jennifer T. Lacey's patient record for information and Appendix A in this *Workbook* to locate the fees to record on the claim, and post them to the financial statement. Date the claim August 15 of the current year. Dr. Caesar is accepting assignment, and the patient's signatures to release information to the insurance company and to have the payment forwarded directly to the physician are on file.

2. Use your CPT code book to determine the correct five-digit code numbers and modifiers for each professional service rendered. Use your HCPCS Level II code book for HCPCS procedure codes and modifiers. Use your ICD-10-CM coding manual to code each active diagnosis. Record the proper information on the financial record and claim form, and note the date that you billed the insurance company.

3. American Commercial Insurance Company sent a check (voucher number 5586) on November 17 in the amount of $880. The patient's responsibility is $220. Post the payment, write off (adjust) the remaining balance, and circle the amount billed to the patient.

PATIENT RECORD NO. T-4

Lacey	Jennifer	T.	11-12-55	F	555-549-0098
LAST NAME	FIRST NAME	MIDDLE NAME	BIRTH DATE	SEX	HOME PHONE

451 Roberts Street	Woodland Hills	XY	12345	
ADDRESS	CITY	STATE	ZIP CODE	

555-443-9899	555-549-0098		lacey@wb.net
CELL PHONE	PAGER NO.	FAX NO.	E-MAIL ADDRESS

430-XX-7709	Y0053498
PATIENT'S SOC. SEC. NO.	DRIVER'S LICENSE

legal secretary	Higgins and Higgins Attorneys at Law
PATIENT'S OCCUPATION	NAME OF COMPANY

430 Second Avenue, Woodland Hills, XY 12345	555-540-6675
ADDRESS OF EMPLOYER	PHONE

SPOUSE OR PARENT	OCCUPATION

		PHONE
EMPLOYER	ADDRESS	

American Commercial Insurance Company, 5682 Bendix Blvd., Woodland Hills, XY 12345	
NAME OF INSURANCE	INSURED OR SUBSCRIBER

5789022	444
POLICY/CERTIFICATE NO.	GROUP NO.

REFERRED BY: Clarence Cutler, MD

Fig. 1

DATE	PROGRESS NOTES No. T-4
8-1-xx	New pt referred by Dr. Cutler, came into office for consultation and additional opinion.
	CC: Full feeling in stomach and low abdominal region.
	Irregular menstruation. Ultrasonic report showed
	leiomyomata uteri and rt ovarian mass; however, visualization of mass poor and type
	cannot be identified. Pap smear Class I. No personal or family hx of CA.
	Comprehensive hx and physical examination performed on healthy appearing white female.
	Wt: 136 lbs. BP 128/60. T 98.6 F. Palpated rt adnexal mass and
	enlarged uterus; vulva and cervix appear normal; LMP 7/16/XX.
	Medical decision making: mod complex
	Tx plan: Adv hospital admit and additional tests to R/O carcinoma.
	Tentatively scheduled abdominal hysterectomy with bilateral salpingo-oophorectomy.
	(M/MDM).
	BC/llf *Bertha Caesar, MD*
8-2-xx	Adm to College Hosp (C HX/PX M/MDM). Scheduled
	surgery at 7:00 A.M. tomorrow.
	BC/llf *Bertha Caesar, MD*
8-3-xx	Perf abdominal
	hysterectomy with bilateral salpingo-oophorectomy.
	BC/llf *Bertha Caesar, MD*
8-4-xx	HV (EPF HX/PX M/MDM) Path report revealed interstitial leiomyomata uteri and corpus
	luteum cyst of rt ovary. Pt C/O PO pain, otherwise doing well.
	BC/llf *Bertha Caesar, MD*
8-5-xx	HV (EPF HX/PX M/MDM). Pt ambulating well, pain decreased. Dressing changed, wound
	healing well.
	BC/llf *Bertha Caesar, MD*
8-6-xx	HV (PF HX/PX SF/MDM). Pain minimal. Pt ambulating without assistance.
	Removed staples, no redness or swelling. Pln DC tomorrow.
	BC/llf *Bertha Caesar, MD*
8-7-xx	Discharge to home; pt doing well. RTO next wk. Disability from 8-1 to 8-23-xx.
	BC/llf *Bertha Caesar, MD*

Fig. 1, cont'd

STATEMENT
COLLEGE CLINIC
4567 Broad Avenue
Woodland Hills, XY 12345-0001
Tel. 555-486-9002
Fax No. 555-487-8976

Acct. No. T-4

Jennifer T. Lacey
451 Roberts Street
Woodland Hills, XY 12345

Phone No. (H)   (555) 549-0098   (W)   (555) 540-6675   Birthdate   11-12-55

Insurance Co.   American Commercial Insurance Company   Policy/Group No.   5789022 / 444

| DATE | REFERENCE | DESCRIPTION | CHARGES | CREDITS | | BALANCE |
				PYMNTS.	ADJ.	
20XX				BALANCE FORWARD ⟶		
8-1-xx		Consult				
8-2-xx		Admit				
8-3-xx		TAH BSO				
8-4-xx		HV				
8-5-xx		HV				
8-6-xx		HV				
8-7-xx		Discharge				

PLEASE PAY LAST AMOUNT IN BALANCE COLUMN

THIS IS A COPY OF YOUR FINANCIAL ACCOUNT AS IT APPEARS ON OUR RECORDS

Fig. 2

Tests

TEST 5: COMPLETE A CMS-1500 CLAIM FORM

Performance Objective

Task: Complete a CMS-1500 claim form for a private case and post transactions to the patient's financial accounting record.

Conditions: Use the patient's record (Fig. 3) and financial statement (Fig. 4), one health insurance claim form, a computer or pen, procedural and diagnostic code books, and Appendixes A in this *Workbook*.

Standards: Claim Productivity Management

Time: _____ minutes

Accuracy: _____

(Note: The time element and accuracy criteria may be given by your instructor.)

Directions

1. Using NUCC guidelines, complete a CMS-1500 claim form and direct it to the private carrier. Refer to Hortense N. Hope's patient record for information and Appendix A in this *Workbook* to locate the fees to record on the claim, and post them to the financial statement. Date the claim July 31 of the current year. Dr. Practon is accepting assignment, and the patient's signatures to release information to the insurance company and to have the payment forwarded directly to the physician are on file.

2. Use your CPT code book to determine the correct five-digit code numbers and modifiers for each professional service rendered. Use your HCPCS Level II code book for HCPCS procedure codes and modifiers. Use your ICD-10-CM coding manual to code each active diagnosis.

3. Record the proper information on the financial record and claim form, and note the date that you billed the insurance company.

PATIENT RECORD NO. T-5

Hope	Hortense	N.	04-12-56	F	555-666-7821
LAST NAME	FIRST NAME	MIDDLE NAME	BIRTH DATE	SEX	HOME PHONE

247 Lantern Pike	Woodland Hills	XY	12345
ADDRESS	CITY	STATE	ZIP CODE

	555-323-1687	555-666-7821	hope@wb.net
CELL PHONE	PAGER NO.	FAX NO.	E-MAIL ADDRESS

321-XX-8809   N0058921
PATIENT'S SOC. SEC. NO.   DRIVER'S LICENSE

Clerk typist   R and S Manufacturing Company
PATIENT'S OCCUPATION   NAME OF COMPANY

2271 West 74 Street, Torres, XY 12349 555-466-5890
ADDRESS OF EMPLOYER   PHONE

Harry J. Hope   carpenter
SPOUSE OR PARENT   OCCUPATION

Jesse Construction Company, 3861 South Orange Street, Torres, XY 12349 555-765-2318
EMPLOYER   ADDRESS   PHONE

Ralston Insurance Company, 2611 Hanley Street, Woodland Hills, XY 12345 Hortense N. Hope
NAME OF INSURANCE   INSURED OR SUBSCRIBER

ATC321458809   T8471811A
POLICY/CERTIFICATE NO.   GROUP NO.

REFERRED BY: Harry J. Hope (husband)

DATE	PROGRESS NOTES
7-1-xx	New F pt comes in complaining of lt great toe pain. Incised, drained, and cleaned area
	around nail on lt great toe. Dx: onychia and paronychia. Started on antibiotic and adv to
	retn in 2 days for permanent excision of nail plate (EPF HX/PX SF/MDM).
	GP/llf *Gerald Practon, MD*
7-3-xx	Pt returns for nail excision. Injected procaine in lt great toe; removed entire toenail.
	Drs applied. PTR in 5 days for PO check.
	GP/llf *Gerald Practon, MD*
7-7-xx	PO check. Dressing changed, nail bed healing well. Pt to continue on AB until gone.
	Retn PRN (PF HX/PX SF/MDM).
	GP/llf *Gerald Practon, MD*

Fig. 3

STATEMENT
Financial Account
COLLEGE CLINIC
4567 Broad Avenue
Woodland Hills, XY 12345-0001
Tel. 555-486-9002
Fax No. 555-487-8976

Hortense N. Hope
247 Lantern Pike
Woodland Hills, XY 12345

Phone No. (H) 555-666-7821 (W) 555-466-5890 Birthdate 4/12/56

Primary Insurance Co. Ralston Insurance Company Policy/Group No. ATC321458809 / T8471811A

Secondary Insurance Co. None Policy/Group No.

DATE	REFERENCE	DESCRIPTION	CHARGES	CREDITS PYMNTS.	ADJ.	BALANCE
20xx		BALANCE FORWARD ➔				
7-1-xx		NP OV				
7-1-xx		I & D lt great toe				
7-3-xx		Excision lt great toenail				
7-7-xx		PO check				

PLEASE PAY LAST AMOUNT IN BALANCE COLUMN

THIS IS A COPY OF YOUR FINANCIAL ACCOUNT AS IT APPEARS ON OUR RECORDS

Fig. 4

Performance Objective

Task: Complete a CMS-1500 claim form and post transactions to the patient's financial accounting record.

Conditions: Use the patient's record (Fig. 5) and financial statement (Fig. 6), one health insurance claim form, a computer or pen, procedural and diagnostic code books, and Appendix A in this *Workbook*.

Standards: Claim Productivity Management

Time: _____ minutes

Accuracy: _____

(Note: The time element and accuracy criteria may be given by your instructor.)

Directions

1. Using NUCC guidelines, complete a CMS-1500 claim form and direct it to your local Medicare Administrative Contractor. Refer to the CMS website to locate your local Medicare Administrative Contractor's address to mail the claim to. Refer to Frances F. Foote's patient record for information and Appendix A in this *Workbook* to locate the fees to record on the claim, and post them to the financial statement. Date the claim October 31 of the current year. Dr. Practon is a participating provider, and the patient's signatures to release information to the insurance company and to have the payment forwarded directly to the physician are on file.

2. Use your CPT code book to determine the correct five-digit code numbers and modifiers for each professional service rendered. Use your HCPCS Level II code book for HCPCS procedure codes and modifiers. Use your ICD-10-CM coding manual to code each active diagnosis.

3. Record the proper information on the patient's financial accounting record and claim form, and note the date that you billed the insurance company.

PATIENT RECORD NO. T-6

Foote	Frances	F.	08-10-32	F	555-678-0943
LAST NAME	FIRST NAME	MIDDLE NAME	BIRTH DATE	SEX	HOME PHONE

984 North A Street	Woodland Hills	XY	12345	
ADDRESS	CITY	STATE	ZIP CODE	

555-443-9908	555-320-7789	555-678-0943		foote@wb.net
CELL PHONE	PAGER NO.	FAX NO.		E-MAIL ADDRESS

578-XX-8924	B4309811
PATIENT'S SOC. SEC. NO.	DRIVER'S LICENSE

retired legal secretary	
PATIENT'S OCCUPATION	NAME OF COMPANY

ADDRESS OF EMPLOYER	PHONE

Harry L. Foote	roofer
SPOUSE OR PARENT	OCCUPATION

BDO Construction Company, 340 North 6th Street, Woodland Hills, XY 12345	555-478-9083
EMPLOYER ADDRESS	PHONE

Medicare	self
NAME OF INSURANCE	INSURED OR SUBSCRIBER

578-XX-8924A	
POLICY/CERTIFICATE NO.	GROUP NO.

REFERRED BY: G. U. Curette, MD, 4780 Main Street, Ehrlich, XY 12350 Tel: 555-430-8788   NPI #34216600XX

DATE	PROGRESS NOTES
10-11-xx	NP pt referred by Dr. Curette with a CC of foot pain centering around rt great toe and
	sometimes shooting up her leg. PF history taken. PF exam revealed severe overgrowth
	of nail into surrounding tissues. AP and lat right foot x-rays taken & interpreted which
	indicate no fractures or arthritis. Pt has had a N workup for gout by Dr. Curette.
	DX: Severe onychocryptosis both margins of rt hallux. Adv to sched. OP surgery at
	College Hospital for wedge resection of skin of nail fold to repair ingrown nail.
	No disability from work (SF/MDM).
	NP/llf *Nick Pedro, MD*
10-13-xx	Pt admitted for OP surgery at College Hospital. Complete wedge resection performed for
	repair of rt hallux ingrown nail. Pt will stay off foot over the weekend and retn next wk for
	PO re ch.
	NP/llf *Nick Pedro, MD*
10-20-xx	PO visit (PF HX/PX SF/MDM). Rt hallux healing well. RTC as necessary.
	NP/llf *Nick Pedro, MD*

Fig. 5

STATEMENT
Financial Account
COLLEGE CLINIC
4567 Broad Avenue
Woodland Hills, XY 12345-0001
Tel. 555-486-9002
Fax No. 555-487-8976

Frances F. Foote
984 North A Street
Woodland Hills, XY 12345

Phone No. (H)   555-678-0943   (W) _____   Birthdate _____ 8/10/32

Primary Insurance Co. _____ Medicare _____   Policy/Group No. ___ 578-XX-8924A

| DATE | REFERENCE | DESCRIPTION | CHARGES | CREDITS | | BALANCE |
				PYMNTS.	ADJ.	
20xx		BALANCE FORWARD ➤				
10-11-xx		NP OV				
10-11-xx		X-rays				
10-13-xx		Wedge excision/skin of nail fold				
10-20-xx		PO				

PLEASE PAY LAST AMOUNT IN BALANCE COLUMN ⇧

THIS IS A COPY OF YOUR FINANCIAL ACCOUNT AS IT APPEARS ON OUR RECORDS

Fig. 6

TEST 7: COMPLETE A CLAIM FORM FOR A MEDICARE/MEDIGAP CASE

Performance Objective

Task: Complete two CMS-1500 claim forms for a Medicare/Medigap case and post transactions to the patient's financial accounting record.

Conditions: Use patient's record (Fig. 7) and financial statement (Fig. 8), two health insurance claim forms, a computer or pen, procedural and diagnostic code books, and Appendix A in this *Workbook*.

Standards: Claim Productivity Management

Time: _____ minutes

Accuracy: _____

(Note: The time element and accuracy criteria may be given by your instructor.)

Directions

1. Using NUCC guidelines, complete two CMS-1500 claim forms and direct them to your local Medicare Administrative Contractor. Refer to the CMS website to locate your local Medicare Administrative Contractor's address to mail the claim to. Refer to Charles B. Kamb's patient record for information and Appendix A to locate the fees to record on the claim, and post them to the financial statement. Be sure to include the Medigap information on the claim form so that it will be crossed over (sent to the Medigap insurance carrier) automatically. Date the claim June 30 of the current year. Dr. Practon is a participating provider with both Medicare and the Medigap program, and the patient's signatures to release information to the insurance companies and to have the payment forwarded directly to the physician are on file.

2. Use your CPT code book to determine the correct five-digit code numbers and modifiers for each professional service rendered. Use your HCPCS Level II code book for HCPCS procedure codes and modifiers. Use your ICD-10-CM coding manual to code each active diagnosis.

3. Record the proper information on the patient's financial accounting record and claim form, and note the date that you billed the insurance company.

PATIENT RECORD NO. T-7

Kamb	Charles	B.	01-26-27	M	555-467-2601
LAST NAME	FIRST NAME	MIDDLE NAME	BIRTH DATE	SEX	HOME PHONE

2600 West Nautilus Street	Woodland Hills	XY	12345
ADDRESS	CITY	STATE	ZIP CODE

			E-MAIL ADDRESS
CELL PHONE	PAGER NO.	FAX NO.	

454-XX-9569	M3200563
PATIENT'S SOC. SEC. NO.	DRIVER'S LICENSE

retired TV actor	Amer. Federation of TV & Radio Artists (AFTRA)
PATIENT'S OCCUPATION	NAME OF COMPANY

30077 Ventura Boulevard, Woodland Hills, XY 12345	555-466-3331
ADDRESS OF EMPLOYER	PHONE

Jane C. Kamb	homemaker
SPOUSE OR PARENT	OCCUPATION

		PHONE
EMPLOYER	ADDRESS	

Medicare (Primary)	self	National Insurance Company (Medigap)
NAME OF INSURANCE	INSURED OR SUBSCRIBER	

454-XX-9569A	Medigap Policy No. 5789002
POLICY/CERTIFICATE NO.	GROUP NO.

REFERRED BY: Mrs. O. S. Tomy (friend)   National PAYRID NAT234567

DATE	PROGRESS NOTES
6-1-xx	New pt comes into ofc to est new PCP in area; recently moved from Ohio. W obese M c/o
	nasal bleeding for two and a half months c̄ headaches and nasal congestion. Pt states he
	has had HBP for 1 yr. Taking med: Serpasil prescribed by dr in Ohio; does not know dosage.
	Took a C HX and performed a C PX which revealed post nasal hemorrhage. Coagulation
	time (Lee and White) and microhematocrit (spun) done in ofc are WNL. BP 180/100.
	Used nasal cautery and post nasal packs to control hemorrhage. Rx prophylactic antibiotic
	to guard against sinusitis NKA. Adv retn tomorrow, bring hypertensive medication.
	Pt signed authorization to request med records from dr in Ohio. D: Recurrent epistaxis
	due to nonspecific hypertension. No disability from work.
	GP/llf *Gerald Practon, MD*
6-2-xx	Pt retns and nasal hemorrhage is reevaluated (PF HX/PX SF/MDM). Postnasal packs
	removed and replaced. BP 182/98. Pt forgot medication for hypertension but states he is
	taking it 2 X d. Adv retn in 1 day, bring medication.
	GP/llf *Gerald Practon, MD*
6-3-xx	Pt retns and nasal hemorrhage is reevaluated (PF HX/PX SF/MDM). Postnasal packs
	removed. BP 178/100. Verified hypertensive medication. Pt to increase dosage to 4 X d.
	Adv retn in 5 days.
	GP/llf *Gerald Practon, MD*
6-8-xx	Pt retns and nasal hemorrhage is reevaluated (EPF HX/PX L/MDM). Prev medical records
	arrived and reviewed. BP 190/102. Pt referred to Dr. Perry Cardi (int) for future care of
	hypertension.
	GP/llf *Gerald Practon, MD*

Fig. 7

STATEMENT
Financial Account
COLLEGE CLINIC
4567 Broad Avenue
Woodland Hills, XY 12345-0001
Tel. 555-486-9002
Fax No. 555-487-8976

Charles B. Kamb
2600 West Nautilus Street
Woodland Hills, XY 12345

Phone No. (H) ___555-467-2601___ (W) __None/retired__ Birthdate ___1-26-27___

Primary Insurance Co. ___Medicare___ Policy/Group No. __454-XX-9569A__

Secondary Insurance Co. _National Insurance Company (Medigap)_ Policy/Group No. __5789002__

DATE	REFERENCE	DESCRIPTION	CHARGES	CREDITS		BALANCE	
				PYMNTS.	ADJ.		
20xx			BALANCE FORWARD		➡		
6-1-xx		NP OV					
6-1-xx		Coagulation time					
6-1-xx		Microhematocrit					
6-1-xx		Post nasal pack/cautery					
6-2-xx		OV					
6-2-xx		Subsequent nasal pack					
6-3-xx		OV					
6-8-xx		OV					

PLEASE PAY LAST AMOUNT IN BALANCE COLUMN ⬆

THIS IS A COPY OF YOUR FINANCIAL ACCOUNT AS IT APPEARS ON OUR RECORDS

Fig. 8

TEST 8: COMPLETE A CLAIM FORM FOR A MEDICAID CASE

Performance Objective

Task: Complete a CMS-1500 claim form for a Medicaid case and post transactions to the patient's financial account-ing record.

Conditions: Use the patient's record (Fig. 9) and financial statement (Fig. 10), one health insurance claim form, a computer or pen, procedural and diagnostic code books, and Appendix A in this *Workbook*.

Standards: Claim Productivity Management

Time: _____ minutes

Accuracy: _____

(Note: The time element and accuracy criteria may be given by your instructor.)

Directions

1. Using NUCC guidelines, complete a CMS-1500 claim form and direct it to the Medicaid fiscal intermediary for your state. Refer to Louise K. Herman's patient record for information and Appendix A to locate the fees to record on the claim, and post them to the financial statement. Date the claim May 31 of the current year.

2. Use your CPT code book to determine the correct five-digit code numbers and modifiers for each professional service rendered. Use your HCPCS Level II code book for HCPCS procedure codes and modifiers. Use your ICD-10-CM coding manual to code each active diagnosis.

3. Record the proper information on the patient's financial accounting record and claim form and note the date that you billed the insurance company.

4. Post the payment of $350 (voucher number 4300), received from the Medicaid fiscal intermediary 40 days after claim submission, and write off (adjust) the balance of the account.

PATIENT RECORD NO. T-8

Herman	Louise	K.	11-04-60	F	555-266-9085
LAST NAME	FIRST NAME	MIDDLE NAME	BIRTH DATE	SEX	HOME PHONE

13453 Burbank Boulevard	Woodland Hills	XY	12345
ADDRESS	CITY	STATE	ZIP CODE

555-466-7003		555-266-9085	herman@wb.net
CELL PHONE	PAGER NO.	FAX NO.	E-MAIL ADDRESS

519-XX-0018	T0943995
PATIENT'S SOC. SEC. NO.	DRIVER'S LICENSE

unemployed budget analyst	
PATIENT'S OCCUPATION	NAME OF COMPANY

ADDRESS OF EMPLOYER	PHONE

Harold D. Herman	retired salesman
SPOUSE OR PARENT	OCCUPATION

EMPLOYER	ADDRESS	PHONE

Medicaid	self
NAME OF INSURANCE	INSURED OR SUBSCRIBER

0051936001X	
MEDICAID NO.	GROUP NO.

REFERRED BY: Raymond Skeleton, MD

DATE	PROGRESS NOTES
5-6-xx	NP pt referred by Dr. Skeleton. CC: Rectal bleeding. Took a comprehensive history and
	performed a comprehensive physical examination. Diagnostic anoscopy revealed
	bleeding int and ext hemorrhoids and 2 infected rectal polyps. Rx antibiotics. Retn in
	2 days for removal of hemorrhoids and polyps (M/MDM)
	RR/llf *Rex Rumsey, MD*
5-8-xx	Pt returned to office for simple internal/external hemorrhoidectomy. Rigid
	proctosigmoidoscopy also perf for removal of polyps using snare technique. Adv. sitz
	baths daily. Continue on AB until gone. Retn in 1 wk.
	RR/llf *Rex Rumsey, MD*
5-15-xx	DNS Telephoned pt and rescheduled.
	Mary Bright, CMA
5-17-xx	PO OV (EPF HX/PX LC/MDM). Pt progressing well. No pain, discomfort or bleeding.
	Discharged from care, retn PRN.
	RR/llf *Rex Rumsey, MD*

Fig. 9

Acct No. __T-8__

STATEMENT
Financial Account
COLLEGE CLINIC
4567 Broad Avenue
Woodland Hills, XY 12345-0001
Tel. 555-486-9002
Fax No. 555-487-8976

Louise K. Herman
13453 Burbank Boulevard
Woodland Hills, XY 12345

Phone No. (H) __555-266-9085__   (W) _____   Birthdate__11/4/60__

Primary Insurance Co. __Medicaid__   Policy/Group No. ___0051936001X___

Secondary Insurance Co._____   Policy/Group No._____

DATE	REFERENCE	DESCRIPTION	CHARGES	CREDITS		BALANCE	
				PYMNTS.	ADJ.		
20xx			BALANCE FORWARD		⟶		
5-6-xx		NP OV					
5-6-xx		Dx anoscopy					
5-8-xx		Int/Ext Hemorrhoidectomy					
5-8-xx		Proctosigmoidoscopy with removal of polyps					
5-17-xx		PO OV					

PLEASE PAY LAST AMOUNT IN BALANCE COLUMN

THIS IS A COPY OF YOUR FINANCIAL ACCOUNT AS IT APPEARS ON OUR RECORDS

Fig. 10

TEST 9: COMPLETE A CLAIM FORM FOR A TRICARE CASE

Performance Objective

Task: Complete a CMS-1500 claim form for a TRICARE case and post transactions to the patient's financial accounting record.

Conditions: Use the patient's record (Fig. 11) and financial statement (Fig. 12), one health insurance claim form, a computer or pen, procedural and diagnostic code books, and Appendix A in this *Workbook*.

Standards: Claim Productivity Management

Time: _____ minutes

Accuracy: _____

(Note: The time element and accuracy criteria may be given by your instructor.)

Directions

1. Using NUCC guidelines, complete a CMS-1500 claim form and direct it to the TRICARE carrier for your area. Refer to Darlene M. Cash's patient record for information and Appendix A to locate the fees to record on the claim, and post them to the financial statement. Date the claim February 27 of the current year. Dr. Cutler is accepting assignment, and the patient's signatures to release information to the insurance company and to have the payment forwarded directly to the physician are on file.

2. Use your CPT code book to determine the correct five-digit code numbers and fees for each professional service rendered. Use your HCPCS Level II code book for HCPCS procedure codes and modifiers. Use your ICD-10-CM coding manual to code each active diagnosis.

3. Record the proper information on the patient's financial accounting record and claim form, and note the date that you billed the insurance company.

PATIENT RECORD NO. T-9

Cash	Darlene	M.	3-15-70	F	555-666-8901
LAST NAME	FIRST NAME	MIDDLE NAME	BIRTH DATE	SEX	HOME PHONE

5729 Redwood Avenue	Woodland Hills	XY	12344	
ADDRESS	CITY	STATE	ZIP CODE	

555-290-5400		555-666-8901	cash@wb.net
CELL PHONE	PAGER NO.	FAX NO.	E-MAIL ADDRESS

298-XX-6754	J3457789
PATIENT'S SOC. SEC. NO.	DRIVER'S LICENSE

teacher	City Unified School District
PATIENT'S OCCUPATION	NAME OF COMPANY

Century High School, 2031 West Olympic Boulevard, Dorland, XY 12345	555-678-1076
ADDRESS OF EMPLOYER	PHONE

David F. Cash	Navy Petty Officer—Grade 8 (active status)
SPOUSE OR PARENT	OCCUPATION

United States Navy	HHC, 2nd Batt, 26th Infantry, APO New York, NY, 10030	
EMPLOYER	ADDRESS	PHONE

TRICARE Standard	David Cash (DOB 4-22-70)
NAME OF INSURANCE	INSURED OR SUBSCRIBER

767-XX-9080	
POLICY/CERTIFICATE NO.	GROUP NO.

REFERRED BY: Hugh R. Foot, MD, 2010 Main St., Woodland Hills, XY 12345   NPI #61 25099XX

DATE	PROGRESS NOTES
1-4-xx	New pt, referred by Dr. Foot comes in complaining of head pain which began yesterday.
	Performed an EPF history and physical exam. Lt parietal area of skull slightly tender,
	some redness of scalp. Pain localized and not consistent with HA syndromes. Rest of
	exam N. Imp: head pain, undetermined nature, possible cyst. Apply hot compresses and
	observe. Take Ibuprofen for pain prn (200 mg up to 2 q. 4 h). Retn in 1 wk, no disability
	from work (SF/MDM).
	CC/llf *Clarence Cutler, MD*
1-11-xx	Pt retns and states that the hot compresses have helped but is concerned with some
	swelling in area. On exam noticed slt elevation of skin in lt parietal area of scalp, no
	warmth over area. Slt pain on palpation. Exam otherwise neg. Imp: Subcutaneous nodule.
	Continue with same tx plan: Hot compresses daily and Ibuprofen prn. Retn in 2 to 3 wks
	if not resolved (PF HX/PX SF/MDM).
	CC/llf *Clarence Cutler, MD*
2-3-xx	Pt retns for reexamination of parietal skull. Elevation of skin still persisting. It has now
	come to a head, is warm to the touch, and consistent with an inflammatory cystic lesion.
	A decision is made to excise the benign lesion. Scalp cyst, 1.5 cm removed under
	procaine block with knife dissection; closed wound with six #000 black silk sutures.
	Adv to retn 1 wk for removal of sutures (EPF HX/PX LC/MDM).
	CC/llf *Clarence Cutler, MD*
2-10-xx	Pt presents for suture removal. Sutures removed and slight oozing occurs in midsection
	of wound. Wound dressed and pt advised to apply antibacterial cream daily. Retn in 4 to
	5 days for final check (PF HX/PX SF/MDM).
	CC/llf *Clarence Cutler, MD*
2-15-xx	Pt presents for PO check of head wound. Parietal area healed well. RTO prn
	(PF HX/PX SF/MDM).
	CC/llf *Clarence Cutler, MD*

Fig. 11

STATEMENT
Financial Account
COLLEGE CLINIC
4567 Broad Avenue
Woodland Hills, XY 12345-0001
Tel. 555-486-9002
Fax No. 555-487-8976

Darlene M. Cash
5729 Redwood Avenue
Woodland Hills, XY 12345

Phone No. (H) ___555-666-8901___ (W) ___555-678-1076___   Birthdate ___3/15/70___

Primary Insurance Co. _TRICARE Standard_____   Policy/Group No. ___767-XX-9080___

Secondary Insurance Co._____   Policy/Group No._____

DATE	REFERENCE	DESCRIPTION	CHARGES	CREDITS PYMNTS.	ADJ.	BALANCE
20xx			BALANCE FORWARD →			
1-4-xx		NP OV				
1-11-xx		OV				
2-3-xx		OV				
2-3-xx		Excision inflammatory cystic scalp lesion				
2-10-xx		OV				
2-15-xx		OV				

PLEASE PAY LAST AMOUNT IN BALANCE COLUMN ⬆

THIS IS A COPY OF YOUR FINANCIAL ACCOUNT AS IT APPEARS ON OUR RECORDS

Fig. 12

TEST 10: COMPLETE TWO CLAIM FORMS FOR A PRIVATE PLAN

Performance Objective

Task: Complete two CMS-1500 claim forms for a private case and post transactions to the patient's financial accounting record.

Conditions: Use the patient's record (Fig. 13) and financial statement (Fig. 14), two health insurance claim forms, a computer or pen, procedural and diagnostic code books, and Appendix A in this *Workbook*.

Standards: Claim Productivity Management

Time: _____ minutes

Accuracy: _____

(Note: The time element and accuracy criteria may be given by your instructor.)

Directions

1. Using NUCC guidelines, complete two CMS-1500 claim forms and direct them to the private carrier. Refer to Gertrude C. Hamilton's patient record for information and Appendix A in this *Workbook* to locate the fees to record on the claim, and post them to the financial statement. Date the first claim August 15 and the second one October 15. Dr. Cardi is accepting assignment, and the patient's signatures to release information to the insurance company and to have the payment forwarded directly to the physician are on file.

2. Use your CPT code book to determine the correct five-digit code numbers and modifiers for each professional service rendered. Use your HCPCS Level II code book for HCPCS procedure codes and modifiers. Use your ICD-10-CM coding manual to code each active diagnosis. Frequently, surgeons wait to receive the pathology report before entering a final diagnosis on the claim form. In this case, the claim was submitted before the pathology report was received.

3. Record the proper information on the financial record and claim form, and note the date that you billed the insurance company.

4. Mrs. Hamilton makes a payment of $200, check number 5362, on her account on October 26. Post the proper entry for this transaction.

357

PATIENT RECORD NO. T-10

Hamilton	Gertrude	C.	03-06-57	F	555-798-3321
LAST NAME	FIRST NAME	MIDDLE NAME	BIRTH DATE	SEX	HOME PHONE

5320 Phillips Street	Woodland Hills	XY	12345
ADDRESS	CITY	STATE	ZIP CODE

555-399-4990	555-312-6677	555-798-3321	hamilton@wb.net
CELL PHONE	PAGER NO.	FAX NO.	E-MAIL ADDRESS

540-XX-7677	D9043557
PATIENT'S SOC. SEC. NO.	DRIVER'S LICENSE

retired secretary	
PATIENT'S OCCUPATION	NAME OF COMPANY

ADDRESS OF EMPLOYER	PHONE

deceased	
SPOUSE OR PARENT	OCCUPATION

EMPLOYER	ADDRESS	PHONE

Colonial Health Insurance, 1011 Main Street, Woodland Hills, XY 12345	self
NAME OF INSURANCE	INSURED OR SUBSCRIBER

540XX7677	4566 (through previous employment)
POLICY/CERTIFICATE NO.	GROUP NO.

REFERRED BY: Gerald Practon, MD, 4567 Broad Avenue, Woodland Hills, XY 12345

Fig. 13

DATE	PROGRESS NOTES No. T-10
7-29-xx	Dr. Practon asked me to consult on this 57-year-old pt adm to College Hosp today.
	Duplex carotid ultrasonography indicates bilateral carotid stenosis. C/HX: Suffered CVA lt
	hemisphere 1 yr prior to adm. Marked rt arm & leg weakness c̄ weakness of rt face and
	slurring of speech. C/PE revealed lt carotid bruit, II/IV, & right carotid bruit, II/IV.
	Performed hand-held Doppler vascular study on bilateral carotids which indicated
	decreased blood flow. Adv brain scan and lt carotid thromboendarterectomy; rt carotid
	thromboendarterectomy at a later date H/MDM.
	PC/llf *Perry Cardi, MD*
7-30-xx	HV (EPF HX/PX MC/MDM). Dr. Practon asked me to take over pt's care. Pt had brain scan
	done today, ECG, and lab work.
	PC/llf *Perry Cardi, MD*
7-31-xx	HV (EPF HX/PX MC/MDM). Brain scan indicates prior CVA; no new findings. ECG, normal
	sinus rhythm with occasional premature ventricular contractions. Lab work WNL.
	Discussed test results with Mrs. Hamilton.
	PC/llf *Perry Cardi, MD*
8-1-xx	HV (PF HX/PX LC/MDM). Decision made for surgery, to be scheduled tomorrow.
	PC/llf *Perry Cardi, MD*
8-2-xx	Pt taken to the operative suite. Performed lt carotid thromboendarterectomy by neck
	incision (see op report). Surgery went as planned, pt in recovery.
	PC/llf *Perry Cardi, MD*
8-3-xx	HV (PF HX/PX SF/MDM). Operative site appears normal. Pt resting comfortably.
	PC/llf *Perry Cardi, MD*
8-4-xx	DC from hosp. Pt to be seen in ofc in 1 week.
	PC/llf *Perry Cardi, MD*
8-12-xx	PO OV (D HX/PX M/MDM). Discussed outcome of surgery. Pt making satisfactory
	progress. Adv rt carotid thromboendarterectomy. Pt would like it done as soon as possible;
	next month if there is an operative time. Scheduled surgery for September 16, 20XX at
	College Hospital.
	PC/llf *Perry Cardi, MD*
9-16-xx	Adm to College Hospital. Performed a D history, D physical examination, and SF medical
	decision making. Rt carotid thromboendarterectomy performed by neck incision.
	DX: Rt carotid stenosis.
	PC/llf *Perry Cardi, MD*
9-17-xx	HV (PF HX/PX SF/MDM). Pt stable and doing well. Operative site looks good. Plan for
	discharge tomorrow.
	PC/llf *Perry Cardi, MD*
9-18-xx	DC from hosp to home. RTC 1 wk.
	PC/llf *Perry Cardi, MD*
9-25-xx	PO visit (PF HX/PX SF/MDM). Pt making satisfactory recovery. Her neighbor will monitor
	BP daily. Retn 1 month.
	PC/llf *Perry Cardi, MD*

Fig. 13, cont'd

STATEMENT

Acct No. __T-10__

COLLEGE CLINIC
4567 Broad Avenue
Woodland Hills, XY 12345-0001
Tel. 555-486-9002
Fax No. 555-487-8976

Gertrude C. Hamilton
5320 Phillips Street
Woodland Hills, XY 12345

Phone No. (H)____(555) 798-3321____ (W) _____ Birthdate____03-06-57_____

Insurance Co____Colonial Health Insurance_____ Policy/Group No._540Xx7677 / 4566__

	REFERENCE	DESCRIPTION	CHARGES	CREDITS		BALANCE	
				PYMNTS.	ADJ.		
20xx			BALANCE FORWARD �				
7-29-xx		Inpatient consult					
7-30-xx		HV					
7-31-xx		HV					
8-1-xx		HV					
8-2-xx		L carotid thromboendarterectomy					
8-3-xx		HV					
8-4-xx		Discharge					
8-12-xx		PO OV					
9-16-xx		Admit					
9-16-xx		R carotid thromboendarterectomy					
9-17-xx		HV					
9-18-xx		Discharge					
9-25-xx		PO OV					

PLEASE PAY LAST AMOUNT IN BALANCE COLUMN

THIS IS A COPY OF YOUR FINANCIAL ACCOUNT AS IT APPEARS ON OUR RECORDS

Fig. 14

A College Clinic Office Policies and Mock Fee Schedule

College Clinic

In this simulation, you are employed as an insurance billing specialist for a group of medical doctors, other allied health specialists, and podiatrists. Each clinic is configured in its own way. The College Clinic has staff physicians who are employed, receive monthly pay checks, and are given Wage and Tax Statements (Form W-2) at the end of the tax year. These doctors are on the staff of a nearby hospital, College Hospital.

Medical practices can have different configurations. For example, individuals or groups can be incorporated. Physicians can be independent contractors, running their own practices outside of the clinic; receive payment by the job and not a salary; and receive a Form 1099 at the end of the tax year.

Reference information to complete insurance claim forms for each assignment follows. Claim forms are to be submitted for the group unless a case involves a physician working as an independent contractor.

Office address:
College Clinic
4567 Broad Avenue
Woodland Hills, XY 12345-0001
Telephone: 555-486-9002

FAX: 555-487-8976
Clinic e-mail: cclinic@cmail.net
Staff e-mail: insert physician's last name followed by a period (.) then cclinic@cmail.net
(example: Pedro Atrics, MD, would have an e-mail address of atrics.cclinic@cmail.net
Group practice, National Provider Identifier (NPI): 3664021CC
Medicare durable medical equipment (DME) supplier number: 3400760001
Group tax ID #: XX12210XX

Hospital address:
College Hospital
4500 Broad Avenue
Woodland Hills, XY 12345-0001
Telephone: 555-487-6789
FAX: 555-486-8900
Hospital NPI: X950731067

College Clinic Staff

Patient records in this *Workbook* include the doctors' names, specialties, subspecialties, and physicians' identification numbers of the College Clinic staff. They are shown in Table 1.

Table 1. College Clinic Staff

Name	Specialty (Abbreviation)	Social Security No.[a]	State License No.	EIN No. or Federal Tax Identification No.	Medicare CMS-Assigned National Provider Identifier (NPI)[b]
Concha Antrum, MD	Otolaryngologist (OTO) or Ear, Nose, and Throat Specialist (ENT)	082–XX–1707	C 01602X	74–10640XX	12458977XX
Pedro Atrics, MD	Pediatrician (PD)	134–XX–7600	D 06012X	71–32061XX	37640017XX
Bertha Caesar, MD	Obstetrician and Gynecologist (OBG)	230–XX–6700	A 01817X	72–57130XX	43056757XX
Perry Cardi, MD	Internist (I) Subspecialty: Cardiovascular Disease (CD)	557–XX–9980	C 02140X	70–64217XX	67805027XX
Brady Coccidioides, MD	Internist (I) Subspecialty: Pulmonary Disease (PUD)	670–XX–0874	C 04821X	75–67321XX	64211067XX
Vera Cutis, MD	Dermatologist (D)	409–XX–8620	C 06002X	71–80561XX	70568717XX
Clarence Cutler, MD	General Surgeon (GS)	410–XX–5630	B 07600X	71–57372XX	43050047XX
Max Glutens, RPT	Physical Therapist (PT)	507–XX–4300	87610X	79–36500XX	65132277XX
Cosmo Graff, MD	Plastic Surgeon (PS)	452–XX–9899	C 08104X	74–60789XX	50307117XX
Malvern Grumose, MD	Pathologist (Path)	470–XX–2301	A 01602X	72–73651XX	
Gaston Input, MD	Internist (I) Subspecialty: Gastroenterologist (GE)	211–XX–6734	C 08001X	75–67210XX	32783127XX
Adam Langerhans, MD	Endocrinologist	447–XX–6720	C 06051X	60–57831XX	47680657XX
Cornell Lenser, MD	Ophthalmologist (OPH)	322–XX–8963	C 06046X	61–78941XX	54037217XX
Michael Menter, MD	Psychiatrist (P)	210–XX–5302	C 07140X	73–66577XX	67301237XX
Astro Parkinson, MD	Neurosurgeon (NS)	210–XX–8533	C 02600X	75–44530XX	46789377XX
Nick Pedro, DPM	Podiatrist	233–XX–4300	E 08340X	62–74109XX	54022287XX
Gerald Practon, MD	General Practitioner (GP) or Family Practitioner (FP)	123–XX–6789	C 01402X	70–34597XX	46278897XX
Walter Radon, MD	Radiologist (R)	344–XX–6540	C 05001X	95–46137XX	40037227XX
Rex Rumsey, MD	Proctologist (Proct)	337–XX–9743	C 03042X	95–32601XX	01999047XX
Sensitive E. Scott, MD	Anesthesiologist (Anes)	220–XX–5655	C 02041X	72–54203XX	99999267XX
Raymond Skeleton, MD	Orthopedist (ORS, Orthop)	432–XX–4589	C 04561X	74–65412XX	12678547XX
Gene Ulibarri, MD	Urologist (U)	990–XX–3245	C 06430X	77–86531XX	25678831XX

[a]Social Security numbers are shown in the table because each individual is issued one and this is a realistic picture because they would be on file.
[b]Providers began using the NPI on May 23, 2007, except for small health plans, whose compliance date was May 23, 2008.

Appendix **College Clinic Office Policies and Mock Fee Schedule**

Abbreviations and Symbols

Abbreviations and symbols may appear on patient records, prescriptions, hospital charts, and patient ledger cards. Abbreviation styles differ, but the current trend is to omit periods in capital letter abbreviations except for doctors' academic degrees. Following is a list of abbreviations and symbols used in this *Workbook* and their meanings.

Abbreviations

A	allergy
AB	antibiotics
Abdom	abdomen
abt	about
a.c.	before meals
Adj[a]	adjustment
adm	admit; admission; admitted
adv	advise(d)
aet	at the age of
agit	shake or stir
AgNO$_3$	silver nitrate
ALL	allergy
AM, a.m.	ante meridiem (time—before noon)
ant	anterior
ante	before
AP	anterior-posterior; anteroposterior
approx	approximate
appt	appointment
apt	apartment
ASA	acetylsalicylic acid (aspirin)
ASAP	as soon as possible
ASCVD	arteriosclerotic cardiovascular disease
ASHD	arteriosclerotic heart disease
asst	assistant
auto	automated, automobile
AV	atrioventricular
Ba	barium (enema)
Bal/fwd[a]	balance forward
BE	barium enema
B/F[a]	balance forward; brought forward
b.i.d.	two times daily
BM	bowel movement
BMR	basal metabolic rate
BP	blood pressure
Brev	Brevital sodium
BX, bx	biopsy
C	cervical (vertebrae); comprehensive (history/examination)
Ca, CA	cancer, carcinoma
c/a[a]	cash on account
CABG	coronary artery bypass graft
CAT	computed axial tomography
cau	Caucasian

CBC	complete blood count
CBS	chronic brain syndrome
cc	cubic centimeter
CC	chief complaint
chr	chronic
ck[a]	check
cm	centimeter
CO, c/o	complains of; care of
compl, comp	complete; comprehensive
Con, CON, Cons	consultation
Cont	continue
CPX	complete physical examination
C&R	compromise and release
Cr[a]	credit
C&S	culture and sensitivity
cs, CS[a]	cash on account
C-section	cesarean section
CT	computed or computerized tomography
CVA	cardiovascular accident; cerebrovascular accident
CXR	chest radiograph
cysto	cystoscopy
D, d	diagnosis; detailed (history/examination); day(s)
D&C	dilatation and curettage
dc	discontinue
DC	discharge
DDS	Doctor of Dental Surgery
def[a]	charge deferred
Del	delivery; obstetrics and gynecology
Dg	diagnosis
dia	diameter
diag	diagnosis; diagnostic
dil	dilate (stretch, expand)
Disch	discharge
DM	diabetes mellitus
DNA	does not apply
DNS	did not show
DPM	Doctor of Podiatric Medicine
DPT	diphtheria, pertussis, and tetanus
Dr	Doctor
Dr[a]	debit
DRG	diagnosis-related group
Drs	dressing
DUB	dysfunctional uterine bleeding
Dx	diagnosis
E	emergency
EC[a]	error corrected
ECG, EKG	electrocardiogram; electrocardiograph
echo	echocardiogram; echocardiography
ED	emergency department
EDC	estimated date of confinement
EEG	electroencephalograph

[a]Bookkeeping abbreviation.

EENT	eye, ear, nose, and throat	IC	initial consultation
EGD	esophagogastroduodenoscopy	I&D	incision and drainage
EKG, ECG	electrocardiogram; electrocardiograph	I/f[a]	in full
E/M	Evaluation and Management (*Current Procedural Terminology* code)	IM	intramuscular (injection)
		imp, imp.	impression (diagnosis)
EMG	electromyogram	incl.	include; including
EPF	expanded problem-focused (history/ examination)	inflam	inflammation
		init	initial (office visit)
epith	epithelial	inj, INJ	injection
ER	emergency room	ins, INS[a]	insurance
Er, ER[a]	error corrected	int	internal
ESR	erythrocyte sedimentation rate	intermed	intermediate (office visit)
est	established (patient); estimated	interpret	interpretation
Ex, exam	examination	IUD	intrauterine device
exc	excision	IV	intravenous (injection)
Ex MO[a]	express money order	IVP	intravenous pyelogram
ext	external	K 35	Kolman (instrument used in urology)
24F, 28F	French (size of catheter)	KUB	kidneys, ureters, and bladder
F	female	L	left; laboratory
FBS	fasting blood sugar	lab, LAB	laboratory
FH	family history	lat	lateral; pertaining to the side
ft	foot, feet	lbs	pounds
FU	follow-up (examination)	LC	low-complexity (decision making)
fwd[a]	forward	LMP	last menstrual period
Fx	fracture	LS	lumbosacral
gb, GB	gallbladder	lt	left
GGE	generalized glandular enlargement	ltd	limited (office visit)
GI	gastrointestinal	L & W	living and well
Grav, grav	gravida, a pregnant woman; used with Roman numerals (I, II, III) to indi- cate the number of pregnancies	M	medication; married
		MC	moderate-complexity (decision making)
		MDM	medical decision making
GU	genitourinary	med	medicine
H	hospital call	mg	milligram(s)
HA	headache	mg/dL	milligrams per deciliter
HBP	high blood pressure	MI	myocardial infarction
HC	hospital call or consultation; high-complexity (decision making)	micro	microscopy
		mL, ml	milliliter
HCD	house call (day)	mo	month(s)
HCN	house call (night)	MO[a]	money order
Hct	hematocrit	N	negative
HCVD	hypertensive cardiovascular disease	NA	not applicable
Hgb	hemoglobin	NAD	no appreciable disease
hist	history	NC, N/C[a]	no charge
hosp	hospital	NEC	not elsewhere classifiable
H&P	history and physical (examination)	neg	negative
hr, hrs	hour, hours	NKA	no known allergies
h.s.	before bedtime	NOS	not otherwise specified
HS	hospital surgery	NP	new patient
Ht	height	NYD	not yet diagnosed
HV	hospital visit	OB, Ob-Gyn	obstetrics and gynecology
HX, hx	history	OC	office call
HX PX	history and physical examination	occ	occasional
I	injection	OD	right eye

---

[a]Bookkeeping abbreviation.

ofc	office	**RBC, rbc**	red blood cell (count)
OP	outpatient	**rec**	recommend
Op, op	operation	**rec'd**	received
OR	operating room	**re ch**	recheck
orig	original	**re-exam**	reexamination
OS	office surgery; left eye	**Reg**	regular
OV	office visit	**ret, retn, rtn**	return
oz	ounce	**rev**	review
PA	posterior-anterior; posteroanterior	**RHD**	rheumatic heart disease
Pap	Papanicolaou (smear, stain, test)	**RN**	registered nurse
Para I	woman having borne one child	**R/O**	rule out
PC	present complaint	**ROA**[a]	received on account
p.c.	after meals	**RPT**	registered physical therapist
PCP	primary care physician	**rt**	right
PD	permanent disability	**RTC**	return to clinic
Pd, PD[a]	professional discount	**RTO**	return to office
PE	physical examination	**RTW**	return to work
perf	performed	**RX, Rx, Rx**	prescribe; prescription; any medication
PF	problem-focused (history/examination)		or treatment ordered
PFT	pulmonary function test	**S**	surgery
PH	past history	**SC**	subcutaneous
Ph ex	physical examination	**sched.**	scheduled
phys	physical	**SD**	state disability
PID	pelvic inflammatory disease	**SE**	special examination
PM, p.m.	post meridiem (time—after noon)	**SF**	straightforward (decision making)
PND	postnasal drip	**Sig**	directions on prescription
PO, P Op	postoperative	**SLR**	straight leg raising
p.o.	by mouth (per os)	**slt**	slight
post	posterior	**Smr**	smear
postop	postoperative	**SOB**	shortness of breath
PPD	purified protein derivative (such as in	**Sp gr**	specific gravity
	tuberculin test)	**SQ**	subcutaneous (injection)
preop	preoperative	**STAT**	immediately
prep	prepared	**strep**	*Streptococcus*
PRN, p.r.n.	as necessary (pro re nata)	**surg**	surgery
Proc	procedure	**Sx**	symptom(s)
Prog	prognosis	**T**	temperature
P & S	permanent and stationary	**T&A**	tonsillectomy and adenoidectomy
PSA	prostate-specific antigen (blood test to	**Tb, tb**	tuberculosis
	determine cancer in prostate gland)	**TD**	temporary disability
Pt, pt	patient	**tech**	technician
PT	physical therapy	**temp**	temperature
PTR	patient to return	**tet. tox.**	tetanus toxoid
PVC	premature ventricular contraction	**t.i.d.**	three times daily
PVT ck[a]	private check received	**TPR**	temperature, pulse, and respiration
PX	physical examination	**Tr, trt**	treatment
q	every	**TURB**	transurethral resection of bladder
qd	one time daily, every day	**TURP**	transurethral resection of prostate
qh	every hour	**TX**	treatment
q.i.d.	four times daily	**u**	units
QNS	quantity not sufficient	**UA, ua**	urinalysis
qod	every other day	**UCHD**	usual childhood diseases
R	right; residence call; report	**UCR**	usual, customary, and reasonable (fees)

[a]Bookkeeping abbreviation.

		Symbols	
UGI	upper gastrointestinal	+	positive
UPJ	ureteropelvic junction or joint	#	pound(s)
UR	urinalysis	c̄, /c	with
URI	upper respiratory infection	s̄, /s	without
Urn	urinalysis	c̄c, c̄/c	with correction (eye glasses)
UTI	urinary tract infection	s̄c, s̄/c	without correction (eye glasses)
W	work; white	-	negative
WBC, wbc	white blood cell (count); well baby care	ō	negative
WC	workers' compensation	!, +	positive
wk	week; work	(L)	left
wks	weeks	(R)	right
WNL	within normal limits	♂	male
Wr	Wassermann reaction (test for syphilis)	♀	female
Wt, wt	weight	—ᵃ	charge already made
X	xray, x-ray(s), times (e.g., 3X means three times)	⊖ᵃ	no balance due
		√ᵃ	posted
XR	xray, x-ray(s)	($0.00) ᵃ	credit
yr(s)	year(s)		

Laboratory Abbreviations

ABG	arterial blood gas(es)
AcG	factor V (AcG or proaccelerin); a factor in coagulation that converts prothrombin to thrombin
ACTH	adrenocorticotropic hormone
A/C ratio	albumin-coagulin ratio
AFB	acid-fast bacilli
AHB	alpha-hydroxybutyric (dehydrogenase)
AHG	antihemophilic globulin; antihemolytic globulin (factor)
ALA	aminolevulinic acid
ALT	alanine aminotransferase (*see* SGPT)
AMP	adenosine monophosphate
APT test	aluminum-precipitated toxoid test
AST	aspartate aminotransferase (*see* SGOT)
ATP	adenosine triphosphate
BSP	bromosulfophthalein (bromsulphalein; sodium sulfobromophthalein) (test)
BUN	blood urea nitrogen
CBC	complete blood count
CNS	central nervous system
CO	carbon monoxide
CPB	competitive protein binding: plasma
CPK	creatine phosphokinase
CSF	cerebrospinal fluid
D hemoglobin	hemoglobin fractionation by electrophoresis for hemoglobin D
DAP	direct agglutination pregnancy (Gravindex and DAP)
DEAE	diethylaminoethanol
DHT	dihydrotestosterone
diff	differential
DNA	deoxyribonucleic acid
DRT	test for syphilis
EACA	epsilon-aminocaproic acid (a fibrinolysin)
EMIT	enzyme-multiplied immunoassay technique (for drugs)
ENA	extractable nuclear antigen

ᵃBookkeeping abbreviation.

esr, ESR	erythrocyte sedimentation (sed) rate
FDP	fibrin degradation products
FIGLU	formiminoglutamic acid
FRAT	free radical assay technique (for drugs)
FSH	follicle-stimulating hormone
FSP	fibrinogen split products
FTA	fluorescent-absorbed treponema antibodies
Gc, Gm, Inv	immunoglobulin typing
GG, gamma G, A, D, G, M	gamma-globulin (immunoglobulin fractionation by electrophoresis)
GG, gamma G E, RIA	immunization E fractionation by radioimmunoassay
GGT	gamma-glutamyl transpeptidase
GLC	gas liquid chromatography
GMP	guanosine monophosphate
GTT	glucose tolerance test
G6PD	glucose-6-phosphate dehydrogenase
HAA	hepatitis-associated agent (antigen)
HBD, HBDH	hydroxybutyrate dehydrogenase
HCT	hematocrit
hemoglobin, electrophoresis	letters of the alphabet used for different types or factors of hemoglobins (includes A_2, S, C, etc.)
Hgb	hemoglobin, qualitative
HGH	human growth hormone
HI	hemagglutination inhibition
HIA	hemagglutination inhibition antibody
HIAA	hydroxyindoleacetic acid (urine), 24-hour specimen
HIV	human immunodeficiency virus
HLA	human leukocyte antigen (tissue typing)
HPL	human placental lactogen
HTLV-III	antibody detection; confirmatory test
HVA	homovanillic acid
ICSH	interstitial cell-stimulating hormone
IFA	intrinsic factor, antibody (fluorescent screen)
IgA, IgE, IgG, IgM	immunoglobulins: quantitative by gel diffusion
INH	isonicotinic hydrazide, isoniazid
LAP	leucine aminopeptidase
LATS	long-acting thyroid-stimulating (hormone)
LDH	lactic dehydrogenase
LE Prep	lupus erythematosus cell preparation
L.E. factor	antinuclear antibody
LH	luteinizing hormone
LSD	lysergic acid diethylamide
L/S ratio	lecithin-sphingomyelin ratio
MC (*Streptococcus*)	antibody titer
MIC	minimum inhibitory concentration
NBT	nitro-blue tetrazolium (test)
OCT	ornithine carbamoyltransferase
PAH	para-aminohippuric acid
PBI	protein-bound iodine
pCO_2	arterial carbon dioxide pressure (or tension)
PCP	phencyclidine piperidine
pcv	packed cell volume
pH	symbol for expression of concentration of hydrogen ions (degree of acidity)
PHA	phenylalanine

PIT	prothrombin inhibition test
PKU	phenylketonuria—a metabolic disease affecting mental development
PO₂	oxygen pressure
P&P	prothrombin-proconvertin
PSP	phenolsulfonphthalein
PT	prothrombin time
PTA	plasma thromboplastin antecedent
PTC	plasma thromboplastin component; phenylthiocarbamide
PTT	prothrombin time; partial thromboplastin time (plasma or whole blood)
RBC, rbc	red blood cells (count)
RIA	radioimmunoassay
RISA	radioiodinated human serum albumin
RIST	radioimmunosorbent test
RPR	rapid plasma reagin (test)
RT₃U	resin triiodothyronine uptake
S-D	strength-duration (curve)
SGOT	serum glutamic oxaloacetic transaminase (*see* AST)
SGPT	serum glutamic pyruvic transaminase (*see* ALT)
STS	serologic test for syphilis
T₃	triiodothyronine (uptake)
TB	tubercle bacillus, tuberculosis
TBG	thyroxine-binding globulin
T&B differentiation, lymphocytes	thymus-dependent lymphs and bursa-dependent lymphs
THC	tetrahydrocannabinol (marijuana)
TIBC	total iron-binding capacity, chemical
TLC screen	thin-layer chromatography screen
TRP	tubular reabsorption of phosphates
UA	urinalysis
VDRL	Venereal Disease Research Laboratory (agglutination test for syphilis)
VMA	vanillylmandelic acid
WBC, wbc	white blood cells (count)

Mock Fee Schedule

Refer to the Mock Fee Schedule (Table 2) to complete the financial accounting statements (ledgers) and claim forms in this *Workbook*. The fees listed are hypothetical and are intended only for use in completing the questions. For the cases that are private, Medicaid, TRICARE, and workers' compensation, use the amounts in the column labeled Mock Fees. For Medicare cases, refer to the three columns pertaining to Medicare and use the amounts in the column labeled Limiting Charge. Follow these instructions unless your instructor wishes you to round out the amounts on the fee schedule to the next dollar.

In a real medical practice, some offices round out the amounts to the next dollar unless the physician is nonparticipating with Medicare, and then according to Medicare regulations, the provider can only bill the exact limiting amount on nonassigned claims. Other offices may have two fee schedules. Schedule B is for Medicare participating physicians, and amounts are listed in dollars and cents. Schedule A is used for other plans, and the amounts are rounded to the next dollar. However, if a fee schedule is sent by the insurance plan, then the medical practice may use the dollars and cents provided.

When completing the insurance claim forms, use the latest edition of *Current Procedural Terminology* (CPT), the professional code book published by the American Medical Association, to find the correct code numbers and modifiers for the services rendered. The Mock Fee Schedule (Table 2) is arranged in the same sequence as the six CPT code book sections (i.e., Evaluation and Management; Anesthesia; Surgery; Radiology, Nuclear Medicine, and Diagnostic Ultrasound; Pathology and Laboratory; and Medicine).

Table 2. Mock Fee Schedule

Code No.	Description	Mock Fees	Medicare[a] Participating	Nonpartici-pating	Limiting Charge	Follow-Up Days
EVALUATION AND MANAGEMENT[b]						
Office						
New Patient						
99201	Level 1 Problem Focused	33.25	30.43	28.91	33.25	
99202	Level 2 Expanded Prob Foc	51.91	47.52	45.14	51.91	
99203	Level 3 Detailed	70.92	64.92	61.67	70.92	
99204	Level 4 Comprehensive	106.11	97.13	92.27	106.11	
99205	Level 5 Comprehensive	132.28	121.08	115.03	132.28	
Established Patient						
99211	Level 1 Nurse Visit	16.07	14.70	13.97	16.07	
99212	Level 2 Problem Focused	28.55	26.14	24.83	28.55	
99213	Level 3 Expanded Prob Foc	40.20	36.80	34.96	40.20	
99214	Level 4 Comprehensive	61.51	56.31	53.79	61.51	
99215	Level 5 Comprehensive	96.97	88.76	84.32	96.97	
Hospital						
Observation Services (new or established patient)						
99217	Observation Care Dischg	66.88	61.22	58.16	66.88	
99218	Dhx/exam SF/LC MDM	74.22	67.94	64.54	74.22	
99219	Chx/exam MC MDM	117.75	107.78	102.39	117.75	
99220	Chx/exam HC MDM	147.48	134.99	128.24	147.48	
Inpatient Services (new or established patient)						
99221	30 min Dhx, Dpx, SF or low MDM	73.00	66.84	63.48	73.00	
99222	50 min Comp/Comp/Moderate	120.80	110.57	105.04	120.80	
99223	70 min Comp/Comp/High MDM	152.98	140.03	133.03	152.98	
Subsequent Hospital Care						
99231	15 min PF, PF, SF MDM	37.74	34.55	32.82	37.74	
99232	25 min EPF, EPF, Moderate	50.85	48.31	55.56		

[a]Some services and procedures may not be considered a benefit under the Medicare program and when listed on a claim form, no reimbursement may be received. However, it is important to include these codes when billing because Medicare policies may change without an individual knowing of a new benefit. For this reason, some of the services shown in this Mock Fee Schedule do not have any amounts listed under the three Medicare columns.

[b]Mock fees for laboratory tests presented in this schedule may not be representative of fees in your region because of the variety of capitation and managed care contracts, as well as discount policies made by laboratories. At the time of this edition, Medicare guidelines may or may not pay for automatic multichannel tests where a large number of tests are performed per panel. Some cases require documentation and a related diagnostic code for each test performed. Provider must have the CLIA level of licensure to bill for tests, and test results must be documented.

Continued

Appendix **College Clinic Office Policies and Mock Fee Schedule**

Table 2. Mock Fee Schedule—cont'd

Code No.	Description	Mock Fees	Medicare[a]			
			Participating	Nonparticipating	Limiting Charge	Follow-Up Days
99233	35 min D, D, HC MDM	76.97	70.45	66.93	76.97	
99238	Discharge <30 min	65.26	59.74	56.75	65.26	
99239	Discharge >30 min					
Consultations						
Office (new or established patient)						
99241	Level 1 PF, PF, SF	51.93				
99242	Level 2 EPF, EPF, SF	80.24				
99243	Level 3 D, D, LC MDM	103.51				
99244	Level 4 C, C, Moderate MDM	145.05				
99245	Level 5 C, C, HC MDM	195.45				
Inpatient (new or established patient)						
99251	Level 1 PF, PF, SF	53.29				
99252	Level 2 EPF, EPF, SF	80.56				
99253	Level 3 D, D, LC MDM	106.10				
99254	Level 4 C, C, Moderate MDM	145.26				
99255	Level 5 C, C, HC MDM	196.55				
Emergency Department (new/established patient)						
99281	PF hx/exam SF MDM	24.32	22.26	21.15	24.32	
99282	EPF hx/exam LC MDM	37.02	33.88	32.19	37.02	
99283	EPF hx/exam MC MDM	66.23	60.62	57.59	66.23	
99284	D hx/exam MC MDM	100.71	92.18	87.57	100.71	
99285	C hx/exam HC MDM	158.86	145.41	138.14	158.86	
Critical Care Services						
99291	First hour	208.91	191.22	181.66	208.91	
99292	Each addl. 30 min	102.02	92.46	87.84	102.02	
Neonatal Intensive Care						
99468	Initial	892.74	817.16	776.30	892.74	
99469	Subsequent unstable case	418.73	383.27	364.11	418.73	
Initial Nursing Facility						
99304	25 min (Low Severity)	64.11	58.68	55.75	64.11	
99305	35 min (Moderate Severity)	90.55	82.88	78.74	90.55	
99306	45 min (High Severity)	136.76	125.18	118.92	136.76	
Subsequent Nursing Facility Care						
99307	PF hx/exam SF DM	37.95	34.74	33.00	37.95	
99308	15 min EPF hx/exam LC DM	55.11	50.44	47.92	55.11	
99309	25 min D hx/exam MC DM	69.61	63.72	60.53	69.61	
99310	35 min C hx/exam HC DM	84.73	77.00	73.14	84.73	
Domiciliary, Rest Home, Custodial Care						
New Patient						
99324	PF hx/exam SF DM	46.10	42.20	40.09	46.10	
99325	EPF hx/exam LC DM	65.02	59.53	56.54	65.02	
99326	D hx/exam MC DM	86.18	78.88	74.94	86.18	
99327	C hx/exam MC DM	107.34	98.23	93.34	107.34	
99328	C hx/exam HC DM	128.50	117.58	111.74	128.50	
Established Patient						
99334	PF hx/exam SF MDM	37.31	34.15	32.44	37.31	
99335	EPF hx/exam LC MDM	49.22	45.05	42.80	49.22	
99336	D hx/exam Moderate MDM	60.61	55.47	52.70	60.61	
99337	C hx/exam M-H DM	72.00	65.89	62.60	72.00	

[a]Some services and procedures may not be considered a benefit under the Medicare program and when listed on a claim form, no reimbursement may be received. However, it is important to include these codes when billing because Medicare policies may change without an individual knowing of a new benefit. For this reason, some of the services shown in this Mock Fee Schedule do not have any amounts listed under the three Medicare columns.

370

Appendix **College Clinic Office Policies and Mock Fee Schedule**   Copyright © 2020 Elsevier, Inc. All Rights Reserved.

Table 2. Mock Fee Schedule—cont'd

Code No.	Description	Mock Fees	Medicare[a] Participating	Nonpartici-pating	Limiting Charge	Follow-Up Days
Home Services						
New Patient						
99341	PF hx/exam SF DM	70.32	64.37	61.15	70.32	
99342	EPF hx/exam LC DM	91.85	84.07	79.87	91.85	
99343	D hx/exam MC DM	120.24	110.06	104.56	120.24	
99344	C hx/exam MC DM	148.63	136.05	129.25	148.63	
99345	C hx/exam HC DM	177.02	162.04	153.50	177.02	
Established Patient						
99347	PF hx/exam SF DM	54.83	50.19	47.68	54.83	
99348	EPF hx/exam LC DM	70.06	64.13	60.92	70.06	
99349	D hx/exam MC DM	88.33	80.85	76.81	88.33	
99350	C hx/exam M-H DM	106.60	97.57	92.70	106.60	
Prolonged Services With Direct (Face-to-Face) Patient Contact (Report in Addition to the Designated E/M Service at Any Level)						
Outpatient						
99354	First hour	96.97	88.76	84.32	96.97	
99355	Each addl. 30 min	96.97	88.76	84.32	96.97	
Inpatient						
99356	First hour	96.42	88.25	83.84	96.42	
99357	Each addl. 30 min	96.42	88.25	83.84	96.42	
Prolonged Services Without Direct Contact						
99358	First hour	90.00				
99359	Each addl. 30 min	90.00				
Physician Standby Service						
99360	Each 30 min	95.00				
Case Management Services						
Team Conferences						
99366		85.00				
99367-99368		105.00				
Telephone Calls						
99441	5–10 min	30.00				
99442	11–20 min	40.00				
99443	21–30 min	60.00				
Care Plan Oversight Services						
99375	30 min or more/month	93.40	85.49	81.22	93.40	
Preventive Medicine						
New Patient						
99381	Infant younger than 1 year	50.00				
99382	1–4 years	50.00				
99383	5–11 years	45.00				
99384	12–17 years	45.00				
99385	18–39 years	50.00				
99386	40–64 years	50.00				
99387	65 years and older	55.00				
Established Patient						
99391	Infant younger than year	35.00				
99392	1–4 years	35.00				

[a]Some services and procedures may not be considered a benefit under the Medicare program and when listed on a claim form, no reimbursement may be received. However, it is important to include these codes when billing because Medicare policies may change without an individual knowing of a new benefit. For this reason, some of the services shown in this Mock Fee Schedule do not have any amounts listed under the three Medicare columns.

Continued

371

Table 2. Mock Fee Schedule—cont'd

Code No.	Description	Mock Fees	Medicare[a] Participating	Nonparticipating	Limiting Charge	Follow-Up Days
99393	5–11 years	30.00				
99394	12–17 years	30.00				
99395	18–39 years	35.00				
99396	40–64 years	35.00				
99397	65 years and older	40.00				
Counseling (new/est pt)						
Individual						
99401	15 min	35.00				
99402	30 min	50.00				
99403	45 min	65.00				
99404	60 min	80.00				
Group						
99411	30 min	30.00				
99412	60 min	50.00				
Other Preventive Medicine Services						
99420	Health hazard appraisal	50.00				
99429	Unlisted preventive med service	Variable				
Newborn Care						
99460	Birthing room delivery	102.50	93.50	88.83	102.15	
99461	Other than birthing room	110.16	100.83	95.79	110.16	
99462	Subsequent hospital care	54.02	49.44	46.97	54.02	
99465	Newborn resuscitation	255.98	234.30	222.59	255.98	
Anesthesiology						

Anesthesiology fees are presented here for CPT codes. However, each case would require a fee for time, e.g., every 15 minutes would be worth $55. This fee is determined according to the relative value system, calculated, and added into the anesthesia (CPT) fee. Some anesthetists may list a surgical code using an anesthesia modifier on a subsequent line for carriers that do not acknowledge anesthesia codes.

Code No.	Description	Mock Fees				
99100	Anes for pt younger than 1 year or older than 70 years	55.00				
99116	Anes complicated use total hypothermia	275.00				
99135	Anes complicated use hypotension	275.00				
99140	Anes complicated emer cond	110.00				
Physician Status Modifier Codes						
P-1	Normal healthy patient	00.00				
P-2	Patient with mild systemic disease	00.00				
P-3	Patient with severe systemic disease	55.00				
P-4	Patient with severe systemic disease that is a constant threat to life	110.00				
P-5	Moribund pt not expected to survive without operation	165.00				
P-6	Declared brain-dead pt, organs being removed for donor	00.00				

[a]Some services and procedures may not be considered a benefit under the Medicare program and when listed on a claim form, no reimbursement may be received. However, it is important to include these codes when billing because Medicare policies may change without an individual knowing of a new benefit. For this reason, some of the services shown in this Mock Fee Schedule do not have any amounts listed under the three Medicare columns.

Table 2. Mock Fee Schedule—cont'd

Code No.	Description	Mock Fees	Medicare[a] Participating	Nonparticipating	Limiting Charge	Follow-Up Days
Head						
00160	Anes nose/sinus (NEC)	275.00				
00172	Anes repair cleft palate	165.00				
Thorax						
00400	Anes for proc ant integumentary system of chest, incl SC tissue	165.00				
00402	Anes breast reconstruction	275.00				
00546	Anes pulmonary resection with thoracoplasty	275.00				
00600	Anes cervical spine and cord	550.00				
Lower Abdomen						
00800	Anes for proc lower ant abdominal wall	165.00				
00840	Anes intraperitoneal proc lower abdomen: NOS	330.00				
00842	Amniocentesis	220.00				
00914	Anes TURP	275.00				
00942	Anes colporrhaphy, colpotomy, colpectomy	220.00				
Upper Leg						
01210	Anes open proc hip joint; NOS	330.00				
01214	Total hip replacement	440.00				
Upper Arm and Elbow						
01740	Anes open proc humerus/elbow; NOS	220.00				
01758	Exc cyst/tumor humerus	275.00				
Radiologic Procedures						
01922	Anes CAT scan	385.00				
Miscellaneous Procedure(s)						
01999	Unlisted anes proc	Variable				
Neurology						
95812	Electroencephalogram	129.32	118.37	112.45	129.32	
95819	Electroencephalogram—awake	126.81	116.07	110.27	126.81	
95860	Electromyography, 1 extremity	88.83	81.31	77.24	88.83	
95864	Electromyography, 4 extremities	239.99	219.67	208.69	239.99	
96101	Psychological testing (per hour)	80.95	74.10	70.39	80.95	
Physical Medicine						
97024	Diathermy	14.27	13.06	12.41	14.27	
97036	Hubbard tank, each 15 min	24.77	22.67	21.54	24.77	
97110	Therapeutic proc, one or more areas, each 15 min	23.89	21.86	20.77	23.89	
97140	Manual therapy (manipulation, traction), one or more regions, each 15 min	16.93	15.49	14.72	16.93	
Special Services and Reports						
99000	Handling of specimen (transfer from Dr.'s office to lab)	5.00				
99024	Postoperative visit (bundled)	No charge				

[a]Some services and procedures may not be considered a benefit under the Medicare program and when listed on a claim form, no reimbursement may be received. However, it is important to include these codes when billing because Medicare policies may change without an individual knowing of a new benefit. For this reason, some of the services shown in this Mock Fee Schedule do not have any amounts listed under the three Medicare columns.

Continued

Appendix **College Clinic Office Policies and Mock Fee Schedule**

Table 2. Mock Fee Schedule—cont'd

Code No.	Description	Mock Fees	Medicare[a] Participating	Nonparticipating	Limiting Charge	Follow-Up Days
99050	Services provided, in the office at times other than regularly scheduled office hours or days when office is normally closed (e.g., holidays, Saturday or Sunday) in addition to basic service	25.00				
99053	Services between 10:00 PM and 8:00 AM in addition to basic service (24 hr facility)	35.00				
99056	Services normally provided in office requested by pt in location other than office in addition to basic service	20.00				
99058	Office services provided on an emergency basis, which causes disruption of other sched svcs.					
99070	Supplies and materials (itemize drugs and materials provided)	10.00				
99080	Special reports: insurance forms					
	Review of data to clarify pt's status	20.00				
	WC reports	50.00				
	WC extensive review report	250.00				
10060	I & D furuncle, onychia, paronychia; single	75.92	69.49	66.02	75.92	10
11042	Débridement; skin, partial thickness	79.32	75.60	68.97	79.32	10
11044	Débridement; skin, subcu. muscle, bone	269.28	246.48	234.16	269.28	10
11100	Biopsy of skin, SC tissue &/or mucous membrane; 1 lesion	65.43	59.89	56.90	65.43	10
11200	Exc, skin tags; up to 15	55.68	50.97	45.42	55.68	10
11401	Exc, benign lesion, 0.6–1.0 cm trunk, arms, legs	95.62	87.53	83.15	96.62	10
11402	1.1–2.0 cm	121.52	111.23	105.67	121.52	10
11403	2.1–3.0 cm	151.82	138.97	132.02	151.82	10
11420	Exc, benign lesion, 0.5 cm or less scalp, neck, hands, feet, genitalia	75.44	69.05	65.60	75.44	10
11422	Exc, benign lesion scalp, neck, hands, feet, or genitalia; 1.1–2.0 cm	131.35	120.23	114.22	131.35	10
11441	Exc, benign lesion face, ears, eyelids, nose, lips, or mucous membrane	119.08	109.00	103.55	119.08	10
11602	Exc, malignant lesion, trunk, arms, or legs; 1.1–2.0 cm dia	195.06	178.55	169.62	195.06	10
11719	Trimming of nondystrophic nails, any number	30.58	27.82	26.33	30.58	0
11720	Débridement of nails, any method, 1–5	32.58	29.82	28.33	32.58	0
11721	6 or more	32.58	29.82	28.33	32.58	0
11730	Avulsion nail plate, partial or complete, simple repair; single	76.91	70.40	66.88	76.91	0
11750	Exc, nail or nail matrix, partial or complete	193.45	177.07	168.22	193.45	10

[a]Some services and procedures may not be considered a benefit under the Medicare program and when listed on a claim form, no reimbursement may be received. However, it is important to include these codes when billing because Medicare policies may change without an individual knowing of a new benefit. For this reason, some of the services shown in this Mock Fee Schedule do not have any amounts listed under the three Medicare columns.

Table 2. Mock Fee Schedule—cont'd

Code No.	Description	Mock Fees	Medicare[a]			
			Participating	Nonpartici-pating	Limiting Charge	Follow-Up Days
11765	Wedge excision of nail fold	57.95	53.04	50.39	57.95	10
12001	Simple repair (scalp, neck, axillae, ext genitalia, trunk, or extremities incl. hands & feet); 2.5 cm or less	91.17	83.45	79.28	91.17	10
12011	Simple repair (face, ears, eyelids, nose, lips, or mucous membranes); 2.5 cm or less	101.44	92.85	88.21	101.44	10
12013	2.6–5.0 cm	123.98	113.48	107.81	123.98	10
12032	Repair, scalp, axillae, trunk (intermediate)	169.73	155.36	147.59	169.73	10
12034	Repair, intermediate, wounds (scalp, axillae, trunk, or extremities) excl hands or feet; 7.6–12.5 cm	214.20	196.06	186.26	214.20	10
12051	Repair, intermediate, layer closure of wounds (face, ears, eyelids, nose, lips, or mucous membranes); 2.5 cm or less	167.60	153.41	145.74	167.60	10
17000	Cauterization, 1 lesion	52.56	48.11	45.70	52.56	10
17003	Second through 14 lesions, each	15.21	17.77	16.88	5.21	
17004	Destruction (laser surgery), 15 or more lesions					10
19020	Mastotomy, drainage/exploration deep abscess	237.36	217.26	206.40	237.36	90
19100	Biopsy, breast, needle	96.17	88.03	83.63	96.17	0
19101	Biopsy, breast, incisional	281.51	257.67	244.79	281.51	10
20610	Arthrocentesis, aspiration or injection major joint (shoulder, hip, knee, or bursa)	52.33	47.89	45.50	52.33	0
21330	Nasal fracture, open treatment complicated	599.46	548.71	521.27	599.46	90
24066	Biopsy, deep, soft tissue, upper arm, elbow	383.34	350.88	333.34	383.34	90
27455	Osteotomy, proximal tibia	1248.03	1142.36	1085.24	1248.03	90
27500	Treatment closed femoral shaft fracture without manipulation	554.90	507.92	482.52	554.90	90
27530	Treatment closed tibial fracture, proximal, without manipulation	344.24	315.09	299.34	344.24	90
27750	Treatment closed tibial shaft fracture, without manipulation	400.94	366.99	348.64	400.94	90
27752	With manipulation	531.63	486.62	462.29	531.63	90
29280	Strapping of hand or finger	35.13	31.36	29.79	35.13	0
29345	Appl long leg cast (thigh to toes)	123.23	112.80	107.16	123.23	0
29355	Walker or ambulatory type	133.75	122.42	116.30	133.75	0
29425	Appl short leg walking cast	102.10	93.45	88.78	102.10	0
30110	Excision, simple nasal polyp	145.21	132.92	126.27	145.21	10
30520	Septoplasty	660.88	604.93	574.68	660.88	90
30903	Control nasal hemorrhage; unilateral	118.17	108.17	102.76	118.17	0

[a]Some services and procedures may not be considered a benefit under the Medicare program and when listed on a claim form, no reimbursement may be received. However, it is important to include these codes when billing because Medicare policies may change without an individual knowing of a new benefit. For this reason, some of the services shown in this Mock Fee Schedule do not have any amounts listed under the three Medicare columns.

Continued

Appendix **College Clinic Office Policies and Mock Fee Schedule**

Table 2. Mock Fee Schedule—cont'd

Code No.	Description	Mock Fees	Medicare[a]			
			Participating	Nonpartici- pating	Limiting Charge	Follow- Up Days
30905	Control nasal hemorrhage, posterior with posterior nasal packs and/or cautery; initial	190.57	174.43	165.71	190.57	0
30906	Subsequent	173.01	158.36	150.44	173.01	
31540	Laryngoscopy with excision of tumor and/or stripping of vocal cords	488.95	447.55	425.17	488.95	0
31541	With operating microscope	428.33	392.06	372.46	428.33	0
31575	Laryngoscopy, flexible fiberoptic; diagnostic	138.48	126.76	120.42	138.48	0
31625	Bronchoscopy with biopsy	312.87	286.38	272.06	312.87	0
32310	Pleurectomy	1234.79	1130.24	1073.73	1234.79	90
32440	Pneumonectomy, total	1972.10	1805.13	1714.87	1972.10	90
33020	Pericardiotomy	1289.25	1180.09	1121.09	1289.25	90
33206	Insertion of pacemaker; atrial	728.42	666.75	633.41	728.42	90
33208	Atrial and ventricular	751.57	687.89	653.50	751.57	90
35301	Thromboendarterectomy, with or with-out patch graft; carotid, vertebral, subclavian, by neck incision	1585.02	1450.82	1378.28	1585.02	90
36005	Intravenous injection for contrast venography	59.18	54.17	51.46	59.18	0
36248	Catheter placement (selective) arterial system, 2nd, 3rd order and beyond	68.54	62.74	59.60	68.54	0
36415	Routine venipuncture for collection of specimen(s)	10.00				
38101	Splenectomy, partial	994.44	910.24	864.73	994.44	90
38220	Bone marrow; aspiration only	73.52	67.29	63.93	73.52	NA
38221	Biopsy, needle or trocar	90.65	82.98	78.83	90.65	NA
38510	Biopsy/excision deep cervical node/s	327.42	299.69	284.71	327.42	10
39540	Hernia repair	1436.50	1314.87	1249.13	1436.50	90
42820	T&A under age 12 years	341.63	312.71	297.07	341.63	90
42821	T&A over age 12 years	410.73	375.96	357.16	410.73	90
43200	Upper GI endoscopy, simple primary exam	201.86	184.77	175.53	201.86	0
43235	Upper GI endoscopy incl. esophagus, stomach, duodenum, or jejunum; complex	238.92	218.69	207.76	238.92	0
43239	Esophagogastro-duodenoscopy, with biopsy, single or multiple	238.92	218.69	207.76	238.92	0
43255	With control of bleeding, any method	281.51	257.67	244.79	281.51	0
43453	Dilation esophagus	254.52	232.97	221.32	254.52	0
43754	Gastric intubation	87.41	80.01	76.01	87.41	
43820	Gastrojejunostomy	971.86	889.58	845.10	971.86	90
44150	Colectomy, total, abdominal	1757.81	108.98	1528.53	1757.81	90
44320	Colostomy or skin level cecostomy	966.25	884.44	840.22	966.25	90
44950	Appendectomy	568.36	520.24	494.23	568.36	90
45308	Proctosigmoidoscopy; removal of polyp	135.34	123.88	117.69	135.34	0
45315	Multiple polyps	185.12	169.44	160.97	185.12	0

[a]Some services and procedures may not be considered a benefit under the Medicare program and when listed on a claim form, no reimbursement may be received. However, it is important to include these codes when billing because Medicare policies may change without an individual knowing of a new benefit. For this reason, some of the services shown in this Mock Fee Schedule do not have any amounts listed under the three Medicare columns.

Appendix **College Clinic Office Policies and Mock Fee Schedule**

Table 2. Mock Fee Schedule—cont'd

Code No.	Description	Mock Fees	Medicare[a]			
			Participating	Nonparticipating	Limiting Charge	Follow-Up Days
45330	Sigmoidoscopy (flexible), diagnostic (with or without biopsy or collection of specimen by brushing or washing)	95.92	87.80	83.41	95.92	0
45333	Sigmoidoscopy (flexible) with removal of polyps	183.99	168.41	159.99	183.99	0
45380	Colonoscopy with biopsy	382.35	349.98	332.48	382.35	0
46255	Hemorrhoidectomy int & ext, simple	503.57	460.94	437.89	503.57	90
46258	Hemorrhoidectomy with fistulectomy	636.02	582.17	553.06	636.02	90
46600	Anoscopy; diagnostic	32.86	30.07	28.57	32.86	0
46614	With control of hemorrhage	182.10	166.68	158.35	182.10	0
46700	Anoplasty, for stricture, adult	657.39	601.73	571.64	657.39	90
47562	Cholecystectomy; laparoscopic	714.99	654.45	621.73	714.99	90
47600	Cholecystectomy; abdominal excision	937.74	858.35	815.43	937.74	90
49505	Inguinal hernia repair, age 5 or over	551.07	504.41	479.19	551.07	90
49520	Repair, inguinal hernia, any age; reducible	671.89	615.00	584.25	671.89	90
50080	Nephrostolithotomy, percutaneous	1323.93	1211.83	1151.24	1323.93	90
50780	Ureteroneocystostomy	1561.23	1429.84	1357.59	1561.23	90
51900	Closure of vesicovaginal fistula, abdominal approach	1196.82	1095.48	1040.71	1196.82	90
52000	Cystourethroscopy	167.05	152.90	145.26	167.05	0
52601	Transurethral resection of prostate	1193.53	1092.47	1037.85	1193.53	90
53040	Drainage of deep periurethral abscess	379.48	347.35	329.98	379.48	90
53060	Drainage of Skene's gland	147.45	134.97	128.22	147.45	10
53230	Excision, female diverticulum (urethral)	859.69	786.91	747.56	859.69	90
53240	Marsupialization of urethral diverticulum, M or F	520.11	476.07	452.27	520.11	90
53270	Excision of Skene's gland(s)	184.39	168.78	160.34	184.39	10
53620	Dilation, urethra, male	100.73	92.20	87.59	100.73	0
53660	Dilation urethra, female	48.32	44.23	42.02	48.32	0
54150	Circumcision	111.78	102.32	97.20	111.78	10
54520	Orchiectomy, simple	523.92	479.56	455.58	523.92	90
55700	Biopsy of prostate, needle or punch	156.22	142.99	135.84	156.22	0
55801	Prostatectomy, perineal subtotal	1466.56	1342.39	1275.27	1466.56	90
57265	Colporrhaphy AP with enterocele repair	902.24	825.85	784.56	902.24	90
57452	Colposcopy	84.18	77.05	73.20	84.18	0
57510	Cauterization of cervix, electro or thermal	115.15	105.40	100.13	115.15	10
57520	Conization of cervix with or without D&C, with or without repair	387.08	354.30	336.59	387.08	90
58100	Endometrial biopsy	71.88	65.79	62.50	71.88	0
58120	D&C, diagnostic and/or therapeutic (non-OB)	272.83	249.73	237.24	272.83	10
58150	TAH w/without salpingo-oophorectomy	1167.72	1068.85	1015.41	1167.72	90
58200	Total hysterectomy, extended, corpus	1707.24	1562.69	1484.56	1707.24	90

[a]Some services and procedures may not be considered a benefit under the Medicare program and when listed on a claim form, no reimbursement may be received. However, it is important to include these codes when billing because Medicare policies may change without an individual knowing of a new benefit. For this reason, some of the services shown in this Mock Fee Schedule do not have any amounts listed under the three Medicare columns.

Continued

Appendix **College Clinic Office Policies and Mock Fee Schedule**

Table 2. Mock Fee Schedule—cont'd

Code No.	Description	Mock Fees	Medicare[a]			
			Participating	Nonpartici-pating	Limiting Charge	Follow-Up Days
58210	Radical abdominal hysterectomy with bilateral total pelvic lymph-adenectomy	2160.78	1977.83	1878.94	2160.78	90
	completed surgically	357.39	327.13	310.77	357.39	90
58300	Insertion of intrauterine device	100.00	93.45	88.78	100.00	0
58340	Hysterosalpingography, inj proc for	73.06	66.87	63.53	73.06	0
58720	Salpingo-oophorectomy, complete or partial, unilateral or bilateral surgical treatment of ectopic pregnancy	732.40	670.39	636.87	732.40	90
59120	Ectopic pregnancy requiring salpingectomy and/or oophorectomy	789.26	722.43	686.31	789.26	90
59121	Without salpingectomy and/or oophorectomy	638.84	584.75	555.51	638.84	90
59130	Abdominal pregnancy	699.12	639.93	607.93	699.12	90
59135	Total hysterectomy, interstitial, uterine pregnancy	1154.16	1056.44	1003.62	1154.16	90
59136	Partial uterine resection, interstitial uterine pregnancy	1154.16	1056.44	1003.62	1154.16	90
59140	Cervical, with evacuation	489.68	448.22	425.81	489.68	90
59160	Curettage postpartum hemorrhage (separate proc)	293.46	268.61	255.18	293.46	10
59400	OB care—routine, incl. antepartum/postpartum care	1864.30	1706.45	1621.13	1864.30	N/A
59510	C-section including antepartum and postpartum care	2102.33	1924.33	1828.11	2102.33	N/A
59515	C-section, postpartum care only	1469.80	1345.36	1278.09	1469.80	N/A
59812	Treatment of incompl. abortion, any trimester	357.39	327.13	310.77	357.39	90
61314	Craniotomy infratentorial	2548.09	2332.35	2215.73	2548.09	90
62270	Spinal puncture, lumbar; diagnostic	77.52	70.96	67.41	77.52	0
65091	Evisceration of eye, without implant	708.22	648.25	615.84	708.22	90
65205	Removal of foreign body, ext eye	56.02	51.27	48.71	56.02	0
65222	Removal of foreign body, corneal, with slit lamp	73.81	67.56	64.18	73.81	0
69420	Myringotomy	97.76	89.48	85.01	97.76	10

RADIOLOGY, NUCLEAR MEDICINE, AND DIAGNOSTIC ULTRASOUND

Code No.	Description	Mock Fees	Participating	Nonpartici-pating	Limiting Charge	Follow-Up Days
70120	X-ray mastoids, less than 3 views per side	38.96	35.66	33.88	38.96	
70130	Complete, min., 3 views per side	56.07	51.33	48.76	56.07	
71010	Chest x-ray, 1 view	31.95	29.24	27.78	31.95	
71045	Chest x-ray, single view	31.95	29.24	27.78	31.95	
71046	Chest x-ray, 2 views	40.97	37.50	35.63	40.97	
71048	Chest x-ray, 4 or more views	54.02	49.44	46.97	54.02	
72100	X-ray spine, LS; 2 or 3 views	43.23	39.57	37.59	43.23	
72114	Complete, incl. bending views	74.97	68.62	65.19	74.97	
73100	X-ray wrist, 2 views	31.61	28.94	27.49	31.61	
73501	Hip x-ray, unilateral 1 view	31.56	28.88	27.44	31.56	

[a]Some services and procedures may not be considered a benefit under the Medicare program and when listed on a claim form, no reimbursement may be received. However, it is important to include these codes when billing because Medicare policies may change without an individual knowing of a new benefit. For this reason, some of the services shown in this Mock Fee Schedule do not have any amounts listed under the three Medicare columns.

Table 2. Mock Fee Schedule—cont'd

Code No.	Description	Mock Fees	Medicare[a]			
			Participating	Nonpartici-pating	Limiting Charge	Follow-Up Days
73502	Hip x-ray, unilateral 2–3 views	37.94	34.73	32.99	37.94	
73590	X-ray tibia & fibula, 2 views	33.35	30.53	29.00	33.35	
73620	Radiologic exam, foot; 2 views	31.61	28.94	27.49	31.61	
73650	X-ray calcaneus, 2 views	30.71	28.11	26.70	30.71	
74241	Radiologic exam, upper gastrointesti-nal tract; with/without delayed films with KUB	108.93	99.71	94.72	108.93	
74245	With small bowel, serial films	161.70	148.01	140.61	161.70	
74270	Barium enema	118.47	108.44	103.02	118.47	
74290	Cholecystography, oral contrast	52.59	48.14	45.73	52.59	
74400	Urography (pyelography), intrave-nous, with or without KUB	104.78	95.90	91.11	104.78	
74410	Urography, infusion	116.76	106.87	101.53	116.76	
74420	Urography, retrograde	138.89	127.13	120.77	138.89	
76805	Ultrasound, pregnant uterus, or real time; complete, first gestation	154.18	141.13	134.07	154.18	
76810	Ultrasound, pregnant uterus, complete: each additional gestation, after first trimester	306.54	280.59	266.56	306.54	
76946	Ultrasonic guidance for amniocentesis	91.22	83.49	79.32	91.22	
77065	Diagnostic mammography; unilateral	62.57	57.27	54.41	62.57	
77066	Diagnostic mammography; bilateral	82.83	75.82	72.03	82.83	
77300	Radiation dosimetry	97.58	89.32	84.85	97.58	
77307	Teletherapy, isodose plan, complex	213.59	195.51	185.73	213.59	
78104	Bone marrow imaging, whole body	230.56	211.04	200.49	230.56	
78215	Liver and spleen imaging	160.44	146.85	139.51	160.44	
78800	Tumor localization, limited area	191.53	175.32	166.55	191.53	

PATHOLOGY AND LABORATORY[1]
ORGAN OR DISEASE-ORIENTED PANELS

Code No.	Description	Mock Fees	Participating	Nonpartici-pating	Limiting Charge	Follow-Up Days
80048	Basic metabolic panel	15.00	14.60	13.87	16.64	
80050	General health panel	20.00	19.20	15.99	21.87	
80051	Electrolyte panel	20.00	19.20	15.99	21.87	
80053	Comprehensive metabolic panel	25.00	20.99	19.94	23.93	
80055	Obstetric panel	25.00	20.99	19.94	23.93	
80061	Lipid panel	30.00	28.60	25.97	32.16	
80074	Acute hepatitis panel	27.00	25.00	20.88	24.88	
80076	Hepatic function panel	27.00	25.00	20.88	24.98	
81000	Urinalysis, nonautomated, with microscopy	8.00	7.44	5.98	8.84	
81001	Urinalysis, automated, with microscopy	8.00	7.44	5.98	8.84	
81002	Urinalysis, nonautomated without microscopy	8.00	7.44	5.98	8.84	
81015	Urinalysis, microscopy only	8.00	7.44	5.98	8.84	
82270	Blood, occult; feces screening 1–3	4.05	3.56	3.31	4.05	
82565	Creatinine; blood	10.00	9.80	8.88	12.03	
82947	Glucose; quantitative	15.00				

[a]Some services and procedures may not be considered a benefit under the Medicare program and when listed on a claim form, no reimbursement may be received. However, it is important to include these codes when billing because Medicare policies may change without an individual knowing of a new benefit. For this reason, some of the services shown in this Mock Fee Schedule do not have any amounts listed under the three Medicare columns.

Continued

Appendix **College Clinic Office Policies and Mock Fee Schedule**

Table 2. Mock Fee Schedule—cont'd

Code No.	Description	Mock Fees	Medicare[a] Participating	Medicare[a] Nonpartici-pating	Medicare[a] Limiting Charge	Follow-Up Days
82951	Glucose tolerance test, 3 spec	40.00	41.00	36.80	45.16	
82952	Each add spec beyond 3	30.00	28.60	25.97	32.16	
83020	Hemoglobin, electrophoresis	25.00	20.00	19.94	23.93	
83700	Lipoprotein, blood; electrophoretic separation	25.00	20.00	19.94	23.93	
84478	Triglycerides, blood	20.00	19.20	15.999	21.87	
84480	Triiodothyronine (T-3)	20.00	19.20	15.99	21.87	
84520	Urea nitrogen, blood (BUN); quantitative	25.00	20.99	19.94	23.93	
84550	Uric acid, blood chemical	20.00	19.20	15.99	21.87	
84702	Gonadotropin, chorionic; quantitative	20.00	19.20	15.99	21.87	
84703	Gonadotropin, chorionic; qualitative	20.00	19.20	15.99	21.87	
85013	Microhematocrit (spun)	20.00	19.20	15.99	21.87	
85025	Complete blood count (hemogram), platelet count, automated, differential WBC count	25.00	20.00	19.94	23.93	
85032	Manual cell count (erythrocyte, leukocyte, or platelet) each	20.00	19.20	15.99	21.87	
85345	Coagulation time; Lee & White	20.00	19.20	15.99	21.87	
86038	Antinuclear antibodies	25.00	20.00	19.94	23.93	
86580	Skin test; TB, intradermal	11.34	10.38	9.86	11.34	
87081	Culture, bacterial, screening for single organisms	25.00	20.00	19.94	23.93	
87181	Sensitivity studies, antibiotic; per antibiotic	20.00	19.20	15.99	21.87	
87184	Disk method, per plate (12 disks or less)	20.00	19.20	15.99	21.87	
87210	Smear, primary source, wet mount with simple stain, for bacteria, fungi, ova, and/or parasites	35.00	48.35	45.93	55.12	
88150	Papanicolaou, cytopath	35.00	48.35	45.93	55.12	
88302	Surgical pathology, gross & micro exam (skin, fingers, nerve, testis)	24.14	22.09	20.99	24.14	
88305	Bone marrow, interpret	77.69	71.12	67.56	77.69	

MEDICINE PROCEDURES

Immunization Injections

Code No.	Description	Mock Fees	Participating	Nonpartici-pating	Limiting Charge	Follow-Up Days
90700	Diphtheria, tetanus, pertussis	34.00				
90703	Tetanus toxoid	28.00				
90712	Poliovirus vaccine, oral	28.00				

Therapeutic Injections

Code No.	Description	Mock Fees	Participating	Nonpartici-pating	Limiting Charge	Follow-Up Days
96372	Therapeutic prophylactic or Dx injection; IM or SC	5.22	4.37	4.15	5.22	
96374	Intravenous push, single or initial substance/drug	21.33	19.53	18.55	21.33	
96379	Intravenous therapeutic prophylactic, or diagnostic	21.33	19.53	18.55	21.33	

Psychiatry

Code No.	Description	Mock Fees	Participating	Nonpartici-pating	Limiting Charge	Follow-Up Days
90832	Individual psychotherapy 20–30 min	60.25	55.15	52.39	60.25	
90853	Group therapy	29.22	26.75	25.41	29.22	

[a]Some services and procedures may not be considered a benefit under the Medicare program and when listed on a claim form, no reimbursement may be received. However, it is important to include these codes when billing because Medicare policies may change without an individual knowing of a new benefit. For this reason, some of the services shown in this Mock Fee Schedule do not have any amounts listed under the three Medicare columns.

Table 2. Mock Fee Schedule—cont'd

Code No.	Description	Mock Fees	Medicare[a] Participating	Medicare[a] Nonparticipating	Medicare[a] Limiting Charge	Follow-Up Days
Hemodialysis						
90935	Single phys evaluation	117.23	107.31	101.94	117.23	
90937	Repeat evaluation	206.24	188.78	179.34	206.24	
Gastroenterology						
91010	Esophageal incubation	69.82	63.91	60.71	69.82	
Ophthalmologic Services						
92004	Comprehensive eye exam	90.86	83.17	79.01	90.86	
92100	Tonometry	47.31	43.31	41.14	47.31	
92230	Fluorescein angioscopy	55.49	50.79	48.25	55.49	
92275	Electroretinography	81.17	74.29	70.58	81.17	
92531	Spontaneous nystagmus	26.00				
Audiologic Function Tests						
92557	Comprehensive audiometry	54.33	49.73	47.24	54.33	
92596	Ear measurements	26.81	24.54	23.31	26.81	
Cardiovascular Therapeutic Services						
93000	Electrocardiogram (ECG)	34.26	31.36	29.79	34.26	
93015	Treadmill ECG	140.71	128.80	122.36	140.71	
93040	Rhythm ECG, 1–3 leads	18.47	16.90	16.06	18.47	
93306	Doppler echocardiography	250.73	229.50	218.03	250.73	
93307	Echocardiography without Doppler	114.60	104.90	99.65	114.60	
Pulmonary						
94010	Spirometry	38.57	35.31	33.54	38.57	
94060	Spirometry before and after bronchodilator	71.67	65.60	62.32	71.67	
94150	Vital capacity, total	13.82	12.65	12.02	13.82	
Allergy and Clinical Immunology						
95024	Intradermal tests; immediate reaction	6.58	6.02	5.72	6.85	
95028	Intradermal tests; delayed reaction	9.32	8.85	10.18	9.32	
95044	Patch tests	8.83	8.08	7.68	8.83	
95115	Treatment for allergy, single inj.	17.20	15.75	14.96	17.20	
95117	2 or more inj.	22.17	20.29	19.28	22.17	
95165	Allergen immunotherapy, single or multiple antigens, multiple-dose vials (professional svcs for preparation supervision)		6.50	6.18	7.11	
Neurology						
95812	Electroencephalogram, 41–60 min	129.32	118.37	112.45	129.32	
95819	Electroencephalogram—awake and	126.81	116.07	110.27	126.81	
95860	Electromyography, 1 extremity	88.83	81.31	77.24	88.83	
96101	Psychological testing (per hour)	80.95	74.10	70.39	80.95	
Physical Medicine						
97024	Diathermy	14.27	13.06	12.41	14.27	
97036	Hubbard tank, each 15 min	24.77	22.67	21.54	24.77	
97110	Physical therapy, initial 30 min	23.89	21.86	20.77	23.89	
97140	Manual therapy (manipulation, traction), one or more regions, each 15 min	16.93	15.49	14.72	16.93	

[a]Some services and procedures may not be considered a benefit under the Medicare program and when listed on a claim form, no reimbursement may be received. However, it is important to include these codes when billing because Medicare policies may change without an individual knowing of a new benefit. For this reason, some of the services shown in this Mock Fee Schedule do not have any amounts listed under the three Medicare columns.

Continued

Appendix **College Clinic Office Policies and Mock Fee Schedule**

Table 2. Mock Fee Schedule—cont'd

Code No.	Description	Mock Fees	Medicare[a]			
			Participating	Nonpartici-pating	Limiting Charge	Follow-Up Days
Chiropractic Manipulative Treatment						
98940	Chiropractic manipulative treatment; spinal 1–2 regions	75.00				
Special Services and Reports						
99000	Handling of specimen (transfer from Dr.'s office to lab)	5.00				
99050	Services provided after office hours, or on Sundays and holidays in addition to basic service in the office	25.00				
99053	Services between 10 PM and 8 AM in addition to basic service	35.00				
99056	Services normally provided in office requested by pt in location other than office	20.00				
99058	Office services provided on an emergency basis	65.00				
99070	Supplies and materials (itemize drugs and materials provided)	25.00				
99080	Special reports:					
	Insurance forms	10.00				
	Review of data to clarify pt's status	20.00				
	WC reports	50.00				
	WC extensive review report	250.00				

[a]Some services and procedures may not be considered a benefit under the Medicare program and when listed on a claim form, no reimbursement may be received. However, it is important to include these codes when billing because Medicare policies may change without an individual knowing of a new benefit. For this reason, some of the services shown in this Mock Fee Schedule do not have any amounts listed under the three Medicare columns.

[b]Data for the surgical follow-up days from St. Anthony's CPT '96 Companion: A Guide to Medicare Billing.

CALIFORNIA
REAL ESTATE PRACTICE

William H. Pivar,
Lowell Anderson,
Daniel S. Otto
with Kartik Subramaniam, Contributing Editor

This publication is designed to provide accurate and authoritative information in regard to the subject matter covered. It is sold with the understanding that the publisher is not engaged in rendering legal, accounting, or other professional advice. If legal advice or other expert assistance is required, the services of a competent professional should be sought.

President: Dr. Andrew Temte
Chief Learning Officer: Dr. Tim Smaby
Executive Director, Real Estate Education: Melissa Kleeman-Moy
Development Editor: Jody Manderfeld

CALIFORNIA REAL ESTATE PRACTICE, NINTH EDITION
©2016 Kaplan, Inc.
Published by DF Institute, Inc., d/b/a Dearborn Real Estate Education
332 Front St. S., Suite 501
La Crosse, WI 54601

Printed in the United States of America
ISBN: 978-1-4754-3575-7

CONTENTS

INTRODUCTION

California Real Estate Practice is the practical application of real estate knowledge to meet the needs of buyers, sellers, lessors, and lessees. It is a course in what to do for success in meeting these needs.

California Real Estate Practice is not a repetition of *California Real Estate Principles*; however, it does cover the practical application of much of what you learned in Principles, as well as the "how" of being a real estate professional.

Note: Every applicant for a real estate salesperson's examination must complete college-level courses in real estate principles and real estate practice, as well as an approved third course, before sitting for the real estate salesperson's examination.

ACKNOWLEDGMENTS

The authors wish to acknowledge the invaluable assistance given to us in this and previous editions from the following professionals and educators:

Thurza B. Andrew, GRI, Mortgage Broker, Chico Valley Mortgage; Associate Professor, Butte Community College; Leonel "Leo" Bello, MBA, City College of San Francisco; Joyce Emory, Real Estate Advisory Council; Ignacio Gonzalez, Mendocino Community College, Ukiah, California; Professor Donna Grogan, El Camino College; Ted Highland, Kaplan Professional Schools; Margaret McCarthy Johnson, CPA; Don Kalal, GRI, California Brokers Institute; Keith H. Kerr, City College of San Francisco; Charles E. Krackeler, CRS, GRI, College of San Mateo; Fred L. Martinez, City College of San Francisco; Judith Meadows; Joe M. Newton, Bakersfield College; Pamela Pedago-Lowe, RE/MAX South County; Ronald Dean Schultz, Diablo Valley College; Nancy E. Weagley, Saddleback College; Evelyn W. Winkel, Esq., Rancho Santiago College; Janet Wright, Place Title Company; and Bud Zeller, GRI, CRS, RIM, ERA Sierra Properties.

It is with fond memories that we acknowledge the contribution of two exceptional real estate educators, Lowell Anderson and Daniel S. Otto, the original authors of this text. They set the direction to produce a working tool for real estate professionals. Their emphasis was to meet the needs of others.

GETTING STARTED IN REAL ESTATE

LEARNING OBJECTIVES

When you have completed this unit, you will be able to

■ explain the effect the real estate industry has, both directly and indirectly, on the economy;

■ describe the unique nature of the real estate marketplace and changes that are taking place within the real estate profession;

■ explain how brokers are compensated and changes taking place as to compensation;

■ list specialties available within or related to the real estate profession;

■ describe the relationship between brokers and salespeople and factors to consider in choosing a broker; and

■ explain the necessity of planning, goal setting, time management, attitude, continued education and training to a real estate career.

KEY TERMS

buyer's market	inventory	personal assistant
California Association of REALTORS®	mentor program	Realtist
	multiple listing service	seller's market
caravans	must-buy buyer	stratified marketplace
completed staff work	must-sell seller	team concepts
daily planning	National Association of REALTORS®	will-buy buyer
e-PRO certification		will-sell seller
employee	office procedures manual	workers' compensation insurance
goal setting		
independent contractor	100% commission office	

WHAT IT MEANS TO BE A REAL ESTATE PROFESSIONAL

It has been said that without the first real estate salesperson, human beings would still be living in caves. This may be an overstatement, but it is true that the real estate profession has played a significant role in improving the living conditions and lifestyles of our citizens.

Although we deal with a product—real estate (namely, the land and that which transfers with it)—the human factor of identifying and fulfilling the needs of others is the dominant emphasis of the real estate profession. We reach success in the real estate profession by first successfully meeting the needs of others. Real estate is, therefore, more a *people* than a *property* profession. Your understanding of people and their motivations will determine your future as a real estate professional. You might consider taking an interest aptitude test to see if you have the *people interests* that fit a career in real estate.

This is a profession that you can be properly proud of, because in its practice you guide buyers in making the largest purchase of their lives, one that will become a significant part of their lives—their homes. You also guide sellers in selling what has likely become more than just real estate but a place of memories. For the buyer as well as the seller, home purchases are important in both emotion and dollars.

REAL ESTATE AND THE ECONOMY

The real estate industry, which includes the production as well as the distribution of real estate, has historically been an engine driving both the California and the U.S. economies.

More jobs have been created in the real estate and related supply, construction, and service industries than from any other source. In addition, the many industries that benefit from a strong real estate market—in new as well as existing proper ties—include those listed below.

Advertising	Escrow
Air-conditioning	Excavating
Aluminum	Fencing
Appliance	Floor coverings
Appraisal	Flooring
Architecture and design	Furniture
Awning	Glass
Banking	Hardware
Bed and bath accessories	Heating
Brick and stone	Home inspection
Cabinetry	Insulation
Carpet cleaning	Insurance
Ceramic	Internet services
Cleaning services	Iron work
Concrete	Landscaping
Construction equipment	Lawn care
manufacture and sales	Lawn equipment and supplies
Construction workers and	Legal
support	Logging
personnel	Lumber
Contracting	Maintenance
Crane service	Millwork
Drywall	Mold abatement
Electrical equipment and	Moving and storage
supplies	Mortgage origination and service
Equipment maintenance	Municipal services

Nursery

Paint

Pest control

Plaster Plastic

Plumbing fixtures

Pools and spas (construction, maintenance and repair)

Portable toilets

Printing

Property inspection

Property management

Remodeling

Road construction

Roofing

Sales (supplies, equipment, and services)

Seal coating

Security (equipment and services)

Septic systems

Service providers

Steel

Stucco

Survey

Textile (fabrics for home furnishings)

Termite

Tile

Title insurance

Tools

Transportation

Vehicle (sales and service)

Wall coverings

Warehousing

Waste removal

Window coverings

Website design

Well (drilling and maintenance)

Real estate salespeople work at the end of the production and marketing pipeline keeping our products moving. If we were unable to effectively market products, the entire process would slow, resulting in increased unemployment that would have been a recessionary effect on our entire economy. The real estate recession of the mid-2000s began with a decrease in lending standards, and the market has been recovering as the remaining toxic inventory moves through the system.

THE REAL ESTATE MARKETPLACE

The real estate marketplace, where you will be aiding buyers and sellers, is generally regarded as an imperfect marketplace. Prices asked for similar properties vary, and the selling price is often less than the asking price. Values generally are set by supply and demand, not by sellers. It is the price a buyer will pay and not the price a seller desires that ultimately determines value. The only constant in the real estate marketplace is change. Inventory and value are not static. The real estate marketplace differs from other commodities. Some of the reasons why the real estate marketplace is unique include the following:

Real estate is not homogeneous

■ **Product differentiation**—Every property is different. No two locations are the same. There are usually differences in square feet, interior design, architectural style, landscaping, decorating, age, maintenance, and other amenities. Because of these differences, it is impossible to determine value scientifically. An appraiser tries to evaluate these differences but only estimates what the sale price should be.

■ **Emotion**—Emotion plays a significant part in a purchase decision. Often a buyer wants just one particular property after having turned down similar offerings without knowing why. This emotional desire can play a significant role in determining what a buyer will pay. Emotion plays a far lesser role for sellers, who are more likely to make their decisions based on logic.

■ **Buyer and seller knowledge**—While internet homesites have resulted in better informed buyers and sellers, the listing prices alone can be misleading. List prices are not sale prices and many listings expire unsold. Location also plays a significant role in determining value. Similar houses on different blocks or different streets can have significantly dissimilar values. In a thin market with few sales for a type of property, the internet data can be especially misleading. Some buyers and sellers in the marketplace have imperfect or erroneous knowledge of prices paid for similar properties. Because of this imperfect knowledge, sellers have sold at what we may consider below-market prices, and sellers have priced their properties so high that buyers show no interest in them. Similarly, imperfect knowledge can result in a buyer paying more than what might be regarded as a reasonable price. The growth of buyer brokerage, where a sole agent represents a buyer, has reduced the likelihood of a buyer overpaying.

■ **Will-sell versus must-sell owners,** and **will-buy versus must-buy buyers**—Buyer and seller motivation play a significant role in what is asked for a property by an owner, what is offered by a buyer, and what an owner will accept. Unmotivated sellers—that is, **will-sell sellers** (those who don't need to sell but who will sell if the price is right)—frequently place property on the market at above-market prices. Sellers who are motivated to sell will be more realistic in their pricing. When a seller is highly motivated or desperate, a **must-sell seller,** the price asked could be less than the sale prices of similarly desirable properties. The degree of seller motivation also will affect the likelihood of a below-list-price offer being accepted. Included in must-sell sellers are those in foreclosure sales to avoid foreclosure as well as short sales and lender dispositions of lender-owned real estate. Lender-owned real estate is usually called REOs (Real Estate Owned). When many such properties are on the market, they have a negative effect on all similar properties in the marketplace. **Will-buy buyers** are buyers who don't really have to buy. Investors and speculators are included in this group. Will-buy buyers generally look for motivated must-sell sellers; in other words, they're often bargain hunters. Investors are usually will-buy buyers. **Must-buy buyers** generally look for properties that meet their specific needs. While even must-buy buyers like bargains, they are more likely to pay a reasonable price. Successful real estate professionals concentrate their time on probabilities rather than possibilities, which means giving priority to must-sell owners and motivated buyers.

■ **Terms**—Because of the dollar value of the purchase, real estate sales tend to be very sensitive to interest rates. Higher interest rates can depress the marketplace because fewer buyers will qualify for loans. Lower rates tend to stimulate the market as more potential buyers qualify for loans. Investors are less likely to borrow money to invest in real property when interest rates are high, because the rate of return on the investment could be disappointing compared with the interest payments the investor would be required to make. By the same token, an investor would be more likely to borrow funds to invest in real property when interest rates are low. If a seller is willing to finance a buyer at a below-market rate of interest, the seller may be able to obtain a premium price for the property. Lower interest rates alone will not stimulate the economy if lenders are reluctant to loan.

> Sale prices in a seller's market may actually be greater than the list price.

The economic forces of **supply and demand** place pressure on prices to rise or fall. In a **seller's market**, buyers must compete among themselves for properties. In a seller's market, there may be multiple offers for a property. Prices will increase in a seller's market. The reverse is true of a **buyer's market**. In a buyer's market, there are many sellers and few buyers, so sellers must compete for the available buyers, which usually means the lowering of prices.

Over the long term, real estate values have tended to increase significantly due to increased demand, which is affected by population movement and growth. However, it is not a truth that real estate values always increase. Economic factors, as well as a perceived desirability, can result in a stable or even declining market. Because price is a function of supply and demand, the areas and properties maintaining the greatest desirability will have the least downward pressure on prices.

A number of factors led to the 2008 meltdown in real estate values. Some of these included the following:

- A rapid rise in real estate values. Where values have increased rapidly, they are likely to show a rapid decline with a change in demand.

- Speculators entering the housing marketplace led to a false sense of actual housing demand. Many developers encouraged multiple sales to speculators, which helped to raise prices. When the market activity slowed, speculators sought to unload their inventory at prices that in many cases were less than what developers were selling the units for. Many speculators defaulted on their loans, resulting in foreclosure sales, which drove prices down further.

- Refinancing of homes became a prime engine of our economy. People were using their homes like credit cards to obtain money for consumer goods. When home values declined, many homeowners realized they were upside down on their loans, meaning that they owed more on their homes than the homes were worth. The result was that many owners walked away, leaving their homes to the lenders.

- Exotic loan types such as option-arms allowed borrowers to qualify for loans with a low monthly payment. When the honeymoon period of low payments ended, the loans required an amortized payment. Payment shock coupled with a declining market encouraged loan defaults.

- No down payment loans or very low down payment loans made from about 2003 until 2007 resulted in many buyers realizing they had no equity in their homes and, in many cases, owed tens or even hundreds of thousands more than similar homes were selling for. This led to a great many loan defaults.

- Lenders who were not keeping the loans but intended to sell them to others became caught up in a "make hay while the sun shines" attitude. Appraisers who did not rubber stamp purchase prices were replaced by those who were more accommodating.

- Ready credit led to developers building more and bigger projects. There was a belief that prosperity for them would never end.

- Rating services gave collateralized mortgage securities investment grade ratings that in retrospect were not justified. The ability to sell these securities fueled the demand for more of them.

- The economies of the world are interrelated and a world downturn led to lower exports, a lack of consumer confidence, lower imports and loss of jobs in both production and services. With two incomes necessary for many families, the loss of an income or even a reduction in hours led to many owners being unable to make mortgage payments.

In the mid- to late- 2000s we had a depressed real estate market, but the market moves in cycles. There was a brisk market in foreclosed properties, fueled both by families seeking homes and by investors. In 2012, several large investment groups entered the marketplace seeking to buy thousands of lender-owned homes. The increased demand resulted in higher prices being paid for distressed properties and was also reflected in higher prices for the resale market. Because few new homes had been built while the market was depressed, the demand for housing, coupled with low interest rates, caused rents to increase and home construction to come back strong. By 2015, home prices in many areas of California had exceeded the highs of 2007. The marketplace corrected itself.

| The real estate market is stratified based on price. |

The real estate marketplace is also a **stratified marketplace**—stratified based on price range. As an example, there might be a seller's market in homes priced under $250,000, with many more buyers than sellers. At the same time, there might be a glut of homes priced between $800,000 and $1,000,000, with few buyers.

The real estate professional helps to bring a measure of order to what could otherwise be a chaotic marketplace. A broker's knowledge, as well as inventory, gives both buyers and sellers comparables and enables the agent to educate them in the realities of the current marketplace. Membership in a **multiple listing service** (MLS) expands the inventory of comparables to provide information on a much broader scale. This information includes more than offering prices, which can be found on the internet; it also includes actual sale prices, special sale conditions, time to sell, as well as property that failed to sell during the listing period.

By serving as a marketing center or clearinghouse for both knowledge and proper ties, real estate brokers can analyze buyer needs and resources to match buyers with properties and guide them to the culminations of sales.

TRENDS IN REAL ESTATE BROKERAGE

The real estate profession has been undergoing significant change in the past few years. This change has included the following:

- Greater emphasis on determining client needs

- Greater interest in single agency buyer representation

- Better-trained and technology-oriented salespeople who regard real estate as a profession

- Buyers and sellers showing greater interest in professional designations, education, and experience of agents

- Expansion of large franchise offices through the absorption of former independent offices (though there will still be a place for small offices specializing in a geographic area or a type of property)

- Growth of the team concept where real estate salespeople form partnerships within a firm

- Greater use of the internet by homebuyers, as well as for marketing

- Decreasing reliance on traditional print advertising

- Increased number of marketing websites

- Growth of personal and office websites

- Increased website sophistication, with virtual tours, movement, and sound

- Use of informative blogs

- Use of social networking sites

- IDX (Internet Data Exchange) cooperation between brokers allows MLS members to display listings of other offices on their websites

- Electronic signatures—by using electronically stored signatures, DocuSign users can annotate and sign electronic documents, allowing for instantaneous transmission of signed documents

- Use of internet-generated forms

- Greater use of email and other cloud-based services to transmit information and contracts

- Mergers of MLSs, providing greater coverage for listings

- Use of smartphones by salespeople, not only to communicate with clients but also to access information

- Increased use of licensed and unlicensed professional assistants

- A change in the role of real estate brokers. With the internet, more buyers are doing their homework and know values and what is available. Agents are being sought to make showings of buyer-selected properties and help finalize a purchase. This has had an impact on fee schedules with the growth of online brokerage firms.

- Growth in one-stop shopping, where real estate firms are able to offer affiliated services

- Growth in number of firms offering lower rates of commissions with lower levels of services

- Increasing number of brokers and salespeople forming limited liability companies (LLC) to protect personal assets. Members have no personal liability for debts of the LLC.

- Increase in marketing efforts for foreign buyers

- Greater importance on marketing to both seniors and singles

- Increased awareness of the diversity of the people being served, which is not limited to race, nationality, culture, or religion. It includes people with handicaps, people in recovery, veterans, victims of domestic violence, et cetera. Understanding their needs and concerns is essential to serving these diverse groups.

■ More negotiation in languages other than English. When the agent does not speak the language, a qualified interpreter should be used (not a minor child).

■ Several states have recently eliminated the real estate salesperson's license and are requiring that all licensees be brokers. The purpose stated by legislators is to enhance consumer protection and increase the professional competence of all licensees. Other states have shown interest in this development, and it could become the norm across the nation. For California to adapt the one-license concept, all licensees would have to meet broker licensing requirements rather than the current lesser educational requirements for salespeople.

■ Changes in broker compensation

The real estate marketplace is constantly undergoing change. Energy and water problems will affect the industry. Political change could include changes in capital gain rates, as well as loss of all or part of homeowner deductions for interest and taxes. Licensees will have to adapt to conditions beyond their control. Licensees realize that the marketplace is dynamic and not static.

BROKER COMPENSATION

Although there are a number of flat-fee brokerage firms, a broker's fee or commission is generally a percentage of the sales price. The fee is negotiable between the broker and the client, although most brokers will stick to the same percentage fee for similar properties. It is an antitrust violation for brokers to agree among themselves as to minimum fees to be charged; however, most major brokerage firms charge similar fees.

There have always been cut-rate or discount brokers that have used their lower fees to market their services. In order to obtain the cooperation of other brokers for sales purposes, many of these discount brokers will have a commission split whereby the sales broker receives a more normal commission and the listing broker takes less. Assume most brokers charge 6% for a residential sale and the normal commission split is 50% to the listing broker and 50% to the selling broker. If a broker took a listing for 5% commission, the broker might agree to give the selling broker the normal

3% and take 2% for his own efforts. A problem with working for a lesser commission is that the listing broker might rely more on other brokers and reduce marketing efforts and expenses.

In a seller's market, with few sellers and many buyers, discount brokerage firms tend to be more successful. In a buyer's market with fewer buyers and many sellers, discount brokers have greater difficulty competing because of the need to increase sales effort while offering to perform for a lesser fee.

Prosperity in the real estate profession (fueled by low interest rates and escalating prices) had resulted in many new entrants into the real estate profession, as well as different approaches to service and pricing. Some brokerage offices charge flat fees rather than a percentage of the sales price. While some discount brokers offer full brokerage services, there has been a growth in limited-services offerings for discount fees. For example, several brokers agree to make a charitable donation to the buyer's or the seller's charity of choice using an agreed portion of fees received. It makes for "feel good" clients without discounting fees.

Some brokers offer MLS access plans, where for a fixed fee they will place the owner's property on an MLS site. The owner will agree to pay a selling broker a fee but will be saving the listing broker's fee. Some brokers offer a choice of plans with various services.

Some limited-service brokers help the owner to sell without an agent. They prepare ads, provide website placement, provide open house material and For Sale signs, and will write up the sales contract should a buyer be procured by the seller.

Some offices have come up with à la carte fee pricing for their services. The owners decides what they want, including MLS placement, placement on additional websites, internet virtual tours, open houses, brochures, and the writing of sales contracts. The owner pays for services selected even if a sale is not completed.

Some buyer agents charge the buyers for their time much as other professionals do. They might provide the first home tour, of up to three hours, at no charge but have an hourly charge thereafter. If the broker shares in a listing agent's commission, then the hourly fee would be reduced or eliminated.

Some buyer agents offer to rebate a portion of the commission received from the sellers to the buyers. They hope that the rebate will increase the number of buyers, which will more than offset the rebate.

Redfin is a lower-rate online brokerage firm that pays its agents a salary rather than a commission. The firm currently charges a listing commission of 1.5% with a minimum of $5,000. The seller pays the selling agent. Typically the seller would pay 1½% to Redfin and 3% to the selling agent, making a total commission of 4½%. Redfin also acts as a buyer's agent, rebating a portion of the commission received to the buyer based on a sliding scale. There are countless variations on the above fee arrangements. When the real estate market declines, the average commission increases. According to *Real Trends*, an industry publication, the average commission jumped from a low of 5.02% in 2005, a time of great sales activity, to 5.4% in 2010. The statistics indicate that brokers are more likely to work for a lower commission when sales are relatively easy than when sales are expected to take greater effort.

Some analysts have predicted that real estate will follow the path of stock broker age with lower and lower fees and clients who make decisions based solely on costs. These fears are unlikely to be realized. While higher property prices, a strong market, and greater competition can be expected to place pressure on fees, real estate buyers require the services that only working face to face with an agent can provide. It takes people skills to understand peoples' needs, and selling is simply satisfying those needs. A property sale cannot be reduced to moving a cursor and pressing an enter key.

The product, or property, is not homogeneous. There are differences, benefits, and possible problems with every property. The real estate market is local in nature and requires in-depth local knowledge. Each buyer is different as to needs, wants, and purchasing ability. The agent must gain the trust of buyers to lead them through what is likely to be the most important purchase of their lives.

AN OVERVIEW OF GENERAL BROKERAGE

Most real estate licensees are engaged in representing buyers or sellers or both buyers and sellers in the sale of residential property. The reason is obvious: most properties that are sold are improved residential properties, and most of these are single-family dwelling units.

Real estate salespeople find owners willing to sell their properties or buyers desiring to buy property and secure agency agreements (listings). They then seek buyers for their property listings or properties for their buyer-agency listings. Real estate brokers and salespeople are able to expand their activities beyond their own listings because of a unique system of cooperation that exists among brokers.

Brokers who are members of an MLS make their sale listings available for other agents to sell. Therefore, any member of an MLS can show and sell a listing of any other member. Even agents who are not members of an MLS service will generally cooperate on their listings. By having access to this huge market inventory, an agent can locate a property that best meets the needs and is within the resources of a prospective buyer. Cooperation is the cornerstone of modern real estate brokerage. Cooperation includes sharing of commission. Members of an MLS system have agreed on sharing arrangements, but agents who are not members should have commission-sharing agreements in writing to avoid misunderstanding.

AREAS OF SPECIALIZATION

There are other areas of activity besides the listing and selling of traditional single-family homes. These areas of real estate activity include the following:

- **Manufactured home sales**—While the industry prefers the term *manufactured home*, most people still refer to these homes, which are transported to a site on their own chassis, as *mobile homes*. Mobile homes differ from other types of housing in that they are normally located on leased sites (mobile home parks). Real estate licensees can list and sell mobile homes that are 8 feet by 40 feet or larger in rental spaces, as well as with the land. Real estate licensees cannot sell new mobile homes without land. These new mobile homes can be sold only through dealers licensed by the Department of Housing and Community Development. Mobile homes fill a significant need for lower-cost housing, as well as a lifestyle need in retirement housing. Many salespeople specialize in mobile home sales.

■ **Tract sales**—Many salespeople like to sell new homes in subdivisions because they like selling a product at a fixed price. Buyers generally arrive at tract sales because of developer promotion.

■ **Residential income property (multifamily residential units)**—Brokers, as well as salespersons, often choose this specialty, although agents who handle primarily single-family home sales can also be involved with this type of income property.

■ **Speculator (flipper) sales**—Distressed or problem properties are sold to investors who intend to resell at a profit rather than hold for income.

■ **Commercial property**—Brokers and salespeople may choose this as a specialty; furthermore, many agents may specialize by type of property. For example, some agents handle only minimalls, while others may specialize in office buildings, retail stores, or warehouses.

■ **Industrial property**—Factory and warehouse specialists make relatively few sales, but the dollar volume in these sales tends to be high. Within this field, there are subspecialties, such as research and development facilities.

■ **Business opportunities**—Businesses are listed and sold with or without real estate. It is a specialized field, and very few residential sales agents ever get involved in a business opportunity sale. Some specialists handle only particular types of businesses, such as taverns, restaurants, or motels.

■ **Land and farm brokerage**—Generally, these specialists cover large geographic areas. Knowledge of farming is an important attribute for these agents. In California, many agents specialize in selling acreage parcels to investors and/or developers.

■ **Lot sales**—Many agents specialize in listing and selling lots for investment purposes, as well as to provide builders with a supply of real estate. General real estate brokerage offices also handle the sale of lots, as well as sales of land parcels of all sizes.

■ **Auction sales**—Auctions are now being used to sell all types of real property. In England and Australia, auctions play a greater role in real estate brokerage activity than in the United States. The importance of auction sales in the United States has been increasing. Many firms hold online auctions. There are a number of firms that deal only in auction sales.

■ **Time-shares**—Besides the sale of new time-shares (which is selling a vacation lifestyle), there is also a growing market in time-share resales.

■ **Counseling**—Some experienced professionals provide expert advice to buyers, sellers, developers, and builders on a fee basis.

■ **Subdividing**—Many real estate professionals have gone into subdividing to provide a stock of parcels for development.

■ **Loan brokerage**—Loan brokers generally find investors for trust deeds and property owners who desire to borrow on their properties. They bring these lenders and borrowers together for a fee.

■ **Mortgage loan activities**—Real estate licensees may act as lenders or agents in making and arranging loans. These activities differ greatly from normal brokerage activities because greater administrative skills are needed. However, both sales and mortgage activities require a strong desire to meet the needs of others. (Mortgage loan activities that require a real estate license are discussed in Unit 12.)

■ **Personal assistants**—Many licensed agents have chosen to work for other agents as salaried assistants. They like the security of a regular paycheck, as well as the chance to use organizational skills. Assistants allow agents to better utilize their time by handling tasks that the agents can delegate. Some agents use virtual assistants for the internet. They update internet information, send additional data to responses, answer email requests, and provide names and information to their employing agent. The National Association of REALTORS® developed a virtual assistants training program for military spouses.

■ **Property management**—As in other specialties, there are subspecialties based on the type of property. (Property management is covered in detail in Unit 15.)

- **Leasing agent**—Leasing agents are not necessarily property managers. They generally charge a fee based on the gross receipts of the lease entered into. There are subspecialties such as residential leasing, industrial leasing, and commercial leasing.

- **Appraisal**—Although a separate license is required, a great many appraisers started out in real estate sales.

BROKER/SALESPERSON RELATIONSHIPS

The real estate broker is almost always an **independent contractor**. According to the *Real Estate Reference Book*, "an independent contractor is one who, in rendering services, exercises an independent employment or occupation and is responsible to the employer only as to the results of his or her work." Very simply, this means that an independent contractor is not under the direction and control of the employer regarding the manner in which work is carried out. The independent contractor is responsible to the employer only for the results. For example, real estate brokers are responsible for results to their principal (employer), who could be a buyer, a seller, a lessor, or a lessee.

Real estate brokers are required to have a written contract with their individual salespeople. Most contracts identify the working relationship of the salesperson as that of an independent contractor (Figure 1.1). California Business and Professions Code Section 10032 allows brokers to hire classified salespersons as employees or independent contractors. Most contracts specify an independent contractor choice because it relieves the broker of unemployment compensation, as well as withholding requirements. The statute provides that obligations to the public (liability) apply to the broker regardless of classification of employee or independent contractor. Section 10177(h) of the Business and Professions Code requires that brokers supervise their salespeople, and exercise of supervision in the performance of work precludes an independent contractor relationship as to liability. Formerly, the broker was required to review contracts prepared by salespersons within five days. This has been replaced by a policy of "reasonable supervision."

FIGURE 1.1:   **Independent Contractor Agreement**

INDEPENDENT CONTRACTOR EMPLOYMENT AGREEMENT
For Sales Agents and Associated Brokers

NOTE: This form is used by an employing broker when entering into an agreement employing a sales agent or a broker on terms calling for the employee to be treated for tax purposes as an independent contractor, to establish the duties of the broker and agent, earned fees and how the fees due the employee will be allocated and shared.

DATE:_____, 20_____, at _____, California.

Items left blank or unchecked are not applicable

FACTS:

1. Broker hereby employs Agent as a real estate sales agent or broker-associate, until terminated by either party, on the following terms.
   1.1   Agent to be treated as an independent contractor for tax purposes.

2. **AGENT** agrees:
   2.1   To maintain a real estate license in the State of California.
   2.2   To provide brokerage services only on behalf of Broker.
   2.3   To follow the Broker's policy manual and any directions orally given by Broker.
   2.4   To use only those real estate forms authorized by Broker.
   2.5   To make complete and immediate disclosure to Broker of any correspondence or document made or received.
   2.6   To immediately deliver and account to Broker for funds received by Agent in the course of this employment.
   2.7   To participate in educational programs and meetings specified by Broker.
   2.8   To visually inspect the physical conditions of any property to be sold or bought for clients.
   2.9   To obligate Broker to no agreement without Broker's prior consent.
   2.10 To expose Broker to no liability to any third party without Broker's prior consent.
   2.11 To furnish their own transportation and carry a liability and property damage insurance policy in an amount satisfactory to Broker with a policy rider naming Broker as a co-insured.
   2.12 To faithfully adhere to the Real Estate Law of the State of California.
   2.13 To file and pay quarterly estimated taxes and self-employment taxes.
   2.14 To contribute to the defense and settlement of litigation arising out of transactions in which Agent was to or shared fees, in an amount equal to Agent's percentage share of the fees.
   2.15 To join and pay fees for membership to professional organizations in which broker is a member.
   2.16 Other _____

3. **BROKER** agrees:
   3.1   To maintain a real estate Broker's license in the State of California.
   3.2   To maintain office(s) with proper facilities to operate a general real estate brokerage business.
   3.3   To maintain membership in the following professional organization(s):
   ☐ Multiple Listing Service
   ☐ Local branch of the California Association of Realtors and National Association of Realtors
   ☐ _____
   3.4   To maintain listings.
   3.5   To provide advertising approved by Broker.
   3.6   To provide worker's compensation insurance for Agent.
   3.7   To file informational tax returns on Agent's fee or other compensation, under State and Federal Tax regulations.
   3.8   To pay Agent as specified in the Broker's fee schedule at section 5.
   3.9   To maintain the following insurance coverage's for Agent:
   ☐ Errors and Omissions   ☐ Life   ☐ Health   ☐ Dental
   3.10 ☐ _____

4. **General Provisions:**
   4.1   Agent has the right to purchase any properties listed by Broker on full disclosure to the Seller of the Agent's activity as a principal, and without diminution of fees to the Broker.
   4.2   Agent is authorized to enter into any documents required to perform any of the services referenced in this agreement.
   4.3   Broker has the right to reject any listing or retainer agreement obtained by Agent.
   4.4   Broker to determine whether any litigation or dispute involving the Broker, or their business and third parties, arising from Agent's activities, will be prosecuted, defended or settled.
   4.5   Arbitration: Any dispute between the Agent and the Broker or with any other Agent employed by Broker that cannot be settled by the Broker, or resolved by the State Labor Commission or by non-binding mediation, will be arbitrated under the rules of the American Arbitration Association.
   4.6   ☐ **See addendum for additional provisions.** [See **RPI** Form 250]

_ _ _ _ _ _ _ _ _ _ _ _ _ _ _ _ PAGE ONE OF TWO — FORM 506 _ _ _ _ _ _ _ _ _ _ _ _ _ _ _ _ _

FIGURE 1.1 (continued):   Independent Contractor Agreement

— — — — — — — — — — — — — — — PAGE TWO OF TWO — FORM 506 — — — — — — — — — — — — — — — — — —

5. Broker's Fee Schedule and Charges:

5.1   Broker is to pay Agent a fee for participating in a sales transaction evidenced by a purchase agreement which confirms the Agent is acting as an agent for Broker and Broker receives a brokerage fee on the transaction.

5.2   The amount of fee due Agent is _____% of the funds remaining from the brokerage fee received by Broker under sections 5.1 or 5.10b after first deducting the following amounts:

   a. Payment to other brokerage offices of sums due them for their participation in the transaction;

   b. Payment to Broker's franchisor of the fee due the franchisor from the transaction;

   c. Payment to Broker of one-half of the then remaining funds if another Agent of Broker is entitled to a fee for negotiating the other end of the transaction;

   d. Other deductions _____.

5.3   From each fee due Agent and before disbursement, Broker will deduct the following amounts and any amounts otherwise due Broker from the Agent:

   a. An advertising or promo charge of $_____.

   b. An errors and omissions insurance coverage charge of $_____.

   c. A charge of $_____ for _____.

   d. Disbursement to another Agent of Broker, transaction coordinator or finder with whom Agent agreed to share the fee due under section 5.2.

5.4   The percentage participation by Agent in the funds remaining under section 5.2 is adjusted to _____% on the following event _____, and will apply until _____.

5.5   Agent is to pay Broker, on the first of each month of employment, a desk fee of $_____.

5.6   Any expenses incurred by Broker in a transaction negotiated by Agent, such as travel expenses, meals, attorney fees, printing, listing service fees, etc., will be deducted from the fee due Agent.

5.7   If all or part of the fee is received in property other than cash, Agent is to obtain Broker's prior approval. In this event, Broker will make one of the following determinations for disposition of the property:

   a. Divide the property between Broker and Agent in kind, based on the fee schedule; or

   b. Pay Agent their dollar share of the fee in cash; or

   c. Retain the property in the names of Broker and Agent, or their trustee, and thereafter dispose of it when on terms Broker and Agent agree to on its acquisition. Any ownership income and expenses will be shared between Broker and Agent in proportion to their share of ownership.

5.8   On termination, Agent to be paid as follows:

   a. Closed Transactions: Agent will receive their share of fees on all transactions which are closed before termination.

   b. Pending Transactions: Agent will receive their share of fees on all pending transactions which close after termination, subject to fee limitations under section 5.9.

   c. Unexpired Listings and Retainers: Agent will receive their share of fees if the client enters into a transaction during the written listing or retainer period. Agent will not earn a fee under any extension of the listing or retainer obtained after termination, subject to fee limitations under section 5.9.

5.9   Fee Limitation: If on termination Agent has pending transactions under section 5.1 or unexpired listings or retainers procured by Agent which require further services normally rendered by Agent, Broker will direct another employed Agent or himself to perform these services. For these services after termination, a reasonable share of the fee will be deducted from the fee due Agent.

5.10 Compensation From Prior Employment: Monies received by Broker from Agent's prior employing brokers representing fees earned by Agent while employed by that broker are to be disbursed by Broker as follows:

   a. ☐ Agent to receive 100% of the monies received by Broker.

   b. ☐ The monies are to be shared with Agent at the percentage set in section 5.2.

   c. ☐ Broker and Agent, respectively, to share the monies _____ : _____.

I agree to render services on the terms stated above.	I agree to employ Agent on the terms stated above.
Date: _____, 20_____	Date: _____, 20_____
Agent's Name: _____	Broker's Name: _____
Agent's Signature: _____	Broker's Signature: _____
Address: _____	Address: _____
_____	_____
Phone: _____	Phone: _____
Cell: _____	Cell: _____
Email: _____	Email: _____

FORM 506	08-15	©2015 **RPI** – **Realty Publications, Inc.** P.O.Box 5707, RIVERSIDE, CA 92517

Brokers and salespeople contract as independent contractors as required by the Internal Revenue Service. The IRS will treat the real estate salesperson as an independent contractor if the following three criteria are met:

1. The salesperson is licensed as a real estate agent.

2. Reimbursement to the salesperson is based solely on sales, not on hours worked.

3. There is a written contract stating that the salesperson will be treated as an independent contractor for tax purposes.

The economic reason a broker wants salespersons to be independent contractors is that if they are independent contractors, the broker is relieved of withholding taxes and Social Security, as well as not contributing to Social Security for the salesperson.

While real estate salespeople are treated as independent contractors for purposes of state and federal income tax reporting and certain other purposes, such as workers' compensation insurance coverage, they are treated as employees in connection with dealing with the public.

Despite the IRS treatment of a real estate salesperson as an independent contractor in California, brokers are responsible for wrongful acts (*torts*) of their salespeople within the course and scope of employment. Because of this potential liability, many brokers require that their salespeople carry high limits of automobile liability insurance and that brokers be named as insured under the policies. If a salesperson has access to the funds of others (such as a property manager who collects rents and deposits), brokers might obtain fidelity bonds to protect themselves from a salesperson's embezzlement. Offices also carry errors and omissions insurance policies that offer liability protection for acts of brokers and agents. Errors and omissions insurance typically does not cover pollution on the property, physical harm to others, or damage to property caused by the insured. Policies typically have deductibles, and the cost of the policy is related to business volume.

FIGURE 1.2:   Employee or Independent Contractor? IRS Considerations

Factors Indicating Control	Employee	Independent Contractor
Is the worker required to comply with employer instructions about when, where, and how work is to be performed?	Yes	No
Is the worker required to undergo training?	Yes	No
Does the worker hire, supervise, and pay others to perform work for which she is responsible?	No	Yes
Must the worker's job be performed during certain set hours?	Yes	No
Must the worker devote full time to the job?	Yes	No
Must the work be performed on the employer's property?	Yes	No
Must tasks be performed in a certain order set by the employer?	Yes	No
Is the individual required to submit regular written or oral reports to the employer?	Yes	No
Is payment by the hour, week, or month?	Yes	No
Is payment in a lump sum?	No	Yes
Are the worker's business and travel expenses paid by the employer?	Yes	No
Does the employer furnish the tools and materials required for the job?	Yes	No
Does the worker rent his own office or working space?	No	Yes
Will the worker realize a profit or loss as a result of her services?	No	Yes
Does the individual work for more than one firm at a time?	No	Yes
Does the worker make his services available to the general public?	No	Yes
Does the employer have the right to fire the worker?	Yes	No
Does the worker have the right to quit the job at any time, whether or not a particular task is complete?	Yes	No

Note: These factors are only possible indicators of a worker's status. Each case must be determined on its own facts, based on all the information.

Brokers must carry **workers' compensation insurance** for salespeople who are considered for this purpose to be employees. Brokers need not carry unemployment insurance coverage because commission salespeople are not eligible for unemployment insurance benefits. Also, because salespeople are paid solely by commission, minimum wage laws do not protect them.

Brokers are required to report the annual earnings of a salesperson to both the licensee and the IRS using IRS Form 1099.

SALESPERSON/SALESPERSON CONTRACTS

Real estate salespeople often team up with one or more other salespeople to form a partnership or selling team. These teams sometimes seem to operate as separate brokerage offices within a brokerage office. The teams are usually organized under written agreements, sometimes for a specified period that provides for renewal by agreement. Team agreements cover adding or termination of team membership. They call for a division of the combined earnings of the group. Commission splits are negotiated within the team. Some teams have a broker who selects the team, supervises all activity, and takes a percentage of total earnings. Other teams have a split based on the role of each agent in a transaction, and they might have a set amount or percentage that goes to the team. Some teams divide duties, such as listing specialist, selling specialist, marketing and office management. Further specialization could be type of property, such as commercial, as well as buyer or seller agents. Advantages of team arrangements are as follows:

- The needs of buyers and sellers are better served because of the greater availability of a team member; someone is always available to help in an area where help is needed.

- Members are motivated because they share in one another's successes.

- Members receive more steady income flow because there is a greater likelihood of income being earned every month.

- Such partnerships better utilize the time, talent, and skills of members and paid assistants.

Teams are likely to have their own websites. The website shown in Figure 4.3 of Unit 4 is the home webpage of a team.

The team must take caution to ensure that members are complying with the Real Estate Commissioner's rules. Because the team is ultimately still operating under the employing broker's license, questions might arise as to the ownership of this team name. From the broker's perspective, they might hold the position that the brokerage owns the team name because it is tied to the broker's personal or corporate broker's license.

The team will naturally dispute the broker's claim of ownership because the salespeople are likely spending their own marketing dollars to promote this team name in print and online. If a salesperson were to move to a different brokerage, that salesperson would want the ability to take the team name with her to the new firm. Additionally, any website domains that the team registers are likely to be done by the team itself and not the broker. Therefore, internet control of the team name would be hard for the broker to enforce. Assembly Bill 2018 (Bocanegra) allows a salesperson to "maintain ownership of a fictitious business name" but still requires that this name be used "subject to the control of a responsible broker."

Despite the fact that the "team name" might be owned by the salesperson according to this bill, it is imperative that brokers supervise and manage exactly how these team names are used.

As an example, section (d) of this bill also requires that

> marketing and solicitation materials, including business cards, print or electronic media and "for sale" signage, using a fictitious business name obtained in accordance with subdivision (a) shall include the responsible broker's identity in a manner equally as prominent as the fictitious business name.

Therefore, it is important that brokers have their teams agree that in any of their marketing, the size and prominence of the team name should not be larger than the broker's to avoid giving the appearance that the team is operating without an employing broker. This is despite the fact that the ownership of the team name could be held by the salesperson and not the broker necessarily.

Fictitious Business Names and Teams

Specifically, AB 2018 defines a "team name" as a professional identity or brand name used by a salesperson, and one or more other real estate licensees, for the provision of real estate licensed services. AB 2018 specifies that

> the use of a team name, as defined above, does not constitute a fictitious business name and would not require a separate license if (1) the name is used by two or more real estate licensees who work together to provide licensed real estate services, or who represent themselves to the public as being a part of a team, group, or association to provide

those services, (2) the name includes the surname (last name) of at least one of the licensee members of the team, group, or association in conjunction with the term "associates," "group," or "team," and (3) the name does not include any term or terms, such as "real estate broker," "real estate brokerage," "broker," or "brokerage" or any other term that would lead a member of the public to believe that the team is offering real estate brokerage services, or imply or suggest the existence of a real estate entity independent of a responsible broker.

Ownership of Team Names

When a team name is tied to a given broker at the California Bureau of Real Estate, a question may arise as to the ownership of the team name. The broker may hold the position that he owns the team name because it is tied to his personal or corporate license at the bureau.

Salespeople will naturally be opposed to this because they are likely spending their own marketing dollars to promote this team name in print and online. If the salespeople were to move to a different brokerage, they would want the ability to take this team name with them to the new firm. Additionally, any website domains that the team registers are likely to be done by the team itself and not the broker. Therefore, internet control of the team name would be hard for the broker to enforce.

AB 2018 (Bocanegra) allows a salesperson to "maintain ownership of a fictitious business name" but still requires that this name be used "subject to the control of a responsible broker."

Despite the fact that the "team name" might be owned by the salesperson, according to 2018, it is imperative that brokers supervise and manage exactly how these team names are used.

If a team or any other sales group operates under a name that does not include the surname of every principal, it must comply with the fictitious name statute, which requires filing the name with the county clerk and complying with advertising requirements.

A partnership or team choice should not be taken lightly. You should choose not only a person or persons you like but those who are similarly dedicated. You want partners you can rely on.

CHOOSING A BROKER

Many people enter the real estate profession thinking it is a certain path to riches. While some real estate sales agents earn over $250,000 per year (about 2%), according to the U.S. Bureau of Labor Statistics (2014) the mean income of a real estate salesperson (average income) was $55,300 per year. The median income was $40,900 (median means half the agents made more than that figure and half made less). You should realize that agents' income tends to increase after the first years, so new agents will likely have lower incomes. The broker you choose to go with can have a significant effect on your income.

At one time, most real estate offices seemed to be running a numbers game. They would take in every real estate licensee willing to come to work for them. Most firms have come to realize that such a practice can be counter-productive in that it can waste both time and money. Today, most offices are interested in agents they believe will fit with their office and either have experience or the drive to learn what is necessary for success. Brokers realize that whom they hire can affect their bottom line—their profit. Direct and indirect costs in hiring an agent who fails to produce can be in the thousands of dollars. Brokers often use the term "desk cost." This is the total office operational overhead divided by the number of salespeople. If a salesperson fails to contribute at least that amount to the **company dollar** (broker's share of commission received), then the agent is a negative factor on earnings.

Expect to be asked direct questions about your past work history, what you expect from being a real estate agent, and what you are willing to give to the job as far as effort and dedication. Your job interview is really a two-way interview, with the broker trying to do what is best for the brokerage firm and with you seeking the firm that will best meet your personal goals.

Because your choice of broker could have a significant effect on your success or failure as a real estate professional, don't jump at the first "come to work for me" offer. You could end up wasting a great deal of what otherwise could be productive time. More important, an initial experience of feeling like a square peg in a round hole could lead you to abandon what would otherwise be a rewarding career.

Before you even think about talking to brokers, you should understand why fewer than 50% of new real estate licensees are still actively engaged in real estate one year after starting work. Your careful initial choice of a broker will reduce your likelihood of becoming a "failure statistic."

A contributing reason for such a high rate of failure is lack of training in what to do to be successful. It's true that some successful agents come into an office absolutely green, observe what successful agents are doing, and then do it themselves, but these agents are the exceptions. In some offices, a new licensee is assigned a desk, provided rudimentary information about using the computer, and will maybe receive a 30-minute briefing. The new agent might be given the task to knock on doors for listings. This can be a frightening task for many new licensees who are not used to rejection. New licensees are often left to learn by osmosis, an approach that is far more likely to result in failure than success.

While many experienced agents generate most of their leads, floor time is important for new licensees. The amount of floor time offered by the broker should be an important consideration in choosing a broker.

Many offices have weekly sales meetings with skill improvement sessions. Some offices use a **mentor program** in which the new hire assists a successful salesperson for several months. This approach can be very good if the mentor is knowledgeable. While some successful agents are not interested in being mentors or are not skilled at training others, many successful agents enjoy working with a *protégé*. They will bring new licensees along on some calls and show them what they are doing and why, as well as answer questions and make suggestions. While some mentors will help you at no cost, they are more likely to expect you to do some work for them. Others might expect a percentage of your deals. There are also professional mentors who have programs with set fees. Before you develop any mentor relationship, check the success of the mentor and others who have been mentored.

Most large offices have a formal training program. Some are excellent, providing motivation and the skills necessary for success. Some offices have training directors who not only conduct training sessions but also work closely with agents to improve their performance. Some offices have extensive CD, video, and audio training libraries, as well as excellent books to augment their training programs and to help develop the skills of success.

Your first few months in real estate are critical because if you can't see success in the near future, you are likely to drop by the wayside and become a failure statistic. You need a broker who will provide you with the training you need for success. When you talk to brokers, find out details about their training programs, what the office does about continuing skill improvement, and what the office has in the way of a library and training aids. Ask to talk to a recent licensee who works in the office. Ask pointed questions about the training and broker assistance. You should be actively interviewing the prospective broker rather than being a passive listener.

Find out about the broker's present employees. How long have they been with the office? If everyone seems to be a relative newcomer, it could indicate a serious problem. Find out about the earnings of the full-time salespersons. This is very important because working around successful people can serve as a great personal motivator. If you are working in the midst of a group of marginal producers, their attitudes, perhaps negative, could make it difficult for you to maintain the positive approach required for your success.

You will likely give your greatest consideration to a broker involved in residential sales because most sales are residential. Commercial or industrial sales might offer huge commissions, but the deals that come together are few and often far apart. As a new licensee, you are unlikely to develop the skills needed to succeed in commercial/industrial selling before financial pressures drive you toward a salaried position. In addition, the background and legal knowledge required for commercial, industrial, and business sales are far different than they are for residential sales and generally require intensive education and training. Keep in mind that the sales skills learned in residential sales can be transferred to other areas of real estate. After you have developed these skills, a number of alternatives will be open to you.

Many real estate boards and associations offer training opportunities. The largest broker organization is the **National Association of REALTORS®** (NAR). The **California Association of REALTORS®** (CAR) is the state organization of NAR. Membership in a local board of REALTORS® automatically includes membership in both CAR and NAR. Among the many advantages of becoming a REALTOR® or REALTOR-Associate® are the training opportunities, legal updates, industry news, access to lockboxes, multiple listing services, legal forms (including computer forms), legal services, and interaction with other professionals guided by the same code of ethics. In addition to the National Association of REALTORs®, there are other organizations of real estate professionals that provide educational services and help their members advance in their profession. They include the National Association of Real Estate Brokers (NAREB), whose members use the Realtist designation; the National Association of Hispanic Real Estate Professionals; and the Asian Real Estate Association of America.

Some of these organizations offer regularly scheduled training sessions; others sponsor special training programs. Many board and association offices have libraries that contain excellent training material, and some have bookstores where training materials and supplies can be purchased. The training publications, along with ideas you gain from your local real estate board or association, can materially affect your future.

If you have already achieved success in real estate, the initial training offered by a broker would not be a major consideration in working for that broker, but other support services and commission arrangements could be very important to you. Some offices offer a sliding commission scale under which the individual salespeople keep a greater portion of the commission dollars as their commissions increase. The purpose of this type of arrangement is to motivate salespeople to achieve greater success, as well as to retain top producers. Health insurance coverage with a broker-paid portion (often related to performance) has been an excellent salesperson retention tool for some brokers.

The salesperson pays the broker in a 100% commission office.

There are a number of **100% commission offices**. In these offices, the salesperson pays a flat desk fee or a desk fee plus a transaction fee to the broker and then keeps all the commissions earned. Desk fees vary based on area, broker's facilities, and support services provided by the broker, such as internet and administrative services and insurance coverage. The desk fee is calculated to cover all office overhead plus provide broker compensation. The broker retains responsibility for the salesperson. Generally, the brokers in 100% offices provide little help to the salespeople, and the salespeople pay for many of their own support services. This type of arrangement is not a good choice for a new licensee, although it can offer benefits for experienced real estate professionals who generate much of their own business. If you are just beginning a real estate career, don't worry about commission splits; 100% of nothing is nothing. Generally, the higher the split, the fewer services provided by the broker to the agent. As a new hire, you want all the help you can get. Figure 1.3 is a worksheet for selecting a broker's office that allows the agent to compare three different brokers.

FIGURE 1.3:   Checklist for Selecting a Broker's Office

Brokers' Names

1. _____
2. _____
3. _____

Benefits provided by the broker	Broker 1	Broker 2	Broker 3
1. New-agent training program			
2. Ongoing training program			
3. Use of a mentor system			
4. Computer training			
5. Quality phone systems (voice mail, call forwarding, etc.)			
6. Fax machine availability			
7. Email address			
8. Office website (grade on a 1 to 10 scale)			
9. Additional websites used			
10. Multiple listing service (MLS)			
11. Success of current sales staff			
12. Computer forms			
13. Open-house signs and flags			
14. Desk fees and MLS board fees			
15. Advertising support			
16. Distribution of leads generated by company websites and relocation websites.			
17. Organized farm for new agents			
18. Weekly meeting and caravans			
19. Broker's interest in you			
20. Can you work with management?			
21. Estimated start-up costs			

How to Choose Where to Work

A new licensee is wise to go to work for an office

- that offers a training program as good as or better than those offered by other area brokers;

- that offers assistance when you need it (for example, an office with a designated person in charge of your training);

- with a good library of books, audiotapes, CDs, and DVDs available for your use;

- that is primarily devoted to the sale of and/or lease in the real estate specialty area you desire to work in;

- where salespeople have good morale, reflected in their length of employment;

- that has a significant proportion of successful agents; and

- that is comfortable for you. You must feel comfortable with the broker, your co-workers, and the operation of the office. If you are uncomfortable, your chances of success are going to be materially diminished.

Because the Bureau of Real Estate will sell lists of real estate applicants, you may be contacted by several local brokers. Friends in the business may also make suggestions. Take your time in your choice because it can have long-lasting implications.

Many enter the real estate profession with the intention of working part time until they learn the business and develop an income. Part-time agents are far less likely to be successful than full-time agents because of the difficulty in being able to serve the needs of buyers and sellers in a timely manner. In addition, few successful brokerage firms will take on a part-time salesperson. Exceptions are time-share sales at special seminars and tract sales.

Brokers compute desk cost as the total office overhead divided by the number of salespersons. Each salesperson's production is expected to cover desk cost, as well as make a contribution to broker profits. A salesperson who, after a training period, consistently fails to produce office revenue sufficient to cover desk cost is unlikely to continue with the brokerage firm.

SUCCESS AND YOUR ATTITUDE

We know that simply moving an agent's desk can change an agent's production. Having successful co-workers around you can serve to generate ideas and motivation to achieve your own success. Unfortunately, the opposite is also true. Having people around you who are unsuccessful or who have a negative attitude can adversely affect your attitude. If they are failures, your chances of failure will be increased. If you associate with successful people, you will likely be associating with people who have a positive attitude. A positive attitude can be infectious, just as the negative attitude of friends and associates can lead you to failure. A negative attitude will lead to a "they aren't really buyers" prejudgment that can make the difference between marginal results and great success.

No one will stand over you in real estate to watch your every move and prod you on. And even though others may reinforce your resolve to succeed, the real motivation for success comes from you. You must be a self-starter who wants to succeed so much that you will continue to strive despite setbacks or the negative attitudes of others. By completing the Success Questionnaire in Figure 1.4, you will gain an understanding of where you are now as well as areas where improvement is needed.

Certainly, motivational seminars, tapes, videos and books help, but these are short-term motivational aids. Long-term success is based on internal motivation to expend the extra effort to learn, to plan, and to practice for your success. Working hard isn't enough. You have to learn to work smart. Think out what needs to be done and why. Plan your work.

You must be interested in people and truly want to help them in meeting their needs. The desire to help and your belief that your product, real estate, offers a solution to their needs will keep you motivated. Use the success of others as a guide to show yourself what can be done. In the same vein, don't become complacent because you are doing better than others. In real estate, don't feel that you are in competition with any other agent. Your only competitor should be yourself. Of course, when you start to realize success, success itself becomes a motivator.

FIGURE 1.4: Success Questionnaire

1. Are you enthusiastic about your work?
   Study the unusually successful people you know and you will find them imbued with an enthusiasm for their work that is contagious. Not only are they excited about what they are doing, but they also get you excited. Remember the maxim: "Enthusiasm is like a contagious disease. It must be caught and not taught."

2. How do you overcome objections?
   Numerous spoken questions and written questions are being fired at you every day. Do you answer them without hesitation, drawing on your reservoir of knowledge? Do you do so to the satisfaction of the client or prospect? Or is there sometimes a hesitation followed by a garbled description that leaves the clients as much in the dark as they were before?

3. Are you self-confident?
   Knowledge gives confidence. A thorough knowledge of both the property in question and the exact advantages that the customer will receive develops this quality of confidence in you, which shows itself in your personality. If the client or customer has confidence in you and your company, a sale may result naturally. The main factor that determines whether customers will have confidence in your product or service is whether they have confidence in you. Your knowledge gives you assurance, a prime factor in assuring others.

4. Do you have the courage of your convictions?
   Many times, we cease to be courageous in the face of opposition. It is a sad commentary, but we live in an era when rapid change breeds fear. Conquer fear! Banish worry, because, as someone once said, worry is the interest you pay on trouble before you get it. Keep your fears to yourself, and share your courage with others. Remember, fear is only in the mind.

5. Are your actions and speech positive?
   A number of years ago there was a popular song with the words "accentuate the positive, eliminate the negative." You need to think and act positively.
   Those who think negatively say, "Business is poor; unemployment rates are more than 9%. That means 9% of the people cannot be considered potential prospects."
   Those who think positively say, "Business is great, with only 9% unemployment. That means 91% of the people are potential prospects." However, being positive does not imply that it gives us the right to be dishonest. But we can state facts positively without being dishonest.

6. Are you persistent?
   Customers admire a salesperson who has developed persistence. No one has respect for a quitter, a person who readily takes no for an answer. If only 1 in 20 presentations results in a sale, your attitude should be: "Thanks for the no. I'm now closer to the yes." (You should of course be considering it a goal to reduce 1 in 20 to 1 in 19.)

7. Are you a problem solver?
   Be a problem solver, not a problem. Problem solvers are people helpers. The basic principles of problem solving are the following:

   ■ Despite any problem, you can persevere, think, and reach a solution.

   ■ Use relentless pressure, persistence, and determination.

   ■ Act as if the problem can be solved. Use the power of positive thinking.

   ■ Remember, you do not sell properties; you sell solutions to people's problems.

   ■ Understand completed staff work. The idea of completed staff work is that you should never present your broker with a problem unless you also present your broker with the possible courses of action to take—your recommendations as to a specific action and why.

8. Are you willing to fail?
   Perhaps this should be phrased as "willing to try, regardless of the chance of failure." Success cannot be achieved without failure. An old story is a good example of this concept: Robert Bruce, King of Scotland, had just been defeated for the 11th time by his enemies, the English. He was dejectedly resting by a tree, ready to give up, when he saw a spider persistently trying to spin a web from one limb to another. After the spider failed to reach its goal 11 times, it finally succeeded on the 12th try. Inspired by this incident, Bruce went forth against his enemy for the 12th time. This time he was victorious, defeating the English at Bannockburn, winning independence for Scotland. To be a successful salesperson, you must be willing to try and perhaps to fail in order to succeed in the end.

We are seeing a change in the way that many successful salespersons do business. Many have significantly reduced the number of hours they spend in the broker's office. With smartphones, email, and fax machines, most of their office time has become home based or car based. With reduced direct contact with brokers and co-workers, self-motivation becomes essential for success.

PROFESSIONAL DESIGNATIONS

The National Association of REALTORS® and numerous other real estate organizations offer myriad professional designations. Some designations relate to general brokerage, while others are for specialized areas of activity. Earning these designations requires a course of study and, in some cases, an examination. Achieving these designations opens up many opportunities because they are regarded highly by others. The Seniors Real Estate Specialist® designation (SRES) will provide the expertise to meet real estate needs of seniors and help you reach this market.

The Association of Energy and Environment Real Estate Professionals offers the Eco Broker designation for agents dedicated to reducing our carbon footprints and protecting the environment. Dealing with an Eco Broker is becoming an important consideration to many buyers. A designation frequently sought is the Graduate, REALTOR® Institute (GRI). Achieving designations such as the GRI will increase your confidence, as well as your sense of self-worth.

CONTINUING TRAINING

Training is not a one-time program. As a real estate professional, you should constantly be improving your skills and increasing your knowledge. The most successful agents continually strive for improvement throughout their careers.

Seek out available training sessions and group-sponsored seminars applicable to your work. *California Real Estate Magazine*, the magazine of the California Association of REALTORS®; *Real Estate Today*, the magazine published by the National Association of REALTORS®; and *REALTOR®*

News, the biweekly newspaper of the National Association of REAL-TORS®, are examples of excellent publications with articles that will help you succeed. Many offices have back issues of these publications in their libraries. In addition, some local associations of REALTORS® have newsletters or publications that discuss local issues. A great many relevant articles and blogs are available on the internet.

When a new idea or approach is proposed during office training sessions, take notes and try to use that idea or approach as soon as possible. Keep in mind that listening may give you ideas, but a demonstration is even better because it shows how to apply the ideas. Using the ideas yourself makes them yours, and they become part of your personal "sales software" to be retained in your memory bank and taken out when a situation warrants their use.

Besides office training sessions, you may have a training supervisor who will critique your efforts. Pay attention. Take criticism as an opportunity for improvement. Criticism is feedback for improvement, not an indication of failure.

Ask questions of the more successful salespeople in your office. Generally, they will share ideas gladly. Consider building a special relationship with a successful agent in your office. In doing so, you will be developing your own mentor. Someone who is supportive of you who possesses both knowledge and experience can be a great help during your first few months in real estate. This is especially important in offices where the broker or office manager has limited time to work with you.

You will find that there are more good ideas for prospecting, listing, and selling than one person could possibly use. By trying various ideas, you will find approaches you feel comfortable with, and you will work these with greater enthusiasm and heighten the likelihood of your success.

Check the course offerings of your local colleges and business schools. Besides specific real estate courses, consider more general business courses in salesmanship, marketing, advertising, and so forth. The knowledge gained in many general courses will have direct application to real estate activities. A number of courses also are offered by correspondence. While some correspondence and online courses are quite good, they lack the insights of an instructor and the give and take of a classroom environment. There is a great deal more to learning than just what is "in the book."

Real estate licensees are required to take continuing education courses for license renewal. Many of these courses will provide you with knowledge directly applicable to your work. Even if you are not required to take a course, you should evaluate what the course can do for you.

WEB LINK

The internet can be a great learning tool. Two of the many websites you should consider visiting are www.relibrary.com and www.realtimes.com.

Many excellent commercial seminars are available to licensees. Besides providing new ideas and approaches, these seminars are motivational in nature. In making decisions about which courses and seminars to attend, ask your broker and/or successful salespeople you know who have attended the courses for their evaluations of the programs.

Self-Training

In your training, you should realize that the quicker you acquire the basic skills needed for success, the greater the likelihood you will remain in the real estate profession. The simple economics of trying to survive a lengthy training period forces many agents to leave real estate when they might otherwise have realized great success. Stated simply, the quicker you learn your survival skills, the more likely you are to survive and succeed.

Therefore, it is important to use every bit of available time toward this goal of self-improvement. As a new licensee, you cannot afford the luxury of relaxing in front of the television after an eight-hour day.

Check your office library, as well as city libraries, for real estate training books and videos. Study them, take notes, and then verbalize (role-play) the approaches presented. Chances are a number of people in your office have trainer material from various seminar presenters. Borrow it; some of the private presenter material is excellent.

Learn the inventory in your market area. Only with product knowledge will you be able to successfully match prospective buyers to properties meeting their needs.

Learn about the facilities within your market area. You want to be able to answer the questions that prospective buyers are likely to ask about schools, parks, transportation, recreational facilities, and so on.

As a word of caution, keep in mind that some of the poorest producers may have excellent resource material available, but if unused it becomes worthless.

Role-Playing

> Role-playing is acting as the person you wish to be.

To communicate effectively with buyers and sellers, you must be able to take your ideas and verbalize them in an effective manner. By using role-playing, you can train yourself to handle telephone inquiries; make listing, showing, and selling presentations; learn to effectively qualify buyers; and learn to overcome both buyer and seller objections. Role-playing can help you overcome the fear that grips many agents when it comes time to ask an owner or a buyer to sign a contract. Role-playing can give you the self-confidence to close (obtain signatures on the contract) in a natural and effective manner.

Role-playing is a mind game. It is also basic acting. In role-playing, you imagine yourself in a situation where you are confronted by unexpected objections of all sorts and then decide on the best way to handle them. (The training material we discussed will provide you with many ideas.) Verbalize your responses before a mirror. Watch your expressions.

Always remember that you are playing the part of a knowledgeable professional. You should constantly strive for improvement. The beauty of role-playing is that you can do it mentally, even when others are present. You can use otherwise nonproductive driving time for role-playing exercises. By role-playing, you will gain confidence and become at ease in dealing with people. An excellent training approach is to role-play with another person with whom you can exchange characters. This really is a team-teaching exercise. Having a third-party observer will increase the effectiveness of this technique and will help keep you focused.

By recording your role-playing presentations, you will hear how you sound. You might feel you need better enunciation or need to speak with greater confidence. Annoying verbal habits become evident, such as verbalizing your pauses with "ahhh" or repeating a phrase such as "you know." If you realize you have problems, you can work to overcome them. Making presentations before a video camera can reveal problems with facial expressions and body language.

After you make any type of presentation, ask yourself, "Could I have handled the situation better?" By thinking about what you should have said, you are actually preparing yourself for future encounters with similar situations. You can thus benefit by failures as well as successes.

Role-playing will improve your communication skills, and as your skills improve, so will your confidence. You will thus overcome fear, a significant factor in the failure of many salespeople. If you fear failure, you are likely to betray your fear by appearing nervous. A prospective buyer or seller is not likely to become convinced to buy or list property by an agent who appears to lack confidence. As you progress, you will become the person you were portraying in your role-playing: a confident, knowledgeable, and caring person interested in fulfilling the needs of others.

Planning

Planning is the process of plotting your course of action to reach specified goals and objectives. It is a blueprint of what you intend to accomplish. Add a timetable, and you also have a tool to evaluate your performance. Planning is never a waste of time. The less time you have to spare, the more important it is to plan your day carefully. Do not forget the oft-repeated statement that 20% of your effort will produce 80% of your results.

Adopt your own system of planning, but be sure to plan. Any system that does away with time-wasters and puts the focus on planning will increase productivity. Self-discipline is the key. If you have it, you will have great success with time management and the other aspects of your life.

Sometimes it may seem that no matter how hard you apply yourself and how efficiently you allocate your time, you have more work to do and more people to see than you can handle satisfactorily. Time management is part of the solution. A good time-management system rounds out your plan and helps you improve efficiency and income. As you refine your techniques of self-management, you may expect a release from the pressures of time as your first dividend.

Time Management

The paradox of time is that "there is never enough, but we have all there is." A time-management authority who conducted a poll of managers found that 90% said they needed more time to get their jobs done right.

Unsuccessful real estate licensees often waste 40% to 50% of every work-day. Just think of your first hour on the job. Are you guilty of the behavior that one time-management expert witnessed? Do you do nothing more than participate in "opening exercises": have a cup of coffee, socialize, read the paper? Little gets done, and that sets a pattern for the day. There's an old proverb that reads as follows: "As the first hour goes, so goes the day."

Time management can make the whole day more productive, allowing you to produce more, get better results, and probably get more rewards as well. Remember, time is capital; know what it is worth.

$$\frac{\text{desired annual earnings}}{1{,}952 \text{ working hours a year}}$$

The figure of 1,952 is based on 244 working days times 8 hours per day.

EXAMPLE Salesperson Graham makes $100,000 per year; his hourly wage is approximately $51 per hour ($100,000 ÷ 1,952 hours = $51, the dollar value of one hour).

Allowing for other activities and unavoidable delays, you will be fortunate to have one-fourth that time (488 hours a year) to actually spend with clients or customers. Thus, the dollar value of your time is even greater than the equation above indicates. To start thinking about how to get the maximum return on your time, ask yourself, "How can I raise the

- number of contacts received and made per week?"
- number of interviews per contact?"
- number of presentations given per interview?"
- number of closes per presentation?"
- number of new prospects per week?"
- number of repeat sales?"
- dollar value of selling time?"

Goal Setting

Can you imagine yourself in a race without a finish line? That is what it is like to work without goals. You can travel a great distance but get nowhere.

Goal setting is a tool for making intelligent decisions. Use the following seven principles to help you set your goals effectively:

1. Goals in real estate selling should be specific rather than abstract. For example:

    ■ Abstract—I will do my best to improve my sales techniques during this week.

    ■ Specific—I will obtain at least one listing and make at least three sales presentations during this week.

    Goals must be measurable. "Doing better" cannot be measured, but giving out 50 calling cards is a measurable goal. If a goal is not measurable, it is not likely to be met.

2. Goals should be in a time frame. Set short-term, intermediate-term, and long-term goals. (The short-term, intermediate-term, and long-term goals listed below are representative only. Goals will vary based on your area of specialization and your geographic area, as well as your individual needs.) For example: Short-term (less than one year)

    ■ I will obtain a minimum of three listings this month.

    ■ This week I will enroll in a college-level course in property management.

    Intermediate-term (one to five years)

    ■ I will complete the required eight broker courses within two years.

    ■ I will obtain the GRI designation within four years.

    Long-term (more than five years)

    ■ I will open my own real estate office within eight years.

    (Your short-term and intermediate-term goals should flow toward meeting your long-term goals.)

3. Goals should be put into writing:

    ■ It is easier to determine your priorities when your goals are written.

    ■ Written goals are easier to examine and revise.

    Translating goals onto paper makes them appear more manageable and helps licensees overcome selling fears.

4. Tell someone, such as your spouse or trusted friend, your goals. Telling another person will serve as motivation to continue striving for your goals. You are now accountable to someone besides yourself.

5. Goals should be reasonably attainable. If your goals are not realistic, you are likely to become discouraged and disappointed.

6. Goals should be adopted only after careful and considerable thought.

    Think about what you really want and why. Reaching goals can take hard work, so you probably will devote time and energy only to those you are really committed to.

7. Goals should not be cast in stone. If interests change, the economy changes, or your needs and desires change, your long-term and intermediate-term goals should change accordingly. If you are no longer motivated to reach a goal, your likelihood of accomplishing that goal will be significantly lessened.

You need action steps to meet goals. In other words, a plan so the goal will be met. As an example, the goal to obtain three listings this month might have the following action plan:

- I will make personal owner contact each week with all for-sale-by-owner ads that include addresses.
- I will check local bulletin boards each week for for-sale-by-owner ads.
- I will mail solicitation material each week to all expired listings.
- I will check the local legal paper for legal notices that could indicate listing opportunities and follow up with personal contacts.

By evaluating yourself, you will discover that wishes can become reality if you have a plan that leads toward their fruition.

Your **daily planning** is the foundation of your goal setting. Your planning for each day should include steps leading to your short-term, intermediate-term, and long-term goals.

Before you start daily planning, precisely log your time for several days. How productive was that 20-minute discussion on the Dodgers? Besides identifying the time-wasters, ask yourself, "Were my efforts devoted more to probabilities rather than mere possibilities?"

Some agents like to divide their activities into A, B, C, and D categories:

> Simply increasing "A" Time will increase productivity.

"A" Time—Time spent making listing presentations and showing properties for sale. This is time spent that can lead directly to a commission.

"B" Time—Time spent in prospecting for buyers and sellers and in preparing for showings

"C" Time—Caravanning, studying inventory, and doing necessary tasks and paperwork in support of "A" Time and "B" Time activities

"D" Time—Time spent for personal and non-work-related activities

This simple rating of time presents a basic truth. If you can double your A" Time, you will double your income, even without any improvement in your skills. When coupled with skill improvement, you can readily see how incomes can soar. Some successful agents hire assistants to take care of a great deal of their "B" Time and "C" Time activities. You can see why a productive salesperson would want to do this.

You are now ready for your daily plan. There are quite a few real estate daily planners available. Consider one for your smartphone and/or computer. Figure 1.5 shows a basic daily planning sheet. By having your planner with you on your smartphone, you can set appointments several days in advance when necessary. A smartphone not only provides planning ability, it also provides much of the information needed to fulfill the tasks in your daily plan.

Just having a planner isn't enough—you must use it. Keep in mind that every activity on your daily plan will not be accomplished. Your schedule will change because of unplanned opportunities. Grab an "A" Time opportunity whenever it comes your way.

At the end of each day, evaluate what you have accomplished. If a task was not accomplished but is still relevant, set it forward to the next day; if not, delete it. If a task is unpleasant but must be done, set it for the beginning of a day. After it is accomplished, you will have a sense of relief rather than worrying about it all day.

If you have a goal to earn $100,000 in one year, you would want to know how many sale and listing transactions would have to be closed to meet that goal. Assume that in your office, the average salesperson's commission per transaction is $5,850. In order to earn $100,000, you would have to close 17.1 transactions per year or 1.42 per month ($100,000 ÷ $5,850). Now you must determine the A, B, C, and D time allocations needed to meet this income goal.

Assistants

Some new licensees will work as salaried **personal assistants** to successful sales agents to gain the experience and confidence necessary for success in sales. While assistants do not make much economic sense for new agents (who must learn before they can train others to help them), they can handle a great deal of a successful agent's B, C, and D time activities, thus allowing for greater "A" Time work. Hundreds of agents in California hire paid full-time or part-time assistants, and one agent we know has a personal staff of four full-time aides. (See Figure 1.6.)

FIGURE 1.5:   Daily Planning Sheet

Source: Jim Loonday, *List for Success: How Real Estate Professionals Make Big Money* (Chicago: Real Estate Education Company®, 1986), 10.

FIGURE 1.6:   **Personal Assistant Contract**

CALIFORNIA
ASSOCIATION
OF REALTORS®

PERSONAL ASSISTANT CONTRACT
(Between Associate-Licensee and Licensed or Unlicensed Assistant)
(C.A.R. Form PAC, Revised 06/12)

This Agreement, dated _____, is between _____,
("Associate-Licensee") and _____ ("Assistant").
Assistant desires to work for Associate-Licensee, and Associate-Licensee desires to use the services of Assistant. In consideration for the covenants and representations contained in this Agreement, Associate-Licensee and Assistant agree as follows:

1. **ASSOCIATE-LICENSEE** is a California real estate licensee with a ☐ salesperson's, or ☐ broker's license. Associate-Licensee is licensed under _____, ("Broker") or ☐ (if checked) works for him/herself.

2. **ASSISTANT REAL ESTATE LICENSE:** Assistant ☐ does, ☐ does not, hold a California real estate license. If Assistant does hold a real estate license, the license must be furnished to Broker immediately upon execution of this Agreement.

3. **EMPLOYER-EMPLOYEE RELATIONSHIP:** Assistant shall be an at-will employee of Associate-Licensee. This means either party may terminate this Agreement at any time with or without cause. As Assistant's employer, Associate-Licensee shall be responsible for compliance with all applicable local, state and federal laws including not limited to minimum wage and overtime pay, timekeeping requirements, income and employment tax withholdings, worker's compensation coverage and compliance with employment discrimination including harassment law. If Associate-Licensee and Assistant desire to enter into a different type of working relationship, such as independent contractor, a separate written agreement must be used. The classification of any person who performs services for an Associate-Licensee as an independent contractor has significant legal consequences for both the Associate-Licensee and the person who performs the services and can result in severe penalties and other adverse consequences if a person is misclassified as an independent contractor. Associate-Licensee and Assistant are advised to seek legal and accounting advice before considering classifying Assistant as an independent contractor.

4. **DUTIES:** Assistant shall assist Associate-Licensee in fulfilling Associate-Licensee's obligations under the Independent Contractor agreement (C.A.R. Form ICA, attached) between Associate-Licensee and Broker. Assistant shall comply with all obligations of Associate-Licensee imposed under the terms of that agreement and any office policy established by Broker. Associate-Licensee shall monitor the work and results of Assistant. If Assistant does not have a real estate license, Assistant shall not engage in any activity for which a real estate license is required. (Assistant may become more familiar with these limitations by reading the "DRE Guidelines for Unlicensed Assistants.") In addition, and more specifically, Assistant shall perform the following activities: _____
   _____
   _____
   _____

5. **COMPENSATION AND BENEFITS:**
   A. **Base Compensation:** Assistant's base compensation is $_____ per **hour** payable in equal bi-weekly installments every other_____(insert day of the week).
   OR ☐ (If checked) Assistant's base compensation is $_____ per **hour** payable in equal semi-monthly installments on the 15th (or_____) and last (or_____) day of the month.
   OR ☐ (If checked) Assistant's base compensation is shown in Exhibit _____ attached hereto an incorporated as a part of this Agreement by reference.
   B. **Expenses:** Assistant shall be reimbursed for reasonable business expenses incurred by Assistant in performing Assistant's duties under this Agreement.
   C. **Advances:** Assistant shall not be entitled to any advance payment from Associate-Licensee upon future compensation, unless specified in a separate written agreement for each such advance. If Associate-Licensee elects to advance funds to Assistant pursuant to a separate written agreement, Associate-Licensee may deduct the amount advanced from any future paycheck due Assistant as specified in the separate written agreement.
   D. **Deductions** authorized by Assistant or required by law (including but not limited to FICA, Medicare and Federal and State income tax) will be with held from Assistant's pay.
   E. **Compensation Review:** Associate-Licensee shall review Assistant's base compensation annually. Associate understands and agrees that any such review is not an express or implied commitment to increase such compensation nor is there any express or implied commitment to maintain Assistant's compensation at any particular level in the future.
   F. **Timekeeping:** Associate-Licensee shall record Assistant's time on a daily basis including starting time, ending time and the beginning and ending time for all meal periods.
   G. **Vacation Policy:** Assistant shall be eligible to accrue vacation at the rate of _____ hours per pay period. The maximum unused vacation benefits Assistant may have at any one time shall equal two year's worth of vacation (or a total of _____ hours) **OR** ☐ as specified in Exhibit _____, attached. If Assistant's earned but unused vacation reaches the maximum accrual amount, Assistant will cease to accrue additional vacation time until Assistant uses enough vacation to fall below the maximum accrual amount. All accrued and unused vacation will be paid to Assistant upon termination of this Agreement as required by law.

Associate Licensee's Initials (_____)(_____)

Assistant's Initials (_____)(_____)

Reviewed by _____ Date _____

EQUAL HOUSING
OPPORTUNITY

PAC REVISED 06/12 (PAGE 1 OF 3) Print Date

PERSONAL ASSISTANT CONTRACT (PAC PAGE 1 OF 3)

Reprinted with permission, California Association of REALTORS®. Endorsement not implied.

FIGURE 1.6 (continued):   **Personal Assistant Contract**

6. **PROPRIETARY INFORMATION AND FILES:**
   A. Assistant acknowledge that as a result of Assistant's employment created by this Agreement, Assistant may given access to, make use of, create, acquire and/or add to non-public proprietary, confidential information of a secret, special and/or unique nature and value to Broker, including without limitation Broker's internal systems, procedures, manuals, confidential reports, client lists and client information, methods, strategies and/or techniques used by Broker, the equipment and methods used and preferred by Broker's clients, the fees paid by clients and any and all other confidential information of Broker (hereafter collectively and individually "Confidential Information"). Assistant further recognizes and acknowledges that all of Broker's Confidential Information which is now or may hereafter be in their possession is the property of Broker and that protection of this Confidential Information against unauthorized disclosure or use is of critical importance to Broker in order to protect Broker from unfair competition. As a material inducement to Associate-Licensee to enter into this Agreement, Assistant covenants and agrees Assistant will not at any time, either while this Agreement is in force or after it is terminated without the prior written consent of Broker make any independent use of such Confidential Information, or disclose the same, directly or indirectly, to any other person, firm, corporation or other entity, for any reason or purpose whatsoever, except as may be required by law provided that Assistant shall cooperate with Broker in taking all necessary and appropriate steps to assure the protection of such Confidential Information from unauthorized use or disclosure outside of any action, proceeding, inquiry or investigation, or except to the extent that any such Confidential Information shall be in the public domain other than by reason of Assistant's breach of this paragraph 6.
   B. All Confidential Information including without limitation files and documents pertaining to listings, leads, transactions and the operation of Broker's real estate brokerage are property of Broker. Assistant shall, on the termination of this Agreement for any reason, immediately surrender to Broker all such Confidential Information including without limitation all documents and files whether in paper or electronic format.
7. **INSURANCE:**
   A. AUTOMOBILE: Assistant shall maintain automobile insurance coverage for liability and property damage in the following amounts $_____ /$_____, respectively. Associate-Licensee and Broker shall be named as additional insured parties on Assistant's policies. A copy of the endorsement showing the additional insured parties shall be provided to Associate-Licensee.
   B. WORKER'S COMPENSATION: Associate-Licensee's Worker's Compensation carrier is _____.
   The contact information for this carrier is as follows: Address:_____
   _____, Telephone:_____
   C. ERRORS AND OMISSIONS INSURANCE: Associate-Licensee represents that (check one):
      (i) ☐ Assistant is covered by errors and omissions insurance obtained by Broker.
      (ii) ☐ Assistant is covered by errors and omissions insurance obtained by Associate-Licensee.
      (iii) ☐ Assistant is not covered by errors and omissions insurance.
8. **COMPLIANCE WITH APPLICABLE LAWS, RULES, REGULATIONS AND POLICIES:** Assistant agrees to comply with all local, state and federal laws and regulations, and any office policy and procedures to which Associate-Licensee is subject as a result of engaging in real estate activity.
9. **NOTICE OF CLAIMS:** Assistant shall immediately notify Associate-Licensee or Broker in writing if Assistant is served with or becomes aware of any lawsuit, claim or proceeding relating to Associate-Licensee or Broker's brokerage business or the performance of this Agreement.
10. **DISPUTE RESOLUTION:** Associate-Licensee and Assistant agree to mediate all disputes and claims between them arising from or connected in any way with this Agreement before resorting to court action. If any dispute or claim is not resolved through mediation, or otherwise, Associate-Licensee and Assistant may agree to submit the dispute to arbitration at, and pursuant to the rules and bylaws of, the Association of REALTORS®.
11. **OTHER TERMS AND CONDITIONS AND ATTACHED SUPPLEMENTS:**
    ☐ Broker and Associate-Licensee Independent Contractor Agreement (C.A.R. Form ICA)
    ☐ Broker/Associate-Licensee/Assistant Three Party Agreement (C.A.R. Form TPA)
    ☐ Broker Office Policy Manual (or, if checked, ☐ available in Broker's office)
    ☐ DRE Guidelines for Unlicensed Assistants
    ☐ California Association of REALTORS® Real Estate Licensing Chart
    _____
    _____
    _____
    _____
    _____
    _____

12. **ATTORNEY FEES:** In any action, proceeding, or arbitration between Associate-Licensee and Assistant arising from or related to this Agreement, the prevailing Associate-Licensee or Assistant shall be entitled to reasonable attorney fees and costs.
13. **ENTIRE AGREEMENT:** This Agreement constitutes the entire Agreement between the parties. Its terms are intended by the parties as a final, complete, exclusive, and integrated expression of their agreement with respect to its subject matter, and may not be contradicted by evidence of any prior agreement or contemporaneous oral agreement. This Agreement may not be amended, modified, altered, or changed except in writing signed by Associate-Licensee and Assistant. If any provision of this Agreement is held invalid and legally unenforceable, the parties agree that such provision shall be deemed amended to the extent necessary to render it and/or the remainder of this Agreement valid and enforceable. Even after termination, this Agreement shall govern all disputes and claims between Associate-Licensee and Assistant connected with their respective obligations under this Agreement, including obligations and liabilities arising from existing and completed listings, transactions and services.

Associate Licensee's Initials (_____)(_____)   Assistant's Initials (_____)(_____)

PAC REVISED 06/12 (PAGE 2 OF 3) Print Date

Reviewed by _____ Date _____

PERSONAL ASSISTANT CONTRACT (PAC PAGE 2 OF 3)

FIGURE 1.6 (continued):   Personal Assistant Contract

Associate-Licensee _____   Date _____
            Signature

Associate-Licensee _____
            Print Name

Address _____   City _____   State _____ Zip _____

Telephone _____   Fax _____   E-mail _____

Associate-Licensee _____   Date _____
            Signature

Associate-Licensee _____
            Print Name

Address _____   City _____   State _____ Zip _____

Telephone _____   Fax _____   E-mail _____

Published and Distributed by:
REAL ESTATE BUSINESS SERVICES, INC.
a subsidiary of the California Association of REALTORS®
525 South Virgil Avenue, Los Angeles, California 90020

Reviewed by _____ Date _____

EQUAL HOUSING
OPPORTUNITY

PAC REVISED 06/12 (PAGE 3 OF 3)

PERSONAL ASSISTANT CONTRACT (PAC PAGE 3 OF 3)

According to the National Association of REALTORS®, 16% of REALTORS® have at least one assistant. While some agents share an assistant, 79% of assistants work for a single agent. Fifty-four percent of personal assistants work part time. Although 48% of assistants are unlicensed, unlicensed assistants are limited in their activities. Some of the activities that might be delegated to assistants include the following:

- Installing signs and lockboxes

- Returning calls and handling correspondence and emails

- Preparing disclosures

- Conducting or assisting in open houses with the consent of the principal

- Financial qualifying of prospective buyers

- Tracking escrows

- Preparing internet listings and updates

- Answering emails within minutes and setting up appointments with prospect

- Preparing property flyers

- Locating property to show

- Contacting owners as to showings

- Managing agent's daily planner

- Handling agent's social media

Unlicensed assistants are prohibited from the following activities:

- Attempting to induce a person to use broker services (prohibits communication with the public in a manner structured for solicitation purposes)

- Showing property, including open houses (simply handing out material is alright)

- Discussing features of a property, unless taken from a data sheet prepared by a licensee

- Discussing terms and conditions regarding a listing or sale

- Discussing property needs with a client

- Discussing contracts or significance of documents with a client

- Participating in any negotiations

The Bureau of Real Estate published guidelines for unlicensed assistants, setting forth what an unlicensed assistant could and could not do; the *Guidelines for Unlicensed Assistants* was published in *Real Estate Bulletin*, Winter 2003, and can be accessed online at www.dre.ca.gov/files/pdf/ guide_unlic_asst.pdf.

WEB LINK

@

ADDITIONAL PREPARATION

Additional preparation will be required to prepare for your career.

When you go to work for an office, you will want to learn about the office **inventory** as soon as possible. This means you must visit office listings. Call ahead if a listing is inhabited. Don't take too much time with each owner, or you will have a long-term job just visiting inventory. In the case of large offices with hundreds of listings, personal visits to each listing would not be possible. As a suggestion, use your office website to review listings and then visit those listings that are in the area, price range, and of the type you feel you would like to concentrate on. You may wish to take digital photographs of features of the property, if they are not covered by your office website or property flyers. Take notes so you don't confuse property features. Until you know the inventory, you will be unable to field inquiries or properly prepare for a showing.

Another benefit of visiting office inventory is that it will give you a sense of area value based on listing prices. You should be able to judge within a relatively short period of time if a listing is priced competitively. Check out homes listed by other offices within the geographic area or specialization area if you have decided to specialize in a particular market segment. In smaller communities, you might be able to see everything that is available, but in larger markets, you will have to be selective and choose homes for which you feel you might have interested buyers.

Of course, you should go on office and board **caravans** of new listings. Avoid visiting properties where you feel the likelihood of your having a buyer is slight. Try to avoid wasting time. Abraham Lincoln said, "A lawyer's time is his stock in trade." It holds true for real estate agents as well as lawyers.

Office Procedure

If your office or company has a **policy manual** (procedures manual), study it. As soon as possible, learn what is expected of you. Know your office meeting and training schedules, and enter them in your daily planner for the month ahead. Find out what the procedure is for depositing customer trust money. You must know what to do when you take a listing or an offer to purchase. Every office is run a little differently from every other office, so be certain you understand what is expected of you.

Be familiar with the forms used by your office so that you will be able to complete them and explain them to others without hesitation. As a personal training exercise, complete a listing for a property you know of, and then complete an offer to purchase for that property. Have both reviewed by another agent.

Find out how to use your office communications systems. What are the procedures for long distance calls and overnight express services? Understand what systems your office provides and how to use them.

Computer Literacy

A 2014 survey by the National Association of REALTORS® (NAR) revealed that

- the internet was used by 92% of buyers and only 30% used newspapers;

- 91% of REALTORS® used social media to some extent; and

- the top three places where REALTORS® placed their listings, besides their own website, were www.Realtor.com, Zillow, and Trulia.

A 2012 NAR survey revealed that

- 90% of buyers used the internet as their first stop in house hunting and

- 80% of buyers contacted a broker from what they saw on the internet.

In today's sales environment, it is readily apparent that you must have computer knowledge. At a minimum, you should be able to use a computer for the following:

- Sending and accessing email

- Searching for available properties from MLS data based on specific criteria (for example: four-bedroom houses in a particular area priced under $400,000)

- Obtaining a printout of houses sold within an area showing features and sale price

- Knowing your office and MLS website and links

- Accessing additional websites covering your market area

- Preparing a listing for website use

- Using word-processing software to produce personalized sales letters and other correspondence

- Producing an attractive property brief (one-page description) for a listing

- Obtaining comparables (listing and sale prices of similar properties) and preparing a comparative market analysis

- Handling loan-qualifying and loan applications online

You should consider **e-PRO certification**. This is the NAR training program to certify real estate professionals as internet professionals. The educational requirements for certification will prepare you for more effective online communications.

Tax Knowledge

You must understand real property taxation and special benefits available for seniors, low-income individuals, and so on. You should also have knowledge of the income tax benefits of home ownership, as well as the tax treatment for investment and income property, including exchanging. (See Unit 14.) Tax knowledge is also important for tracking your own expenses for income tax preparation. What you can deduct will significantly affect your net income.

Sales Equipment

You must be equipped to be a successful real estate salesperson. You should consider the following:

iPad or other tablet device. Many real estate agents are relying on iPads or other tablet devices, such as those that run on the Android operating system, to conduct their real estate sales business. Most MLS interfaces are optimized to display on tablet devices. Other agents are using their tablets to generate and sign contracts through applications designed for this purpose.

Wireless printers. Wireless printers are available starting at about $100. The printers can be mounted in your vehicle and used in conjunction with your netbook or laptop to print out information on properties as well as contracts. With a wireless printer, you can turn your vehicle into a mobile office.

Smartphone. Over 80% of real estate agents now use smartphones. They do so to increase agent efficiency. Consider a smartphone such as an Apple iPhone with the following features and real estate apps:

- All phone services, including caller ID, call waiting, and recording
- Wireless email
- Daily planning
- Storing of addresses and telephone numbers
- Managing contacts for return calls, action, et cetera.
- Making to-do lists
- Taking notes
- Writing memos
- Amortization schedule
- Doing financial calculations (closing costs, payments, etc.)
- Retrieving and sending emails
- Downloading MLS information and other data from the internet

- Available For Sale by Owner properties

- Zillow value estimates

- Transferring data to and from desktop computers

- Setting an alarm for appointment reminders

- Entering business-related expenses for tax purposes

- Using universal connectors for add-ons, such as portable keyboard, modems, and more

- Accessing a global positioning system (GPS) for driving instructions to addresses from your location; Waze is a community-based traffic navigation system that saves both time and gas.

- Open House Pro is an open house management system that helps follow up leads on walk-ins

- Dropbox is a free service that allows you to bring photos, documents, and videos anywhere. Any file you place in Dropbox is accessible.

- AroundMe identifies where you are and all businesses in the category that you type in

- Camera

- Customizing for specific needs

- Security. Red Alert is a security app that can contact 911 if you are in danger; it also features a built-in alarm.

A 2008 CAR survey revealed that 27% of respondents felt that a hands-free cell phone was their most important business upgrade in the past 12 months. A survey today would reveal that cell phone to be a smartphone with a real estate app. The real estate app gives the agent information on local listing and area information. The NAR has apps that will show sold homes on map zones, price-reduced properties, and foreclosed properties, as well as customized searches. In California, you cannot use a hand-held cell phone while driving.

Using a search engine, you will find App stores that offer a variety of apps, with many designed for real estate agents.

Business cards.   Your license number must be printed on your business card. You should also include your email address and your cell phone number. If you are fluent in another language or languages and are targeting persons who speak that language, then your business card should indicate your language fluency. Your name must appear as it is on your real estate license. A nickname may be highlighted to indicate it is not the salesperson's legal name. The name of your employing broker must be in at least eight-point type. Your photo on your card will help contacts identify you. A fold-out card might be required to provide all pertinent data.

Some brokers do not want photos used on business cards because of agent safety. Brokers feel that "glamour photos" might cause contacts with the agent other than real property–related business. Other brokers fear the photos could encourage racial or ethnic discrimination. You should be aware of these concerns. However, the author believes tasteful business card photos are proper, as well as being a positive business practice.

Electronic business cards have seen increased use by real estate professionals. While they may look like ordinary cards, when they are inserted into a computer, they can provide videos, resumes, and links to social networking, as well as your office site.

A QR code (quick response code) is a bar code readable by smartphones. One phone scans the other for data transfer. Use of a QR code can mean a paperless electronic card.

Your car.   Your car should be kept clean at all times. Avoid smoking in your car because many people are offended by the smell of tobacco. You might want to use an air freshener. If you are going to purchase a car, consider a full-size four-door model or SUV for ease in entering and exiting. This is of particular value when dealing with older prospective buyers. To test for comfort, sit in the rear seat of the vehicle before you decide to purchase.

Carry the following items in the trunk, glove box, or under the seat:

1. A plastic bag with extra forms and pens

2. A flashlight

3. A For Sale sign and stake. Large For Sale signs erected on heavy posts are generally installed by a crew hired by the broker. Many offices install small signs until the large sign can be erected. In addition, many communities limit the size of For Sale signs, so smaller signs must be used.

4. Basic tools (hammer, screwdriver, pliers, assorted nails, screws, nuts, and bolts) for setting or repairing firm signs

5. A 50-foot tape measure (and/or an electronic measuring device)

6. A small tape recorder to record your thoughts or ideas if your smartphone does not have this capability

7. A supply of business cards

8. Maps showing school districts, public transportation, recreational areas, et cetera. (Use colored marking pens.)

9. A digital camera with a minimum of 14 megapixels for clarity

If your office does not have an 800 number and your buyers come primarily from outside your local calling area, you might consider your own 800 number. An 800 number is available at a very reasonable cost. Many independent providers offer these services.

Computer. As you gain experience and knowledge, you will find that you will be spending more time away from your office. Your office will become more of a place to meet clients than a workstation. Your own computer to access your office computers and MLS services is a necessity. A computer offers the benefit of a larger monitor than a smartphone's screen. Your home office should also include a printer, scanner, fax, and copier (now available as 4-in-1 machines). You will need them. Having a home office will reduce wasted time and allow you to utilize spare time at home. You can track contact information and activities with contact management software. You can even set alarms as to contacts.

Note: You should be aware that a home office may qualify as an IRS tax deduction if the space is used exclusively and regularly as your principal place of business. You should check with your accountant to determine if your home office expenses qualify as tax deductions.

WEB LINK

Specialty items.   There are a number of sources for real estate signs, flags, cards, newsletters and give-away advertising items. Many boards of REALTORS® have stores. In addition there are a number of providers on the internet such as www.sanzospecialties.com.

You.   You want to dress as a professional within your area would dress. Your clothes reflect the image you want to convey, that of a person who feels competent in her role. Avoid trendy fashions; conservative is best. Avoid overly flashy or expensive jewelry; you don't want to divert attention from what you are saying. Use cologne or aftershave lotion sparingly. If people can smell you coming, chances are you overdid it.

Learn to smile. Smile while you are on the telephone and when you talk to people. An upbeat person can make others feel good and can set an upbeat mood for a sale.

Take care of yourself. Your body is the only one you have. Watch your diet, get adequate sleep, and exercise on a regular basis. A healthy body will be reflected in your energy and productivity.

Recordkeeping.   Keep records of all written communications and notes of any problems. Do not make verbal promises. Follow up communications with an email. Contemporaneous dated notes are important. Records can be kept electronically. Many of the problems you will encounter are based on understanding later what was communicated. Good records can avoid legal disputes and serve to reinforce your position if disputes do occur.

SUMMARY

Real estate professionals deal in the fulfillment of needs. The product that fulfills these needs is real estate.

Real estate activity can be an important engine for economic growth because more people are employed in real estate and construction-related jobs than in any other industry.

Competition has changed the way many brokers charge for their services.

Real estate professionals work in an imperfect and changing marketplace. The reasons for this imperfection include product differentiation, emotions, imperfect buyer and seller knowledge, buyer and seller motivation, and the differing terms of the sale. The real estate professional brings a degree of order to this marketplace.

Real estate is changing with new technology, as well as with better-educated and trained professionals. Changes are also taking place because of competition.

Most real estate agents are engaged in listing and selling single-family residences. Other areas of activity or specialization include the following:

- Mobile home sales

- Residential income property

- Commercial property

- Industrial property

- Business opportunities

- Land and farm brokerage

- Lot sales

- Auction sales

- Loan brokerage

- Land development

- Property management

- Leasing

The real estate salesperson is considered by real estate law to be an employee of the broker but for tax purposes usually is contractually designated as an independent contractor.

If the salesperson meets the IRS criteria as an independent contractor, withholding tax is not deducted from the salesperson's commission checks. Also, the employer need not contribute to the salesperson's Social Security.

Choosing a broker is an extremely important decision. A new licensee should be particularly interested in the aid and training provided by the broker. Brokers want to hire salespersons who will succeed, and salespersons want a broker who can meet their needs.

Your attitude can be a significant factor in your success. A negative attitude will be reflected in your production.

Working for a REALTOR® or a Realtist will give you the advantage of a broad educational program, as well as access to publications. Keep in mind that training is a career-long activity and is an integral part of your career as a real estate professional. You must equip yourself with the basic tools of the real estate profession and know how to use them. Besides office training and boards of REALTORS® sessions, engage in self-training. This includes reading books and periodicals, using available videos, and, most important, role-playing to prepare yourself to handle any conceivable situation.

Establish goals for yourself. These should include short-term, intermediate-term, and long-term goals. You need a plan to meet these goals. Your planning will reduce wasted time and lead to realization of your goals. The basic building block of your planning is a daily plan.

One of your first steps toward success in a new office is learning your inventory. You must learn office procedures, acquire basic computer literacy, and have basic knowledge of property and income taxes as they relate to real estate sales activities. You must also acquire some basic tools so you can perform as a real estate professional. Keep records of what was communicated and when. Good records can avoid problems.

Of course, you want to personally convey the image of a professional in your dress and manner. Take care of yourself because your health is related to your productivity.

CLASS DISCUSSION TOPICS

1. Describe your local market area and evaluate it. Is your local market stratified? How? If you were to choose an area of specialization, what would it be? (Consider both geographic area and activity.) Justify your choice.

2. Describe the training programs provided by local offices.

3. What are your long-term goals? What short-term and intermediate-term goals would help in meeting these long-term goals?

4. What training material is available for your use in your office?

5. What training material and course offerings are available through your board or association of REALTORS®?

6. Prepare a daily plan in advance. How was your time actually spent on that day? Discuss deviations from the plan and the reasons for the deviations. Were they justified?

7. Evaluate your average day. What percentage of your time is spent in "A" Time activities? "B" Time activities? "C" Time activities? "D" Time activities?

8. What could you do now to increase the percentage of your time spent on "A" Time activities?

9. Do you know of any real estate firms in your area that have merged? If so, what benefits do you feel resulted from the merger?

10. Are there brokers in your area offering lower fees than their competition?

11. Are they providing similar services to those offered by their higher priced competitors?

12. Discuss what you consider to be a successful team. How are team members compensated? What are the benefits of team members?

13. For class discussion, bring to class one current-events article dealing with some aspect of real estate practice.

UNIT 1 QUIZ

1. The real estate marketplace could *BEST* be described as being
    a. homogeneous.
    b. stratified.
    c. perfect.
    d. uninfluenced by emotion.

2. *MOST* real estate agents are primarily engaged in which area of activity?
    a. Residential property
    b. Raw land and lots
    c. Commercial property
    d. Development

3. The IRS will treat real estate salespeople as independent contractors if three criteria are met. Which is *NOT* one of the criteria?
    a. The salesperson's reimbursement is solely based on sales, not hours worked.
    b. The salesperson represents himself as an independent contractor when dealing with third parties.
    c. There is a written contract stating that the salesperson will be treated as an independent contractor for tax purposes.
    d. The salesperson is licensed as a real estate agent.

4. A broker ordinarily would be liable to salespeople for
    a. unemployment compensation.
    b. workers' compensation.
    c. Social Security contributions.
    d. none of these.

5. In choosing a broker, a new licensee should be *LEAST* interested in an office that
    a. has a high percentage of successful salespeople.
    b. has a good library of books, tapes, and videos for training.
    c. offers 100% commission.
    d. is a member of a local multiple listing service.

6.   The *BEST* way to learn is to
   a.   listen to what others say.
   b.   read instructional material.
   c.   watch what others are doing.
   d.   use the ideas you observe or read about.

7.   Which of the following statements regarding role-playing is *TRUE?*
   a.   Role-playing situations are limited only by our own imagination.
   b.   Role-playing can be verbalized or nonverbalized.
   c.   Role-playing exercises can involve more than one person.
   d.   All of these.

8.   Which statement is an example of a specific goal?
   a.   I will work harder next week.
   b.   I will improve my listing presentation.
   c.   I will make 10 calls tomorrow on for-sale-by-owner ads and schedule three property showings by Sunday.
   d.   I will learn by observing successful agents.

9.   All of the following will aid you in goal achievement *EXCEPT*
   a.   that goals should be attainable.
   b.   that goals should be based on what you really want.
   c.   that goals should be kept to yourself because they are personal.
   d.   that goals should be exact so that you can measure their attainment.

10.   Proper daily planning means that you should endeavor to
   a.   reduce "D" Time activities.
   b.   increase "A" Time activities.
   c.   place more emphasis on probabilities than on possibilities.
   d.   accomplish all of these.

UNIT TWO

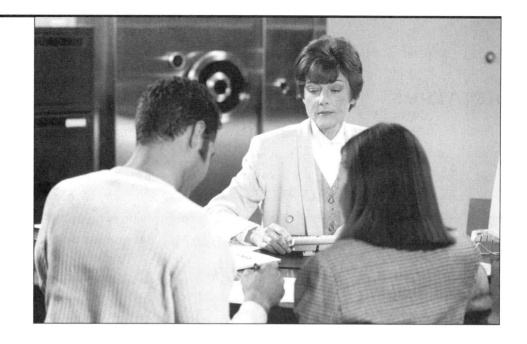

ETHICS, FAIR HOUSING, TRUST FUNDS, AND OTHER LEGAL ISSUES

LEARNING OBJECTIVES

When you have completed this unit, you will be able to

- define ethics and explain how to evaluate an act as ethical or unethical,

- understand federal and state fair housing laws and regulations and how they relate to real estate practice,

- explain the antitrust provision of the Sherman Antitrust Act and the applicability of the act to real estate practice, and

- understand real estate professionals' responsibility regarding sexual harassment and the handling of trust funds.

KEY TERMS

Americans with
  Disabilities Act
blockbusting
Civil Rights Act of
  1866
Civil Rights Act of
  1870
Civil Rights Act of
  1964
Civil Rights Act of
  1968
commingling
conversion

diversity training
Dred Scott decision
ethics
Fair Employment and
  Housing Act
familial status
Golden Rule
group boycotting laws
market allocation
place of public
  accommodation
price-fixing
readily achievable

REALTORS® Code of
  Ethics
redlining
Rumford Act
sexual harassment
Sherman Antitrust
  Act
steering
tie-in agreements
trust funds
Unruh Act

WHAT IS ETHICS?

The word **ethics** comes from the Greek *ethikos*, meaning *moral*, and *ethos*, meaning *character*. Ethics is a moral standard for life, and the test for that standard is quite simple. It is the **Golden Rule**: "Do unto others as you would have them do unto you." To evaluate conduct to determine whether it is ethical, simply ask yourself, "If the roles were reversed, would I consider the conduct I am contemplating to be proper?"

While no person is perfect, real estate professionals should strive for fair and honest dealings with all parties. If they do so, they will be acting in an ethical manner.

Ethics and the Law

> The best test of ethics is the Golden Rule.

You should do right not because of a fear of punishment or exposure but because the reward is the conduct itself. George Bernard Shaw stated, "You cannot believe in honor until you have achieved it." Similarly, you cannot truly understand why you should be a moral person until you become such a person.

The fact that everyone is doing an unethical act does not make it right. Nor does the fact that if you didn't do it someone else would.

Ethics has nothing to do with legality or illegality. **Laws** set minimum standards for what a society regards as acceptable behavior. Violation of the law is an illegal act for which the state has set penalties. Laws can change: what is illegal today could be legal tomorrow, and what is legal today could be illegal tomorrow. Similarly, a legal act could be unethical, and an illegal act could be ethical. As an example, adultery may be legal because it may not violate the law, but being unfaithful to a spouse would be considered unethical behavior because it does not pass the test of the Golden Rule. Similarly, failing to have a current dog license would violate the law, but it would not be unethical behavior based on the Golden Rule.

Ethics deals in what is right, not in minimum standards. While laws change to accommodate current attitudes, ethics remains constant. If conduct is wrong, based on the application of the Golden Rule, it remains wrong, even though others may engage in such conduct.

| Ethics goes beyond the law. | Ethics tends to precede the law. For instance, in the early 1980s, there was a rash of home purchases with loans being assumed and sellers carrying the balance of the purchase price using a second trust deed. These no-down-payment purchasers would rent the homes, pocket the rent receipts, and then not make payments on either the first or second trust deed, a practice called *rent skimming*. Some purchasers were able to delay foreclosure for more than a year. |

Though this practice was not at the time a violation of the law, if you apply the Golden Rule to this conduct, it is reprehensible and, of course, unethical. Statutes were later enacted that made rent skimming illegal.

Gray Ethical Areas

Ethics is not an exact science. What is ethical or unethical is not always clear. Our sense of right and wrong is based on our experiences. If in your heart you believe an action is proper, then it is ethical to you. However, if you have to ask someone if an action is legal, then you clearly feel there is something questionable in the action.

If you would not want others to know what you have done, then it is also clear that you feel the action is tainted. Or if you feel you have to justify an action with a defense such as "If I didn't do it, someone else would," it is clear that you know the action is wrong. Shakespeare said it best over 400 years ago: "To thine own self be true, and it must follow, as the night the day, thou canst not then be false to any man."

Ethics and Motive

Your motive for an action could determine whether the action is ethical or unethical. For example, while on a caravan visiting new listings, you notice several building code violations in one of the properties and you notify the county authorities of the violations. If you did so because you felt the violations presented a real danger to present occupants and any future buyers, then your action would have to be viewed as ethical. But if safety was not a concern, and you reported the violations solely because of animosity toward the listing agent, then your action would clearly be viewed as unethical because you were intentionally trying to hurt another without any redeeming reason.

Ethics and Your Career

Ethics is not incompatible with good business practices. Successfully meeting the needs of buyers and sellers will reinforce your self-esteem and serve as a motivator for further success. Over the long haul, an ethical professional will be rewarded with a loyal clientele and a steady stream of referrals. Most successful real estate salespeople obtain the greater portion of their business from referrals from people with whom they have worked in the past. If you want long-term success, you must earn the trust of others. From a pragmatic viewpoint, good ethics is good business.

Do not fall into the trap of measuring your success by dollars earned rather than by how you have successfully helped others. If you measure success solely in dollars, it becomes easy to take a pragmatic approach to real estate. You can lead yourself to believe that because the end—dollars—is important, the means to reach it are of less importance. You could find yourself acting in a self-serving manner, placing your own interests above the best interests of those you are serving. In short, it can be easy to become an unethical real estate salesperson or broker. Unfortunately, some real estate agents take a pragmatic approach based on "What will it do for me *now?*" A great many real estate license revocations have been the result of this "me" attitude.

CODES OF ETHICS

REALTORS®

A number of professional organizations have codes of ethics. The **REALTORS® Code of Ethics** is based on the Golden Rule and is an excellent guide to ethical behavior. The word *REALTOR®* denotes a member of the National Association of REALTORS® (NAR). But even if you are not a member of the NAR, you should read this code and use it as a guide in your relations with others.

Realtists

At one time, African Americans were excluded from just about every professional business group. In 1947, a group of African American brokers founded the National Association of Real Estate Brokers (NAREB) and adopted the word *Realtist* to designate their members. The NAREB, like the NAR, is constantly striving to increase the professionalism of the real estate industry.

California Code of Ethics

In 1979, former Real Estate Commissioner David Fox expressed a need for a California Code of Ethics. This code was known as the *Commissioner's Code of Ethics*. Because it was a repetition of conduct made illegal by other sections of the law, it was repealed in 1996. While illegal conduct is generally unethical, this code failed to carry ethics beyond the law. Legality or illegality of an act does not make it ethical or unethical. The real estate commissioner has, however, adopted the National Association of REALTORS® Code of Ethics.

The real estate commissioner has issued suggestions for professional conduct in sale, lease, and exchange transactions and suggestions for professional conduct when negotiating or arranging loans secured by real property or the sale of a promissory note secured by real property. These comprise Figure 2.1.

FAIR HOUSING AND ANTIDISCRIMINATION LEGISLATION

Fair housing legislation and practices involve almost every activity in real estate. The federal and state governments have passed legislation in the areas of fair housing and antidiscriminatory practices. Material regarding housing discrimination also appears in the real estate commissioner's Rules and Regulations and in the Business and Professions Code.

Federal Laws

Real estate brokers and salespeople should heed these laws in every stage of the real estate process. An understanding of the history of antidiscrimination laws will help you understand the need for this legislation.

FIGURE 2.1:   Suggestions for Professional Conduct

The Real Estate Commissioner has issued "Suggestions for Professional Conduct in Sale, Lease, and Exchange Transactions" and "Suggestions for Professional Conduct When Negotiating or Arranging Loans Secured by Real Property or Sale of a Promissory Note Secured by Real Property."

The purpose of the Suggestions is to encourage real estate licensees to maintain a high level of ethics and professionalism in their business practices when performing acts for which a real estate license is required.

The Suggestions are not intended as statements of duties imposed by law nor as grounds for disciplinary action by the Bureau of Real Estate but as suggestions for elevating the professionalism of real estate licensees.

As part of the effort to promote ethical business practices of real estate licensees, the real estate commissioner has issued the following Suggestions for Professional Conduct:

(a) Suggestions for Professional Conduct in Sale, Lease, and Exchange Transactions. In order to maintain a high level of ethics and professionalism in their business practices, real estate licensees are encouraged to adhere to the following suggestions in conducting their business activities:

  (1) Aspire to give a high level of competent, ethical, and quality service to buyers and sellers in real estate transactions.
  (2) Stay in close communication with clients or customers to ensure that questions are promptly answered and all significant events or problems in a transaction are conveyed in a timely manner.
  (3) Cooperate with the California Bureau of Real Estate's enforcement of, and report to that Bureau evident violations of, the Real Estate Law.
  (4) Use care in the preparation of any advertisement to present an accurate picture or message to the reader, viewer, or listener.
  (5) Submit all written offers in a prompt and timely manner.
  (6) Keep oneself informed and current on factors affecting the real estate market in which the licensee operates as an agent.
  (7) Make a full, open, and sincere effort to cooperate with other licensees, unless the principal has instructed the licensee to the contrary.
  (8) Attempt to settle disputes with other licensees through mediation or arbitration.
  (9) Advertise or claim to be an expert in an area of specialization in real estate brokerage activity (e.g., appraisal, property management, industrial siting, mortgage loan, etc.), only if the licensee has had special training, preparation, or experience in such areas.
  (10) Strive to provide equal opportunity for quality housing and a high level of service to all persons regardless of race, color, sex, religion, ancestry, physical handicap, marital status, or national origin.
  (11) Base opinions of value, whether for the purpose of advertising or promoting real estate brokerage business, upon documented objective data.
  (12) Make every attempt to comply with these Suggestions for Professional Conduct and the Code of Ethics of any organized real estate industry group of which the licensee is a member.

FIGURE 2.1 (continued):   Suggestions for Professional Conduct

(b)   Suggestions for Professional Conduct When Negotiating or Arranging Loans Secured by Real Property or Sale of a Promissory Note Secured by Real Property. In order to maintain a high level of ethics and professionalism in their business practices when performing acts within the meaning of subdivision (d) and (e) of Section 10131 and Sections 10131.1 and 10131.2 of the Business and Professions Code, real estate licensees are encouraged to adhere to the following suggestions, in addition to any applicable provisions of subdivision (a), in conducting their business activities:

(1)   Aspire to give a high level of competent, ethical, and quality service to borrowers and lenders in loan transactions secured by real estate.

(2)   Stay in close communication with borrowers and lenders to ensure that reasonable questions are promptly answered and all significant events or problems in a loan transaction are conveyed in a timely manner.

(3)   Keep oneself informed and current on factors affecting the real estate loan market in which the licensee acts as an agent.

(4)   Advertise or claim to be an expert in an area of specialization in real estate mortgage loan transactions only if the licensee has had special training, preparation, or experience in such area.

Suggestions for Professional Conduct

(5)   Strive to provide equal opportunity for quality mortgage loan services and a high level of service to all borrowers or lenders regardless of race, color, sex, religion, ancestry, physical handicap, marital status, or national origin.

(6)   Base opinions of value in a loan transaction, whether for the purpose of advertising or promoting real estate mortgage loan brokerage business, on documented objective data.

(7)   Respond to reasonable inquiries of a principal as to the status or extent of efforts to negotiate the sale of an existing loan.

(8)   Respond to reasonable inquiries of a borrower regarding the net proceeds available from a loan arranged by the licensee.

(9)   Make every attempt to comply with the standards of professional conduct and the code of ethics of any organized mortgage loan industry group of which the licensee is a member.

The conduct suggestions set forth in subsections (a) and (b) are not intended as statements of duties imposed by law nor as grounds for disciplinary action by the Bureau of Real Estate, but as guidelines for elevating the professionalism of real estate licensees.

Although the Declaration of Independence originally contained language condemning slavery, that language was removed shortly before the document was signed to ensure the consensus of all the states. However, the Declaration of Independence did retain the following statement: "We hold these truths to be self-evident, that all men are created equal, that they are endowed by their Creator with certain Inalienable Rights, that among these are Life, Liberty, and the pursuit of Happiness." There was also an attempt to outlaw slavery when the U.S. Constitution was written. Because of strong opposition, wording that would outlaw slavery was not included based on "practical" considerations.

While there was strong antislavery sentiment in the northern states, by the mid-1800s, the South's economy had become dependent on slave labor. The invention of the cotton gin and the Industrial Revolution had made cotton growing very lucrative. In 1820, the Missouri Compromise allowed Missouri to enter the Union without restrictions as to slavery, while Maine would enter as a free state. The western territories were to be free.

In 1857, the U.S. Supreme Court issued the *Dred Scott* **decision** that basically ordered the federal government to keep out of the slavery issue because it was a matter for the states to decide. The court held that only a state could exclude slavery and that Congress had exceeded its authority by prohibiting slavery in the territories. The Missouri Compromise was thus held unconstitutional.

The Declaration of Independence Is Not Law

While inspiring, the Declaration of Independence is not law. Had it been law, there likely would not have been the necessity for most of the federal and state antidiscrimination laws. An attempt to include antislavery language in the Constitution failed. In fact, the Constitution provided that a slave should be considered as being only three-fifths of a person in determining the congressional representation of a state.

The court also made clear that "Negroes" were not entitled to rights as U.S. citizens and had "no rights which any white man was bound to respect." The court pointed out that slaves were property and that the U.S. Constitution guaranteed property rights.

The *Dred Scott* decision was received with anger in the North. It led to sectionalism that divided the nation and was a prime cause of the Civil War.

Thirteenth Amendment.   The Thirteenth Amendment to the Constitution abolished slavery, but it did not specifically address the rights of former slaves.

Civil Rights Act of 1866.   The **Civil Rights Act of 1866** was intended to provide equal treatment for former slaves. It states that "all citizens of the United States shall have the same rights in every state or territory as is enjoyed by white citizens thereof to inherit, purchase, lease, sell, hold, and convey real and personal property."

The Civil Rights Act of 1866 had no exceptions.

While this act was broad in its protection, it applied only to race. There were exceptions to the act, which could be enforced by any individual who was discriminated against. Remedies included injunction and compensatory and punitive damages.

Fourteenth Amendment. The Fourteenth Amendment to the Constitution was passed after the Civil Rights Act of 1866. Supporters of the amendment pointed out that it would protect the rights granted in the 1866 act by providing protection in the U.S. Constitution. This would prevent a later Congress or court from taking away these rights.

The Fourteenth Amendment states the following:

> All persons born or naturalized in the United States, and subject to the jurisdiction thereof, are citizens of the United States and of the State wherein they reside. No State shall make or enforce any law which shall abridge the privileges or immunities of citizens of the United States; nor shall any State deprive any person of life, liberty, or property, without due process of law; nor deny any person within its jurisdiction the equal protection of the laws.

Obviously, the Fourteenth Amendment did not limit itself to race. A reasonable interpretation of the above quote would be that the Fourteenth Amendment offered comprehensive civil rights protection.

Civil Rights Act of 1870. Some attorneys were of the opinion that because the Fourteenth Amendment was passed after the Civil Rights Act of 1866, that act had been effectively replaced and was no longer law. So to protect against later courts taking away the remedies granted by the 1866 act, the following statement was tacked onto a voting rights act in 1870 (**Civil Rights Act of 1870**):

> (A)nd be it further enacted that the act to protect all persons in the United States in their civil rights and furnish the means of their vindication, passed April nine, eighteen hundred and sixty-six, is hereby re-enacted.

Thus, the Civil Rights Act of 1866 was passed twice to make certain it would withstand possible future challenges in the courts. However, the act was effectively gutted by state court decisions and failure of the federal courts to enforce the act. The act, as well as the Fourteenth Amendment, was ineffective in providing equal rights for approximately 100 years.

Executive Order 11063. On November 21, 1962, President John F. Kennedy issued an order that prohibited discrimination in housing wherever federal funds were involved. The order affected property sales involving FHA and VA loans, as well as other government-subsidized programs. It stated that

> the executive branch of the government, in faithfully executing the laws of the United States which authorize federal financial assistance, directly or indirectly for the provision, rehabilitation, and operation of housing and related facilities, is charged with an obligation and duty to assume that the laws are fairly administered and that benefits there under are made available to all Americans without regard to their race, color, creed, or national origin.

Civil Rights Act of 1964. The **Civil Rights Act of 1964** made the 1962 executive order law and is considered among the first of the modern civil rights acts. While it prohibited discrimination in all federally assisted programs, prior and later acts are far more comprehensive.

Jones v. Mayer. In the same year that the Civil Rights Act of 1968 was passed (below), the Supreme Court decided the case of *Jones v. Mayer*, which involved a seller who refused to sell a home to an African American. Both the district court and the court of appeals ruled that the Civil Rights Act of 1866 prohibited discrimination by the state but not by individuals. The Supreme Court reversed, ruling that the Civil Rights Act of 1866 applied to private property and could be enforced by the party discriminated against. The court based its decision on the 13th Amendment because the act was passed before passage of the 14th Amendment..

Jones v. Mayer upheld the Civil Rights Act of 1866.

Civil Rights Act of 1968. The **Civil Rights Act of 1968** prohibited discrimination in housing based on national origin, race, religion, and color. (Sexual discrimination was added in 1974.) The act prohibits the following:

- Discrimination by brokers toward clients and customers
- Refusal to show, rent, or sell through the false representation that a property is not available
- Discrimination as to access to multiple listing services
- Discriminatory sales or loan terms

Steering is directing based on a group.

Blockbusting is inducing panic selling.

Redlining is refusal to loan in designated areas.

- **Steering**, the act of directing people of different races, religions, et cetera, away from or toward particular areas

- **Blockbusting**, the process of inducing panic selling by representing that prices will drop or crime will increase because of the possible entrance of minority group members to the area

- **Redlining**, the refusal to loan within an area

- Retaliatory acts against persons making fair-housing complaints and intimidation to discourage complaints

- Discriminatory advertising, which is prohibited even when related to activities exempt from the act

There has been a great deal of concern as to what advertising might be considered discriminatory. Advertising that a property is close to a particular house of worship or a place that has a racial connotation (such as "Martin Luther King Hospital") has been held to be discriminatory, as have ads that indicate a preference for a particular race or marital status or ads that indicate a member of a protected category is not welcome.

Advertising Terms Acceptable by HUD

HUD has indicated that use of the following terms and phrases are not discriminatory: master bedroom, rare find, desirable neighborhood, kosher meals available, apartment complex with chapel, Santa Claus, Easter Bunny, St. Valentine's Day, Merry Christmas, Happy Easter, mother-in-law suite, bachelor apartment, great view, fourth-floor walkup, walk-in closets, jogging trails, walk to bus stop, nonsmoking, sober, two-bedroom, family room, no bicycles allowed, and quiet streets.

There is still a great deal of confusion as to what HUD will consider discriminatory advertising. Several groups have published lists of terms that are acceptable, that are to be used with caution, or that are to be regarded as discriminatory. However, clearance through one of these lists does not mean that HUD will not regard the language as discriminatory. One problem is that words have different connotations within different groups, as well as regions in the country. HUD has indicated it will not approve any of the published lists. (See Unit 8 for more details.)

There are some exemptions to the Civil Rights Act of 1968. The following exemptions apply to the Civil Rights Act of 1968 but are not exemptions under the Civil Rights Act of 1866 or under California fair housing laws:

- Religious groups, which can discriminate in providing nonprofit housing, provided that the religion is open to all, regardless of race, sex, color, or national origin

- Private clubs, which can discriminate or give preference to members when selling or leasing housing for noncommercial purposes

- Owners of single-family homes, who can discriminate when selling or renting without an agent, provided that they do not own more than three such homes and are not in the business of renting

- Owners of one-to-four-residential-unit buildings who occupy a unit and who can discriminate if an agent is not used in renting

> The 1988 Fair Housing Amendments Act extended protection in regard to familial status and the handicapped.

1988 Fair Housing Amendments Act.   This important law extended federal protection against housing discrimination to include **familial status** and handicapped persons. It also strengthened the enforcement mechanisms and gave HUD greater enforcement power. Familial status protection refers to persons under age 18 living with a parent or guardian, persons in the process of obtaining legal custody, and pregnant persons.

The real estate agent should also be aware that adult-only designations are no longer possible, although there are exceptions to this rule. Operators of projects can either set up a community in which all residents must be at least age 62 or in which 80% of the units are occupied by at least one person age 55 years or older.

Even if an apartment complex has a family section, designation of an all-adult area still is prohibited. Steering prospective tenants toward a particular area in an apartment complex and away from another area also violates the act.

Apartments can have rules for children's use of facilities when there is a nondiscriminatory reason for the difference in rules. The Civil Rights Act of 1968 does not prohibit owners from setting maximum occupancy of units as long as the rule is enforced without discrimination. (It is likely that unreasonably limited occupancy rules would be unenforceable because they would discriminate against families with children.)

Discrimination against the handicapped is prohibited. The term *handicapped* refers to both mentally and physically handicapped persons. AIDS is considered a handicap under the act, so landlords and sellers cannot discriminate against a person with AIDS or HIV infection. The law specifically prohibits discrimination against guide dogs and support animals. Landlords cannot require additional security deposits because of these animals.

Property managers should be aware that the handicapped must be allowed to alter their units and common areas if such alterations are necessary for reasonable use and enjoyment of the premises. The property manager cannot increase the security deposit because of these alterations. However, the landlord *can* require that the tenant agree to put the premises back as they originally were if an able-bodied person would not wish the alterations to remain.

Brokers should prominently display the Equal Housing Opportunity poster (Figure 2.2) in all rental offices. Failure of the broker to post this poster in the place of business can shift the burden of proof to the broker to prove that an act was nondiscriminatory under federal law, should a complaint be made.

Advertising residential financing must contain an Equal Housing Opportunity logo, slogan, or statement advising the homeseeker that financing is available to all persons regardless of race, color, religion, sex, handicap, familial status, or national origin.

Americans with Disabilities Act. The **Americans with Disabilities Act (ADA)** prohibits discrimination that would deny the equal enjoyment of goods, services, facilities, and accommodations in any existing place of public accommodation, based on an individual's physical or mental disabilities. A **"place of public accommodation"** applies to stores, offices, and other nonresidential commercial facilities open to the public.

Owners and operators of such establishments (including property management firms) must make the facilities accessible to the extent *readily achievable*. (See Figure 2.3.) **"Readily achievable"** is defined as "easily accomplished without a great deal of expense." This would be based on the cost of compliance related to property values and on the financial abilities of the person(s) involved. New construction must be readily accessible unless it is structurally impractical.

The ADA also applies to employment discrimination. Employers having 15 or more employees must alter their workplaces to provide reasonable accommodations for handicapped employees unless it creates an undue hardship on the business. Compliance for a real estate office might consist of designating parking spaces for the handicapped, ramping curbs, adding railings on steps, lowering counters, creating wider aisles between desks, et cetera.

The act provides for civil penalties of $75,000 for the first discriminatory act and $150,000 for each subsequent violation, including compensatory damages and attorneys' fees. Because of the substantial penalties, owners and property managers should be aware that a cottage industry has evolved of handicapped persons and attorneys who seek out properties with handicapped-access deficiencies to sue for damages. Several handicapped individuals have brought legal action against more than 100 businesses. Businesses usually agree to a settlement rather than a costly trial and possible penalties.

Equal Credit Opportunity Act. This federal act prohibits credit discrimination because of sex, marital status, age, race, religion, national origin, or because the income of a credit applicant is from public assistance.

FIGURE 2.2:   Equal Housing Opportunity Poster

U. S. Department of Housing and Urban Development

**EQUAL HOUSING
OPPORTUNITY**

We Do Business in Accordance With the Federal Fair Housing Law

(The Fair Housing Amendments Act of 1988)

It is illegal to Discriminate Against Any Person Because of Race, Color, Religion, Sex, Handicap, Familial Status, or National Origin

---

■ In the sale or rental of housing or residential lots

■ In advertising the sale or rental of housing

■ In the financing of housing

■ In the provision of real estate brokerage services

■ In the appraisal of housing

■ Blockbusting is also illegal

Anyone who feels he or she has been discriminated against may file a complaint of housing discrimination:
     1-800-669-9777 (Toll Free)
     1-800-927-9275 (TTY)
     www.hud.gov/fairhousing

U.S. Department of Housing and Urban Development
Assistant Secretary for Fair Housing and Equal Opportunity
Washington, D.C. 20410

Previous editions are obsolete   form HUD-928.1 (6/2011)

California fair housing laws.   California has several fair housing laws, as well as administrative regulations dealing with discrimination. A single act could be a violation of more than one state or federal law or regulation, or both.

Unruh Act.   The **Unruh Act** prohibits discrimination in all business establishments. The Unruh Act applies to real estate brokers, salespeople, and anyone managing an apartment building or other business establishment. Business discrimination includes housing discrimination based on sex, race, color, religion, ancestry, national origin, disability, medical condition, marital status, familial status, and sexual orientation. ADA provisions have been incorporated into the act.

FIGURE 2.3:   Reasonable Modifications to Public Facilities or Services

Provide doors with automatic opening mechanisms

Provide menus (and real estate listings) in a large-print or braille format

Install an intercom so customers can contact a second-floor business in a building without an elevator

Lower public telephones

Add grab bars to public restroom stalls

Permit guide dogs to accompany customers

Provide a shopper's assistant to help disabled customers

Provide ramps in addition to entry stairs

A violation of the Unruh Act, can result in a court award of a maximum of three times actual damages but not less than $4,000. In addition, the violation could result in a civil penalty up to $25,000.

The Unruh Act applies to business discrimination.

The act has been expanded to apply to age discrimination in rental apartments and condominium properties. Housing developed and designed for the special needs of senior citizens is exempt from this act.

Rumford Fair Housing Act.   The **Fair Employment and Housing Act**, also known as the **Rumford Act** (Government Code Sections 12900 et seq.), prohibits discrimination in supplying housing accommodations on the basis of sex, color, race, religion, marital status, family status, sexual orientation, disability, source of income, ancestry, or national origin. Anyone selling, renting, leasing, or financing housing must comply with the Rumford Act.

While the Unruh Act applies to discrimination by businesses, the Rumford Act applies to all housing discrimination by individuals and businesses. Unlike the Unruh Act, it applies only to housing.

At Home With Diversity

In today's market, the average real estate agent no longer reflects the typical buyer. In recognition of our rapidly changing national demographics, the National Association of REALTORS® and the U.S. Department of Housing and Urban Development created the At Home with Diversity program to expand home ownership opportunities for more Americans by training real estate professionals to actively and aggressively seek out potential homebuyers from all racial and cultural backgrounds. Licensees who take this **diversity training** program, sponsored by the NAR, will learn how attending diverse cultural and community events can expand their client base, find out how simple multicultural etiquette can lead to success with new clients and customers, and develop sound diversity strategies to incorporate into their overall business plan.

An individual violating any part of this act may be reported to the Department of Fair Employment and Housing within one year of the occurrence. The Rumford Act predated the Civil Rights Act of 1968. Rumford Act violations are also violations of the federal act.

Business and Professions Code

The California Business and Professions Code governs real estate licensees' behavior, in addition to federal and state fair housing laws. The code provides detailed antidiscrimination material, including a definition of the term *discrimination* as used in the code, and sections detailing behavioral guidelines for licensees and grounds for disciplinary action in cases of noncompliance.

Section 125.6: Disciplinary Provisions for Discriminatory Acts

Under Section 125.6, persons who hold a license under the provisions of the code are subject to disciplinary action if they refuse to perform a licensed activity or make any discrimination or restriction in the performance of the licensed activity because of an applicant's race, color, sex, religion, ancestry, physical handicap, or national origin.

Section 10177(l): Further Grounds for Disciplinary Action

Discrimination occurs

> if a licensee solicited or induced the sale, lease, or listing for sale or lease, of residential property on the ground, wholly or in part, of loss of value, increase in crime, or decline of the quality of the schools, due to the presence or prospective entry into the neighborhood of a person or persons of another race, color, religion, ancestry, or national origin.

Regulations of the Real Estate Commissioner
Section 2780: Discriminatory Conduct as the Basis for Disciplinary Action

Prohibited discriminatory conduct by real estate licensees based on race, color, sex, religion, physical handicap, or national origin includes:

a. refusing to negotiate for the sale, rental, or financing;

b. refusing or failing to show, rent, sell, or finance;

c. discriminating against any person in the sale or purchase, collection of payments, or performance of services;

d. discriminating in the conditions or privileges of sale rental or financing;

e. discriminating in processing applications, referrals, or assigning licenses;

f. representing real property as not available for inspection;

g. processing an application more slowly;

h. making any effort to encourage discrimination;

i. refusing to assist another licensee;

j. making an effort to obstruct, retard, or discourage a purchase;

k. expressing or implying a limitation, preference, or discrimination;

l. coercing, intimidating, threatening, or interfering;

m. soliciting restrictively;

n. maintaining restrictive waiting lists;

o. seeking to discourage or prevent transactions;

p.   representing alleged community opposition;

q.   representing desirability of particular properties;

r.   refusing to accept listings;

s.   agreeing not to show property;

t.   advertising in a manner that indicates discrimination;

u.   using wording that indicates preferential treatment;

v.   advertising selectively;

w.   maintaining selective pricing, rent, cleaning, or security deposits;

x.   financing in a discriminatory manner;

y.   discriminating in pricing;

z.   discriminating in services;

aa.   discriminating against owners, occupants, or guests;

ab.   bb. making an effort to encourage discrimination;

cc.   implementing discriminatory rule in multiple listings and other services; and

dd.   assisting one who intends to discriminate.

Section 2781: Panic Selling

Section 2781 prohibits discriminatory conduct that creates fear or alarm to induce sale or lease because of the entry into an area of people of another race, color, sex, religion, ancestry, or national origin.

Section 2782: Duty to Supervise

Brokers must take reasonable steps to be familiar with, and to familiarize their salespeople with, the federal and state laws pertaining to prohibition of discriminatory process.

Holden Act (Housing Financial Discrimination Act of 1977). The Holden Act prohibits financial institutions from engaging in discriminatory loan activities or practices. Activities covered under this act include awarding building, improvement, purchase, or refinancing loans using the criteria of race, color, national origin, ancestry, sex, religion, or marital status. Discrimination based on the ethnic composition of the area surrounding a property (redlining) is also illegal.

California Omnibus Housing Nondiscrimination Act. This act makes all California's nondiscrimination acts consistent with the California Fair Employment and Housing Act as to coverage. All the acts apply to discrimination on the basis of national origin, ancestry, race, color, gender, religion, marital status, familial status, disability, source of income, and sexual orientation.

COMMISSIONER'S RULES AND REGULATIONS

Article 10 of the Real Estate Commissioner's Rules and Regulations concerns the discriminatory activities of real estate licensees. Regulations 2780, 2781, and 2782, contained within Article 10 (summarized above), list unacceptable discriminatory practices by licensees. Regulation 2780 indicates that discriminatory conduct by real estate licensees is a basis for disciplinary action by the Commissioner.

Licensees must be color-blind in their relations with owners and prospective buyers and tenants. Anything less is a violation of the law, as well as just "bad business."

SEXUAL HARASSMENT

In today's workplace, you must be cognizant of what could be regarded by others as **sexual harassment**. Charges of sexual harassment could result in legal expenses and significant damage awards or settlement costs, as well as being time consuming to resolve. Sexual harassment can be defined by how your actions are viewed by others, not necessarily by your intent.

Besides the costs involved, a claim of sexual harassment can adversely affect your working relationship with others. This would include co-workers, agents in other offices, and buyers and sellers.

Always conduct yourself in a businesslike manner. The only needs of others that you try to fulfill must be those relating to real estate.

Jokes, remarks, and touching might be regarded by others as sexual harassment.

In general, observe the following:

- Avoid sexually oriented jokes and anecdotes. Don't use "cute," double-meaning terms. Never discuss your love life or that of others in the workplace.

- Avoid patting, hugging, and touching others. What you might regard as a sign of "friendship" might be regarded differently by others.

- Allow others space. While in some cultures it is acceptable to talk to others with your face just inches from the other person, many people regard this closeness as intimidating and/or sexual harassment.

- Avoid romantic overtures or entanglements in the workplace.

- Avoid asking a co-worker for a date. If repeated on numerous occasions, it could be regarded as harassment. If a romantic relationship gets started in the workplace, a difficult working relationship will normally be the result should the romantic relationship end.

- Whenever possible, avoid one-on-one encounters in other than an open area. Some problem tenants have made multiple claims of sexual harassment by owners and property managers.

If a buyer or a seller seems to be inviting sexual advances, ignore the signals. You could be wrong, and if you are, you could find yourself facing a charge of sexual harassment.

SHERMAN ANTITRUST ACT

The **Sherman Antitrust Act** is a federal act to protect consumers from businesses that conspired to control prices and/or competition. Penalties for violation can include imprisonment. The act prohibits the following:

- **Price-fixing** (brokers cannot agree on minimum fees to be charged) Prudent brokers will add a statement in bold to the listing advising the seller of the negotiability of real estate commissions. This is an important aspect of strengthening the industry's compliance with this rule.

- **Market allocation** (it's illegal to divide a marketplace geographically or by type of service because it reduces competition)

- **Group boycotting** (firms may not agree to refuse to do business with a firm or individual)

- **Tie-in agreements** (agreements that require a client to buy additional goods or services as a condition of doing business or cooperating)

In September 2005, the Department of Justice filed a lawsuit alleging that a REALTOR® policy allowing brokers to block their listings from being displayed on other broker websites is a restraint on competition. An antitrust settlement between the National Association of REALTORS® and the

Justice Department in May 2008 prohibits REALTOR® rules that block listings of homes from being displayed on other brokers' websites.

A violation of the Sherman Act is likely to also violate California antitrust laws allowing for damages for injuries suffered.

OTHER LAWS AND REGULATIONS

Besides civil rights and antitrust legislation, there are numerous other federal and state statutes that apply to real estate transactions.

The Real Estate Settlement Procedures Act (RESPA) prohibits kickbacks from service providers to brokers. It makes illegal what was a common but unethical practice of "taking care" of agents who steered business to service providers. By accepting kickbacks of any sort, the agent feels an obligation to the service provider to steer business to that service provider when the agent's obligations should be to best serve the interests of the principal. Kickbacks prohibited by RESPA include cash, free business equipment, nonbusiness meals, tickets to events, and recreation fees.

California regulations include Sections 1000 through 10581 of the Business and Professions Code, which regulates real estate licensing, and Sections 11000 through 11030 of the Code, which regulates real estate licensees.

TRUST FUNDS

Trust funds refer to money or anything of value received by an agent, but not belonging to the agent, and held for the benefit of another. When a broker receives funds for a transaction, the broker must, within three days of receipt of the funds, do one of the following:

- Give the funds to the principal.

- Deposit the funds directly into escrow.

- Place the funds in the broker's trust account. (A broker who does not receive funds in trust does not need to have a trust account.)

Commingling is the mixing of property of another (trust funds) with property of the broker. Commingling is a violation of the Commissioner's Regulations and subject a broker to severe disciplinary action. Holding the funds without authorization is **commingling**. (The broker can hold a check uncashed at the direction of the buyer before acceptance of an offer and at the direction of the seller after acceptance.)

Should a broker misappropriate trust funds for personal or any other use than what was designated, the act would be considered **conversion**, which is a criminal offense.

It is important that **trust funds** be handled properly. Improprieties regarding trust funds are the number one reason for disciplinary action against real estate licensees. Some general rules for trust funds include the following:

- Trust accounts must be in the name of the broker as trustee.

- Unless otherwise agreed, in cooperative sales, listing brokers deposit the funds in their trust account.

- In the absence of written permission from the client, a broker may not receive a commission or consideration of any kind for placement of the trust monies.

- A separate record must be kept of all trust funds received that are not deposited in a trust account (example: checks returned to offeror when offer is rejected). Accounts must be balanced daily and reconciled with bank records monthly.

- Accounts must be demand deposits (non-interest-bearing that can be withdrawn without notice) with the exception that accounts may be kept in a separate interest-bearing account with a federally insured lender at the direction of the owner of the funds. The broker may not benefit from any interest earned. Drawing interest on trust funds for the benefit of the principal can cause an accounting challenge. Interest earned must be prorated if one trust account contains funds for multiple beneficiaries.

- A broker may keep no more than $200 of broker funds in the trust account.

- This is to cover bank charges. Any greater amount of nontrust money in the account would subject the broker to disciplinary action.

■ Earned commissions must be withdrawn from the account within 30 days.

■ Columnar records must be kept (double entry) with separate records for each beneficiary and transaction.

■ The account must be open for inspection by the Bureau of Real Estate.

■ Should a BRE audit reveal a violation of the law, the broker will be assessed the cost of the audit, as well as be subject to disciplinary action, which could result in revocation of the broker's license.

■ The broker can designate another person to withdraw trust funds from the trust account, but if that person is not licensed, a bond is required. However, the broker bears liability for any improper action.

■ Records must be kept for three years.

■ Computer programs are available for trust fund accounting. See Figure 2.4 for a sample Trust Bank Account Record for Trust Funds Deposited and Withdrawn.

There are additional regulations and reporting requirements for trust monies received by mortgage loan brokers.

Penalties for trust fund violations include the following:

■ A financial penalty

■ Suspension or revocation of license

■ Imprisonment

FIGURE 2.4: **Trust Bank Account Record for All Trust Funds Deposited and Withdrawn**

CALIFORNIA
ASSOCIATION
OF REALTORS

**TRUST BANK ACCOUNT RECORD FOR ALL TRUST FUNDS
DEPOSITED AND WITHDRAWN**
(C.A.R. Form TAA, Revised 11/07)

Broker: _____

Address: _____

DATE	DEPOSIT (Received From)	OR	WITHDRAWAL (Paid To)	AMOUNT	BALANCE
					If applicable, forward from previous page $
	Name: _____ ☐ check ☐ cash ☐ _____ For: _____		Name: _____ Check # _____ For: _____	$	$
	Name: _____ ☐ check ☐ cash ☐ _____ For: _____		Name: _____ Check # _____ For: _____	$	-$
	Name: _____ ☐ check ☐ cash ☐ _____ For: _____		Name: _____ Check # _____ For: _____	$	$
	Name: _____ ☐ check ☐ cash ☐ _____ For: _____		Name: _____ Check # _____ For: _____	$	$
	Name: _____ ☐ check ☐ cash ☐ _____ For: _____		Name: _____ Check # _____ For: _____	$	$
	Name: _____ ☐ check ☐ cash ☐ _____ For: _____		Name: _____ Check # _____ For: _____	$	$
	Name: _____ ☐ check ☐ cash ☐ _____ For: _____		Name: _____ Check # _____ For: _____	$	$
	Name: _____ ☐ check ☐ cash ☐ _____ For: _____		Name: _____ Check # _____ For: _____	$	$
	Name: _____ ☐ check ☐ cash ☐ _____ For: _____		Name: _____ Check # _____ For: _____	$	$
	Name: _____ ☐ check ☐ cash ☐ _____ For: _____		Name: _____ Check # _____ For: _____	$	$

SAMPLE

THIS FORM HAS BEEN APPROVED BY THE CALIFORNIA ASSOCIATION OF REALTORS® (C.A.R.). NO REPRESENTATION IS MADE AS TO THE LEGAL VALIDITY OR ADEQUACY OF ANY PROVISION IN ANY SPECIFIC TRANSACTION. A REAL ESTATE BROKER IS THE PERSON QUALIFIED TO ADVISE ON REAL ESTATE TRANSACTIONS. IF YOU DESIRE LEGAL OR TAX ADVICE, CONSULT AN APPROPRIATE PROFESSIONAL.

This form is available for use by the entire real estate industry. It is not intended to identify the user as a REALTOR®. REALTOR® is a registered collective membership mark which may be used only by members of the NATIONAL ASSOCIATION OF REALTORS® who subscribe to its Code of Ethics.

The copyright laws of the United States (Title 17 U.S. Code) forbid the unauthorized reproduction of this form, or any portion thereof, by photocopy machine or any other means, including facsimile or computerized formats. Copyright © 1992-2008, CALIFORNIA ASSOCIATION OF REALTORS®, INC. ALL RIGHTS RESERVED.

REBS INC.
Published and Distributed by:
REAL ESTATE BUSINESS SERVICES, INC.
a subsidiary of the California Association of REALTORS
525 South Virgil Avenue, Los Angeles, California 90020

TAA REVISED 11/07 (PAGE 1 OF 1)   Print Date

Reviewed by _____ Date _____

EQUAL HOUSING OPPORTUNITY

Reprinted with permission, California Association of REALTORS®. Endorsement not implied.

CASE EXAMPLES

The following case examples are included to help you understand how ethics applies to you and to help you recognize your responsibilities regarding fair housing.

Case Example 1

Broker McIntosh realized that Henry Higgins was extremely naive about financial matters. While McIntosh usually charged a 6% commission for similar residential properties, when she filled out the listing for Higgins's home, she wrote "11%" in the commission block. She did, however, explain to Higgins that her fee was 11% and provided Higgins an estimate of what he would receive based on a sale at the list price, which was realistically set. Analyze McIntosh's actions from an ethical perspective.

Analysis 1

Legally, McIntosh did nothing wrong. Commissions are negotiable, and she simply negotiated to her advantage. Ethically, there are some problems. McIntosh charged almost twice her customary fee for the service, not because of problems the property presented but because she thought she could. This action certainly would not pass the test of the Golden Rule. How do you suppose McIntosh would feel if she found that a mechanic charged her an exorbitant fee for a simple adjustment to her vehicle because she was naive about mechanical matters?

A more interesting ethical question arises regarding other owners who have listed similar properties with McIntosh for a 6% commission. McIntosh is likely to give priority to selling the 11% listing over other listings, which would work to the detriment of other owners who expected the best efforts from McIntosh. Similarly, if McIntosh customarily split commissions with selling agents, other agents would likely give similar preferences. Therefore, applying the Golden Rule from the perspective of other owners also indicates that the 11% commission is unethical.

There could be circumstances, however, in which a higher-than-normal commission is justified. These could include property that requires greater sales effort or situations in which a quick sale is essential to protect the owner's interests (for example, a pending foreclosure).

Case Example 2

Tom Huang wanted to buy a lot in Sunrise Estates. While there were several dozen vacant lots in the subdivision, none currently had For Sale signs. Huang contacted Omni Realty and met with salesperson Upton. Upton told Huang that if a lot could be purchased in Sunrise Estates, she would find it.

Using tax records, Upton contacted owners of the vacant lots and asked them if they wanted to sell their lots. Owner Pike was receptive to the idea of a sale and indicated he would sell if he could net $100,000. Upton knew the lots were worth between $150,000 and $175,000, so she purchased it for $100,000. She then contacted Huang and told him about the lot and that she was now the owner. Huang was delighted and agreed to buy the lot for $160,000. Upton never revealed the transaction to her broker. What ethical problems are raised by this case?

Analysis 2

Tom Huang could reasonably assume that Upton was working on his behalf when she agreed to locate a lot for him. Instead, Upton acted on her own behalf and purchased a lot for herself, which she offered to Huang at a higher price as a principal.

While Huang may have been comfortable with Upton's purchase and may not have objected to the price, what started as a clear buyer's agency relationship was unilaterally changed by Upton to her own benefit. Huang paid more for the lot than he should have, had Upton been properly serving him. Upton had no duty to disclose to Pike that she felt the price was too low or that she had a buyer whom she believed would pay more money. Upton was not Pike's agent.

Although Huang had contacted Upton through Omni Realty, Upton turned what was originally contemplated as a brokerage situation into her own purchase and sale for profit. She in fact deprived her broker of a commission by her self-serving actions. Application of the Golden Rule would indicate unethical conduct on the part of Upton.

Case Example 3

Broker Zwerik was a member of a listing service. While Zwerik usually submitted his listings to the service, whenever he took a high-value listing that was also highly salable, he would recommend to the owner that for the owner's protection it would be best that Zwerik Realty be the only firm allowed to show the property. He would then cross out the listing authorization to cooperate with other agents and to give the listing to a listing service. He had the owner initial these modifications.

When other agents called Zwerik about his signs or ads on the property, Zwerik told them that the owner had specified in writing that only his firm would be allowed to show the property and that the listing information should not be given to any other agent. Was Zwerik's conduct proper?

Analysis 3

Broker Zwerik wants to be able to sell other office listings and wants other offices to help in the sale of most of his listings. But when he takes a listing that offers a substantial commission and is exceptionally desirable, the spirit of cooperation ends. The reason he persuades owners that he alone be allowed to show the property is based solely on the value and salability of the listing, not on the owner's best interests. Apply the Golden Rule: Would Zwerik want other brokers to withhold their better listings from him and give him only properties less likely to be sold? The answer is obvious. Broker Zwerik is guilty of unethical conduct.

In addition, keeping a listing off a listing service reduces the likelihood of a sale. Even for a highly salable listing, it is unethical because it is not in the best interest of Zwerik's client. Zwerik clearly misrepresented the reason to exclude other agents. The owner could have a cause of action against Zwerik.

Case Example 4

Mr. and Mrs. Jones and their two small children call your office inquiring about a three-bedroom condominium that you have advertised for sale. The unit is in a six-unit complex and is four years old. While you had intended to show the prospective buyers other units as well, it's love at first sight and they want to buy the unit advertised. You know that Tom Sinn lives in the unit next to the unit that is for sale. Sinn's well-publicized child molestation conviction was recently set aside by a higher court that ruled the photos taken from Sinn's home were illegally obtained and should not have been allowed admissible as evidence. What should you do?

Analysis 4

Because the conviction was set aside, Sinn is not a convicted sex offender, so even if the buyers checked the Megan's Law website, they would not learn of the allegations made against Sinn.

You have a duty to disclose any detrimental information you know of concerning a property. There is no question that a buyer who has small children would consider this information detrimental.

To fail to inform Mr. and Mrs. Jones about their next-door neighbor could subject their children to danger. Application of the Golden Rule would require disclosure, even though disclosure may not be required by law. Even if the prospective buyers had no children, it's possible that visitors might.

There is another problem as to the agent's duty to the owners. The owners must be told if you will be disclosing information as to the neighbor and why. Because disclosure might materially affect the chances of a sale or the sales price, you should consider offering the owners the opportunity to cancel the listing.

Case Example 5

Salesperson Garcia was contacted by a representative of an organization for the developmentally disabled. The representative was looking for a group home with at least five bedrooms on a large lot. Checking the multiple listings, Garcia discovered that three homes were available that met the location, price, and size criteria of the organization. One of these homes was on the same block as the home of Garcia's broker, Douglas LaRue. Garcia contacted LaRue, who told her to show the other two homes to her prospect but not the home on his block because he thought he had a buyer for it. What ethical issues are raised by this case?

Analysis 5

Garcia should have treated the prospective buyer as any other buyer. By contacting her broker before she showed the properties, Garcia was, in effect, saying, "What do I do if they want to live near you?" She was assuming that these citizens should be treated differently from other buyers, for example, a large family looking for a large house. Garcia's conduct does not pass the test of the Golden Rule.

If broker LaRue did not want the house shown because he felt that it could take away a sale he was going to make, then LaRue is not treating Garcia fairly. The Golden Rule would seem to dictate that until sold, everyone should have an equal opportunity to sell it. There is also an ethical problem as to the owner in that LaRue is withholding a potential buyer from the property. It is in the owner's best interests that the property be available to all prospective buyers.

If Broker LaRue directed that the home on his block not be shown because he believed that the presence of developmentally disabled citizens would be a detriment to the neighborhood, it would clearly be unethical because he is willing to locate them close to someone else and to profit on the sale. This certainly would not pass the test of the Golden Rule.

LaRue and Garcia were likely in violation of the 1988 Amendment to the Civil Rights Act of 1968 in discriminating against the disabled by refusing to tell the organization about an available home they knew could meet the buyer's needs. This action also would be considered steering.

Case Example 6

Henrietta Jackson, a single African American woman, inquired about an apartment with a For Rent sign. The manager showed her a vacant three-bedroom, two-and-a-half-bath unit. The manager told her the rent was $1,850 per month. She was told to think it over, and if she decided that she wanted the apartment, she should contact the manager, who would give her a rental application.

Gomer Clyde, a single white male, inquired about apartments one hour after Henrietta Jackson left. He was shown the three-bedroom apartment, which he was told was the only current vacancy. He was informed that in four days a studio apartment would be available at $700 per month and a one-bedroom apartment would be available in about 40 days for $1,100 per month. The manager took Clyde back to her office, where she showed him diagrams of the floor plans of the two additional apartments.

She asked Clyde which of the three apartments best met his needs. When Clyde indicated that he liked the studio apartment best, the manager handed him an application and said, "Fill out this application now and give me a deposit check for $100. I will call you tomorrow to let you know if your application has been approved." Is there a problem with the actions of the manager?

Analysis 6

It appears that the apartment manager violated the Unruh Act (discrimination by a business), the Rumford Act, probably the Civil Rights Act of 1866, certainly the Civil Rights Act of 1968, and the Commissioner's Regulations.

The two prospective renters were treated differently. Whether the discrimination was because she was a single woman or because she was African American, Jackson was discriminated against. It was illegal as well as unethical. While Jackson was not denied a rental, she was also not told about upcoming vacancies that would better meet her needs. This information was volunteered to Clyde, a single white male.

Jackson was told to think about the unit and contact the manager about a rental application if she was interested. The manager not only did not try to sell her on the units, but the manager's conduct was likely to discourage a rental application. On the other hand, the manager used good sales techniques to get Clyde to submit an application and pay his deposit on the first visit.

The discrimination in this case is certainly subtler than that encountered by African Americans and single women in the past, disparate treatment is still discrimination.

Case Example 7

A country home had been the scene of horrible crimes that had drawn national attention. The home had been boarded up for a number of years, but the present owner had just finished decorating the home and had placed it on the market through your firm. Your broker tells all the agents, "The law does not require disclosure of a death from any cause after three years," implying that the crime need not be mentioned to prospective buyers.

You show the house to a family that is moving to the area due to a job transfer. They have three small children, and they love the huge yard and bright and cheery rooms. Because of the very reasonable list price, they want to put in an offer right away. What do you do?

Analysis 7

This is an example of "when in doubt—disclose." While California law does not mandate a disclosure after three years, place yourself in the shoes of the buyers. Consider how it would affect your peace of mind as well as that of your children (if any) when you learned the history of the house. The application of the Golden Rule clearly indicates that while nondisclosure is legal, in this case it may be unethical.

If you were acting as a buyer's agent or dual agent, you would likely have a duty to disclose what would be regarded by most buyers as material information. This breach of fiduciary duty could result in agent liability for damages.

The owner should have been informed at the time of listing that your office would disclose the crime to any prospective buyers before an offer was taken. The broker's action seemed to encourage nondisclosure by relying on the letter of the law. In this case, such action appears unethical.

Case Example 8

Henry Shibata of Shibata Realty managed a small commercial building in a stable neighborhood of middle-class homes. The building had been vacant for more than six months, and the owner was concerned about the loss of income.

Shibata received a deposit and a lease from Ms. Corcoran, who wished to lease the building for 10 years. The rent specified was higher than the rent being asked for the property. Shibata knew that Corcoran was one of the largest owner/operators of adult bookstores in the region. The lease provision regarding use read "any legal purpose." An adult bookstore was not in violation of the current zoning codes, although there were no such stores within a 3-mile radius of the property. What should Shibata do?

Analysis 8

Shibata must inform the owner about the lease and about the proposed tenant. He can point out that the presence of an adult bookstore might create a great deal of animosity toward the owner, as well as have a possible negative effect on area property values.

If Shibata believes the lease would be detrimental to the community and the owner wants to accept it, an ethical approach would be to ask to be relieved from the management contract. However, if he believes that even though the presence of the business would hurt the area, First Amendment rights of free speech should be paramount and Corcoran should not be stifled, then handling the lease would be ethical conduct.

Case Example 9

The best friend of broker Kritski was Timothy Plunk, a home inspector. Plunk was well qualified as an inspector and had an excellent reputation. Kritski customarily recommended Plunk to buyers, telling them only that he regarded Plunk as being extremely competent. Kritski's buyers were pleased with Plunk.

Every Christmas, Kritski and Plunk exchanged gifts. Plunk would give Kritski a case of his favorite single-malt Scotch whisky, and Kritski would give Plunk a tie. Is there any ethical problem with their relationship?

Analysis 9

There is nothing unethical about recommending a friend for services; however, the close personal relationship should have been revealed. A buyer might feel that the friendship could influence what the inspection disclosed.

The apparent disparity in the value of the gifts exchanged creates, at the very least, an appearance of a kickback for recommending Plunk. The broker should have realized this and either refused the gift or increased the value of his gift to negate the disparity in value. As presented, it appears to be both unethical and illegal conduct.

Case Example 10

Broker Esposito has his office in the small town where he lives. The local high school recently was destroyed by fire. Because the structure was supposed to be "fireproof," the school board had no insurance on the structure. The students are now being bused to five other community high schools. The bus rides for the students range from 40 minutes to almost two hours each way.

A special bond election is coming up for a citizens' vote to provide funds for a new high school. The additional tax burden on the largely low-income and middle-income residents will be significant. Esposito has talked to several retirees who have indicated that they will have to sell their homes and move elsewhere if the bond passes.

The local real estate association has asked for a vote to assess members a special fee to fight against the bond issue because it feels the issue will depress local property values, cause people to move to nearby lower-taxed communities, and increase residential and commercial vacancies. Esposito voted to assess members and to fight the bond issue. Were his actions ethical?

Analysis 10

This case is unusual because a vote either way could be ethical or unethical, based on the reasons for the vote. If Esposito's vote were based on the fact that a bond issue would personally hurt his business, although he believed it was necessary for the long-term growth of the community, then his vote would be ethically wrong. If he voted for the assessment because he felt that the damage to retirees and the community as a whole outweighed having a community high school and the long bus rides, then such a vote would be ethically correct.

Similarly, if Esposito had opposed the assessment, the ethics of his opposition would be based on his reasons. As an example, if Esposito believed the bond issue would be bad for the community and create hardships far beyond the benefits but favored a bond because he had nine children in school, then his decision would be self-serving, and voting against the assessment could be unethical. Esposito could also have ethically voted against an assessment or bond position based on the belief that the real estate association should not be involved in local political decisions.

Case Example 11

LaMont, a mortgage broker, has 14 licensees working at his firm. Most of the loans arranged by LaMont are with a particular institutional lender. The lender currently requires that the borrower pay one point to obtain the quoted rate. LaMont is allowed to keep any overage that he is able to obtain. LaMont splits the overage equally with his salespeople. To determine how he could maximize income, LaMont analyzed loans arranged over the past six months. He discovered that points charged for loans averaged out as follows:

- Loans over $500,000 = 1.1 points

- Loans for $250,000 to $500,000 = 1.35 points

- Loans under $250,000 = 1.64 points

He also discovered that points paid by borrowers varied by race. LaMont's results indicated the following:

- Caucasians = 1.17 points

- Mexican Americans = 1.62 points

- African Americans = 1.73 points

Do these results indicate any ethical problems?

Analysis 11

From the facts, it appears that LaMont's staff is targeting minorities and less-affluent borrowers for disparate treatment. They appear to be taking advantage of these borrowers by quoting and insisting on more points than others are paying. Apparently, LaMont's employees are taking the position that "we will get what the market will bear."

A person applying for a loan would ordinarily believe that the terms quoted are the same for everyone and are not based on race or other factors. The fact that this is not a level playing field does not pass the test of the Golden Rule. Obtaining a loan should not be like buying a used car. Buyers of used cars know that everything is negotiable. Most borrowers wrongfully believe that they are required to pay what is quoted. Borrowers could assume that the loan officer is acting for them in an agency capacity. The borrower could have a cause of action against the loan broker as to a breach of an implied agency. While the agents' intent may not have been to discriminate, that is the result.

Case Example 12

Broker Thall owns Thall Mortgage Company. About 20% of his loans failed to close because of appraisals that were significantly below the purchase prices. The broker for Big Realty Company, which gave Thall Mortgage Company about one-half of its business by referrals, told Thall that the appraiser would have to do better or he would find a more cooperative mortgage company.

Thall told his appraiser, Adam Fine, that appraisals had to more realistically reflect the marketplace. There were too many appraisals below the purchase prices. Fine told Thall that what a single buyer was willing to pay did not change the fair market value. He indicated that he had data to strongly support all of his valuations and had followed the *Uniform Standards of Professional Appraisal Practice (USPAP)*.

Thall stopped using Fine and now uses Willard Fast for the appraisals. For 132 appraisals over the past two-year period, not one came in under the contract purchase price. What, if any, are the problems in this case?

Analysis 12

The broker for Big Realty acted unethically in trying to induce Thall to act in an unethical and illegal manner. Thall and the broker for Big Realty violated Section 2785 of the Real Estate Commissioner's Regulations that prohibit a real estate licensee from improperly influencing or attempting to influence a real estate appraiser. Big Realty also disregarded the interests of its buyers. (If there were a buyer agency or dual agency, they would have breached that agency to the buyer.)

In trying to influence Fine, Thall was encouraging appraisals related to con-tract prices, not necessarily fair market value. This could be a fraud on both the borrower and the lender, who would be led to believe that the appraisal fairly reflected fair market value. If the lender were federally insured, it would be a federal crime. Foreclosures could result in lender losses because of inflated appraisals and loans.

Willard Fast apparently understood the game that was being played and had agreed to do what was expected of him instead of following the *USPAP*.

SUMMARY

Ethics is fair and honest dealing.

Ethics differs from the law because the law sets minimum standards of acceptable conduct, whereas ethics deals in what is right. The test for determining whether an action is ethical is the Golden Rule.

The National Association of REALTORS® and the National Association of Real Estate Brokers have developed ethical codes to promote profession-alism in the real estate industry.

Federal fair housing legislation began with the Civil Rights Act of 1866, which applied to racial discrimination. The Civil Rights Act of 1870 reiter-ated the 1866 act. The Civil Rights Act of 1964 elevated a 1962 executive order into law. The act prohibited housing discrimination when there was any government assistance or involvement. The Civil Rights Act of 1968 expanded discriminatory protection to include national origin, color, and religion, as well as race. By amendment, the act was extended to sex, physical handicaps, and familial status. The act specifically prohibits steering (that is, directing persons to housing based on race), blockbusting (obtaining listings or sales based on the fear of loss in value because minority group members are entering the area), and redlining (refusing to loan within a certain area).

The Americans with Disabilities Act requires that owners and operators of places of public accommodations make the premises accessible to the extent readily achievable.

Diversity training programs aid licensees in understanding the customs and culture of other peoples, as well as the motivations in their decision-making processes. The National Association of REALTORS® has developed a diversity training program.

The Unruh Act is a California act that prohibits discrimination by a business establishment. The Rumford Act is considered California's fair housing act.

The Holden Act prohibits financial institutions from engaging in discriminatory practices, and the California Business and Professions Code and the Real Estate Commissioner's Rules and Regulations provide details regarding discriminatory practices of California real estate licensees. The Omnibus Housing Nondiscrimination Act makes all California nondiscrimination acts consistent in coverage with the California Fair Employment and Housing Act.

You must be cognizant of the fact that what you regard as innocent conduct could be regarded by others as sexual harassment. You should always conduct yourself in a businesslike manner. An allegation of sexual harassment could be expensive in dollars and time.

The Sherman Antitrust Act prohibits brokers from price-fixing, using a group boycott, and engaging in tie-in sales.

Trust funds must be protected and kept separate from broker funds. Records must be kept for each beneficiary and transaction.

CLASS DISCUSSION TOPICS

1. Without giving names, discuss any ethical problems you have observed in the real estate industry.

2. You have just brought in a cash deposit for which your broker gives you a receipt. Later, you find a duplicate cash deposit slip on the floor for that exact amount for deposit into a personal account of your broker. What should you do?

3. Salesman Rutkowski was showing a couple homes in a beautiful subdivision. Rutkowski took a route to the property that added 3 miles to the trip in order to avoid driving through a racially mixed housing area that contained many structures in need of repair. Discuss the ethics of Rutkowski's actions.

4. Broker Shimato was handling the grand opening of Big Town Estates. To emphasize the desirability of the property, Shimato sent out a press release indicating that 71 of the 400 homes to be built were sold before the grand opening. At the grand opening, the model of the subdivision showed sold flags on a large number of sites. Actually, Shimato had only three advance sales. Analyze Shimato's actions from an ethical standpoint.

5. Salesperson Sven Petersen took a listing for $389,500, although his comparative market analysis indicated a sales price between $295,000 and $310,000. Peterson's broker, Olaf Petersen, told Peterson to "start working on the owner to reduce the price." He told Peterson, "It isn't a good listing now, but it will be one in a few months. Anyway, any listing is better than no listing." Discuss ethical problems raised by this case, if any.

6. In Britain, the National Association of Estate Agents (a real estate professional organization) considers it an unethical practice to contact bereaved relatives of a deceased person in order to obtain a listing. Do you agree? Why?

7. Billie Bob Smith built a model home for his new subdivision. His newspaper ads showed an artist's rendering that made the home appear much larger than it was. In small letters the ad stated "Not to Scale." The price printed next to the drawing was $289,500. The small asterisk at the bottom of the page said "Plus Lot." The

model itself, which had a sign that said "From $289,500," included upgraded carpets, tile, cabinetry, landscaping, patio, et cetera. If a prospect wanted a home just like the model, the price would be $370,450 plus a lot starting at $140,000. Discuss the ethical problems, if any, of Smith's advertising and model home.

8. You are presenting an offer to owners represented by another agent. The offer requires that the owner carry back a second trust deed for $209,000. The other agent tells the owner that the buyer has "ace-high credit, and he has an excellent employment history." You are the selling agent, and you know from prequalifying the buyer that he has had prior credit problems owing to a lengthy period of unemployment; however, he has been working steadily for the past two years and is now up to date on all payments. What should you do?

9. While on caravan viewing new listings, you see another agent from your office, who is a close friend, slip a small Dresden figurine into her purse. What should you do?

10. Figure 2.5 is a list of the most common real estate licensee violations. Which of these reasons are clearly unethical and which could be ethical?

11. Give an example of a broker violation. Using Figure 2.5, what code section was violated?

12. Bring to class one current-events article dealing with some aspect of real estate practice for class discussion.

FIGURE 2.5:   Top Enforcement Violations

The following is a list of the top violations of the real estate law that are filed by the Bureau of Real Estate against real estate licensees. All references refer to sections of the California Business and Professions Code and the Regulations of the Real Estate Commissioner.

(1) Trust Fund Record Keeping

   Section 10145 – General statute governing the handling of trust funds. Regulation 2831 – Maintaining columnar records for trust funds received. Regulation 2831-a – Maintaining separate records for each beneficiary. Regulation 2831.2 – Performing monthly reconciliation of trust fund accounts.

   Regulation 2834 – Allowing unlicensed and unbonded signatories on a trust account.

(2) Trust Fund Shortages

   Section 10145 – General statute governing the handling of trust funds. Regulation 2832 – Trust fund handling.

   Regulation 2832.1 – Trust fund shortages.

(3) Failure to Supervise

   Section 10177 (h) – Failure to reasonably supervise activities of salesperson.

(4) Unlicensed Activity Violations

   Section 10130 – Act as a real estate licensee without first obtaining a license.

   Section 10137 – Unlawful employment or payment to unlicensed individual or salesperson not employed by broker.

(5) Misrepresentation Violations

   Section 10276-a – Substantial misrepresentation in a real estate transaction in which a license is required.

UNIT 2 QUIZ

1. Three brokers agreed that they would not let a third broker show any of their listings. This action would be regarded as
    a. a group boycott.
    b. price-fixing.
    c. market allocations.
    d. a tie-in agreement.

2. Ethics' relationship to law is that
    a. if an act is illegal it is also unethical.
    b. ethics tends to precede the law.
    c. ethics and the law both set minimum standards for behavior.
    d. what is ethical is legal.

3. Which of the following phrases would be considered nondiscriminatory in an advertisement for a rental?
    a. Christian family
    b. Prefer working married couple
    c. Just two blocks to St. Michael's
    d. None of these

4. A broker with a disabled employee widened the doorway to the restroom to accommodate a wheelchair. This work was performed to comply with the
    a. Civil Rights Act of 1866.
    b. Americans with Disabilities Act.
    c. Rumford Act.
    d. Fair Housing Amendment Act of 1988.

5. The Civil Rights Act of 1866 specifically covers what type of discrimination?
    a. Sex
    b. Marital status
    c. Age
    d. Race

6. A broker showed African American prospective buyers homes in African American and racially mixed neighborhoods. He would show African American prospects homes in predominantly Caucasian areas only if the prospects specifically requested to see homes in those areas. The broker's action would described as
    a. illegal.
    b. unethical.
    c. steering.
    d. all of these.

7. A broker refused to show a young Hispanic family of five a condominium about which they had inquired. The broker's action would be proper if
    a. the broker considered the unit too small for the family.
    b. there were no other children in the development.
    c. the development has an age exemption because all occupants are 55 years of age or older.
    d. 70% of the units are occupied by elderly.

8. A landlord can properly refuse to accept an applicant because the applicant
    a. has a guide dog and the apartment is on the fourth floor.
    b. is a single but obviously pregnant woman.
    c. appears to be gay and the landlord is afraid of catching AIDS.
    d. None of these

9. The state act that specifically prohibits discrimination in business establishments is the
    a. Unruh Act.
    b. Rumford Act.
    c. Holden Act.
    d. Civil Rights Act of 1968.

10. Which of the following actions dealing in trust funds would be a violation of the law?
    a. Giving trust funds received to a principal
    b. Placing depository trust funds directly into escrow
    c. Placing trust funds in a trust account
    d. Placing trust funds in the personal care of a bonded employee

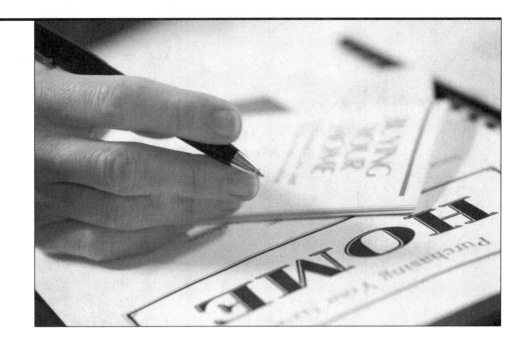

UNIT THREE

3

MANDATORY DISCLOSURES

LEARNING OBJECTIVES

When you have completed this unit, you will be able to

■ explain fiduciary- and agency-related disclosures, real estate transfer disclosure, agent's inspection disclosure, disclosure of death or AIDS, and natural and environmental hazards disclosures;

■ describe subdivision and common interest development disclosures; and

■ explain financing-related and other mandatory disclosures.

KEY TERMS

adjustable-rate loan
  disclosure
advisability of title
  insurance
agency
agency disclosure
Agent's Inspection
  Disclosure
AIDS disclosure
associate licensee
blanket encumbrance
  disclosure
brownfields
buyer's agent
California Land
  Project
carbon monoxide
  detector notice
common interest
  subdivision
Consumer Caution
  and Home
  Ownership
  Counseling Notice
controlled business
  arrangement
designated agent
dual agency
Easton v. Strassburger
elder abuse law
Environmental
  Hazards Disclosure
farming area disclosure

fiduciary responsibility
fire hazard areas
flood hazard areas
Gas or Hazardous
  Liquid Transmission
  Lines Disclosure
hazardous waste
  disclosure
Home Energy Rating
  System (HERS)
home inspection
  notice
*Homeowner's Guide to
  Earthquake Safety*
industrial/airport
  disclosure
Integrated Closing
  Disclosure
interstate land sales
landslide inventory
  report
Loan Estimate
material facts
Megan's Law
Mello-Roos bonds
methamphetamine
  contamination order
military ordnance
  location
Mining Operations
  Notice
nonresidential energy
  use disclosure

public report
Real Estate Transfer
  Disclosure
  Statement (TDS)
red flag
rescission rights
renter notice of
  foreclosure
Residential
  Earthquake Hazards
  Report
seller's agent
seller financing
  addendum and
  disclosure
septic system
  disclosure
sick building syndrome
single agency
smoke detector
  disclosure
stigmatized property
structural pest control
  inspection
Subdivided Lands Law
toxic mold
Truth-in-Lending
  Disclosure
water-conserving
  fixtures
water heater bracing
window security bars

UNDERSTANDING DISCLOSURES

Real estate agents used to say that the three main factors in real estate were "location, location, location." Today, they are "disclosure, disclosure, disclosure." Although the concept of *caveat emptor,* or "let the buyer beware," has been around for centuries, in the past several decades, California legislators, courts, and the Bureau of Real Estate (BRE) have been pushing enactment of disclosure laws. Although many agents think these laws are new, in reality, real estate law has always stressed full disclosure. However, in the past, some agents did not understand what full disclosure meant or when it was necessary to disclose certain circumstances. As a result, buyers and sellers began to take agents to court for nondisclosure. Such court cases became so numerous in certain areas that California legislators and the BRE worked to enact laws and regulations to force agents to disclose certain items. These laws and regulations have led to increased paperwork for real estate transactions, so agents must be familiar with all aspects of disclosure to complete transactions properly.

The disclosure laws discussed in this unit primarily involve 1-4-unit residential real property. Often, commercial buyers are deemed to be more sophisticated than buyers of residential real estate. Therefore, many of the disclosures that a homebuyer would get are absent from a commercial transaction. Also, the information given here is general in nature. In situations involving specific facts, consult your attorney concerning your specific case. To help avoid future disputes and litigation, always disclose the issue in question.

> A material fact is any fact that, if disclosed, could affect the decision of an entity in completing the transaction.

Full disclosure means disclosing, or giving notice of, all **material facts** in a transaction. A *material fact* is any fact that, if disclosed, could affect the decision of an entity (person or persons) in completing (to buy, to sell, etc.) a transaction. Many facets of a property might need to be disclosed to a prospective seller, buyer, or borrower to complete a transaction legally and to secure the financing necessary to purchase the property. The disclosure laws impose obligations not only on real estate licensees but also on the principals to the transaction. This is why the agent must consider all the material facts.

Full disclosure will

- protect the principals (buyers and sellers),

- establish and build trust and confidence between the licensee and principals, and

- satisfy the law.

The agent must not only disclose the information but also make certain that the principal understands the information and the importance of the information disclosed. Disclosures should be in writing to protect all parties involved.

Certain disclosures are mandated. A *mandated disclosure* is an item of information required by law to be conveyed from one entity involved in a real estate transaction to another entity in the same transaction. *Information* means some type of material data, facts, news, or figures. The phrase *required by law* means some obligation imposed by a legal authority, such as the BRE, the state legislature, or a court. *Convey* means to present from one entity (person or persons) to another entity. Thus, a mandated disclosure is simply a material fact obligated by law to be disclosed.

While the latest California Association of REALTORS® forms, as well as the forms from other California forms publishers, provide for most mandatory disclosures, outdated forms (as well as forms produced for national use) can result in a failure to properly disclose. You are not excused from disclosure because a form you used did not include or reference the disclosure.

Disclosure obligations in residential real estate sales of 1–4-unit properties are many and varied. Some are mandatory for real estate agents, some for sellers, some for both licensees and principals. At times, every agent will be in doubt about exactly what to disclose. The general rule is, "When in doubt on a particular issue, always disclose."

FIDUCIARY RESPONSIBILITY AND DISCLOSURES

An agent is one who represents another. When a principal appoints an agent, the principal assumes **vicarious liability** for the act of the agent within the scope of the agency. Of course agents would also be liable for their wrongful or negligent acts. The agency relationship demands that the agent use best efforts to protect the interests of the principal and to carry out the agency responsibilities.

When a real estate broker acts as an agent of only the seller or only the buyer, this is called a **single agency**. The **dual agency** may be used only if the buyer and the seller are both aware of the situation and approve of the arrangements. In many states, dual agency is not allowed because of the problems inherent in conflicting interests. Although this type of agency is in common use, many attorneys look on this arrangement as a conflict of interest ripe for lawsuits. Real estate agents often carry errors and omissions insurance to help protect against this problem. An agent who represents both the buyer and the seller without the approval of both is guilty of an undisclosed *divided* or dual agency and is in violation of the real estate law (Business and Professions Code 10176(d)).

An agent's **fiduciary responsibility** to the principal is one of *trust*. The duties include the following:

- Loyalty

- Obedience

- Confidentiality

- Disclosure

- Accounting

The agent must be *loyal* to the principal, placing the principal's interests above those of the agent. An agent's actions, therefore, cannot be inconsistent with the principal's interests. The agent cannot act in a self-serving manner to the detriment of the principal. As an example, assume a buyer's agent, in seeking a property for a buyer, discovered a property meeting the buyer's needs that was bargain priced. If the broker purchased the property to resell at a profit, the broker would be competing with the principal. This would be a breach of fiduciary duty.

Fiduciary duty is one of good faith and trust.

Duty to Other Party (Nonagency)

> The listing agent has a duty to conduct a diligent visual property inspection.

In dual agency situations, caution must be exercised so that aiding one principal is not detrimental to the other principal.

One duty of the agent to the principal is *obedience*. The agent must obey the principal's *lawful directions*. A principal direction to discriminate or fail to disclose a material fact could not be followed, and the principal should be so advised. These are not lawful directions. Agents also have a duty of *skill* and *diligence* and must diligently exercise their skills in the performance of agency duties.

Their duty of trust prohibits agents from revealing confidential information about the principal to others without the consent of the principal. For example, if a seller's agent revealed to a prospective buyer, without the principal's permission, that the principal was in serious financial straits, the agent's action would be a violation of the duty of trust. This information could seriously reduce the principal's bargaining ability. It could also encourage an offer at a lower price than was originally intended. Similarly, a buyer's agent could not inform a seller that the buyer had a particular need for the seller's property or that the buyer considered the seller's asking price to be extremely low.

The fiduciary duty of the agent includes full disclosure of material facts discovered by the agent that the principal would reasonably want to know in making decisions. Full disclosure would likely include the duty to warn a principal of any known dangers, such as possible problems relating to an offer, a lease, or an option. It also includes a duty to fully and honestly convey information concerning value and market conditions. Again, if there is any doubt as to the material nature of information, disclose.

An agent of a seller would not have a duty to tell a buyer that the agent would receive a greater commission or a bonus if the agent were able to sell a particular property, but if the agent were a buyer's agent, then such a disclosure would be required because failure to do so could create the appearance of a conflict of interest. It is a material fact that the buyer, as principal, would want to know.

The agent must account for all monies received and disbursed. Reasonable records must be kept.

When dealing with third parties, you are not held to the degree of fiduciary duties to a principal; nevertheless, you have duties of fairness, honesty, and disclosure. You must disclose to the buyer any detrimental information you know concerning a property that might affect its value or desirability to the buyer.

If you realize a buyer is mistaken about a property, you have a duty to let the buyer know the facts. Suppose, for example, that a buyer indicates he wants a site for an automobile repair facility. If you know that the current zoning precludes this use, you have a duty to inform the buyer about the zoning restriction.

If you have knowledge of a problem concerning the property before an offer, your disclosure must be made before the purchase offer. Your duty of disclosure, however, extends beyond the offer and acceptance of the offer. As an example, if you discover a serious structural problem after acceptance of an offer, you have a duty to inform the buyer, as well as the owner, of the problem.

For 1–4-unit residential properties, you have an actual duty to conduct a reasonably diligent visual inspection of the property. (See *Agent's Inspection Disclosure* later in this unit.) While the law does not require a visual inspection for other than 1–4-unit residential properties, you still have a duty to disclose known detrimental information to the buyer.

Facilitators and Designated Agents

When dealing with a broker in another state, California agents should understand that there could be differences in types of agency relationships and duties. Though not allowed in California, real estate brokers in some states are allowed to work as facilitators or intermediaries. These are third parties who are not agents of either the buyer or the seller; instead, they assist the buyer and the seller in the transference of real property ownership. They do, however, have a duty to treat all parties fairly and must disclose known defects in a property.

A number of states allow a broker to designate one salesperson as a principal's sole agent. When the listing broker is also the selling broker, the selling salesperson would then be the buyer's sole agent. An advantage of the **designated agent** concept lies in the fact that it is used to avoid problems often associated with conflicting duties of dual agency. Both buyer and seller have separate agency representation. However, both agencies are under the supervision of a single broker, so an appearance of a conflict of interest is still present. This type of agency relationship has not been adopted in California.

AGENCY DISCLOSURE

Civil Code Sections 2373–2382, which deal with agency relationships in real estate transactions involving 1–4-unit residential properties, became law on January 1, 1988. Any licensee in a transaction involving residential real property of 1–4 units must disclose agency. In 2015, mandatory written agency disclosure was extended to commercial transactions. Agents must disclose their exact agency role in all transactions.

To understand **agency disclosure**, brokers and salespersons must understand the term *agency*. An agent is one who represents another, called the **principal**, in dealings with a third person or persons. Such a representation is called agency. The agency disclosure form defines agency as

> a person acting under provisions of this title in a real property transaction, [including] a person who is licensed as a real estate broker under Unit 3 (commencing with Section 10130) of Part 1 of Division 4 of the Business & Professions Code, and under whose license a listing is executed or an offer to purchase is obtained.

The word *agent* is synonymous with *employing broker*. Though it is common in the real estate industry for salespeople to call themselves *real estate agents*, it is important to understand that there is only one agent in a company, the real estate broker, and all agency comes under that person. The law now uses the term **associate licensee**, defined as "a person who is licensed as a real estate salesperson or broker who is either licensed under a broker or has entered into a written contract with a broker to act as the broker's agent and to function under the broker's supervision." There is but one broker of record or responsible broker per company, and all associate licensees (salespeople) are **subagents** of that broker.

Brokers and salespeople should understand the various ways the word *agent* can be used in a real estate transaction. The licensee who lists the seller's home is called the *listing agent* or seller's agent. The licensee who brings the buyer into the transaction is called the buyer's agent or selling agent. An agent who represents the seller is called the **seller's agent**, and the agent who represents the buyer is called the **buyer's agent**. At one time, selling agents were considered subagents of the listing broker, so they represented the seller and the buyer had no representation. This has changed dramatically.

As previously stated, when an agent represents only a buyer *or* a seller, it is considered a single agency, and when an agent represents both buyer *and* seller, it is known as a dual agency.

Some brokerage offices have elected single agency. *Single agency* means that they will represent the buyer or the seller but not both. Their reason is that they feel duties to both principals in a transaction can create the appearance of a conflict of interest. This can result in lawsuits because of the perception of the parties. Single agency, representing one party to the transaction, reduces the likelihood of misunderstandings.

While the listing agent for a property could be either a seller's sole agent or a dual agent, the selling agent could be a buyer's agent (representing the buyer alone), a seller's agent (representing the seller alone), or a dual agent (representing both buyer and seller) with the knowledge and consent of both.

Even in a large company with multiple offices, there still is only one broker. For example, Bigtime Real Estate Company has an office in Los Angeles and another in San Francisco. If the agent from the Los Angeles office lists a property for sale and the agent from the San Francisco office brings in a buyer, whom does each agent represent or owe a fiduciary responsibility to? Does the listing agent exclusively represent the seller, and the selling agent exclusively represent the buyer? The agents are under the same employing broker (agency), so either both agents represent the seller or both agents represent both the seller *and* the buyer (dual agency).

Note: An agent (broker), however, is supposed to get the best and most honest deal for his principal. In a dual agency situation, the agent is compelled to obtain the highest price and best terms for the seller and also the lowest price and best terms for the buyer. In court, it is often hard to convince the jury that a dual agent has accomplished that. This is why full disclosure is extremely important.

FIGURE 3.1: **Disclosure Regarding Real Estate Agency Relationships**

AGENCY LAW DISCLOSURE

Disclosure Regarding Real Estate Agency Relationships

Prepared by: Agent _____ Phone _____

Broker _____ Email _____

NOTE: This form is used by agents as an attachment when preparing a seller's listing agreement, a purchase agreement or a counteroffer on the sale, exchange or lease for more than one year of residential property, nonresidential property or mobilehomes to comply with agency disclosure law controlling the conduct of real estate licensees when in agency relationships. [Calif. Civil Code §§2079 et seq.]

DATE: _____, 20_____, at _____, California.

TO THE SELLER AND THE BUYER: _____

1. **FACTS:** When you enter into a discussion with a real estate agent regarding a real estate transaction, you should, from the outset, understand what type of agency relationship or representation you wish to have with the agent in the transaction.

2. **SELLER'S AGENT:** A Seller's Agent under a listing agreement with the Seller acts as the Agent for the Seller only. A Seller's Agent or a subagent of that Agent has the following affirmative obligations:
   2.1   To the Seller:
       a.   A fiduciary duty of utmost care, integrity, honesty and loyalty in dealings with the Seller.
   2.2   To the Seller and the Buyer:
       a.   Diligent exercise of reasonable skill and care in performance of the Agent's duties.
       b.   A duty of honest and fair dealing and good faith.
       c.   A duty to disclose all facts known to the Agent materially affecting the value or desirability of the property that are not known to, or within the diligent attention and observation of the parties.
   2.3   An Agent is not obligated to reveal to either party any confidential information obtained from the other party which does not involve the affirmative duties set forth above.

3. **BUYER'S AGENT:** A Selling Agent can, with a Buyer's consent, agree to act as the Agent for the Buyer only. In these situations, the Agent is not the Seller's Agent, even if by agreement the Agent may receive compensation for services rendered, either in full or in part, from the Seller. An Agent acting only for a Buyer has the following affirmative obligations:
   3.1   To the Buyer:
       a.   A fiduciary duty of utmost care, integrity, honesty and loyalty in dealings with the Buyer.
   3.2   To the Seller and the Buyer:
       a.   Diligent exercise of reasonable skill and care in performance of the Agent's duties.
       b.   A duty of honest and fair dealing and good faith.
       c.   A duty to disclose all facts known to the Agent materially affecting the value or desirability of the property that are not known to or within the diligent attention and observation of the parties. An Agent is not obligated to reveal to either party any confidential information obtained from the other party which does not involve the affirmative duties set forth above.

4. **AGENT REPRESENTING BOTH THE SELLER AND THE BUYER:** A Real Estate Agent, either acting directly or through one or more associate licensees, can legally be the Agent of both the Seller and the Buyer in a transaction, but only with the knowledge and consent of both the Seller and the Buyer.
   4.1   In a dual agency situation, the Agent has the following affirmative obligations to both the Seller and the Buyer:
       a.   A fiduciary duty of utmost care, integrity, honesty and loyalty in the dealings with either the Seller or the Buyer.
       b.   Other duties to the Seller and the Buyer as stated above in their respective sections.
   4.2   In representing both the Seller and the Buyer, the Agent may not, without the express permission of the respective party, disclose to the other party that the Seller will accept a price less than the listing price or that the Buyer will pay a price greater than the price offered.

5. The above duties of the Agent in a real estate transaction do not relieve a Seller or a Buyer from the responsibility to protect their own interests. You should carefully read all agreements to assure that they adequately express your understanding of the transaction. A Real Estate Agent is a person qualified to advise about real estate. If legal or tax advice is desired, consult a competent professional.

6. Throughout your real property transaction, you may receive more than one disclosure form depending upon the number of Agents assisting in the transaction. The law requires each Agent with whom you have more than a casual relationship to present you with this disclosure form. You should read its contents each time it is presented to you, considering the relationship between you and the Real Estate Agent in your specific transaction.

7. This disclosure form includes the provisions of §2079.13 to §2079.24, inclusive, of the Calif. Civil Code set forth on the reverse hereof. Read it carefully.

| (Buyer's Broker) | Date | (Buyer's Signature) | Date |

| (Associate Licensee Signature) | Date | (Buyer's Signature) | Date |

| (Seller's Broker) | Date | (Seller's Signature) | Date |

| (Associate Licensee Signature) | Date | (Seller's Signature) | Date |

-------------------- PAGE 1 OF 2 — FORM 305 --------------------

©2015 RPI — Realty Publications, Inc.

FIGURE 3.1 (continued): Disclosure Regarding Real Estate Agency Relationships

-- PAGE 2 OF 2 — FORM 305 --

2079.13. As used in Sections 2079.14 to 2079.24, inclusive, the following terms have the following meanings:

a. " Agent" means a person acting under provisions of Title 9 (commencing with Section 2295) in a real property transaction, and includes a person who is licensed as a real estate broker under Chapter 3 (commencing with Section 10130) of Part 1 of Division 4 of the Business and Professions Code, and under whose license a listing is executed or an offer to purchase is obtained.

b. "Associate licensee" means a person who is licensed as a real estate broker or salesperson under Chapter 3 (commencing with Section 10130) of Part 1 of Division 4 of the Business and Professions Code and who is either licensed under a broker or has entered into a written contract with a broker to act as the broker's agent in connection with acts requiring a real estate license and to function under the broker's supervision in the capacity of an associate licensee.

The agent in the real property transaction bears responsibility for his or her associate licensees who perform as agents of the agent. When an associate licensee owes a duty to any principal, or to any buyer or seller who is not a principal, in a real property transaction, that duty is equivalent to the duty owed to that party by the broker for whom the associate licensee functions.

c. "Buyer" means a transferee in a real property transaction, and includes a person who executes an offer to purchase real property from an agent through an agent, or who seeks the services of an agent in more than a casual, transitory, or preliminary manner, with the object of entering into a real property transaction. " Buyer" includes vendee or lessee.

d. "Commercial real property" means all real property in the state, except single-family residential real property, dwelling units made subject to Chapter 2 (commencing with Section 1940) of Title 5, mobilehomes, as defined in Section 798.3, or recreational vehicles, as defined in Section 799.29.

e. "Dual agent" means an agent acting, either directly or through an associate licensee, as agent for both the seller and the buyer in a real property transaction.

f. "Listing agreement" means a contract between an owner of real property and an agent, by which the agent has been authorized to sell the real property or to find or obtain a buyer.

g. "Listing agent" means a person who has obtained a listing of real property to act as an agent for compensation.

h. "Listing price" is the amount expressed in dollars specified in the listing for which the seller is willing to sell the real property through the listing agent.

i. "Offering price" is the amount expressed in dollars specified in an offer to purchase for which the buyer is willing to buy the real property.

j. "Offer to purchase" means a written contract executed by a buyer acting through a selling agent that becomes the contract for the sale of the real property upon acceptance by the seller.

k. "Real property" means any estate specified by subdivision (1) or (2) of Section 761 in property that constitutes or is improved with one to four dwelling units, any commercial real property, any leasehold in these types of property exceeding one year's duration, and mobilehomes, when offered for sale or sold through an agent pursuant to the authority contained in Section 10131.6 of the Business and Professions Code.

l. "Real property transaction" means a transaction for the sale of real property in which an agent is employed by one or more of the principals to act in that transaction, and includes a listing or an offer to purchase.

m. "Sell," "sale," or "sold" refers to a transaction for the transfer of real property from the seller to the buyer, and includes exchanges of real property between the seller and buyer, transactions for the creation of a real property sales contract within the meaning of Section 2985, and transactions for the creation of a leasehold exceeding one year's duration.

n. "Seller" means the transferor in a real property transaction, and includes an owner who lists real property with an agent, whether or not a transfer results, or who receives an offer to purchase real property of which he or she is the owner from an agent on behalf of another. "Seller" includes both a vendor and a lessor.

o. "Selling agent" means a listing agent who acts alone, or an agent who acts in cooperation with a listing agent, and who sells or finds and obtains a buyer for the real property, or an agent who locates property for a buyer or who finds a buyer for a property for which no listing exists and presents an offer to purchase to the seller.

p. "Subagent" means a person to whom an agent delegates agency powers as provided in Article 5 (commencing with Section 2349) of Chapter 1 of Title 9. However, "subagent" does not include an associate licensee who is acting under the supervision of an agent in a real property transaction.

§2079.14. Listing agents and selling agents shall provide the seller and buyer in a real property transaction with a copy of the disclosure form specified in Section 2079.16, and, except as provided in subdivision (c), shall obtain a signed acknowledgment of receipt from that seller or buyer, except as provided in this section or Section 2079.15, as follows:

a. The listing agent, if any, shall provide the disclosure form to the seller prior to entering into the listing agreement.

b. The selling agent shall provide the disclosure form to the seller as soon as practicable prior to presenting the seller with an offer to purchase, unless the selling agent previously provided the seller with a copy of the disclosure form pursuant to subdivision (a).

c. Where the selling agent does not deal on a face-to-face basis with the seller, the disclosure form prepared by the selling agent may be furnished to the seller (and acknowledgment of receipt obtained for the selling agent from the seller) by the listing agent, or the selling agent may deliver the disclosure form by certified mail addressed to the seller at his or her last known address, in which case no signed acknowledgment of receipt is required.

d. The selling agent shall provide the disclosure form to the buyer as soon as practicable prior to execution of the buyer's offer to purchase, except that if the offer to purchase is not prepared by the selling agent, the selling agent shall present the disclosure form to the buyer not later than the next business day after the selling agent receives the offer to purchase from the buyer.

§2079.15. In any circumstance in which the seller or buyer refuses to sign an acknowledgment of receipt pursuant to Section 2079.14, the agent, or an associate licensee acting for an agent, shall set forth, sign, and date a written declaration of the facts of the refusal.

§2079.17. (a) As soon as practicable, the selling agent shall disclose to the buyer and seller whether the selling agent is acting in the real property transaction exclusively as the buyer's agent, exclusively as the seller's agent, or as a dual agent representing both the buyer and the seller. This relationship shall be confirmed in the contract to purchase and sell real property or in a separate writing executed or acknowledged by the seller, the buyer, and the selling agent prior to or coincident with execution of that contract by the buyer and the seller, respectively.

b. As soon as practicable, the listing agent shall disclose to the seller whether the listing agent is acting in the real property transaction exclusively as the seller's agent, or as a dual agent representing both the buyer and seller. This relationship shall be confirmed in the contract to purchase and sell real property or in a separate writing executed or acknowledged by the seller and the listing agent prior to or coincident with the execution of that contract by the seller.

c. The confirmation required by subdivisions (a) and (b) shall be in the following form:

_____[Do not fill out]_____ is the agent of (check one):
(Name of the Seller's Agent)
☐ the seller exclusively; or
☐ both the buyer and seller.

_____[Do not fill out]_____ is the agent of (check one):
(Name of the Buyer's Agent if not the same as the Seller's Agent)
☐ the buyer exclusively; or
☐ the seller exclusively; or
☐ both the buyer and seller.

d. The disclosures and confirmation required by this section shall be in addition to the disclosure required by Section 2079.14.

§2079.18. No selling agent in a real property transaction may act as an agent for the buyer only, when the selling agent is also acting as the listing agent in the transaction.

§2079.19. The payment of compensation or the obligation to pay compensation to an agent by the seller or buyer is not necessarily determinative of a particular agency relationship between an agent and the seller or buyer. A listing agent and a selling agent may agree to share any compensation or commission paid, or any right to any compensation or commission for which an obligation arises as the result of a real estate transaction, and the terms of any such agreement shall not necessarily be determinative of a particular relationship.

§2079.20. Nothing in this article prevents an agent from selecting, as a condition of the agent's employment, a specific form of agency relationship not specifically prohibited by this article if the requirements of Section 2079.14 and Section 2079.17 are complied with.

§2079.21. A dual agent shall not disclose to the buyer that the seller is willing to sell the property at a price less than the listing price, without the express written consent of the seller. A dual agent shall not disclose to the seller that the buyer is willing to pay a price greater than the offering price, without the expressed written consent of the buyer.

This section does not alter in any way the duty or responsibility of a dual agent to any principal with respect to confidential information other than price.

§2079.22. Nothing in this article precludes a listing agent from also being a selling agent, and the combination of these functions in one agent does not, of itself, make that agent a dual agent.

§2079.23. A contract between the principal and agent may be modified or altered to change the agency relationship at any time before the performance of the act which is the object of the agency with the written consent of the parties to the agency relationship.

§2079.24. Nothing in this article shall be construed to either diminish the duty of disclosure owed buyers and sellers by agents and their associate licensees, subagents, and employees or to relieve agents and their associate licensees, subagents, and employees from liability for their conduct in connection with acts governed by this article or for any breach of a fiduciary duty or a duty of disclosure.

| FORM 305 | 09-14 | ©2014 **first tuesday**, P.O. BOX 5707, RIVERSIDE, CA 92517 (951) 781-7300 |

Franchise offices are usually independently owned, with a different broker for each independently owned office. Thus, different agents from different offices may not be under the same agency (the same broker). Because the listing associate licensee is from a different office (different agency), the licensee can exclusively represent the seller, and the selling licensee can create an exclusive agency with the buyer. However, under the law of disclosing agency, all types of agency must be disclosed.

Any associate licensee who acts on behalf of others in selling, buying, exchanging, or leasing real estate creates agency for her broker (the agent).

An agent can receive a commission from a seller but still be the buyer's agent. Agency has nothing to do with who pays the commission (California Civil Code 2079.19). Buyer's agents customarily receive their compensation from the sellers.

Agency relationships can be either *implied* or *express*. Formalities are not necessarily required to create an agency relationship; the licensee can create an implied agency with a buyer or a seller simply through the words used when talking to prospective clients. For example, a court might determine that an implied agency is created when a licensee says to a buyer on the phone, "I have time today to look for property for your specific needs, to help you solve your housing problems." Agency can also be created by an express contract, such as a listing agreement. (See Unit 6.) Remember, once this agency relationship is created, the licensee has a fiduciary relationship with the principal. A fiduciary incurs the highest obligations under the law.

The Disclosure Process

The three-step process of disclosing agency can be remembered by using the acronym *DEC*.

Step 1: Disclose. This step will be in writing. Using a prescribed disclosure form (Figure 3.1), the licensee must educate the principal about the three different types of agents—seller's agent, buyer's agent, and dual agent—and how they operate. After this full disclosure, it is necessary to obtain the principal's signature. In dealing with consumers (buyers), the broker should educate the buyer about agency relationships as soon as possible, provide the potential buyer with the disclosure regarding agency relationships, and obtain the buyer's signature.

Step 2: E̲lect.   In this step, the agent and the principal decide which type of agency will be used. Because circumstances can change with each transaction, it is imperative that the principal and the agent thoroughly understand the implications of the agency roles they agree on and elect. Nothing has to be signed in this step, but care must be taken that both principal and agent enjoy full understanding (disclosure) of the agency elected.

> The three steps of the disclosure process are Disclose, Elect, and Confirm.

Step 3: C̲onfirm.   The confirmation of the type of agency elected in step 2 must be in writing. The agent and the principal(s) must sign the confirmation statement. Usually this confirmation is included as part of the purchase contract (also known as a *deposit receipt*), but it is also available as a separate document. If dual agency is elected, the agent must disclose that fact to both the buyer and the seller because a dual agent needs the consent of both. Because the broker is the agent, it is the broker's responsibility to make certain that proper disclosures have been made.

The selling agent should confirm the agency with the buyer, even if the buyer is not to be represented by an agent.

Timing of Disclosure

When should an agent disclose agency? The Bureau of Real Estate mandates disclosure "as soon as possible" when more than a casual relationship exists, and most offices have a policy manual that addresses the requirement of prompt disclosure. The three steps in the process may be taken at different times. Below are some general ideas on when to disclose, when to elect, and when to confirm.

Listing agents not selling their own listings.   In these cases, agents should provide the disclosure to the seller before entering into the listing agreement, elect as soon as is practical, and confirm the agency before or coincident with the seller's acceptance of the purchase contract.

Listing agents selling their own listings (in-house). In this case, the agent should disclose (that she is either the seller's exclusive agent or a dual agent of both seller and buyer), elect, and confirm to the seller and the buyer as in the preceding transaction.

Selling agents working with a buyer. Selling agents who are not listing agents always should disclose as soon as is practical and before a buyer's making an offer. As above, they should also elect as soon as is practical and confirm before or coincident with a buyer's and a seller's execution of the purchase contract.

Selling agents working with a seller. Selling agents who are not listing agents should remember to disclose to sellers as soon as is practical. They should elect as soon as is practical and confirm before or coincident with a buyer's and a seller's execution of the deposit receipt.

The chart in Figure 3.2 sums up the important information on agency disclosure that will be found in many offices' policy manuals.

REAL ESTATE TRANSFER DISCLOSURE

Under current law (California Civil Code Sections 1.102–1.102.14), the purchaser of residential real property (including residential stock cooperative housing) of four units or less is entitled to a **Real Estate Transfer Disclosure Statement (TDS)** from the seller. The term *transfer* refers to sale, exchange, real property sales contract (installment land sales contract), option, lease option, and so forth. Since January 1, 1987, any seller, whether represented by an agent or not, has been required to give the buyer a written disclosure statement of the condition of the property. The disclosure statement must identify

- items in the home and whether these items are operational (part A);

- significant defects of the home, if any (part B); and

- all information regarding improvements and alterations, concerns with neighbors and the neighborhood, zoning, a homeowners association, and other possible problem areas (part C).

FIGURE 3.2:   Agency Law Summary Chart

Listing Agent (Representing Seller Only)

What?	Who?	When?	How?	Law
Disclose	Provide disclosure form to seller.	Prior to entering into the listing agreement.	Obtain signed copy of disclosure form (C.A.R. Form AD).	Cal. Civ. Code §§ 2079.14, 2079.16
Confirm	Confirm in writing with the seller and buyer that you are seller's agent exclusively.	Prior to or same time as Seller's Execution of Purchase Agreement (last party to sign purchase contract).	In Purchase Agreement (C.A.R. Form RPA-CA) or another writing signed by buyer, seller, and listing agent (C.A.R. Form AC-6).	Cal. Civ. Code § 2079.17

Dual Agent (Office Represents Seller and Buyer)
For an office selling their own listing, in ADDITION to the above, the office MUST do the following:

What?	Who?	When?	How?	Law
Disclose	Provide disclosure form to buyer.	ASAP before buyer executes offer.	Obtain signed copy of Disclosure Form (C.A.R. Form AD)	Cal. Civ. Code §§ 2079,14, 2079.16
Confirm	Confirm in writing with seller and buyer that your office is the dual agent. (Note: Office is dual agent even if one salesperson in office represents the seller and another salesperson in the same office represents the buyer.)	Prior to or same time as Seller's Execution of Purchase Agreement (last party to sign purchase contract).	In the Purchase Contract (C.A.R. Form RPA-CA) or another writing signed by buyer, seller, and listing agent (C.A.R. Form AC-6).	Cal. Civ. Code § 2079.17

Selling Agent (Representing Buyer Only)

What?	Who?	When?	How?	Law
Disclose	Provide disclosure form to buyer.	ASAP before buyer executes offer (i.e., after more than a casual, transitory, or preliminary inquiry).	Obtain signed copy of disclosure form (C.A.R. Form AD).	Cal. Civ. Code §§ 2079,14, 2079.16
Disclose	Provide disclosure form to seller.	ASAP before presenting seller with offer.	(1) Obtain signed copy directly from seller or through listing agent or (2) provide by certified mail to seller (C.A.R. Form AD – may use new AD form or same form already signed by buyer).	Cal. Civ. Code §§ 2079,14, 2079.16
Confirm	Confirm in writing with buyer and seller whether you are buyer's agent exclusively.	Prior to or same time as seller's execution of purchase contract (last party to accept contract)	In the purchase contract (C.A.R. Form RPA-CA) or another writing signed by buyer, seller, and selling agent (C.A.R. Form AC-6).	Cal. Civ. Code § 2079.17

A copy of the form must be delivered to the buyer. If only one agent is involved, that agent must deliver it to the buyer. If two agents are involved, it is the responsibility of the selling agent (the agent who obtained the offer) to deliver it to the buyer. If the seller has not filled out the disclosure statement, the buyer should be notified in writing of the buyer's right to receive such a statement.

Seller Disclosure Exemptions

Exempted from disclosure are transfers

- requiring public report,
- pursuant to court order,
- by foreclosure,
- by a fiduciary,
- from one co-owner to one or more co-owners,
- between spouses or to a direct blood relative,
- between spouses in connection with a dissolution,
  - by the state controller,
- as a result of failure to pay property taxes,
- to or from any government entity (including exchanges), and
  - from probate.

Right of Termination

The disclosure statement should be delivered as soon as practical and before the execution of the offer to purchase. If the statement is not delivered before the execution, or is later amended, the buyer has the right to cancel the offer within three days after delivery (five days if mailed). To cancel the offer, the buyer must write a notice of termination and deliver it to the seller or the seller's agent. Failure to provide a transfer disclosure statement will not invalidate a closed transaction, but failure to comply could result in liability for damages. The transfer disclosure form is shown in Figure 3.3.

FIGURE 3.3:   Real Estate Transfer Disclosure Statement

THIS FORM FOR USE
IN CALIFORNIA ONLY

Real Estate Forms
Since 1966

REAL ESTATE TRANSFER DISCLOSURE STATEMENT
(Statutory Form)

THIS DISCLOSURE STATEMENT CONCERNS THE REAL PROPERTY SITUATED IN THE CITY OF _____,
COUNTY OF _____, STATE OF CALIFORNIA, DESCRIBED AS _____

THIS STATEMENT IS A DISCLOSURE OF THE CONDITION OF THE ABOVE DESCRIBED PROPERTY IN COMPLIANCE WITH SECTION 1102 OF THE CIVIL CODE AS OF (DATE) _____. IT IS NOT A WARRANTY OF ANY KIND BY THE SELLER(S) OR ANY AGENT(S) REPRESENTING ANY PRINCIPAL(S) IN THIS TRANSACTION, AND IS NOT A SUBSTITUTE FOR ANY INSPECTIONS OR WARRANTIES THE PRINCIPAL(S) MAY WISH TO OBTAIN.

I. COORDINATION WITH OTHER DISCLOSURE FORMS

This Real Estate Transfer Disclosure Statement is made pursuant to Section 1102 of the Civil Code. Other statutes require disclosures, depending upon the details of the particular real estate transaction (for example: special study zone and purchase-money liens on residential property).

Substituted Disclosures: The following disclosures and other disclosures required by law, including the Natural Hazard Disclosure Report/Statement that may include airport annoyances, earthquake, fire, flood, or special assessment information, have or will be made in connection with this real estate transfer, and are intended to satisfy the disclosure obligations on this form, where the subject matter is the same:

☐ Inspection reports completed pursuant to the contract of sale or receipt for deposit.
☐ Additional inspection reports or disclosures: _____

II. Seller's information

The Seller discloses the following information with the knowledge that even though this is not a warranty, prospective Buyers may rely on this information in deciding whether and on what terms to purchase the subject property. Seller hereby authorizes any agent(s) representing any principal(s) in this transaction to provide a copy of this statement to any person or entity in connection with any actual or anticipated sale of the property.

THE FOLLOWING ARE REPRESENTATIONS MADE BY THE SELLER(S) AND ARE NOT THE REPRESENTATIONS OF THE AGENT(S), IF ANY. THIS INFORMATION IS A DISCLOSURE AND IS NOT INTENDED TO BE PART OF ANY CONTRACT BETWEEN THE BUYER AND SELLER.

Seller ☐ is, ☐ is not occupying the property.

A.   The subject property has the items checked below (read across): *

☐ Range	☐ Oven	☐ Microwave
☐ Dishwasher	☐ Trash Compactor	☐ Garbage Disposal
☐ Washer/Dryer Hookups		☐ Rain Gutters
☐ Burglar Alarms	☐ Carbon Monoxide Device(s)	☐ Fire Alarm
☐ T.V. Antenna	☐ Satellite Dish	☐ Intercom
☐ Central Heating	☐ Central Air Conditioning	☐ Evaporator Cooler(s)
☐ Wall/Window Air Conditioning	☐ Sprinklers	☐ Public Sewer System
☐ Septic Tank	☐ Sump Pump	☐ Water Softener
☐ Patio/Decking	☐ Built-in Barbecue	☐ Gazebo
☐ Sauna		
☐ Hot Tub ☐ Locking Safety Cover	☐ Pool ☐ Child Resistant Barrier	☐ Spa ☐ Locking Safety Cover
☐ Security Gate(s)	☐ Automatic Garage Door Opener(s)	☐ Number Remote Controls _____
☐ Garage: ☐ Attached	☐ Not Attached	☐ Carport
☐ Pool/Spa Heater: ☐ Gas	☐ Solar	☐ Electric
☐ Water Heater: ☐ Gas		
☐ Water Supply: ☐ City	☐ Well	☐ Private Utility, or
☐ Gas Supply: ☐ Utility	☐ Bottled	Other _____
☐ Window Screens	☐ Window Security Bars,	☐ Water-Conserving Plumbing Fixtures
	☐ Quick Release Mechanism on Bedroom Windows	

Exhaust Fan(s) in _____ 220 Volt Wiring in _____ Fireplace(s) in _____
Gas Starter _____ Roof(s): Type: _____ Age: _____ (approx.)
Other: _____
Are there, to the best of your (Seller's) knowledge, any of the above that are not in operating condition? ☐ Yes ☐ No. If yes, then describe.
(Attach additional sheets if necessary.): _____

* Installation of a listed appliance, device, or amenity is not a precondition of sale or transfer of the dwelling. The carbon monoxide device, garage door opener, or child-resistant pool barrier may not be in compliance with the safety standards relating to, respectively, carbon monoxide device standards of Chapter 8 (commencing with Section 13260) of Part 2 of Division 12 of, automatic reversing device standards of Chapter 12.5 (commencing with Section 19890) of Part 3 of Division 13 of, or the pool safety standards of Article 2.5 (commencing with Section 115920) of Chapter 5 of Part 10 of Division 104 of, the Health and Safety Code. Window security bars may not have quick-release mechanisms in compliance with the 1995 edition of the California Building Standards Code. Section 1101.4 of the Civil Code requires all single-family residences built on or before January 1, 1994, to be equipped with water-conserving plumbing fixtures after January 1, 2017. Additionally, on and after January 1, 2014, a single-family residence built on or before January 1, 1994, that is altered or improved is required to be equipped with water-conserving plumbing fixtures as a condition of final approval. Fixtures in this dwelling may not comply with Section 1101.4 of the Civil Code.

Buyer acknowledges receipt of a copy of this page. [_____] [_____] Date _____

Page 1 of 3
FORM 110.21 CAL (01-2012) COPYRIGHT BY PROFESSIONAL PUBLISHING CORP., NOVATO, CA

PROFESSIONAL PUBLISHING

Form generated by: TrueForms™   www.TrueForms.com   800-499-9612

FIGURE 3.3 (continued):   Real Estate Transfer Disclosure Statement

Property Address _____

B. **Are you (Seller) aware of any significant defects/malfunctions in any of the following?** ☐ Yes ☐ No. **If yes, check appropriate box(es) below.**

☐ Interior Walls ☐ Ceilings ☐ Floors ☐ Exterior Walls ☐ Insulation ☐ Roof(s) ☐ Windows ☐ Doors ☐ Foundation ☐ Slab(s) ☐ Driveways ☐ Sidewalks ☐ Walls/Fences ☐ Electrical Systems ☐ Plumbing/Sewers/Septics ☐ Other Structural Components (Describe: _____

_____).

If any of the above is checked, explain. (Attach additional sheets if necessary):

_____
_____
_____
_____
_____
_____
_____
_____
_____

C. **Are you (Seller) aware of any of the following:**

1. Substances, materials, or products which may be an environmental hazard such as, but not limited to, asbestos, formaldehyde, radon gas, lead-based paint, mold, fuel or chemical storage tanks, and contaminated soil or water on the subject property . . . . ☐ Yes ☐ No
2. Features of the property shared in common with adjoining landowners, such as walls, fences, and driveways, whose use or responsibility for maintenance may have an effect on the subject property . . . . ☐ Yes ☐ No
3. Any encroachments, easements or similar matters that may affect your interest in the subject property . . . . ☐ Yes ☐ No
4. Room additions, structural modifications, or other alterations or repairs made without necessary permits . . . . ☐ Yes ☐ No
5. Room additions, structural modifications, or other alterations or repairs not in compliance with building codes . . . . ☐ Yes ☐ No
6. Fill (compacted or otherwise) on the property or any portion thereof . . . . ☐ Yes ☐ No
7. Any settling from any cause, or slippage, sliding, or other soil problems . . . . ☐ Yes ☐ No
8. Flooding, drainage or grading problems . . . . ☐ Yes ☐ No
9. Major damage to the property or any of the structures from fire, earthquake, floods, or landslides . . . . ☐ Yes ☐ No
10. Any zoning violations, nonconforming uses, violations of "setback" requirements . . . . ☐ Yes ☐ No
11. Neighborhood noise problems or other nuisances . . . . ☐ Yes ☐ No
12. CC&R's or other deed restrictions or obligations . . . . ☐ Yes ☐ No
13. Homeowners' Association which has any authority over the subject property . . . . ☐ Yes ☐ No
14. Any "common area" (facilities such as pools, tennis courts, walkways, or other areas co-owned in undivided interest with others) . . . . ☐ Yes ☐ No
15. Any notices of abatement or citations against the property . . . . ☐ Yes ☐ No
16. Any lawsuits by or against the Seller threatening to or affecting this real property, including any lawsuits alleging a defect or deficiency in this real property or "common areas" (facilities such as pools, tennis courts, walkways, or other areas co-owned in undivided interest with others) . . . . ☐ Yes ☐ No
17. Any Mello-Roos special tax levy lien or fixed lien assessment pursuant to Improvement Bond Act of 1915 on subject property. (If yes, disclosure notice should be obtained from levying agency.) . . . . ☐ Yes ☐ No
18. Any former federal or state ordnance locations (as defined in C.C. 1102.15) within one mile of the subject property ☐ Yes ☐ No
19. Whether subject property is affected by or zoned to allow certain manufacturing or commercial or airport use as set forth in CCP 731a . . . . ☐ Yes ☐ No
20. An order from a local health officer prohibiting the use or occupancy of portions of the property contaminated by methamphetamine. (If so, a copy of the order must be delivered to any prospective purchaser.) . . . . ☐ Yes ☐ No

If the answer to any of these is yes, explain. (Attach additional sheets if necessary.): _____

_____
_____

D. 1. The Seller certifies that the property, as of the close of escrow, will be in compliance with Section 13113.8 of the Health and Safety Code by having operable smoke detectors(s) which are approved, listed, and installed in accordance with the State Fire Marshal's regulations and applicable local standards.

2. The Seller certifies that the property, as of the close of escrow, will be in compliance with Section 19211 of the Health and Safety Code by having the water heater tank(s) braced, anchored, or strapped in place in accordance with applicable law.

Seller certifies that the information herein is true and correct to the best of the Seller's knowledge as of the date signed by the Seller.

Seller _____ Date _____ Seller _____ Date _____

Buyer acknowledges receipt of a copy of this page. [_____] [_____] Date _____

PROFESSIONAL PUBLISHING

Form generated by: TrueForms™   www.TrueForms.com   800-499-9612

FIGURE 3.3 (continued):   Real Estate Transfer Disclosure Statement

Property Address _____

III. **AGENT'S INSPECTION DISCLOSURE** (Listing Agent)
(To be completed only if the Seller is represented by an agent in this transaction.)
THE UNDERSIGNED, BASED ON THE ABOVE INQUIRY OF THE SELLER(S) AS TO THE CONDITION OF THE PROPERTY AND BASED ON A REASONABLY COMPETENT AND DILIGENT VISUAL INSPECTION OF THE ACCESSIBLE AREAS OF THE PROPERTY IN CONJUNCTION WITH THAT INQUIRY, STATES THE FOLLOWING:
☐ Agent notes no items for disclosure.
☐ Agent notes the following items:

_____
_____
_____
_____
_____
_____
_____

Agent (Broker
Representing Seller) _____ By _____ Date _____
　　　　　　　　　(Please Print)　　　　　　　　(Associate Licensee or Broker Signature)

IV. **AGENT'S INSPECTION DISCLOSURE** (Selling Agent)
(To be completed only if the agent who has obtained the offer is other than the agent above.)
THE UNDERSIGNED, BASED ON A REASONABLY COMPETENT AND DILIGENT VISUAL INSPECTION OF THE ACCESSIBLE AREAS OF THE PROPERTY, STATES THE FOLLOWING:
☐ Agent notes no items for disclosure.
☐ Agent notes the following items:

_____
_____
_____
_____
_____
_____

Agent (Broker
Obtaining the Offer) _____ By _____ Date _____
　　　　　　　　　(Please Print)　　　　　　　　(Associate Licensee or Broker Signature)

V. **BUYER(S) AND SELLER(S) MAY WISH TO OBTAIN PROFESSIONAL ADVICE AND/OR INSPECTIONS OF THE PROPERTY AND TO PROVIDE FOR APPROPRIATE PROVISIONS IN A CONTRACT BETWEEN BUYER(S) AND SELLER(S) WITH RESPECT TO ANY ADVICE /INSPECTIONS/DEFECTS.**

I/WE ACKNOWLEDGE RECEIPT OF A COPY OF THIS STATEMENT.

Seller _____ Date _____   Buyer _____ Date _____

Seller _____ Date _____   Buyer _____ Date _____

Agent (Broker
Representing Seller) _____ By _____ Date _____
　　　　　　　　　(Please Print)　　　　　　　　(Associate Licensee or Broker Signature)
Agent (Broker
Obtaining the Offer) _____ By _____ Date _____
　　　　　　　　　(Please Print)　　　　　　　　(Associate Licensee or Broker Signature)

SECTION 1102.3 OF THE CIVIL CODE PROVIDES A BUYER WITH THE RIGHT TO RESCIND A PURCHASE CONTRACT FOR AT LEAST THREE DAYS AFTER THE DELIVERY OF THIS DISCLOSURE IF DELIVERY OCCURS AFTER THE SIGNING OF AN OFFER TO PURCHASE. IF YOU WISH TO RESCIND THE CONTRACT, YOU MUST ACT WITHIN THE PRESCRIBED PERIOD.

A REAL ESTATE BROKER IS QUALIFIED TO ADVISE ON REAL ESTATE. IF YOU DESIRE LEGAL ADVICE, CONSULT YOUR ATTORNEY.

Page 3 of 3
FORM 110.23 CAL (01-2012) COPYRIGHT BY PROFESSIONAL PUBLISHING CORP., NOVATO, CA

PROFESSIONAL PUBLISHING

Form generated by: TrueForms™   www.TrueForms.com   800-499-9612

AGENT'S INSPECTION DISCLOSURE

Whenever agents take listings on 1–4-unit residential properties, they should fill out a Real Estate Transfer Disclosure Statement. Even if the seller is exempt from the transfer disclosure statement requirements—for example, if the property is being sold to a co-owner—the agent is responsible for conducting an investigation and inspection independent of the seller and for filling out a transfer disclosure statement. The agent uses the same disclosure statement as that in Figure 3.3. Section III of that disclosure statement, the **Agent's Inspection Disclosure**, is to be completed if the seller is represented by a listing agent.

On May 31, 1984, the California State Supreme Court refused to hear the *Easton v. Strassburger* ([1984] 152 Ca.3d 90) case, making the decision of the appellate court case law in California final. Under *Easton*, a real estate agent was deemed responsible not only for what was known or accessible only to the agent or the principal but also for what the agent "should have known," following a reasonably competent and diligent inspection. This court case has been codified in the Civil Code, beginning with Section 2079, and became effective January 1, 1986. It requires that all real estate agents conduct a competent and diligent visual inspection of all accessible property areas in a real estate sale involving 1–4-unit residential properties and disclose to the prospective buyer all material facts affecting the value or desirability of the property. There are no exceptions to or exemptions from this law. If an agent does not comply with this code section, the statute of limitations for bringing suit is two years.

A difficulty with this section of code is that it does not tell agents what to inspect or how. The following suggestions may help agents find physical problems and fundamental defects in the home. The major factors contributing to defects in homes are structural failure, material deterioration, water damage, mold, and insect infestation. When one of these factors is found in a home, some or all of the other factors often are present.

Structural Failure

Structural failure can be caused by environmental extremes, poor design, material deterioration, water, or insects. When inspecting for structural failure, agents should look for the following:

- Cracks in structural walls, beams, and columns (outside and inside), particularly foundations, or in corners of walls and around doors and windows (large V-shaped cracks may indicate settlement, upheaval, or lateral movement of soil; minor cracking is normal)

- Severe bulging in floors or structural walls

- Floors that slope

- Excessive deflection of girders and joists evidenced by a caved-in and creaky floor

- Doors that fail to close or that have been trimmed to close

- A roof ridgeline that is not straight

- Instability in any structural member

Material Deterioration

Material deterioration can be produced by substandard material or construction procedures. A moist environment can produce damp rot (a decaying fungus), one of the most severe types of material damage. Principal items to look for when inspecting for material deterioration include the following:

- Decay or warping of wood members (porches are a prime candidate)

- Rotting, cracking, or warping—check around doors and windows especially

- Erosion of concrete, masonry units, or mortar

Water Problems

Water problems can be caused by faulty plumbing, a rising ground water level, seepage, improper drainage, or condensation from inadequate ventilation. Water is a common enemy of a house. Principal items to look for when inspecting for water problems include the following:

- Water stains on ceilings that may be coming from leaky plumbing or a leaky roof

- Mold, mildew, and rust—be particularly alert for black mold

- Loose or warped wood members

- Rotted wood

- Cracked, chipped, or curled tile

- Premature interior paint deterioration—check for peeling and flaking

- Roof defects

Toxic Mold

Sellers of 1–4-unit residential property must disclose in the Real Estate Transfer Disclosure Statement if the owner is aware of mold on the premises.

The presence of **toxic mold** can have serious health effects. It is caused by damp conditions. Solving mold conditions can require walls being torn open. In some cases, buildings have been razed because the cost to cure the problem was too great. If a house has a dampness problem or has a musty odor, you should recommend to a buyer that the home inspector test for mold. Mold detection kits are available at hardware and building supply stores as well as through the internet. Some kits are priced less than $10.

Carpenter ants and subterranean termites are the most damaging of all insects. Both attack wooden structures internally and might leave few visible signs of infestation on the surface, making their presence virtually impossible to detect.

Insect Infestation

Undetected and therefore untreated insect infestation could make the home structurally unsound over time. The following are some insect signs to look for:

- Carpenter ants: wood shavings near wood members

- Termites: earth and wood droppings, which look like sawdust and mud tubes leading from ground to wood or marks where mud tubes were removed

With regard to termite infestation, companies are licensed by the Structural Pest Control Board in California. Copies of termite reports conducted within the last two years are available for a fee to anyone who requests them.

There are two sections to termite reports:

- Section 1 is for what is commonly called active infestation. The industry standard is that the seller would pay for this termite damage.

- Section 2 is for what is generally a condition that could lead to a future problem. Examples of conditions noted in section 2 would be plumbing leaks or excessive moisture conditions. Generally, the buyer would pay to correct section 2 problems.

There are too many possible defects to mention here, but agents have developed inspection techniques to detect some of the more common problems. For example, defective wood framing can be detected after a few years by uneven floors and window sills. If an uncarpeted floor looks uneven, a simple test is to place a marble at several places on the floor; rolling marbles may indicate a problem. Resawn doors or doorjambs reworked because they were no longer perpendicular to the floor signify a structural defect. Sticking doors and windows can indicate green lumber, sloppy workmanship, foundation settling, or imperfect framing. Ceiling stains generally indicate a past or current roof problem. A **red flag** is anything that indicates a possible problem. Any red-flag information should be conveyed to the purchaser with a warning that it could indicate a problem. Remember, agents' legal responsibility extends only to a visual inspection of reasonably accessible areas.

A *red flag* is a visual sign or indication of a defect.

Many agents today use the following three techniques to help protect them in the area of inspection disclosure:

1. Have the buyer pay for a home inspection, whereby a professional inspector examines the property, verifies defects on the transfer disclosure statement, and points out any defects that are not on the statement

2. Obtain a home warranty. The purchase contract may call for the seller to pay the cost, typically between $250 and $400 for one-year coverage. Coverages vary but generally include appliances and electrical, plumbing, heating, and cooling systems. Some brokers offer home warranty protection on all their sales. Buyers often purchase the coverage if not otherwise provided.

3. Have the seller supply the buyer with a pest control inspection report

Real estate agents are required only to visually inspect one-to-four residential units.

Even if any one or all of these techniques are used, the agent is still responsible for inspecting the home and retains liability for any undisclosed defects that the agent knew about or should have discovered with a reasonably diligent visual inspection.

In addition to physical problems of the property itself, the agent must disclose anything else that might affect the buyer's decision to buy the property. These factors range from the property's being in a flood zone or on or near an earthquake fault to the presence of a nearby nuclear power plant. The agent needs to learn as much as possible about the house and the area around it.

SELLER'S PROPERTY QUESTIONNAIRE

This form is required and is not a substitute for the Real Estate Transfer Disclosure Statement. The seller completes the form to provide additional information about a property.

DISCLOSURE OF DEATH OR AIDS

While the Civil Code does not specifically require disclosure of a death upon the property, Section 1710.2 provides that the agent is not liable for failure to disclose to the buyer any deaths that occurred on the property more than three years before offers to purchase or lease the property. There is, therefore, an understanding that known deaths that occurred within the past three years should be disclosed. **AIDS disclosure** is unnecessary. An agent does not have to disclose that a former owner or resident ever had AIDS or died of AIDS. However, if a buyer asks a direct question concerning cause of deaths, the statute does not protect an agent from misrepresentation.

Stigmatized Property

Stigmatized property is property that may be perceived as undesirable for other than physical or environmental reasons. Besides murder or suicide, a house could be stigmatized by the fact that molestations occurred in the home, that the property has a reputation of being haunted, that satanic rituals had taken place there, or that the property has the reputation of being unlucky because of calamities that befell previous residents.

Because we don't know what a court will say should have been disclosed, as well as because disclosure is the right thing to do, if a fact or reputation could conceivably affect a buyer's decision, disclose it.

Licensed Care Facilities

Opinion 95-907 of the California Attorney General's Office makes it clear that a real estate agent need not disclose the location of a licensed care facility that serves six or fewer people. (A larger facility close to a property being sold would likely require disclosure.)

NATURAL HAZARDS DISCLOSURE

Earthquake Safety

As of January 1, 1993, the state law requires that when selling 1–4-unit residential properties built before January 1, 1960, you must disclose whether the dwelling has earthquake weaknesses. The California Seismic Safety Commission has published *The Homeowner's Guide to Earthquake Safety*, a booklet intended to help buyers, sellers, and real estate agents recognize some of the weaknesses in houses that affect earthquake safety. The buyers should sign that they have received the guide (Figure 3.4).

For all houses sold in California, an earthquake safety disclosure statement must be filled out and signed by the buyer and the seller. This disclosure statement is called the **Residential Earthquake Hazards Report** (Figure 3.5). The agent should prepare to answer the following seven questions, which are answered in the booklet on the pages noted:

1. What is a braced water heater? (page 6)

A braced water heater is one that has metal strips to attach it to the wall.

2. Is the house bolted to the foundation? (page 7)

If the house has a crawl space, you should be able to see the tops of the anchor bolts every 4 to 6 feet along the sill plate.

3. What is a cripple wall? (pages 8 and 9)

A cripple wall is a short wood wall on top of the foundation that creates a crawl space.

4. Is the foundation made of unreinforced masonry? (page 10)

Most brick and stone foundations are unreinforced. For concrete block, check the blocks on the top of the foundation. If they are hollow, the foundation probably is not reinforced. (Generally, steel rods are embedded in grout in the cells if the foundation is reinforced.)

FIGURE 3.4:   Earthquake Safety Client Card

To Whom It May Concern:
I have received a copy of "The Homeowner's Guide to Earthquake Safety."

Date: _____   (Signature) _____

Time: _____   (Printed Name) _____

Date: _____   (Signature) _____

Time: _____   (Printed Name) _____

FIGURE 3.5: Residential Earthquake Hazards Report

RESIDENTIAL EARTHQUAKE HAZARDS REPORT

Prepared by: Agent _____ Phone _____
Broker _____ Email _____

NOTE: This form is used by a seller's agent on the sale of a one-to-four unit residential property built prior to 1960 to disclose to a buyer, together with a copy of the "Homeowner's Guide to Earthquake Safety," any potential earthquake weaknesses the property may have. [See ft Form 316-1; Calif. Government Code §§8897 et seq.]

Name _____ Assessor's Parcel No. _____
Street Address _____ Year Built _____
City _____, County _____, Zip Code _____

Answer these questions to the best of your knowledge. If you do not have actual knowledge as to whether the weakness exists, answer "Don't Know." If your house does not have the feature, answer "Doesn't Apply." The page numbers in the right-hand column indicate where in the "Homeowner's Guide to Earthquake Safety" you can find information on each of these features.

	Yes	No	Doesn't Apply	Don't Know	See Page
1. Is the water heater braced, strapped, or anchored to resist falling during an earthquake.	☐	☐	☐	☐	12
2. Is the house anchored or bolted to the foundation?	☐	☐	☐	☐	14
3. If the house has cripple walls:					
3.1 Are the exterior cripple walls braced?	☐	☐	☐	☐	16
3.2 If the exterior foundation consists of unconnected concrete piers and posts, have they been strengthened?	☐	☐	☐	☐	18
4. If the exterior foundation, or part of it, is made of unreinforced masonry, has it been strengthened?	☐	☐	☐	☐	20
5. If the house is built on a hillside:					
5.1 Are the exterior tall foundation walls braced?	☐	☐	☐	☐	22
5.2 Were the tall posts or columns either built to resist earthquakes or have they been strengthened?	☐	☐	☐	☐	22
6. If the exterior walls of the house, or part of them, are made of unreinforced masonry, have they been strengthened?	☐	☐	☐	☐	24
7. If the house has a living area over the garage, was the wall around the garage door opening either built to resist earthquakes or has it been strengthened?	☐	☐	☐	☐	26
8. Is the house outside an Alquist-Priolo Earthquake Fault Zone (zones immediately surrounding known earthquake faults)?	*Lines 8 and 9 to be reported on the Natural Hazards Disclosure Report*				36
9. Is the house outside a Seismic Hazard Zone (zone identified as susceptible to liquefaction or land sliding)?					36

If any of the questions are answered "No," the house is likely to have an earthquake weakness. Questions answered "Don't Know" may indicate a need for further evaluation. If you corrected one or more of these weaknesses, describe the work on a separate page. [See ft Form 250]

As Seller of the property described herein, I have answered the questions above to the best of my knowledge in an effort to disclose fully any potential earthquake weaknesses it may have.

EXECUTED BY:

_____ _____ _____, 20____
(Seller) (Seller) (Date)

I acknowledge receipt of this form, completed and signed by Seller. I understand that if Seller has answered "No" to one or more questions, or if Seller has indicated a lack of knowledge, there may be one or more earthquake weaknesses in this house.

_____ _____ _____, 20____
(Buyer) (Buyer) (Date)

This earthquake disclosure is made in addition to the standard real estate transfer disclosure statement also required by law. [See ft Forms 314 and 304]

FORM 315   06-14   ©2014 **first tuesday**, P.O. BOX 5707, RIVERSIDE, CA 92517 (800) 794-0494

©2015 RPI — Realty Publications, Inc.

5. If the house is on a hillside, two questions need to be answered: (1) Are the exterior tall foundation walls braced? (2) Were the tall posts or columns either built to resist earthquakes or have they been strengthened? (page 11)

If wall studs are without plywood sheathing, diagonal wood bracing, or steel bracing, the wall is not braced. Consult an engineer to determine if posts or unbraced walls need strengthening.

6. Are the exterior walls strengthened? (page 12)

If the house was built before 1940, walls are most likely not reinforced. You can check the house plans, which are probably on file with the building department. Otherwise, it could be difficult to determine if walls are reinforced. There are professional testing services that can determine the presence of steel in the walls.

7. If the house has a living area over the garage, was the wall around the garage door strengthened or built to resist earthquakes? (page 13) Check if there are braces or plywood panels around the garage-door opening. If the garage-door opening is in line with the rest of the house, additional bracing is probably not needed.

If these questions cannot readily be answered by a cursory inspection, the services of a professional inspector or engineer may be required.

Commercial Property Earthquake Hazards

Sellers or sellers' agents must give buyers a copy of the *Commercial Property Owner's Guide to Earthquake Safety* for sales or exchanges of any real property built of precast concrete or reinforced masonry walls with wood frame floors or roofs built before January 1, 1975, unless such property falls within an exemption category.

Natural Hazard Disclosure Statement

The Natural Hazards Disclosure Statement sets forth the following additional natural hazard disclosures that must be made on a statutory form when the property lies within one or more state mapped hazard zones. If the property is within a seismic hazard zone as shown by the state geologist, the fact must also be disclosed. Although sellers can take it upon themselves to make such disclosures, many transactions involve a third-party provider such as Property I.D. (www.propertyid.com) or Disclosure Source (www.disclosuresource.com) that interprets the maps for the sellers and makes the statutorily required disclosures to the buyer. These reports cost between $80 and $120, on average. (See Figure 3.6.)

- **Special flood hazard areas—Flood hazard areas** are indicated on maps published by the Federal Emergency Management Agency (FEMA). (Maps may be purchased from FEMA by calling 1-800-358-9616.) The seller's agent must disclose this to the buyer if the agent has knowledge that the property is in such a zone or if a list of areas has been posted in the county recorder's office, county assessor's office, and county planning agency.

FIGURE 3.6: **Natural Hazard Disclosure Statement**

NATURAL HAZARD DISCLOSURE STATEMENT

Prepared by: Agent _____ **Phone** _____
Broker _____ **Email** _____

NOTE: The seller's listing broker (and the seller) must prepare a Natural Hazard Disclosure (NHD) and deliver it to prospective buyers of any property prior to making a purchase agreement offer and indicate compliance in the purchase agreement or a counteroffer. If not so disclosed, the buyer has the right to cancel the purchase agreement within three days of delivery of the disclosure in person. [Calif. Civil Code §1103.3]

DATE:_____, 20_____, at_____, California.

This disclosure statement is prepared for the following:

☐ Seller's listing agreement

☐ Purchase agreement

☐ Counteroffer

☐ _____

dated _____, 20_____, at _____, California,

entered into by _____, as the _____,

regarding real estate referred to as _____

_____.

Natural Hazard Disclosure Statement:

Seller and Seller's Agent(s) or a third-party consultant disclose the following information with the knowledge that even though this is not a warranty, prospective buyers may rely on this information in deciding whether and on what terms to purchase the subject property.

Seller hereby authorizes any agent(s) representing any principal(s) in this action to provide a copy of this statement to any person or entity in connection with any actual or anticipated sale of the property.

THE FOLLOWING ARE REPRESENTATIONS MADE BY SELLER AND SELLER'S AGENT(S) BASED ON THEIR KNOWLEDGE AND MAPS DRAWN BY THE STATE AND FEDERAL GOVERNMENT. THIS INFORMATION IS A DISCLOSURE AND IS NOT INTENDED TO BE PART OF ANY CONTRACT BETWEEN BUYER AND SELLER.

THIS REAL PROPERTY LIES WITHIN THE FOLLOWING HAZARDOUS AREA(S): (Check appropriate response)

1. A SPECIAL FLOOD HAZARD AREA (Any type Zone "A" or "V") designated by the Federal Emergency Management Agency.

    Yes_____ No_____ Do not know/information not available from local jurisdiction_____

2. AN AREA OF POTENTIAL FLOODING shown on an inundation map pursuant to Section 8589.5 of the Government Code.

    Yes_____ No_____ Do not know/information not available from local jurisdiction_____

3. A VERY HIGH FIRE HAZARD SEVERITY ZONE pursuant to Section 51178 or 51179 of the Government Code. The owner of this property is subject to the maintenance requirements of Section 51182 of the Government Code.

    Yes_____ No_____

4. A WILDLAND AREA THAT MAY CONTAIN SUBSTANTIAL FOREST FIRE RISKS AND HAZARDS pursuant to Section 4125 of the Public Resources Code. The owner of this property is subject to the maintenance requirements of Section 4291 of the Public Resources Code. Additionally, it is not the state's responsibility to provide fire protection services to any building or structure located within the wildlands unless the Department of Forestry and Fire Protection has entered into a cooperative agreement with the local agency for those purposes pursuant to Section 4142 of the Public Resources Code.

    Yes_____ No_____

5. AN EARTHQUAKE FAULT ZONE pursuant to Section 2622 of the Public Resources Code.

    Yes_____ No_____

— — — — — — — — — — — — — — — — — — — PAGE ONE OF TWO — FORM 314 — — — — — — — — — — — — — — — — — — —

FIGURE 3.6 (continued):   Natural Hazard Disclosure Statement

— — — — — — — — — — — — — — — *PAGE TWO OF TWO — FORM 314* — — — — — — — — — — — — — — —

6. A SEISMIC HAZARD ZONE pursuant to Section 2696 of the Public Resources Code.

Yes (Landslide Zone)_____   Yes (Liquefaction Zone)_____

No_____   Map not yet released by state_____

THESE HAZARDS MAY LIMIT YOUR ABILITY TO DEVELOP THE REAL PROPERTY, TO OBTAIN INSURANCE OR TO RECEIVE ASSISTANCE AFTER A DISASTER.

THE MAPS ON WHICH THESE DISCLOSURES ARE BASED ESTIMATE WHERE NATURAL HAZARDS EXIST. THEY ARE NOT DEFINITIVE INDICATORS OF WHETHER OR NOT A PROPERTY WILL BE AFFECTED BY A NATURAL DISASTER. BUYER(S) AND SELLER(S) MAY WISH TO OBTAIN PROFESSIONAL ADVICE REGARDING THOSE HAZARDS AND OTHER HAZARDS THAT MAY AFFECT THE PROPERTY.

Check only one of the following:

☐ Seller and their agent represent that the information herein is true and correct to the best of their knowledge as of the date signed by Seller and Seller's Agent.

☐ Seller and their agent acknowledge that they have exercised good faith in the selection of a third-party report provider as required in Civil Code Section 1103.7, and that the representations made in this Natural Hazard Disclosure Statement are based upon information provided by the independent third-party disclosure provider as a substituted disclosure pursuant to Civil Code Section 1103.4. Neither Seller nor their agent has independently verified the information contained in this statement and report or is personally aware of any errors or inaccuracies in the information contained on the statement. This statement was prepared by

Third-Party Disclosure Provider_____ Date _____

Date:_____, 20_____   Date:_____, 20_____

Seller: _____   Seller's
Broker: _____BRE #_____

Seller: _____   Agent: _____BRE #_____

Buyer represents that he has read and understands this document. Pursuant to Civil Code Section 1103.8, the representations made in this Natural Hazard Disclosure Statement do not constitute all of Seller's or Seller's Agent's disclosure obligations in this transaction.

Buyer:_____ Date: _____

Buyer:_____ Date: _____

FORM 314   11-13   ©2013 **first tuesday**, P.O. BOX 5707, RIVERSIDE, CA 92517 (800) 794-0494

©2015 RPI — Realty Publications, Inc.

■ **Areas of potential flooding**—These areas are subject to possible flooding, as shown on a dam failure map. Disclosure must be made if the seller or the seller's agent has knowledge of the designation or a list of properties, including seller's property, has been posted at the county recorder's office, county assessor's office, and county planning agency. (**Note:** If an owner has received federal flood disaster assistance, then the seller must notify the purchaser of the requirement to obtain and maintain flood insurance.)

■ **Very high fire hazard zones**—The state has imposed in these **fire hazard areas** fire protection requirements that subject owners to property maintenance requirements.

■ **State fire responsibility areas**—These are areas where the state not only sets protection requirements but also has primary firefighting responsibility. This disclosure must be made if the seller or the seller's agent has actual knowledge of this designation or the local agency has a map that includes the seller's property that has been posted at county recorder's office, assessor's office, and planning agency.

■ **Wildland area that may contain substantial fire risks and hazards**—Unless the Department of Forestry enters into a cooperative contract, the state is not responsible for fire protection services within wildland areas. The seller must make this disclosure if the seller or the seller's agent has knowledge that the property is in a designated area or if maps showing the property to be in such an area is posted at the office of the country recorder, county assessor, and county planning agency.

WEB LINK

■ **Earthquake fault zone as indicated on maps**—Maps can be obtained online through www.consrv.ca.gov/CGS.

■ **Seismic hazard zone**—An earthquake in such a zone could result in strong shaking, soil liquefaction, or landslides. The seller or the seller's agent must disclose to the buyer that the property is in such a zone if the seller or the seller's agent has actual knowledge that the property is in such a zone or that maps showing the property is in such a zone have been posted at the offices of the county recorder, county assessor, and county planning agency. **Note:** If upon looking at a map, a reasonable person cannot tell with certainty if a property is within a designated area, then the Natural Hazards Disclosure Statement should be marked "Yes."

Landslide Inventory Report

A California Geological Survey developed highway corridor landslide hazard maps. The maps provide an inventory of hillside activity along selected corridors. Maps may be downloaded from www.conservation.ca.gov/cgs/rghm/landslides. While there is not a specific requirement for this report, because the potential for landslides or mudflows is a material fact, these potential dangers should be revealed to prospective buyers.

ENVIRONMENTAL HAZARDS DISCLOSURE

California legislation mandates **environmental hazards disclosure** (Civil Code 25417) to inform homeowners and prospective homeowners about environmental hazards located on and affecting residential property. The seller seldom knows if there are any environmental hazards. Thus, a statement that the seller is unaware of environmental hazards is not a guarantee that the property is free of such hazards. It is in the seller's and the future buyer's interest to know what hazards are common, where they might be found, and how they might be alleviated.

California's Environmental Hazards Booklet

The Real Estate Transfer Disclosure Statement specifies environmental hazards. By providing the booklet *Environmental Hazards: A Guide for Homeowners, Buyers, Landlords, and Tenants*, neither the seller nor the seller's agent need furnish the buyer any more information concerning hazards unless the seller or the agent have actual knowledge of environmental hazards concerning the property.

Hazardous Substances Released

Health and Safety Code Section 25359.7(a) requires **hazardous waste disclosure**. Owners of nonresidential property must give prior notice to buyers or lessees if they know of the release of hazardous substances on the property or if they have reasonable cause to believe hazardous substances exist on or beneath the property. *Brownfields* is a term used to describe contaminated soil.

Tenants are required to notify landlords (both residential and nonresidential) of hazardous substances that they know have been released or believe to exist on or beneath the property. Failure to disclose constitutes a default under the lease.

Lead-Based Paint

The seller or the lessor of residential property built before 1978 must deliver to prospective buyers or tenants the booklet ***Protect Your Family from Lead in Your Home***, which was prepared by the federal Environmental Protection Agency.

Providing the California booklet *Environmental Hazards: A Guide for Homeowners, Buyers, Landlords, and Tenants* meets the federal requirement.

Owners must disclose to their agents, as well as prospective buyers and tenants, the presence of known lead-based-paint hazards. Any available records or reports as to lead-based paint must be provided.

Landlords who receive any federal subsidies or have federally related loans, when confronted with deteriorating paint in a pre-1978 housing unit, must alert tenants to the possible health dangers and use government-certified workers and special containment practices to minimize risk of public exposure. As it relates to lead-based paint, the EPA started enforcement of a new rule on October 1, 2010. This new rule requires that contractors and maintenance professionals working in pre-1978 housing be certified, that their employees be trained, and that they follow protective work practice standards.

This applies to renovation, repair, or painting activities affecting more than 6 square feet of lead-based paint in a room or more than 20 square feet of lead-based paint on the exterior.

WEB LINK

Visit www.epa.gov/lead for more information.

Environmental Hazards Booklet

The Bureau of Real Estate and the Department of Health Services have prepared a booklet for homeowners and buyers called *Residential Environmental Hazards*. This booklet is distributed by the California Association of REALTORS®, as well as other form providers, for use by real estate agents to fully disclose environmental hazard issues to prospective buyers. The booklet contains approximately38 pages to be read by buyers, who should sign a form signifying that they have received the booklet. Inside the back cover is a tear-out sheet (Figure 3.7) to be signed by the buyer(s) and retained in the broker's files.

Under the mandated disclosure of environmental hazards, it is important for brokers to have copies of these tear-outs in their files. Sales agents should make their own photocopies to keep in their personal escrow files. The booklet is divided into six sections and two appendixes. The sections are as follows:

- Asbestos

- Formaldehyde

- Lead

- Radon

- Hazardous Waste

- Household Hazardous Wastes

The appendixes contain the following:

- A list of federal and state agencies

- A glossary of terms

All agents should obtain copies of this booklet and familiarize themselves with the six basic topics. You will be asked questions by your buyers and sellers, and every buyer must be given a copy of the booklet.

(**Note:** The above could place a significant financial burden on an owner, and this burden is not limited to 1–4-unit residential properties.)

FIGURE 3.7:   Environmental Hazards Client Card

To Whom It May Concern:

I have received a copy of "Environmental Hazards: A Guide for Homeowners, Buyers, Landlords, and Tenants" from the Broker(s) in this transaction.

Date:	(Signature)
Time:	(Printed Name)
Date:	(Signature)
Time:	(Printed Name)

Water Contamination

Well water has been seriously contaminated in many areas of California by industrial, agricultural, farming, and military operations. Many wells have been capped. Besides arsenic from mining, there are countless insecticides and chemicals of all types that were not known to be harmful when discharged.

Perchlorate, the primary ingredient of solid rocket fuel, is believed to be particularly dangerous to health. It alters hormonal balances (thyroid) and impedes metabolism and brain development. The EPA has urged the Pentagon to conduct widespread testing, but the Defense Department has resisted.

If an agent knows of problems in a water supply or a house has its own well in an area where water contamination has been found, then the broker has a duty to provide the information to a prospective buyer.

Sick Building Syndrome

Many modern commercial buildings have sealed windows and receive fresh air through their ventilation systems. Some of these buildings have developed what is known as **sick building syndrome (SBS)**. Common tenant complaints include headaches; eye, nose, and throat irritations; dry cough; dry or itchy skin; dizziness; nausea; difficulty concentrating; fatigue; and sensitivity to odors. The problems relate to time spent in the building, and most sufferers report relief soon after leaving the building.

SBS problems may be located in the entire building or just in one area. A problem with SBS is that a specific cause is not known, although it appears to be related to inadequate ventilation. Corrective action has been to increase ventilation and to clean the ventilation system.

If an agent knows that a property has a reputation as a sick building, the agent should reveal this fact. Failure to do so could expose the agent to significant liability. However, specific SBS disclosure is not mandated by law.

SUBDIVISION DISCLOSURE

There are a number of disclosures that relate to subdivisions.

Public Report

The purpose of the California Subdivided Lands Law is to protect purchasers in new subdivisions from fraud. A disclosure known as a **public report** must be provided to purchasers, who must sign that they have received and accepted the report before they are bound to complete the purchase. The California Real Estate Commissioner must approve the public report, which simply discloses information on the project such as location, size of the offering, identity of the subdivider, the interest to be conveyed, and provisions for handling deposits, purchase money, taxes, and assessments. Also included are use restrictions, unusual costs that a buyer will have to bear at time of purchase, hazards, adverse environmental findings, special permits required, utility availability, and so forth. A public report is good up to five years from date of issuance.

The Real Estate Commissioner may issue a preliminary public report that is good for one year or until the public report is issued, whichever occurs first. A subdivider can accept a deposit with a reservation if there is a preliminary public report, but the purchaser is not obligated until signing that he accepts the public report.

A conditional public report that allows the subdivider to enter into a binding contract can be issued, but the escrow cannot be closed until issuance of the public report. The conditional public report period cannot exceed six months and may be renewed for one six-month period. If the public report is not issued within this period or if the purchaser is not satisfied with the final public report because of material changes, the purchaser is entitled to the full refund of any deposit.

COMMON INTEREST SUBDIVISION

A **common interest subdivision** is a subdivision in which owners own or lease a separate lot or unit together with an undivided interest in the common areas of the project. These common areas usually are governed by a **homeowners association (HOA)**.

In the sale of a common interest subdivision, along with the public report, the purchaser must be given a brochure published by the Bureau of Real Estate titled *Common Interest Development General Information*. In addition, and before transfer of title, owners of condominiums, community apartment projects, cooperatives, and planned unit developments must provide purchasers with a copy of the covenants, conditions, and restrictions; bylaws; and articles of incorporation, plus an owners association financial statement, including the current assessments, late charges, plans on change in assessments, and any delinquent assessments and costs. (A homeowners association must furnish the owner a copy of the latest version of documents within 10 days of request by the owner. Only a reasonable fee beyond actual costs may be charged for this.)

Upon request, HOAs must provide an estimate of the fee for providing prospective buyers with governance documents and required disclosures. The fee must be based on actual costs to the HOA, which cannot bundle nonmandatory documents with the required documents to increase the fee. There cannot be an additional fee for electronic delivery of documents. In addition to required disclosures, 12 months of minutes of the HOA meetings must be supplied upon request.

> For common interest subdivisions, buyers must be provided information about restrictions and the homeowners association (HOA).

If there is an age restriction, a statement must be included that it is only enforceable to the extent permitted by law (citing applicable law).

If there is a drought state of emergency declared by the governor or local government, a homeowners association may not fine a homeowner for reduced watering or ceasing to water plants. If recycled water is used, the association can still fine the owner for not keeping up landscaping. HOA prohibitions on replacing turf with low-water-use plants are void and unenforceable.

Homeowners associations cannot prohibit an owner from keeping one pet (subject to reasonable restrictions), nor can they prohibit solar panels or enforce any prohibition on water-efficient plantings.

Homeowners associations, as well as landlords, cannot prohibit tenants from personal agriculture in portable containers but can specify container requirements.

Civil Code Section 1360.2 requires sellers of common interest developments to disclose whether rental restrictions exist. The code also prohibits an HOA from placing rental restrictions that limit existing owners. Restrictions added to the CC&Rs can apply only to subsequent buyers.

If the association plans to sue or has commenced an action against the developer for damages, the construction defects must be listed. If a settlement has been reached regarding construction defects, the defects to be corrected must be described, and an estimate of when the work will be completed, as well as status of other defects, must be provided to the buyer.

Homeowners associations can record a lien against a member's property for unpaid assessments if the amount exceeds $1,800. There is a 90-day redemption period after lien foreclosure.

Condominium Conversion Notice

When a developer intends to convert an apartment to individual ownership, the developer must notify current and prospective tenants of the intent, the public hearings, and the right to purchase their unit.

Interstate Land Sales Full Disclosure Act

This federal act requires disclosures for interstate sale of remote unimproved lots for subdivisions of 25 or more parcels. The act, which was enacted to prevent fraud, requires disclosures as to title, location, facilities, utilities availability and charges, and soil conditions. After receiving a copy of the property report, the prospective purchaser has a seven-calendar-day *cooling-off period* in which to cancel the transaction.

California Land Project

Similar to the Interstate Act, the California Act applies to 50 or more unimproved parcels in low population density areas. The purchaser must be informed of the 14-day right to cancel the purchase (seven days for federal).

FINANCING DISCLOSURE

There are a number of broker, as well as lender, disclosures relating to financing.

Seller Financing Disclosure

Financial disclosure involving seller carryback financing of 1–4-unit residential properties was one of the first mandated disclosures. In the 1970s, the term *creative financing* became very popular, and in most cases, it meant the seller was to *carry back* (accept a note for part of the purchase price secured by a wraparound or junior mortgage, deed of trust, or contract for deed) a second or third trust deed on the property just sold. Although much of this creative financing was an honest attempt to sell the seller's property and provide a win-win situation for both the buyer and the seller, some agents were not prudent in their judgment. If the seller had to foreclose on the buyer, the payments on the home often were so high that the seller could not handle the foreclosure and would lose the equity in the note she was carrying.

Unethical or unsophisticated agents and buyers developed *walk-away financing* in the late 1970s and early 1980s. An unethical purchaser would convince the seller and his agent to let the purchaser buy the property with a low down payment and then borrow on the property and let the buyer pull cash out. The buyer would make no payments on the property and would let the seller and the lenders reclaim the overencumbered property. Of course, the seller would be on the "short end of the stick."

This kind of financing and the complaints stemming from the victims helped enact Civil Code Sections 2956–2967, which became law on July 1, 1983. These statutes require disclosure of seller carryback financing on 1–4 unit residential property in the **Seller Financing Addendum and Disclosure Statement**. The disclosure must be made to both the buyer and the seller, and the units do not have to be owner-occupied for the statute to govern.

Many items and facts must be disclosed, including these major items:

- The terms of the note, such as original loan amount, interest rate, and term (number of payments)

■ All other liens on the property: the original loan amount, current balance, interest rate and any provisions for variations in the interest rate, term, balloon payments, maturity date, and whether any payments are currently in default

■ That the note, if not fully amortized, will have to be refinanced at maturity and that this might be difficult or impossible to accomplish in the conventional marketplace (If balloon payments are called for, the seller [holder of the note] must notify [send or deliver to] the buyer not less than 60 days or more than 150 days before the due date of the note. The notice must specify to whom payment is due, the due date, and the exact amount due [or a good-faith estimate], including the unpaid balance, interest, and other allowable charges.)

■ That loans have or will have negative amortization, or that deferred interest ARMs (adjustable-rate mortgages) could have negative amortization, must be clearly disclosed and its potential effects explained (negative amortization means that the monthly payments are less than the monthly interest on the loan, with the result that the borrower ends up owing more than the original loan amount)

■ Who is liable for the payoff of the underlying loan in an all-inclusive trust deed (AITD) if the lender accelerates the loan

■ The buyer's creditworthiness (credit report, job verification, etc.)

■ A request for notice of default filed and recorded for the seller to help protect the seller in case any senior loans are foreclosed

■ That a title insurance policy will be obtained and furnished to both buyer and seller

■ That a tax service has been arranged to notify the seller whether property taxes have been paid on the property and who will be responsible for the continued service and compensation of the tax service, and that arrangements have been made to notify the seller if the casualty insurance payments are being paid

■ That the deed of trust securing the note will be recorded, thus avoiding the problems of not recording the trust deed

■ The amount, source of funds, and purpose of the funds when the buyer is to receive cash from the proceeds of the transaction

Remember that the items above represent only a condensed version of the financing disclosure law. How disclosure must be made on the forms is shown in California Civil Code Sections 2956-2967.

Adjustable-Rate Loan Disclosure

Lenders offering an adjustable-rate residential mortgage must provide prospective borrowers the most recent copy of the Federal Reserve publication *Consumer Handbook on Adjustable-Rate Mortgages*.

Blanket Encumbrance Disclosure

If there is an underlying blanket encumbrance that affects more than one parcel, the buyer's funds should be protected unless the unit can be released from the blanket encumbrance. The borrower must be made aware of and sign a notice that her interests could be lost if the holder of the blanket encumbrance forecloses, even though the borrower is current on his or her obligations.

Mortgage Loan Disclosure Statement

When a real estate broker solicits or negotiates loans that are not federally related on behalf of lenders or borrowers, the broker must deliver a mortgage loan disclosure statement (MLDS) to the borrower within three business days of receiving the borrower's written loan application. For federally related loans, the Real Estate Settlement Procedures Act (RESPA) disclosures apply.

Lender/Purchaser Disclosure

This disclosure applies to private-party lenders and pension plans that make or purchase loans through a broker. The broker must provide a disclosure statement as to loan terms and loan status, as well as information about the property securing the loan and other encumbrances.

Borrower's Right to Copy of Appraisal

If the borrower paid for the appraisal, a lender must notify the borrower that the borrower can request and receive a copy of the appraisal report.

TILA-RESPA Rule

The Real Estate Settlement Procedures Act applies to federally related loans for 1–4-unit residential properties. The lender must furnish the buyer with a **Loan Estimate** form showing estimated closing and loan costs within three days of receiving the application and not less than seven days prior to consummation, as well as a booklet called *Your Home Loan Toolkit* within three days of application. Federally related loans include loans made by federally regulated lenders, lenders having federally insured deposits, loans that will be federally insured or guaranteed, and loans that are to be resold to Fannie Mae or Freddie Mac. There must be a justifiable service for every charge made. An administrative fee cannot be charged because it is not for a service performed.

RESPA allows a **controlled business arrangement** where a broker has a financial interest in a service provider. However, the relationship of the broker and the service provider must be fully disclosed, and the buyer must be free to use providers of other service, such as escrow services and loan brokerage services.

Integrated Disclosures

A number of disclosures have been combined as a result of requirements of the Dodd-Frank Wall Street Reform and Consumer Protection Act of 2010 to simplify RESPA and truth-in-lending disclosures. The disclosures have been combined into the following two forms, which are covered in Unit 12:

1. Loan estimate

2. Closing Disclosure

Lender Compensation Disclosure

A broker must reveal to all parties to a transaction if the broker is to receive any compensation from a lender before the transaction closes escrow. **Note:** California law prohibits a broker from receiving referral fees from service providers.

Notice of Transfer of Loan Servicing

For loans secured by 1–4-unit residential properties, the borrower must be notified when the loan servicing function (collection) is transferred.

Consumer Caution and Home Ownership Counseling Notice

This notice must be given to applicants for a covered loan no later than three days before signing loan documents. It warns borrowers they are placing a lien on their home and could lose their home and all their equity. A covered loan is a consumer loan for a 1-4 residential unit building that is the principal residence of the consumer and where the original principal balance does not exceed the current conforming loan (loans that can be purchased by Freddie Mac or Fannie Mae)

Truth in Lending Act (Regulation Z)

This federal consumer protection act requires advertising disclosure of finance charges. Interest expressed as an annual percentage rate (APR) and terms of credit, if trigger terms, are used in the advertisement (see Unit 8). Before a borrower is obligated to complete designated loans, there must be full credit disclosure.

Notice of Adverse Action (Equal Credit Opportunity Act)

When a creditor denies a loan applicant, the creditor must provide a statement of reason for the denial or the applicant's right to obtain such a statement. Generally, this must be provided within 30 days of loan application.

Holden Act Disclosure

At the time of the loan application, borrowers must be notified of the prohibition against lender discriminatory practices and their rights under the law. The act prohibits refusing to lend in designated areas (redlining).

OTHER DISCLOSURES

Methamphetamine Contamination Order

Sellers or landlords must provide buyers and tenants with a copy of the cleanup order for contaminated structures. (**Note:** the cleanup order, not the fact of the contamination, must be disclosed.)

Megan's Law

WEB LINK

Megan's Law provides for registration of sex offenders and public availability of knowledge regarding the location of these offenders. Now, every sales contract or lease of 1–4-unit residential properties must include a notice informing buyers or lessees of the public availability of this information on the database website, www.meganslaw.ca.gov.

Elder Abuse Disclosure

California's Elder Abuse Law requires that escrow holders, realty agents, and others report elder financial abuse, fraud, or undue influence. The county public guardian is authorized to take control of the elder's assets to prevent abuse. If an agent feels that an elderly person is being financially abused, reporting the abuse is mandatory.

Mello-Roos Bond Disclosure

Mello-Roos bonds are municipal-type bonds issued to fund streets, sewers, and so forth for a new development. The bonds shift the expenses from the developer to each homebuyer, who must pay an assessment to retire the bond. The net effect is higher taxes for the homebuyer.

A broker must disclose to a buyer that a project is subject to a Mello-Roos levy for a sale or lease for more than five years. Failure to give notice before signing the sales contract (or lease) gives the buyer or the tenant a three-day right of rescission after receipt of the notice.

Structural Pest Control Inspection and Certification Reports

While the law does not require a **structural pest control inspection**, if required by contract or lender, a copy must be delivered to the buyer, and a copy must be filed with the state Structural Pest Control Board. Section 1 of the report covers visible evidence of active termite infestation, while section 2 covers conditions likely to lead to infestation. (When lender requires clearance, it refers to section 1.)

Septic System Disclosure

The disclosure is required when property is not presently connected to a sewer. The purchaser is alerted to the fact that an inspection may not discover latent defects. The buyer is also made aware of the fact that should a sewer connection be required in the future, the owner will have additional expenses.

Energy Conservation Retrofit and Thermal Insulation Disclosures

Some communities require energy retrofitting as a condition of sale. The seller or the agent should disclose the requirements of local statutes. New-home sellers must disclose in their sales contracts the type, thickness, and R-value of the insulation.

Foreign Investment Real Property Tax Act

The buyer must be informed about the IRS withholding requirement of 10% of the gross sales price when the seller is a foreign person. (See Unit 14 for exemptions.)

The buyer must be informed about the California requirement to withhold 31/3% of the total sale price paid as state income tax. (See Unit 14 for details about this requirement and its exemptions.)

Notice Regarding Advisability of Title Insurance

If no title insurance is to be issued through an escrow, the buyer must receive a separate notice about the advisability of obtaining title insurance. (See Civil Code Section 1057.6.)

Importance of Home Inspection Notice

For the sale of 1–4-unit residential properties (including mobile homes) involving FHA financing or HUD-owned property, the borrower must sign a **home inspection notice** titled The Importance of a Home Inspection.

Smoke Detector Notice

A buyer of a single-family home must receive a **smoke detector disclosure** written statement indicating that the property is in compliance with current California law regarding the presence of smoke detectors. The issuance of a building permit triggers a requirement to update smoke detectors (10 year nonremovable battery).

Carbon Monoxide Detector Notice

Every residential unit that has fossil-fuel heating must have a carbon monoxide detector, and a seller disclosure of the presence or absence of a detector is required.

Window Security Bars

A seller must disclose, on the Real Estate Transfer Disclosure Statement, the presence of **window security bars** and any safety release mechanism on the bars.

Water Heater Bracing

Sellers of real property must certify to prospective purchasers that the **water heater bracing** has been properly installed.

Water Conservancy Plumbing Fixtures

By 2017, single-family residences built before 1994 must be equipped with water conservancy fixtures. By 2019, all multifamily units must have water conservancy fixtures. For property altered or improved after 2014, water conservancy fixtures must be a condition of final permit approval (low-flow toilets, showerheads, and faucets).

Starting in 2017, sellers of single-family residences must disclose to buyers the requirements of plumbing fixtures and whether or not the unit includes noncompliant plumbing. For multifamily units, the disclosure requirement begins in 2019.

Home Energy Rating System (HERS)

The homeseller or the broker must inform the buyer of the existence of the California Whole-House Home Energy Rating Program. Providing the Home Energy Rating System booklet meets the disclosure requirements.

Nonresidential Energy Use Disclosure

To encourage energy efficiency use, owners must disclose the energy consumption to prospective buyers, lessers, and lenders.

Supplemental Tax Bill Disclosure

Residential sellers must disclose to buyers in writing to expect supplemental tax reassessment bills.

Industrial/Airport Disclosure

Sellers of 1–4-unit residential properties must disclose any actual knowledge of airport or industrial use or zoning that could affect the property. Airport noise disclosure has been added to the California Transfer Disclosure Statement.

Farming Area Disclosure

Developers and residential sellers must disclose if property is within 1 mile of a farming operation.

Notice of Mining Operation

If property is within 1 mile of a mining operation, notice must be given.

Gas or Hazardous Liquid Transmission Lines

The sale of 1-4 residential units requires the disclosure of gas or hazardous liquid transmission lines in the vicinity.

Military Ordnance Location

If a transferor has knowledge that a property is within 1 mile of a former **military ordnance location** (military training ground) that may contain explosives, the transferor must disclose in writing that these former federal or state locations may contain potentially explosive ammunition. (the buyer has a statutory right of rescission.)

Commissions

A notice must be given to the party paying any real estate commission that commissions are negotiable. This notice must be in a font not less than 10 points and in bold typeface.

Renter Notice of Foreclosure

Civil Code Section 2924.85 requires that rental applicants be given notice that the owner has received a notice of default and that there is a pending foreclosure.

RIGHT OF RESCISSION

For detailed California disclosure requirements, check the Bureau of Real Estate website: www.bre.ca.gov.

There are statutory **rescission rights** for a number of transactions. Buyers (or borrowers) must be informed of their rights. Failure to disclose rights of rescission extends this right.

Truth in Lending Act—When a loan for consumer credit is secured by a borrower's residence, a rescission right exists until midnight of the third business day following the completion of the loan.

Interstate Land Sales Full Disclosure Act—This federal act calls for a disclosure statement, known as a *property report*, for subdivisions of 25 or more unimproved residential properties of less than 5 acres each that are sold in interstate commerce. Besides the required disclosures to the purchasers, the purchasers have a seven-day right of rescission.

California land projects—Have a 14-day right of rescission.

Time-share—Because of abusive sales tactics of many time-share developers, purchasers of time-shares now have a rescission right of three days after signing the contract.

Undivided interest subdivision—An undivided interest subdivision is one where the owners are tenants in common with the other owners but don't have an exclusive possessory interest in a particular unit or space. An example is a campground where owners have a right to use a space if available. Purchasers in undivided interest subdivisions have a three-day right of rescission following the day the agreement is signed.

Home equity sales—Because of fraud and unfair dealings by home equity purchasers, a homeowner has a rescission right when selling her equity interest in a residence in foreclosure. There is a right to cancel any contract with an equity purchaser until midnight of the fifth business day following the sales agreement or until 8 am on the day of the sale, whichever occurs first.

Mello-Roos disclosure—Failure to disclose the fact that a property is in a Mello-Roos district would allow the transferee a three- to five-day right of rescission.

BRE DISCLOSURE BOOKLET AND CALIFORNIA ASSOCIATION OF REALTORS® DISCLOSURE CHART

To aid members in understanding the numerous disclosure obligations that real estate professionals should be aware of, the California Association of REALTORS® has prepared a California Real Estate Law Disclosure Chart. This chart is included as Figure 3.8.

California Bureau of Real Estate Disclosure Booklet—The Bureau of Real Estate publishes a booklet titled *Disclosures in Real Property Transactions*. It may be purchased from the BRE or viewed and downloaded free at www.dre.ca.gov/files/pdf/re6.pdf. In Unit 10, you will find that the purchase contract includes many of the required disclosures.

WEB LINK

FIGURE 3.8:   List of Disclosures

(The following form is copyrighted by the California Association of REAL-TORS®, © 2014, and is reprinted under a limited license with permission. Photocopying or any other reproduction, whether electronic or otherwise, is strictly prohibited.)

CALIFORNIA
ASSOCIATION
OF REALTORS®

Summary Disclosure Chart

Member Legal Services
Tel (213) 739-8282
Fax (213) 480-7724
December 19, 2014 (revised)

The Summary Disclosure Chart is designed to provide REALTORS® and their clients with an easy-to-use reference guide for determining the applicability of the state and federal laws to real estate transactions most commonly handled by real estate licensees.

The Summary Disclosure Chart provides a disclosure "trigger" as well as a brief summary of the disclosure requirement, but does not cover all disclosures required by law. More detailed information regarding disclosure and other legal topics is available to C.A.R. members on car.org.

For a quick answer to required disclosures based on the type of property (residential one-to-four units, residential five or more units, commercial property or vacant land, and manufactured or mobile homes, see the **Sales Disclosure Chart**. For information on lease and rental transactions, please refer to the legal chart, **Lease/Rental Disclosure Chart**. For the disclosure requirements involving homes in a new subdivision, please refer to legal chart, **New Home Disclosure Chart**. For the disclosure requirements for foreclosure sales or sales of REO property, see the legal chart, **REO Disclosure Chart**.

For additional disclosure requirements when selling a property in a common interest development, please refer to legal article, **Condominium or Other Common Interest Development Disclosures**.

SUBJECT	DISCLOSURE TRIGGER	DISCLOSURE REQUIREMENT (Brief Summary) FORM	C.A.R. INFORMATION SOURCE LAW CITATION
Advisability of Title Insurance	An escrow transaction for the purchase or simultaneous exchange of real property where a policy of title insurance will <u>not</u> be issued to the buyer.	The buyer must receive the statutory notice. The law does not specify who is responsible for providing this notice. Typically handled by escrow agent.	Cal. Civ. Code § 1057.6.

FIGURE 3.8 (continued): **List of Disclosures**

SUBJECT	DISCLOSURE TRIGGER	DISCLOSURE REQUIREMENT (Brief Summary) FORM	C.A.R. INFORMATION SOURCE LAW CITATION
Agency Disclosure (Education Form) and **Agency Confirmation (Who Represents Each Party)**	Sale[2] of residential real property of 1-4 units and mobile homes, commercial, vacant land and industrial property, but not residential income of 5 units or more; lease for a term of over one year on the above referenced property.	The buyer must receive the agency disclosure form (AD) from the buyer's agent prior to signing the offer. The seller must receive the agency disclosure form (AD) from the seller's agent prior to signing the listing contract and must receive another agency disclosure form (AD) from the buyer's agent prior to accepting the buyer's offer. The agency confirmation form must be given to the buyer and seller "as soon as practicable." This can be accomplished either by having the language in the purchase agreement or by using a separate form (AC-6). C.A.R. forms AD (disclosure) and AC-6 (confirmation).	Legal Q&As, **Agency Disclosure and Confirmation**, and **Agency Laws Summary Chart** Cal. Civ. Code §§ 2079.13 *et seq.*
Airport in Vicinity	NHD report is completed by third-party disclosure company	The NHD expert must determine if the property is located within an "airport influence area" as defined in Business & Professions Code § 1010(b). If so, the report must contain a statutory statement, *Notice of Airport in Vicinity.*	Cal. Civ. Code § 1103.4(c)(1).
Area of Potential Flooding (in the event of dam or reservoir failure)	Sale of all real property if the seller or the seller's agent has actual knowledge or a list has been compiled by parcel and the notice posted at a local county recorder, assessor and planning agency. Also applies to manufactured homes and personal property mobile homes.	The seller's agent or the seller without an agent must disclose to the buyer if the property is in this Area of Potential Flooding as designated on an inundation map, if a parcel list has been prepared by the county and a notice identifying the location of the list is available at the county assessor, county recorder or county planning	Legal Q&A, **Natural Hazard Disclosure Statement** Cal. Gov't Code §§ 8589.4, 8589.5; Cal. Civ. Code § 1103.

FIGURE 3.8 (continued):   List of Disclosures

SUBJECT	DISCLOSURE TRIGGER	DISCLOSURE REQUIREMENT (Brief Summary) FORM	C.A.R. INFORMATION SOURCE LAW CITATION
		commission office, or if the seller or seller's agent has actual knowledge that the property is in an area. If a TDS is required in the transaction, either C.A.R. Form NHD, *Natural Hazard Disclosure Statement* or an updated Local Option disclosure form must be used to make this disclosure.	
Broker's Statutory Duty to Inspect Property	Sale [3] of all residential real property of 1-4 units (No exemptions except for never-occupied properties where a public report is required or properties exempt from a public report pursuant to Business & Professions Code § 11010.4) Also applies to manufactured and personal property mobile homes.	A real estate licensee must conduct a reasonably competent and diligent visual inspection of the property; this inspection duty does not include areas which are reasonably and normally inaccessible, off the site, or public records or permits concerning the title or use of the property; this inspection duty includes only the unit for sale and not the common areas of a condo or other common interest development. There is no requirement that the inspection report be in writing; however, it is recommended that all licensees put it in writing. C.A.R. Form TDS (or for mobile homes and manufactured housing, C.A.R. Form MHTDS) may be used. If the seller is exempt from the TDS, then C.A.R. Form AVID may be used by the agent.	Legal Q&A, **Real Estate Licensee's Duty to Inspect Residential Property** Cal. Civ. Code §§ 2079 *et seq.*
Carbon Monoxide Detector Disclosure & Compliance	The Carbon Monoxide Poisoning Prevention Act of 2010 requires a carbon monoxide detector device (battery or hard-wired) to be	The C.A.R. Forms TDS and MHTDS add a disclosure regarding these devices. No separate disclosure form is required.	Cal. Civ. Code §§ 1102.6, 1102.6d. Note: Installation is not a precondition

FIGURE 3.8 (continued):   **List of Disclosures**

SUBJECT	DISCLOSURE TRIGGER	DISCLOSURE REQUIREMENT (Brief Summary) FORM	C.A.R. INFORMATION SOURCE LAW CITATION
	installed in all dwelling units. Existing single-family units must have the device installed on or before July 1, 2011 and all other existing dwelling units must have the device installed by Jan. 1, 2013. See manufacturer instructions for the number of devices and location of installation.		of sale or transfer of the dwelling.
Commercial Property Owner's Guide to Earthquake Safety	<u>Mandatory delivery:</u> Sale, transfer, or exchange of <u>any</u> real property or manufactured home or mobile home if built of precast concrete or reinforced/unreinforced masonry with wood frame floors or roofs and built before Jan. 1, 1975, located within a county or city, if not exempt. Almost same exemptions as from Transfer Disclosure Statement.[11] Additional exemption if the buyer agrees, in writing, to demolish the property within one year from date of transfer. <u>Voluntary delivery:</u> Transfer of [4] <u>any</u> real property.	<u>Mandatory delivery:</u> The transferor/transferor's agent must give the transferee a copy of *The Commercial Property Owner's Guide to Earthquake Safety*. [5] <u>Voluntary delivery:</u> If the *Guide* is delivered to the transferee, then the transferor or broker is not required to provide additional information concerning general earthquake hazards. Known earthquake hazards must be disclosed whether delivery is mandatory or voluntary.	Cal. Bus. & Prof. Code § 10147; Cal. Gov't Code §§ 8875.6, 8875.9, 8893.2, 8893.3; Cal. Civ. Code § 2079.9.
Death (in last 3 years)	Sale , lease, or rental of <u>all</u> real property.	The transferor/agent has no liability for not disclosing the fact of any death which occurred more than 3 years prior to the date the transferee offers to buy, lease, or rent the property. Any death which has occurred within a 3-year period should be disclosed if deemed to be "material." Affliction with AIDS or death from AIDS, no matter when it occurred, need not be voluntarily disclosed. However, neither a seller nor	Legal Q&A, **Disclosure of Death and AIDS and the Prohibition Against Discrimination on the Basis of AIDS** Cal. Civ. Code § 1710.2.

FIGURE 3.8 (continued): **List of Disclosures**

SUBJECT	DISCLOSURE TRIGGER	DISCLOSURE REQUIREMENT (Brief Summary) FORM	C.A.R. INFORMATION SOURCE LAW CITATION
		seller's agent may make an intentional misrepresentation in response to a direct question concerning AIDS/death from AIDS on the property. An agent may simply respond that discussing such information is an invasion of privacy.	
Earthquake Fault Zone′	Sale of <u>all</u> real property which does contain or will eventually contain a structure for human occupancy and which is located in an earthquake fault zone (special studies zone) as indicated on maps created by the California Geological Survey.[8] Also applies to manufactured and personal property mobile homes.	The seller's <u>agent</u> or the seller without an agent must disclose to the buyer the fact that the property is in an earthquake fault zone (special studies zone), if maps are available at the county assessor, county recorder, or county planning commission office, or if the seller or seller's agent has actual knowledge that the property is in the zone. If the map is not of sufficient accuracy or scale to determine whether the property is in the zone, then either the agent indicates "yes" that the property is in the zone or the agent may write "no" that the property is <u>not</u> in this zone, but then a report prepared by an expert verifying that fact must be attached to C.A.R. Form NHD. If a TDS is required in the transaction, either C.A.R. Form NHD, *Natural Hazard Disclosure Statement*, or an updated local option disclosure form must be used to make this disclosure.	Legal Q&A, **Natural Hazard Disclosure Statement** Cal. Pub. Res. Code §§ 2621 *et seq.;* Cal. Civ. Code § 1103.
Energy Use Report	Sale of commercial building, lease of entire commercial building or loan application to finance entire commercial	The owner shall disclose energy use report no later than 24 hours prior to execution of sales or lease contract, or submittal of the	Public Resources Code 25402.10. 20 CCR §§ 1680-

FIGURE 3.8 (continued):   List of Disclosures

SUBJECT	DISCLOSURE TRIGGER	DISCLOSURE REQUIREMENT (Brief Summary) FORM	C.A.R. INFORMATION SOURCE LAW CITATION
	building. The effective date of the law depends on the size of the building. For buildings with sq. ft. 50,000 or more, it is January 1, 2014. For buildings with sq. ft. 10,000 to 50,000, it is January 1, 2014. For buildings with sq. ft. 5,000 to 10,000 it is July 1, 2014.	loan application. An account with the EPA's Energy Star program must be opened or updated 30 days before disclosure is made.	1684.
Farm or Ranch Proximity	NHD report is completed by third-party disclosure company	The NHD expert must determine if the property is located within one mile of real property designated as farm or ranch land on a GIS map. If so, the report must contain a statutory statement, *Notice of Right to Farm*.	Cal. Civ. Code § 1103.4(c)(3).
FHA/HUD Inspection Notice	Sale of HUD-owned residential real property of 1-4 units, including mobile homes on a permanent foundation, or properties which involve FHA loans.	For all existing properties except those "under construction," the borrower must receive from the lender the notice: "For Your Protection: Get a Home Inspection." C.A.R. Form HID.	HUD Mortgagee Letter 06-24

6

FIGURE 3.8 (continued):   List of Disclosures

SUBJECT	DISCLOSURE TRIGGER	DISCLOSURE REQUIREMENT (Brief Summary) FORM	C.A.R. INFORMATION SOURCE LAW CITATION
Federal Withholding (FIRPTA) and California Withholding Tax	Federal withholding: All sales, including installment sales, exchanges, foreclosures, deeds in lieu of foreclosure and other transactions by a "foreign person." CA withholding: Any "disposition of a California real property interest" (includes sales, exchanges, foreclosures, installment sales, and other types of transfers). See the Legal Q&As for the exemptions.	Federal: Buyers must withhold 10% of the gross sales price and send it to the IRS. If the seller is not a "foreign person," he or she may complete the affidavit of non-foreign status. CA: Buyers must withhold 3 1/3 percent of the gross sales price on any sale of California real property interests, unless an exemption applies, and send it to the FTB. C.A.R. form AS may be used, if applicable, to avoid withholding at time of transfer.	Legal Q&As, **Federal Withholding: The Foreign Investment in Real Property Tax Act (FIRPTA),** and **California Withholding on the Sale of Real Property** 42 U.S.C. § 5154a. Cal. Rev. & Tax Code §§ 18662(e)(f).
Flood Disaster Insurance Requirements (Applicable for any flood disaster[10] declared after Sep. 23, 1994)	Any transfer [6] of personal (e.g., mobile homes), residential, or commercial property where the owner received federal flood disaster assistance conditioned on the owner subsequently obtaining and maintaining flood insurance.	The transferor must notify the transferee in writing on a document "evidencing the transfer of ownership of the property" about the requirement to obtain and maintain flood insurance in accordance with applicable Federal law. Failure to notify the transferee means that in the event the transferee fails to maintain the required flood insurance and the property is damaged by a flood disaster requiring Federal disaster relief, the transferor will be required to reimburse the Federal government. The law is unclear as to what document(s) should contain this notice. C.A.R. Forms RPA-CA and NHD may be acceptable, but technically are not documents that "evidence the transfer of	Legal Q&A, **Federal Flood Insurance Disclosure** 42 U.S.C. § 5154a.

FIGURE 3.8 (continued): **List of Disclosures**

SUBJECT	DISCLOSURE TRIGGER	DISCLOSURE REQUIREMENT (Brief Summary) FORM	C.A.R. INFORMATION SOURCE LAW CITATION
		ownership." Clearly, a grant deed is such a document.	
Gas and Hazardous Liquid Transmission Pipeline Notice	Every Contract for sale of residential real property.	The Notice informs the buyer that information about the general location of these pipelines is available to the public on line via the National Pipeline Mapping System (NPMS) and provides the web address. The following C.A.R. forms contain this statutory notice: RPA-CA, RIPA, NCPA, NODPA, MHPA.	Cal. Civ. Code § 2079.10.5
Home Energy Ratings System (HERS) Booklet (Optional Disclosure) (Booklet Now Available)	Transfer [9] or exchange of <u>all</u> real property. Also applies to manufactured and personal property mobile homes.	If an energy ratings booklet is delivered to the transferee, then a seller or broker is not required to provide additional information concerning the existence of a statewide energy rating program. *Home Energy Rating System (HERS) Booklet (*part of *Combined Hazards* booklet)	Cal. Civ. Code § 2079.10; Cal. Pub. Res. Code §§ 25402.9, 25942.
Homeowner's Guide to Earthquake Safety Booklet and Residential Earthquake Hazards Report (form in booklet)	<u>Mandatory delivery:</u> Transfer of residential real property of 1-4 units, manufactured homes, and mobile homes, of conventional light frame construction, and built prior to Jan. 1, 1960, if not exempt (almost same exemptions as for the Transfer Disclosure Statement[11]). Additional exemption if the buyer agrees, in writing, to demolish the property within one year from date of transfer. <u>Voluntary delivery:</u> Transfe [6] of <u>any</u> real property.	<u>Mandatory delivery:</u> The licensee must give the transferor the booklet *The Homeowner's Guide to Earthquake Safety*[12] and the transferor must give this booklet to the transferee. Known structural deficiencies must be disclosed by the transferor to the transferee and the form in the booklet entitled *Residential Earthquake Hazards Report* may be used to make this disclosure. <u>Voluntary delivery:</u> If the *Guide* is delivered to	Cal. Bus. & Prof. Code § 10149; Cal. Gov't Code §§ 8897.1, 8897.2, 8897.5; Cal. Civ. Code § 2079.8.

FIGURE 3.8 (continued): List of Disclosures

SUBJECT	DISCLOSURE TRIGGER	DISCLOSURE REQUIREMENT (Brief Summary) FORM	C.A.R. INFORMATION SOURCE LAW CITATION
		the transferee, then the transferor or broker is not required to provide additional information concerning general earthquake hazards.

Known earthquake hazards must be disclosed whether delivery is mandatory or voluntary. | |
| **Industrial Use Zone Location** | Transfer[6] or exchange of residential real property of 1-4 units. | The seller of real property subject to the TDS law must disclose "actual knowledge" that the property is affected by or zoned to allow an industrial use of property (manufacturing, commercial, or airport use) as soon as possible before transfer of title.

C.A.R. Form SSD or SPQ may be used. | Cal. Civ. Code § 1102.17; Cal. Code Civ. Proc. § 731a. |
| **Lead-Based Paint Pamphlet and Form** | Sale or lease of all residential property, built before Jan. 1, 1978, except as indicated below.

Also applies to manufactured homes and personal property mobile homes.

Exemptions:

• foreclosure or trustee's sale transfer (REO properties and deed-in-lieu of foreclosure are NOT exempt!)
• zero-bedroom dwelling (loft, efficiency unit, dorm, or studio)

• short-term rental (100 or fewer days) | The seller/lessor must provide the buyer/lessee with a lead hazard information pamphlet, disclose the presence of any known lead-based paint and provide a statement signed by the buyer that the buyer has read the warning statement, has received the pamphlet, and has a 10-day opportunity to inspect before becoming obligated under the contract.

The purchaser (not lessee) is permitted a 10-day period to conduct an inspection unless the parties mutually agree upon a different time period.

The agent, on behalf of the seller/lessor, must ensure compliance with the | Legal Q&As, **Federal Lead-Based Paint Hazard Disclosures**, and

Federal Lead-Based Paint Renovation Rule

Residential Lead-Based Paint Hazard Reduction Act of 1992, 42 U.S.C. § 4852d. |

9

FIGURE 3.8 (continued): **List of Disclosures**

SUBJECT	DISCLOSURE TRIGGER	DISCLOSURE REQUIREMENT (Brief Summary) FORM	C.A.R. INFORMATION SOURCE LAW CITATION
	• housing for elderly or handicapped (unless children live there) • rental housing certified free of lead paint	requirements of this law. C.A.R. pamphlet, *Protect Your Family From Lead in Your Home*, and C.A.R. form FLD satisfy these requirements (except for sales of HUD properties— then HUD forms required). The C.A.R. Combined Hazards booklet may be used in lieu of the pamphlet mentioned above.	
Material Facts	Any transfer of real property or manufactured homes or mobile homes. No exemptions.	A seller (transferor) or real estate agent involved in the transaction must disclose any <u>known material facts</u> that affect the value or desirability of the property. Whether or not something is deemed material is determined by case law. C.A.R. Form SSD or SPQ may be used.	Case law: *Nussbaum v. Weeks* (1990) 214 Cal. App. 3d 1589 (seller's duty); *Easton v. Strassburger* (1984) 152 Cal. App. 3d 90 (agent's duty); Cal. Civ. Code § 2079 *et seq.*
Megan's Law Disclosure (Registered Sex Offender Database)	Sale[13] or lease/rental of all residential real property of 1-4 units (No exemptions except for never-occupied properties where a public report is required or properties exempted from a public report pursuant to Bus. & Prof. Code § 11010.4)	Every lease or rental agreement and every sales contract is required to include a statutorily-defined notice regarding the existence of public access to database information regarding sex offenders. The following C.A.R. forms contain this statutory notice: RPA-CA, RIPA, PPA, NCPA, NODPA, MHPA, LR, IOA, RLAS	Legal Q&A, **Megan's Law: Disclosure of Registered Sex Offenders** Cal. Civ. Code § 2079.10a.

10

FIGURE 3.8 (continued):   **List of Disclosures**

SUBJECT	DISCLOSURE TRIGGER	DISCLOSURE REQUIREMENT (Brief Summary) FORM	C.A.R. INFORMATION SOURCE LAW CITATION
Mello-Roos, 1915 Bond Act Assessments, and voluntary contractual assessment.	Transfer[6] or exchange of residential real property of 1-4 units subject to a continuing lien securing the levy of special taxes pursuant to the Mello-Roos Community Facilities Act or the 1915 Bond Act. Same exemptions as for the Transfer Disclosure Statement except that new subdivisions are not exempt.	The transferor must make a good faith effort to obtain a disclosure notice concerning the special tax or assessment from each local agency that levies a special tax or assessment and deliver the notice(s) to the prospective transferee. Transferors may comply with this law by using a third-party disclosure company. The transferee has a 3 or 5-day right of rescission. There is no affirmative duty by an agent to discover a special tax or district or assessment not actually known to the agent.	Legal Q&A, **Mello-Roos District Disclosure Requirements** Cal. Civ. Code § 1102.6b; Cal. Gov't Code § 53340.2 (Mello-Roos Form), § 53341.5 (new subdivisions), § 53754 (bond), Cal. Str. & H. Code § 5898.24.
Meth Lab Clean-Up Order **(Release of Illegal Controlled Substance Remediation Order)**	Transfer by "purchase, exchange, gift, lease, inheritance, or legal action" of any "parcel of land, structure, or part of a structure" where the manufacture of methamphetamine or storage of methamphetamine or a prohibited hazardous chemical occurred.	In the event that toxic contamination by an illegal controlled substance has occurred on a property and upon receipt of a clean-up order from the Dept. of Toxic Substances Control (DTSC) or a Local Health Officer, the transferor must provide a copy of this order to the transferee. In the case of rental property, the landlord must give a prospective tenant a copy of this order which must be attached to the rental agreement. Non-compliance with this law permits the tenant to void the rental agreement. C.A.R. Form SSD, SPQ or MCN may be used.	Cal. Health & Safety Code § 25400.28 (disclosure), § 25400.36 (definitions).

FIGURE 3.8 (continued): **List of Disclosures**

SUBJECT	DISCLOSURE TRIGGER	DISCLOSURE REQUIREMENT (Brief Summary) FORM	C.A.R. INFORMATION SOURCE LAW CITATION
Military Ordnance Location (former military munitions site)	Transfer [6] or exchange of residential real property of 1-4 units and lease of any residential dwelling unit. Same exemptions as for the Transfer Disclosure Statement.	Disclosure is required when the transferor/lessor has actual knowledge that a former military ordnance location (military training grounds which may contain explosives) is within one mile of the property. The transferor/lessor must disclose in writing to the transferee/lessee, that these former federal or state military ordnance locations may contain potentially explosive munitions. The transferee has a 3 or 5-day right of rescission. C.A.R. Form SSD or SPQ may be used.	Cal. Civ. Code §§ 1102.15, 1940.7.
Mining Operation	NHD report is completed by third-party disclosure company	The NHD expert must determine if the property is located within one mile of a mine operation as reported by the Office of Mine Reclamation map. If so, the report must contain a statutory statement, Notice of Mining Operation.	Cal. Civ. Code § 1103.4 (c)(3).
Mold (Disclosure of Excessive Mold or Health Threat)	Sale, lease, rental, or other transfer of any commercial, industrial or residential property	There are no current disclosure requirements until after the Dept. of Health Services (DHS) develops permissible exposure limits for mold and a consumer booklet. The TDS has been modified to include the word "mold" in paragraph II.C.1. As always, any transferor must disclose actual knowledge of toxic mold on	Legal Q&A, **Mold and Its Impact on Real Estate Transactions** Cal. Health & Safety Code §§ 26100 *et seq.*, §§ 26140, 26141, 26147, 26148.

FIGURE 3.8 (continued):   **List of Disclosures**

SUBJECT	DISCLOSURE TRIGGER	DISCLOSURE REQUIREMENT (Brief Summary) FORM	C.A.R. INFORMATION SOURCE LAW CITATION
		the property. C.A.R. Form RGM may be used (optional).	
Natural Hazard Disclosure Statement (Form)	Transfer[14] of residential real property of 1-4 units if the property is located in one or more of the following hazard zones: Special Flood Hazard Area, Area of Potential Flooding, Very High Fire Severity Zone, Earthquake Fault Zone, Seismic Hazard Zone, or State Responsibility Area Also applies to manufactured homes and personal property mobile homes. See the Legal Q&A for the list of exemptions.	The seller and the listing agent must sign the statutory form or a substantially equivalent form (provided by a disclosure company or other) to be provided to the buyer. C.A.R. Form NHD (statutory form).	Legal Q&A, **Natural Hazard Disclosure Statement** Cal. Civ. Code §§ 1103 *et seq.*
Pest Control Inspection Report and Certification **(wood destroying pests or organisms)**	Transfer of title of any real property or the execution of a real property sales contract, as defined in Civil Code Section 2985, <u>only if</u> required by contract or the transferee's lender.	The transferor, fee owner, or his/her agent, must deliver to the transferee a copy of a structural pest control inspection report and certification if any remediation work is required, as soon as practical, before close of escrow or execution of a real property sales contract (land sale contract). Delivery to a transferee means delivery in person or by mail to the transferee him/herself or any person authorized to act for him/her in the transaction or to such additional transferees who have requested such delivery from the transferor or his/her agent in writing. Delivery to either husband or wife will be deemed delivery to a	Cal. Civ. Code § 1099.

FIGURE 3.8 (continued):   List of Disclosures

SUBJECT	DISCLOSURE TRIGGER	DISCLOSURE REQUIREMENT (Brief Summary) FORM	C.A.R. INFORMATION SOURCE LAW CITATION
		transferee, unless the contract affecting the transfer states otherwise.	
Private Transfer Fee	Transfer[6] or exchange of residential real property of 1-4 units. Same exemptions as for the Transfer Disclosure Statement.	If the property being transferred is subject to a transfer fee, as defined in Section 1098, the transferor must provide, at the same time as the TDS, a transfer tax disclosure statement. C.A.R. Form NTF may be used.	Cal. Civ. Code §§ 1102.6e, 1098, 1098.5.
Residential Environmental Hazards Booklet (Optional Disclosure)	Transfer[15] or exchange of all real property. Also applies to manufactured homes and personal property mobile homes.	If a consumer information booklet[16] is delivered to the transferee, then a seller or broker is not required to provide additional information concerning common environmental hazards. Although highly recommended, delivery is voluntary. However, known hazards on the property must be disclosed to the transferee. C.A.R. *Combined Hazards* booklet may be used.	Cal. Civ. Code § 2079.7.
Seismic Hazard Zones	Sale of all real property which does contain or will eventually contain a structure for human habitation and which is located in a seismic hazard zone as indicated on maps created by the California Division of Mines and Geology. Also applies to manufactured homes and personal property mobile homes.	The seller's agent or the seller without an agent must disclose to the buyer the fact that the property is in a seismic hazard zone if maps are available at the county assessor, county recorder, or county planning commission office, or if the seller or seller's agent has actual knowledge that the property is in the zone. If the map is not of sufficient accuracy or scale to determine whether the property is in the zone,	Legal Q&A, **Natural Hazard Disclosure Statement** Cal. Pub. Res. Code § 2690 *et seq.*, § 2694; Cal. Civ. Code § 1103.

FIGURE 3.8 (continued):   List of Disclosures

SUBJECT	DISCLOSURE TRIGGER	DISCLOSURE REQUIREMENT (Brief Summary) FORM	C.A.R. INFORMATION SOURCE LAW CITATION
		then either the agent indicates "yes" that the property is in the zone or the agent may write "no" that the property is <u>not</u> in this zone, but then a report prepared by an expert verifying that fact must be attached to C.A.R. Form NHD. If a TDS is required in the transaction, either C.A.R. Form NHD, "Natural Hazard Disclosure Statement" or an updated local option disclosure form must be used to make this disclosure.	
Smoke Alarms Must Be In Compliance	All existing real property dwelling units must have a smoke alarm centrally located outside each sleeping area (bedroom or group of bedrooms). All used manufactured homes, used mobile homes, and used multi-family manufactured housing must have a smoke alarm in each room designed for sleeping. However, as point of sale requirement for single family properties and duplexes, the exemptions are the same under the TDS law. Except that, transfers to or from governmental entities, and transfers of property acquired by a beneficiary after a foreclosure or trustee's sale, or after a deed in lieu, which are exempt under the TDS law, are not exempt from compliance as a point of sale requirement. In addition, new real property construction with a permit after Aug. 14, 1992 must have a hard-wired smoke alarm in each bedroom. Any additions, modifications, or repairs to real property (after Aug. 14, 1992) exceeding $1,000 for which a permit is required or the addition of any bedroom will also trigger the requirement of a smoke alarm in each bedroom. (These may be battery operated.)	**LOCAL LAW MAY BE MORE RESTRICTIVE! Check with the local City or County Department of Building and Safety.** See next section for Disclosure requirement.	Legal Q&A, **Smoke Alarm Requirements** Cal. Health & Safety Code §§ 13113.7, 13113.8, 18029.6.

15

FIGURE 3.8 (continued):   **List of Disclosures**

SUBJECT	DISCLOSURE TRIGGER	DISCLOSURE REQUIREMENT (Brief Summary) FORM	C.A.R. INFORMATION SOURCE LAW CITATION
Smoke Alarm Written Statement of Compliance	The seller of a single family or two-unit dwellings, factory-built housing, a used manufactured home, used mobile home or used multi-unit manufactured housing must provide the buyer with a written statement indicating that the property is in compliance with current California law. Same exemptions for real property as from the TDS law. However, transfers to or from any governmental entity, and transfers by a beneficiary or mortgagee after foreclosure sale or trustee's sale, which are exempt under the TDS law, are <u>not</u> exempt from this law.	C.A.R. Forms TDS and MHTDS now include a statement of compliance. C.A.R. Form WHSD may be used when no TDS is used in the transaction. HCD Declaration must be used for used mobile homes, used manufactured homes, and used multi-unit manufactured housing, and be given to the buyer within 45 days prior to the transfer of title.	Legal Q&A, **Smoke Alarm Requirements** Cal. Health & Safety Code §§ 13113.8, 18029.6; 25 Cal. Code Regs. § 5545.
Special Flood Hazard Area	Sale of real property located in Zone "A" or " V" as designated by FEMA and if the seller or the seller's agent has actual knowledge <u>or</u> a list has been compiled <u>by parcel</u> and the notice posted at a local county recorder, assessor and planning agency. Also applies to manufactured homes and personal property mobile homes.	The seller's <u>agent</u> or the seller without an agent must disclose to the buyer if the property is in this Special Flood Hazard Area, if a parcel list has been prepared by the county and a notice identifying the location of the list is available at the county assessor, county recorder or county planning commission office, or if the seller or seller's agent has actual knowledge that the property is in an area. If a TDS is required in the transaction, either C.A.R. Form NHD, "Natural Hazard Disclosure Statement" or an updated Local Option disclosure form must be used to make this disclosure.	Legal Q&A, **Natural Hazard Disclosure Statement** Cal. Civ. Code § 1103; Cal. Gov't Code § 8589.3.

FIGURE 3.8 (continued):   List of Disclosures

SUBJECT	DISCLOSURE TRIGGER	DISCLOSURE REQUIREMENT (Brief Summary) FORM	C.A.R. INFORMATION SOURCE LAW CITATION
State Responsibility Area (Fire Hazard Area)	Sale of <u>any</u> real property located in a designated state responsibility area (generally a "wildland area") where the state not local or federal govt. has the primary financial responsibility for fire prevention. The California Department of Forestry provides maps to the county assessor of each affected county.[17] Also applies to manufactured homes and personal property mobile homes.	The seller must disclose to the buyer the fact that the property is located in this zone, the risk of fire, state-imposed additional duties such as maintaining fire breaks, and the fact that the state may not provide fire protection services. The disclosure must be made if maps are available at the county assessor, county recorder or county planning commission office, or if the seller has actual knowledge that the property is in the zone. If the map is not of sufficient accuracy or scale to determine whether the property is in this Area, then either the agent indicates "yes" that the property is in this Area or the agent may write "no" that the property is <u>not</u> in this Area, but then a report prepared by an expert verifying that fact must be attached to C.A.R. Form NHD. If a TDS is required in the transaction, either C.A.R. Form NHD, "Natural Hazard Disclosure Statement" or an updated local option disclosure form must be used to make this disclosure.	Legal Q&A, **Natural Hazard Disclosure Statement** Cal. Pub. Res. Code §§ 4125, 4136; Cal. Civ. Code § 1103.
Supplemental Property Tax Notice	Transfer[6] of residential real property of 1-4 units. Same exemptions as for the Transfer Disclosure Statement.	The seller or seller's agent must deliver to the buyer the statutory notice. C.A.R. Form SPT may be used.	Cal. Civ. Code § 1102.6c.

17

FIGURE 3.8 (continued): **List of Disclosures**

SUBJECT	DISCLOSURE TRIGGER	DISCLOSURE REQUIREMENT (Brief Summary) FORM	C.A.R. INFORMATION SOURCE LAW CITATION
Subdivided Lands Law	Sale, leasing, or financing of new developments (condos, PUDs) or conversions consisting of 5 or more lots, parcels, or interests. However, a transfer of a single property to 5 or more unrelated people (unless exempt) may also trigger this law. There are exemptions too numerous to discuss in this chart.	The owner, subdivider, or agent, prior to the execution of the purchase contract or lease, must give the buyer/lessee a copy of the final public report (FPR), preliminary public report (PPR), or the conditional public report (CPR) issued by the DRE. No offers may be solicited until the DRE has issued one of these three reports. If the DRE has issued a CPR or PPR, then offers may be solicited, but close of escrow is contingent upon issuance of the FPR. Contracts entered into pursuant to a PPR may be rescinded by either party; contracts entered into pursuant to a CPR are contingent upon satisfaction of certain specified conditions.	Legal Q&As, **Subdivided Lands Law**, and **Subdivision Applicability Chart** Cal. Bus. & Prof. Code §§ 11018.1, 11018.12; 10 Cal. Code Regs. § 2795. See generally, Cal. Bus. & Prof. Code §§ 11000 *et seq.*; 10 Cal. Code Regs. §§ 2790 *et seq.*
Subdivision Map Act	Any division of real property into 2 or more lots or parcels for the purpose of sale, lease, or financing. There are exemptions too numerous to discuss in this chart.	The owner/subdivider must record either a tentative and final map, or a parcel map (depending on the type of subdivision). Escrow on the transfer cannot close until the appropriate map has been recorded.	Legal Q&A, **Subdivision Applicability Chart** Cal. Gov't Code §§ 66426, 66428. *See generally*, Cal. Gov't Code §§ 66410 *et seq.*
Transfer Disclosure Statement	Transfer[6] of residential real property of 1-4 units. Also applies to manufactured homes and personal property mobile homes.	Sellers and real estate agents must complete a statutory disclosure form. C.A.R. Form TDS (statutory form for real property); C.A.R. Form MHTDS (statutory form for personal property mobile homes)	Legal Q&As, **Transfer Disclosure Statement Law**, and **Transfer Disclosure Statement**

FIGURE 3.8 (continued):   List of Disclosures

SUBJECT	DISCLOSURE TRIGGER	DISCLOSURE REQUIREMENT (Brief Summary) FORM	C.A.R. INFORMATION SOURCE LAW CITATION
			Exemptions Cal. Civ. Code §§ 1102 *et seq.*
Very High Fire Hazard Severity Zone	Sale of any real property. Also applies to manufactured homes and personal property mobile homes.	The seller must disclose the fact that the property is located within this zone and whether it is subject to the requirements of Gov't Code Section 51182 (e.g., clear brush, maintain fire breaks). The disclosure must be made if maps are available at the county assessor, county recorder or county planning commission office, or if the seller has actual knowledge that the property is in the zone. If the map is not of sufficient accuracy or scale to determine whether the property is in this zone, then either the agent indicates "yes" that the property is in this zone or the agent may write "no" that the property is <u>not</u> in this zone, but then a report prepared by an expert verifying that fact must be attached to C.A.R. Form NHD. If a TDS is required in the transaction, either C.A.R. Form NHD, "Natural Hazard Disclosure Statement" or an updated local option disclosure form must be used to make this disclosure.	Legal Q&A, **Natural Hazard Disclosure Statement** Cal. Gov't Code §§ 51178, 51183.5; Cal. Civ. Code § 1103.
Water Conserving Fixtures Compliance	Applies only to real property built on or before Jan. 1, 1994 containing water fixtures. Effective date of law for single-family residential real property is Jan. 1, 2017. Effective date for two or more	Noncompliant plumbing fixtures (defined in Section 1101.3(c)) must be replaced by water conserving plumbing fixtures.	Legal Q&A, Water-Conserving Plumbing Fixtures Cal. Civ. Code § 1101.1 *et seq.*

19

FIGURE 3.8 (continued):   List of Disclosures

SUBJECT	DISCLOSURE TRIGGER	DISCLOSURE REQUIREMENT (Brief Summary) FORM	C.A.R. INFORMATION SOURCE LAW CITATION
	unit resid. real prop. and commercial real prop is Jan. 1, 2019. Effective date where some types of permitted types of permitted improvements are made is Jan. 1, 2014. Exemptions: • Registered historical sites. • Certified not technically feasible by licensed plumber. • Water service disconnected.		
Water Conserving Fixtures Disclosure	Applies only to real property built on or before Jan. 1, 1994 containing water fixtures. Effective date of law for single-family residential real property is Jan. 1, 2017. Effective date for two or more unit residential real prop. and commercial real prop. is Jan. 1, 2019. Exemptions: • Registered historical sites. • Certified not technically feasible by licensed plumber. • Water service disconnected.	The seller or transferor must disclose in writing to the prospective transferee that the law requires that noncompliant plumbing fixtures must be replaced with water-conserving plumbing fixtures and the required date, and also whether the real property includes any noncompliant plumbing fixtures (Cal. Civ. Code § 1101.4(c) single family and Cal. Civ. Code § 1101.5(a) multi-family and commercial).	Cal. Civ. Code § 1101.1 et seq.
Water Heater Bracing Statement of	All real property with any standard water heater with a	All owners of new or replacement water heaters	Legal Q&A, Water Heater Bracing and

FIGURE 3.8 (continued):   **List of Disclosures**

SUBJECT	DISCLOSURE TRIGGER	DISCLOSURE REQUIREMENT (Brief Summary) FORM	C.A.R. INFORMATION SOURCE LAW CITATION
Compliance	capacity of not more than 120 gallons for which a pre-engineered strapping kit is readily available. Legislative intent suggests this law applies only to residential properties, but the language of the statute does not limit the requirement to residential properties. All used mobile homes, used manufactured homes, and used multi-family manufactured housing with a fuel gas-burning water heater.	and all owners of existing residential water heaters must brace, anchor or strap water heaters to resist falling or horizontal displacement due to earthquake motion. Water heaters located in closets are also subject to this law. The seller of real property must certify in writing to a prospective purchaser that he has complied with this section and applicable local code requirements. C.A.R. Forms TDS and MHTDS now include a statement of compliance. C.A.R. Form WHSD may be used when no TDS is used in the transaction. HCD Declaration must be used for used mobile homes, used manufactured homes, and used multi-unit manufactured housing, and be given to the buyer within 45 days prior to the transfer of title.	Disclosure Requirements Cal. Health & Safety Code §§ 19211, 18031.7; 25 Cal. Code Regs. § 4102.

ENDNOTES

1. It is imperative to check local disclosure requirements. Local law may be more stringent than state law in certain areas or there may be additional disclosures required.

2. "Sale" includes exchanges of real property and installment land sale contracts (also called real property sales contracts) (Cal. Civ. Code 2079.13(l)).

3. This provision also applies to leases with an option to purchase, ground leases of land improved with 1-4 residential units, and real property installment sales contracts (Cal. Civ. Code § 2079.1).

4. Transfers which can be made without a public report pursuant to Section 11010.4 of the Business and Professions Code are exempt from a TDS but not from the Homeowner's Guide.

5. This Guide is available from C.A.R. and/or local Boards/Associations.

6. "Transfer" for the purposes of this law means transfer by sale, exchange, lease with option to purchase, purchase option, ground lease coupled with improvements, installment land sale contract, or transfer of a residential stock cooperative (Cal. Civ. Code § 1102).

FIGURE 3.8 (continued):   List of Disclosures

7. These zones were formerly called, "Special Studies Zones." Some maps may still refer to the old name.

8. The maps may be purchased from BPS Reprographics by calling (415) 512-6550 with the names of the required maps. Special Publication 42 indicates the names of the maps of the Earthquake Fault Zones. This publication is available from the California Geological Survey (formerly the California Division of Mines and Geology) by calling (916) 445-5716.

9. Transfers which can be made without a public report pursuant to Section 11010.4 of the Business and Professions Code are exempt from a TDS but not from the Homeowner's Guide.

10. "Flood disaster area" means an area so designated by the U.S. Secretary of Agriculture or an area the President has declared to be a disaster or emergency as a result of flood conditions.

11. Transfers which can be made without a public report pursuant to Section 11010.4 of the Business and Professions Code are exempt from a TDS but not from the Homeowner's Guide.
12. This Guide is available from C.A.R. and/or local Boards/Associations.

13. This provision also applies to leases with an option to purchase, ground leases of land improved with 1-4 residential units, and real property installment sales contracts (Cal. Civ. Code § 2079.1).

14. "Transfer" for the purposes of this law means transfer by sale, exchange, lease with option to purchase, purchase option, ground lease coupled with improvements, installment land sale contract, or transfer of a residential stock cooperative (Cal. Civ. Code § 1103).

15. Transfers which can be made without a public report pursuant to Section 11010.4 of the Business and Professions Code are exempt from a TDS but not from the Homeowner's Guide.

16. The consumer information booklet entitled *Environmental Hazards, A Guide for Homeowners and Buyers* is available from C.A.R. and/or local Boards/Associations.

17. The Department of Forestry's telephone number is (916) 653-5121.

California law sometimes requires that a specific form (or exact language) be used. Examples are the AD, FLD, TDS, MHTDS, and the NHD. Others times, the law requires a disclosure but doesn't mandate that particular language be used. However, C.A.R. provides forms for that purpose--indicated in this chart by the words "may be used." The law doesn't require the use of these forms. Examples are the AVID, MCN, NTF, SBSA, SSD, SPQ, AS, AB, WHSD, REO, and REOL.

This chart is just one of the many legal publications and services offered by C.A.R. to its members. For a complete listing of C.A.R.'s legal products and services, please visit car.org.

Readers who require specific advice should consult an attorney. C.A.R. members requiring legal assistance may contact C.A.R.'s Member Legal Hotline at (213) 739-8282, Monday through Friday, 9 a.m. to 6 p.m. and Saturday, 10 a.m. to 2 p.m. C.A.R. members who are broker-owners, office managers, or Designated REALTORS® may contact the Member Legal Hotline at (213) 739-8350 to receive expedited service. Members may also submit online requests to speak with an attorney on the Member Legal Hotline by going to http://www.car.org/legal/legal-hotline-access/. Written correspondence should be addressed to:

CALIFORNIA ASSOCIATION OF REALTORS®
Member Legal Services
525 South Virgil Ave.
Los Angeles, CA 90020

22

FIGURE 3.8 (continued):   **List of Disclosures**

The information contained herein is believed accurate as of December 19, 2014. It is intended to provide general answers to general questions and is not intended as a substitute for individual legal advice. Advice in specific situations may differ depending upon a wide variety of factors. Therefore, readers with specific legal questions should seek the advice of an attorney.

SUMMARY

The purpose of the disclosure requirements in real estate practice is fairness. Parties deserve to have the facts before they make decisions. These facts include detrimental facts known by the agent that the buyer or the seller would likely consider in decision making. The duty of disclosure is inherent in an agency. The fiduciary duty of the agent requires full disclosure. There is also a duty to nonagency third parties to disclose known *detrimental information.*

To avoid misunderstandings, agents must explain the various agency options to both buyer and seller. The agent makes a selection, and the parties confirm the selection.

The seller has disclosure duties to the buyer. For 1–4-unit residential properties, the seller must complete a Real Estate Transfer Disclosure Statement. The agent must also provide the results of his visual inspection to the owner.

An agent need not disclose a death on the premises after three years. An agent also need not disclose that a former resident was afflicted with or died of AIDS. Stigmatized property should be disclosed if a buyer would reasonably want to know about it.

When there is seller financing, a seller financing addendum and disclosure is required. Buyers must be warned of any dangers.

For 1–4-unit residential properties built before January 1, 1960, the agent must disclose whether the dwelling has earthquake weaknesses. This is accomplished with a Residential Earthquake Hazards Report. For commercial property of specified construction, the seller or the seller's agent must give the buyer a copy of the *Commercial Property Owner's Guide to Earthquake Safety.*

Other required natural hazard disclosures are for the following: special flood hazard area, area of potential flooding, very high fire hazard severity zone, wildlife area that may contain substantial forest fire risks and hazards, earthquake fault zone, seismic hazard zone, and landslide inventory report.

These disclosures are made in a statutory form, the Natural Hazard Disclosure Statement.

Homeowners must be informed about environmental hazards on or affecting their property. The broker must provide a booklet to buyers on environmental hazards. Buyers and lessees also must be informed about hazardous substances released on or believed to be present on a property. Tenants must inform landlords if they release hazardous substances on the property.

For 1–4-unit residential properties built before 1978, purchasers must be given a *Protect Your Family from Lead in Your Home* booklet. Giving the buyers the California booklet, *Environmental Hazards: A Guide for Homeowners, Buyers, and Tenants*, also satisfies the federal requirement.

Prospective purchasers must be notified if a property is within 1 mile of a former military ordnance site where explosives might be located. Known water contamination must also be disclosed.

Subdivision disclosures include the public report and common interest information. Notices must also be provided to tenants of their rights when apartments are converted to common interest developments.

The Interstate Land Sales Act is a disclosure act governing sales of unimproved lots in interstate commerce. Its purpose is to prevent fraud. California has similar state disclosure requirements.

For common interest subdivisions, purchasers must be provided an information booklet on common interest subdivisions, as well as a copy of the CC&Rs, articles of incorporation, bylaws, rules and regulations, financial statement including changes, and plans for changes in assessments.

When there is seller financing, a seller financing addendum and disclosure is required. Buyers must be warned of any dangers.

Both federal and state laws require disclosures that must be made where applicable.

There are statutory rights of rescission for a number of disclosures.

CLASS DISCUSSION TOPICS

1. A property you have for sale is about two blocks from a park frequented by homeless people and prostitutes. So as not to offend prospective buyers, you avoid this area by a roundabout drive. Have you acted in a proper manner?

2. A buyer offers to trade 50 emeralds for a home you have listed. What, if any, are your obligations?

3. What environmental hazards would likely be present in your community?

4. Are there agents in your area who operate solely as buyer's agents? What are the advantages to a buyer in dealing with such an agent?

5. You receive what appears to be a fair offer from a prospective buyer; however, you know the buyer has sued sellers after purchasing several other properties. What do you tell your seller?

6. Evaluate your own home for possible environmental hazards.

7. Complete a Real Estate Transfer Disclosure Statement as if you were the seller of the property where you presently live.

8. Bring to class one current-events article dealing with some aspect of real estate practice for class discussion.

UNIT 3 QUIZ

1. Which of the following statements regarding an agent's duty in a real estate transaction is *TRUE*?
   a. An agent has a fiduciary duty to the principal.
   b. An agent must disclose any known detrimental information to a buyer, even when the agent represents the seller.
   c. Any material facts the agent becomes aware of must be disclosed to the principal.
   d. All of these are true.

2. Which of the following statements regarding agency disclosure is *TRUE*?
   a. An agent need not provide a seller of a commercial building with an agency disclosure.
   b. The listing agent cannot elect to be only a buyer's agent.
   c. Both of these are true.
   d. Neither of these is true.

3. Which of the following statements regarding agency disclosure is *TRUE*?
   a. The confirmation of agency must be in writing.
   b. The three steps of the disclosure process are disclose, elect, confirm.
   c. The selling agent must confirm the agency before the buyer makes an offer.
   d. All of these are true.

4. Which seller(s) must provide a Real Estate Transfer Disclosure Statement?
   a. The seller of a lot
   b. The seller of a 4-unit apartment building
   c. The seller of a 16-unit apartment building
   d. All of these

5. Under *Easton*, an agent's duty of inspection and disclosure covers
    a. all types of property.
    b. accessible and inaccessible areas.
    c. a visual inspection and known or should have known defects.
    d. none of these.

6. Which statement regarding earthquake safety disclosure is *TRUE*?
    a. It applies to 1–4-unit residential properties.
    b. It applies only to homes built before 1930.
    c. The buyer can waive her right to a hazards report.
    d. Delivery of a copy of *The Homeowner's Guide to Earthquake Safety* is evidenced by an affidavit from the agent.

7. The buyers sign that they have received a booklet relating to
    a. environmental hazards.
    b. floods, tornados, and earthquakes.
    c. foreclosure rights.
    d. rescission rights.

8. *Brownfields* is a term related to
    a. insect infestation.
    b. soil contamination.
    c. undeveloped acreage.
    d. seller financing.

9. The purpose of the Subdivided Lands Law is to
    a. prohibit premature subdivisions.
    b. set minimum physical standards.
    c. protect purchasers from fraud.
    d. allow for a uniform growth pattern.

10. A right of rescission is provided by law for purchase agreements involving all *EXCEPT*
    a. 1–4-unit residential properties.
    b. time-shares.
    c. undivided interest subdivisions.
    d. both b and c.

UNIT FOUR

PROSPECTING AND BUSINESS DEVELOPMENT

LEARNING OBJECTIVES

When you have completed this unit, you will be able to

- define prospecting and explain the importance of attitude in prospecting,

- describe methods of prospecting and sources of leads,

- understand regulations affecting prospecting, and

- explain the importance of the internet, farming, and a prospecting plan.

KEY TERMS

bird dogs   door-to-door   niche marketing
CAN-SPAM Act   canvassing   nongeographic farm
centers of influence   endless chain   prospecting
contact management   farming   real estate owned
    system   geographic farm   (REO)
do-not-call registry   megafarming   telephone canvassing
                                       networking

WHAT IS PROSPECTING?

Prospecting is the process of locating owners who are interested in selling property and prospective buyers who are interested in purchasing property.

> Prospecting is locating potential buyers and sellers.

Without prospecting, you would have much less inventory and fewer buyers. Real estate professionals know that even when buyers and sellers seek them out, it is often the result of prior prospecting or successfully helping someone they know.

Successful real estate agents understand that prospecting is an important element in their success. It is a continuing process of being aware of what is happening around them, organizing their efforts, being persistent, and developing problem-solving and time-management skills. Not only must licensees constantly prospect, they must have the proper attitude toward prospecting. A professional attitude includes considering prospecting a challenge and being positive and enthusiastic in speech and action. The author recommends the SSS system: *see* the people, *serve* the people, *sell* the people.

Develop the Proper Attitude

Prospecting is any method of exposure to people who can buy or sell real estate; hence, it is a major challenge to every licensee. The following questions will help you evaluate your own attitude toward prospecting:

■ **Do you consider prospecting a major challenge?** Successful real estate selling entails countless hours and considerable expenditure of energy to keep up with a highly competitive market. Your attitude is the key to your success.

- **Do you recognize the urgency to maintain a constant supply of new prospects?** It is absolutely necessary to provide yourself with a constant supply of customers. Prospects may be found most anywhere; they are all around you.

- **Do you have a well-organized system to use in prospecting?** Because of the many prospect sources available and the necessity of assigning priorities to these sources, advance planning is essential. To get the best results from your prospecting, an effective and well-organized prospecting system is essential.

- **Are you afraid of rejection?** Prospecting is searching for the one among many who needs your services. Therefore, you will encounter rejection more often than success. Fear of being rejected is one of the contributing factors to failure of new licensees. You must take rejection professionally and not personally.

Many successful agents use licensed assistants to aid them in prospecting. When an assistant locates prospective buyers or sellers, the agent then takes over. This frees the agent for "A" Time activities (Unit 1).

METHODS OF PROSPECTING

The successful salesperson is always prospecting. A good prospector knows and accepts that different groups of people have not only varying interests and motivations but also substantially different political, social, philosophical, and economic views. Prospecting is less a matter of getting listings and sales than it is a matter of developing sources for listings and sales. A licensee's ability to do this is limited only by imagination and commitment.

The prospecting method that will produce the best results varies according to the agent and the situation. The broker or the salesperson should choose a method or methods based on the following:

- Type of property involved
- Period of time planned for

- Types of prospects

- Neighborhood and property characteristics, including the properties themselves (number of bedrooms and baths, etc.), income characteristics of the neighborhood (income, family, and social interests), changes taking place (such as a changeover from single-family to multiple-family dwellings), special advantages of the location (schools, shopping centers, recreation areas, and so forth), and special interests and groups to which the agent belongs

After taking these factors into consideration, licensees also should review their own sales skills and personality and choose methods that emphasize their strengths and minimizes their weaknesses. The following material covers just a few of the methods for prospecting. Real estate salespersons should consult with their brokers as to the selection and implementation of prospecting methods.

Door-to-Door Canvassing

While shunned by some real estate agents, **door-to-door canvassing** can be an excellent way to cover a geographic area. Successful canvassers know the number of people they must contact to obtain one good lead. They set goals of a particular number of contacts to achieve the number of leads they desire. They treat a rejection as one contact closer to another lead.

The best times to canvass are obviously when residents are home. With the large percentage of two-income families, early evenings or Saturday mornings are effective times. In retirement areas, daytime canvassing between 9 am and 11 am and between 2 pm and 4 pm could be effective. Do not canvass door to door after dark.

Canvassing an area having many retirees can be particularly beneficial, because many people welcome someone to talk to and can offer valuable information as to needs of neighbors.

When you canvass door to door, step back from the door after you ring the bell so you won't appear menacing. Don't carry a briefcase because this also can be menacing. A notepad or a clipboard is far less intimidating. Smile when you talk, and keep in mind that you must get the homeowner's attention within the first 20 seconds. In some areas, more doors will be opened to women than to men. Women are generally considered less intimidating.

Published reverse directories giving occupants' names from the address are now available in only a few areas. However, internet sites such as www.whitepages.com/ reverse can provide occupants' names from an address. This is particularly valuable when approaching a for sale by owner.

A sample approach for door-to-door canvassing would be as follows:

- Introduce yourself and give your broker affiliation.

- Explain why you are at their front door. An excellent reason is to ask if they can help find a home for a particular family. People often like to help specific persons but have little interest in people in general. Never use a fictitious family. Simply describe one of the people you are working with to find a home. Never give out names or personal information about prospective buyers without their permission. Let the property owner know why you are interested in the specific area, such as a particular school, park, transportation, employment, et cetera.

- Ask if they know of anyone in the area who is planning to move or has had a change in family circumstances that might cause the person to contemplate a move. Also ask owners about their own specific plans. Ask owners if they or any of their neighbors might have any real estate purchase or sale plans for a home, second home, or investment property.

- Ask whether they would like to receive free (monthly) emails or newsletters showing the number of properties in the area that are on the market, the average listing price per square foot, and similar sale information.

- Thank the owner, leave your card, and jot down responses for future reference.

After a home has been sold by you or your office, a door-to-door canvass of the neighborhood can be especially effective. Consider the following approach, replacing the words in brackets with words that fit your situation:

> Good morning [Mrs. Smith]. I am [Jane Thomas] from [Uptown Realty]. We have just sold the [Kowalski] home at [211 Elm down the block; the house with the large pine tree in the front yard]. The new owners are [Mr. and Mrs. Collins. He is an engineer, and she teaches first grade at Sunnyside School. They have one daughter, Mary Ann, who is nine years old]. I hope you will welcome them to your neighborhood.
>
> As you undoubtedly realize, you live in a desirable area. In advertising the [Kowalski] home, we were contacted by a number of families whose needs we were unable to meet. Right now, I am looking for a home for a very fine family. [He is an accountant who is being transferred to our area from Ohio. They have two sons, ages three and six.] I need help in finding them a home. Do you know anyone who is planning to move? Has anyone in the area recently had a change in family size because of marriage, divorce, birth, or death, or has anyone recently retired? (Again, never give out personal information without approval. You want to present the prospective buyer as someone who would be welcome as a neighbor.)

Note: You first showed your competence by a sale, gave them information about a new neighbor, and then asked them for help for a particular family.

Consider visiting the clubhouse or pool of common-interest developments. You will often find people who are not only willing but eager to talk to you. This is especially true in retirement communities. By asking questions, you may get referrals of possible sellers or buyers. When you contact these referrals, it is not really a cold call because they were recommended to you by a friend.

Besides canvassing for listings, you can canvass for buyers. By working an area around a new listing, you can approach owners with information about the listing and ask their help in choosing their new neighbors. Most people like their neighborhood and will tell you if they have any friends or acquaintances who might be considering relocating.

When canvassing around a listing, you should tell the party about the home that is available and ask whether they have a friend, family member, or coworker who might like to move to the area. You are giving them an opportunity to help pick their new neighbors.

Canvassing rentals around a new listing can be an effective method of securing buyers.

> (Good Morning) I am _____ from (Realty). We have just listed a (3BR, 2 bath Cape Cod home) on (Sycamore Street) just (2 blocks) from here. I can show you how ownership can be a reality not just a dream. Would you rather remain here as a renter or own your own (single) family home?

With currently rising rents and relatively low interests, home payments are likely to be in line with or lower than rent. If you can get renters to listen to how they can be owners, you will have prospects to work with.

In some areas, agents like to canvass in teams, with each agent taking every other house. Team canvassing can help keep agents motivated to complete the goal you jointly set. A team approach also gives a canvasser a feeling of greater security.

Note: In some communities, door-to-door canvassing is not allowed or might require a permit.

Telephone Canvassing

The Federal Communications Commission has established the National Do Not Call Registry to protect consumers from unwanted commercial solicitations. Landline, as well as all telephone numbers, may be registered. The fine for calling someone whose name appears in the **do-not-call registry** is up to $16,000 per call.

WEB LINK

If you make calls seeking buyers, sellers, lessees, or lessors of property or to solicit any services, you should do so only after checking the registry. For detailed information about accessing the registry and exemptions, it is suggested that you check www.donotcall.gov.

There is a relatively simple solution that avoids paging through huge lists. It is the use of a software program that scrubs the number of people who are on the do-not-call registry. There are now dozens of such programs available, such as www.scrubdnc.net/faq.aspx and www.safecaller.com.

WEB LINK

WEB LINK

Brokers who do not use a scrubber program can request an account number, which can be given to agents. Agents can then access the registry by area code on the internet at https://www.telemarketing.donotcall.gov. A broker can obtain access to five area codes at no charge, but there is a charge for additional area codes.

Telephone solicitors often use automatic dialers in conjunction with scrubbers. Automatic dialers are prohibited as to cellphone numbers.

The following are some exceptions to the do-not-call rules:

Do-not-call lists are available from the Federal Trade Commission by area code, and up to five area codes will be provided free of charge. Each additional area code requires a $25 fee. It is necessary to check the updates on the registry at least every 90 days. For greater details, visit the website, *https:// www.donotcall.gov*.

- You may call a listed party if you have an existing business relationship (within 18 months of a purchase, sale, or lease).

- You may call a party within three months of an inquiry the party made.

- You may call people who have given you written permission to call.

- You may call commercial numbers (the registry only applies to residential phones).

- You may call the numbers on for-sale-by-owner ads or signs as a buyer representative, but not for the purpose of obtaining seller representation.

- You may call for survey purposes, but no solicitation for representation can be included in the call.

Because of the restrictive do-not-call rules, you should obtain written permission to make further calls when working with buyers, sellers, and even visitors to open houses.

Direct Mail Canvassing

Direct mail is an expensive way to canvass but with do-not-call restrictions, besides direct contact, it is the only way to reach many parties. Because of cost, agents should carefully plan their mailings and keep track of response rates from different mailings. To be effective, a mailing must get attention and result in action. (See Figures 4.1 and 4.2.)

FIGURE 4.1: **Sample Mailing**

UR

H O M E   R E A L T Y

_____ ⟵——— _Date and address_
_____
_____
_____

Dear _____:

Can You Help a Neighbor?

We need a 3-bedroom home in your neighborhood for a [young family]. [The husband is an engineer and the wife is a schoolteacher. They have an 11-year-old son and a daughter who is 7. They would like to relocate prior to school in September and desire a home within walking distance of Midvale School.]

[1. I will be calling you in a few days to determine 2. Please call me] if you know of anyone in the neighborhood who might consider selling their home to this fine family.

Sincerely,

_____

Enclosure: ⟵——— _Card_

Note: While positive-appearing personal information can be an inducement to help a family, never include personal information without specific permission from the family.

Some general rules for direct mail canvassing include the following:

- Use a #10 plain envelope; don't use a window envelope.

- Don't use a mailing label; type or, preferably, hand-address the envelope.

- Consider first-class stamps (preferably commemorative stamps). If your letter looks like junk mail, it will likely be treated in that manner.

- Don't try to indicate that your letter is something it is not, such as by trying to give it the appearance of a government letter.

- If you get the reader's attention in the first few lines, the letter will be read in its entirety.

- If you indicate you will be contacting the recipient, you force them to consider your message. When you come to the owners' door, they will know why you are there.

- Never send out a mass mailing without test marketing the mailing piece.

- By keeping track of responses to different mailing pieces, you can eliminate ineffective mailings.

- Offering a premium such as a Dodger baseball cap for filling out a questionnaire can be effective in gaining information.

FIGURE 4.2: **Sample Mailing**

UR
HOME REALTY

_____ ◄—— *Date and address*

Dear _____:

I Apologize

If you want to buy a home in [Claridge Estates], I don't really have much to show you. There has been a terrific demand, and the few owners who have taken advantage of the market quickly sold their homes. However, if you really want to buy, call me and I will put your name on my list of buyers, and I will call or e-mail you as soon as properties come on the market.

Now if you are interested in selling, that's a different story! I can prepare a report for you of recent comparable sales indicating the price range we can anticipate from a sale in the current market. This service is at no cost or obligation to you.

Want to take advantage of our offer? Call or e-mail me today.

Yours truly,

_____

P.S. If you would like to be on our e-mail list to receive new listing and sales information in your neighborhood, please sign up on our site, [www.ur-home.net].

If you have already listed your home for sale with another broker, please disregard this letter.

Enclosure: ◄——— *Card*

Email Solicitation

CAN-SPAM is an acronym for Controlling the Assault of Non-Solicited Pornography and Marketing.

To protect consumers from being assaulted by misleading unsolicited email messages, unsolicited emails must include the following:

- Opt-out mechanism where the recipient can indicate no more emails are to be sent

- Functioning return email address

- Valid subject line indicating a message is an advertisement

- Legitimate physical address of the mailer

It is a misdemeanor to send spam with falsified header information. Each violation is subject to a fine of up to $16,000.

Email solicitations are effective for both seller and buyer. A subject header such as "New Listing Edgemont Estates" or "No Down Payment— 4 Bedrooms" will likely get the email opened if it addresses a need or interest of the recipient. For potential sellers, receiving an email heading such as "Real Estate Sales Activity -Edgemont Estates" can be effective. A monthly email showing the number of listings and sales, average price, price per square foot, as well as high and low prices for both listings and sales is of interest to many owners. Many of the same firms that provide mailing lists for areas also provide email addresses by zip code. Because of low costs and a greater consumer reliance on the internet, internet solicitations are playing a significant role in prospecting.

While email solicitations are low cost, you should realize that an estimated 70 to 80% of email real estate solicitations never get opened. Consider using an email distribution program to manage lists and generate reports as related to your email campaigns.

Building an Email Database

An often overlooked aspect of marketing for real estate agents is the amount of people they meet each and every day that could be added to an email database. New agents should make a conscious effort to put every person who comes into an open house, or every prospect they meet, into an email database to receive marketing material from them. Because the sales cycle for real estate can be quite long, staying at the top of a potential client's mind is crucial to getting the deal at the right time.

In terms of for sale by owners and expired listings, we might want to let readers know where they can purchase these leads. If not where, we should probably let them know that they can buy these leads if they want to. The most popular and commonly used are sites such as www.theredx.com and www.landvoice.com.

WEB LINK

Fax Solicitations

The federal Telephone Consumer Protection Act and FCC regulations prohibit sending unsolicited advertisements and solicitations to a fax machine. Permission to send a fax message can be granted only by a signed statement that includes the fax number to which the fax may be sent. This requirement rules out fax messages for initial contacts for real estate solicitation purposes. A penalty of $1,500 may be assessed for each unsolicited fax.

Newsletters

Many brokers have successfully used newsletters as a prospecting tool. Newsletters are more likely to be read if they include local information about events and people, local athletic team event dates and results, recipes, and important local telephone numbers, as well as real estate information such as mortgage rates and market sales data. A number of vendors supply newsletters, some of which can be readily customized. Members of the California Association of REALTORS® have access to a free newsletter that can be personalized by accessing www.car.org and checking on the newsletter sign-up balloon and then selecting Homeowner's Guide. Newsletters can be mailed, emailed, and left in clubhouses and other public places.

WEB LINK

EXPIRED LISTINGS

Never contact owners before their listing has expired. Attempting to solicit a listing away from another REALTOR® is a violation of the NAR Code of Ethics. When contacting the owners, you want to find out immediately if they have relisted the property with their agent or another agent. If they have, wish them well and end the discussion.

When a listing contract expires, it means the listing office was unsuccessful in procuring a buyer for a property during the contract period. Owners will likely sign a new listing contract with their agent if they are satisfied with the efforts of that agent. If not, the owners may try to sell their property without an agent. But, in most cases, they will list their property with another office. Your approach should be low key. You should realize that the owners are likely frustrated and even distrustful of agents. They may have heard a very positive presentation and assurances of success that did not materialize. If you can convince owners that you know why their property didn't sell and show them a plan likely to lead to success, you have a good chance at the listings.

> If you can show why a property failed to sell and how you can succeed, you have an opportunity to list the property.

The reason a property failed to sell could be related to an agent who failed to market it properly. More likely, however, it relates to the price asked and/or the appearance of the property (exposure). Very simply, a home must be competitive in its marketplace to sell. When there are many sellers and few buyers, being competitive is not enough. A home must appear and be priced in such a manner that it stands out above the competition as a "best buy."

If owners are negative or antagonistic during a front-door approach, consider asking for a glass of water. Chances are you won't be refused because the simple act of helping you puts the owners in a better mood. Frustrated sellers need and want to be heard. Let the sellers go on about the failure of their last agent to secure a buyer and be empathetic toward them.

Then ask three questions:

1. Why do you think your home failed to sell?

2. What could have been done better?

3. Would you like to hear my analysis of why there isn't a Sold sign on your home right now?

An advantage of working expired listings is that owners generally now have more realistic expectations than they had when their property was originally listed for sale.

NEWSPAPER LEADS

Newspapers can provide a number of sources of buyers and sellers. When checking newspapers for leads, don't forget that there are other papers besides the large daily papers. There are "shoppers," or throwaway papers, usually devoted entirely to ads; there are papers for groups, such as for mobile home owners; and there is a wide variety of ethnic and foreign language papers. All of these papers contain leads.

For Sale by Owner (FSBO)

A major reason owners try to sell without an agent is that they feel they are saving a commission. Another reason could be related to a prior unpleasant experience with an agent. The owners must be shown that working with an agent is in their best interests, and that the agent will in fact be earning the compensation.

A simple way to get to talk to a for sale by owner (FSBO) is to visit the home and tell the owner about one of the buyers you are working with and then ask, "If I had an offer from this buyer, would you want to see it?"

Because few people would not want to see an offer, the answer likely will be in the affirmative. Of course, this gives you the opportunity to view the home. You could then ask for a one-party short-term listing if you feel you have a prospective buyer who would be interested in the property.

Another approach after introducing yourself might be to ask, "Would you be offended if I asked to see your home?" Most owners will answer in the negative, because, again, to say otherwise would be implying that they are offended.

When viewing a for-sale-by-owner property, you want to come across to the owners as a person they could like. Compliment them on noteworthy things, ask questions, and show you are interested. Make suggestions that will help them sell. Ask how they are advertising the property, what the response has been, their reason for selling, what they will do when they sell, et cetera. Answers can be listing ammunition.

An excellent approach to owners who are advertising their own homes is a front-door offer of a for-sale-by-owner kit:

> [Mr. Chan], I am [Gary Frank from Canyon Realty]. I can help you sell your home without any agent fees. Our office has put together a for-sale-by-owner kit that contains a For Sale sign, contracts, loan contacts, required disclosures, instructions for open houses, and a lot more information. We provide these kits absolutely free as a goodwill gesture. Of course, we hope that if you decide later you want professional assistance, you will consider [Canyon Realty]. I can give you one of these free kits now and show you how to use the forms, although it will take close to an hour to cover the forms and disclosures. Will you [and your wife] be home at seven tonight, or would eight be more convenient?

Your kit should be everything you discussed and more. Put warning labels on sheets that talk about subordination clauses, contingencies, owner points, and so on.

When you meet with the owners, give them the For Sale signs and ask to sit down to go over the forms. Suggest the kitchen table, because it is a non-threatening environment and allows for a physical closeness. Go over the forms, explaining the clauses, the importance of disclosures, and anything else your experience tells you is important for this seller to know. By the time you finish your presentation, the owners will probably be wondering if a sale without an agent is really as simple as they had imagined.

Ask the owner how he or she arrived at the price.

Next, ask, "May I inquire what you're asking for your home? How did you arrive at that price?"

The owners' price likely is based on a single sale or what they would like to get for the property. Continue with, "It would be presumptuous of me to tell you if the price is high or low, but our firm can prepare a comparative market analysis from our computer data. I would like to do a comparative market analysis on your home. This is, of course, provided at no charge."

Chances are the owners will accept your offer. They have already received valuable material, and you have likely sold yourself as a professional. Your appointment to present the market analysis should be on the next day.

After you present the market data analysis, ask the owners if you could just take a few minutes to express why you feel they should consider having an agent. After giving them all this valuable material, the owners will feel obligated to answer in the affirmative. You can then go into a listing presentation. (See Units 5 and 6.)

A variation of the this approach is to offer the owners the use of Open House signs and banners. Use the presence of signs and banners as a reason to follow up with the seller. "How's our sign holding up, Mr. Johnson?" "Is there anything else I can help you with?" These questions provide the agent a reason to continue to follow up with the for sale by owner. Generally, most for sale by owners either end up listing with an agent or taking the property off the market. Consistent follow-up will put you in the front running when the seller does decide to list.

Rental Ads

When a single-family or a mobile home is advertised for rent, it may be a case of an owner who really wants to sell but who needs income for payments. If the owners indicate they will give a tenant an option to purchase, you know they want to sell. Telephone numbers outside the area are more likely than local numbers to signify owners highly motivated to sell. Owner contact can be made face to face or by letter.

Whenever you receive a rental inquiry at your office or through canvassing, don't dismiss the prospect because you don't have any rentals. Prospective renters can frequently be turned into buyers with just a few questions: "Have you considered buying?" "Would you be interested in buying if you could buy with no or very little down payment and have monthly payments similar to what you would pay in rent?"

If you can show prospective renters how they can be buyers, you gain a lead for your existing listings and increase the likelihood of closing a sale. If a prospective renter was formerly an owner, chances are she is not going to be happy as a renter.

Trades

People advertising willingness to trade usually want to sell. By explaining delayed exchanges (see Unit 14), you can show owners how they can sell and still have their trade. Keep in mind that some people advertising trades may be dealers.

Marriage and Engagement Announcements

These announcements can be a source of leads. Perhaps the couple getting married have one or more previous residences each that they want to sell. The couple may also be looking to purchase a new residence. It is also possible that parents of the couple may be wishing to downsize or relocate. These are all prospects worth talking to.

Birth Announcements

Birth announcements could be leads to listings of condominiums or mobile homes and even to sales of single-family homes.

Legal Notices

Notices of legal action can be an excellent source of leads for motivated buyers and sellers. Rather than checking through county records, consider subscribing to a legal notice newspaper in your county.

Foreclosure.   When a notice of default is recorded, it indicates an owner is in trouble. Often the only help is a speedy sale. Keep in mind that just because a property is in foreclosure does not mean it is a good listing opportunity. Before listing, obtain a property profile from a title company. (A *property profile* is a computer printout showing the owner of the property and the liens against the property. It is a free service that title companies provide to the real estate profession.) Keep in mind that even if the liens against the property could exceed the property value, a short sale might be possible.

Legal notices indicate problems and problems = opportunities.

Probate.   Heirs who inherit property often prefer cash. In other cases, the property must be sold to pay debts of the estate or to carry out the wishes of the deceased. Contact the executor or administrator of the estate for a listing.

Divorce. The largest asset of most families is their home. Because California is a community property state, divorce often means that a home must be sold so the assets can be divided.

Bankruptcy. In California, owners in bankruptcy may be able to keep their homes because of their homestead exemption. However, many people in bankruptcy seek a new start and often wish to relocate. A sale listing may therefore be possible. Keep in mind that based on when the listing is taken, the bankruptcy court may need to approve the listing contract and subsequent payment of commissions.

Death notices. Although death of a spouse frequently means a sale, it can be difficult to solicit a listing after a death. We recommend that no approach be made for at least one month after a death, and then the approach could be to ask the homeowner's help in locating a home in the area for a particular family. An owner who is at all interested in relocating will bring it up.

Evictions. An eviction means an owner with a problem. When owners of income property don't have problems, they are not likely to be highly motivated to sell. When owners have problems, motivation to sell increases in relation to the seriousness of the problems. Eviction notices are a good source of motivated sellers.

Building permits. An individual who takes out a building permit could still own another home. Because of the length of the building period, that individual might intend to place the other home on the market later. When the building permit is taken out in the name of the builder, it could mean that a home is being built for speculation. In either case, building permit calls might produce excellent listings.

Code violations. Notices of code violations and/or fines indicate an owner with a problem property. Owners who don't want to deal with these problems can be motivated sellers.

Tax delinquencies. Owners delinquent in taxes might have financial problems. The solution to their problem could be a sale. These notices can be an excellent listing source.

When owners have legal problems or personal or family problems, the best approach is to ask the owner's help in meeting the needs of another. Any indication that you are contacting them because they are in serious difficulty would likely result in a defensive and negative reaction.

OTHER PROSPECTING METHODS

Advertising

Besides using it as a selling tool, advertising can be used to obtain listings.

Roy Brooks was a legendary estate agent in England. He gained celebrity status because of his unusual and very effective ads. He found that an advertisement for property to sell that was like everyone else's ads made his ad just one among many. He realized that ads for listings had to stand out from the others. To do this, he advertised for particular prospective buyers. One of the ads Roy Brooks used was the following:

> WE HAVE A RATHER REPULSIVE OLD MAN who, with his child-wife, is looking for an elegant town res. pref. Belgravia, Chelsea, or S. Ken. Price not important but must be realistic as he has, at least, his head screwed on the right way. Usual scale of commission required. ROY BROOKS.

Make your ad stand out.

Note: Before you use an ad such as this, get permission from the "repulsive old man and his child-wife."

Look for Problems

As you drive around, look for problem properties: properties in need of repair, overgrown landscaping, properties obviously vacant, and properties that have had rental signs up for a long time. Also watch for For Sale by Owner signs.

Visible problems usually mean the need for a change in ownership, a problem you, as a real estate professional, are prepared to solve. You can locate the owners of these properties by checking with the county tax assessor's office or a title company.

Internet Site

California Association of REALTORS® surveys illustrate the growing use of the internet by homebuyers. Only 28% of buyers utilized the internet in 2000. In 2005, 62% of homebuyers indicated that the internet was an integral part of their homebuying process, up from 56% in 2004, and by 2007, the number increased to 72%. A 2009 REALTOR® study in Massachusetts revealed that 90% of homebuyers utilized the internet in the buying process, and in 2014 it had risen to 92%.

Studies indicate that internet buyers devoted more time to research before working with an agent and spent just two weeks looking with an agent and viewed just 6.2 homes. Buyers who did not use the internet spent an average of seven weeks working with an agent and viewed 14.5 homes before making a purchase.

The growing importance of the internet reinforces the need for brokers to use internet sites to achieve maximum benefits. An office website or personal website should be referenced on all of your cards, ads, and letters. Such a site could show your success in an area, as well as any value changes in the area. One way to show success is a "success list" of properties sold. The site also could show advantages of low interest rates, indicating that the time to sell or buy couldn't be better.

The design of an internet site is not the place for economy. While there are self-help books and computer programs for designing your own site, and designers who advertise that they will prepare your site for $200 or less, site preparation is not the place for bare-bones economy. Many sites use motion and sound to keep the prospect watching. View a variety of sites, including those of other brokers, and strive for a site designer who will better your competition. The prevalence of IDX searches allows MLS data to be displayed on the agent's website directly. This can be a cost-effective solution and gives the agent the ability to tell a buyer or a seller to search the MLS directly from the agent's website.

We have included a sample home page (Figure 4.3) to give you ideas for what can be done. While there is motion on this site, it doesn't appear in print. The main picture changes with views of Sun City as well as offerings.

Some brokers have home pages on their sites where a viewer can click "find a home" or "What does (Jones Realty) have to offer?" The latter sells your firm's competence and integrity.

The "find a home" portion of your site can result in calls from "half-sold" buyers you didn't know existed but who had visited your firm on a website.

FIGURE 4.3:   Bob & Michael Horne WEBSITE

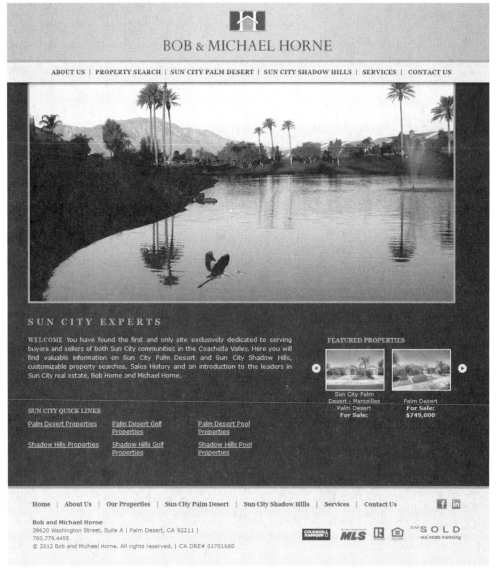

Used with the permission of Bob and Michael Horne.

WEB LINK

A single property can be presented on numerous separate websites. As an example, a home located in the Coachella Valley could be presented on www.Realtor.com and other national sites. It could also be on an area site. In addition, if the broker belongs to a relocation service or a franchise, or both, property could be presented on additional sites. General websites such as www.craigslist.com attract millions of viewers. Many brokers realize that these sites can be especially productive. It is not unusual for a broker-age firm to have their offerings on from 6 to 10 websites, including their own firm's site.

By checking competitors' internet presentations of their listings, you will see a significant variance. Some properties indicate "picture not available," while others not only have an attractive exterior photo but also allow the viewer to click on additional photos, a detailed property description, and possibly even a virtual tour.

A visitor to your website might not be interested in your offerings and go elsewhere. You want to know who that visitor was and what his interests are. You can get this information with a nonthreatening offer of help. Offering to provide emails of new listings before they are even advertised is a great hook, because most buyers are interested in a first chance, especially in an active market. The visitor would then fill in price parameters, must-have and would-like features, and finally their name and email address.

You can also prospect for both buyers and sellers by using mailings or ads offering to supply owners with details of sales (by email), so that they can understand area values. They would register on your site, giving details of a home that they want comparables for. The emails they would receive would include photos and details, as well as sale prices of similar home sales. Because you are providing an owner with information of interest, a personal contact should result in a positive response.

Just as classified ads (discussed in Unit 8) are in competition with other classified ads, your internet property presentations are in competition with many others. (It is important that you incorporate what you will learn in Unit 8 into your website.)

WEB LINK

Websites of others can also be a source for leads. By checking www.forsale-byowner.com, you might find homes in your area that you might not have known were on the market. There are a number of other sites that include for-sale-by-owner listings, such as www.craigslist.org, forsalebyowner.com, www.homepointe.com, www.owners.com, FSBO.com and HomesByOwner.com.

In Unit 8, you will learn many ways to use the internet, including social media sites and blogs.

Check Interested Parties

Property neighbors. When you have a listing of land or income property, contact adjoining property owners, as well as owners of similar property in the area. Neighbors are a source of both buyers and sellers. For residential property, the approach to neighbors could be "Would you like to help choose your new neighbor?" When neighbors have an interest in an outcome, they can be an effective source of prospects.

For income property, as well as farms and raw land, adjoining property owners are good buyer candidates. All many people want is "What's mine and what's next to mine."

Investors and speculators. When an investment property is sold, find out who the buyer is. The same holds true for lots and fixer-uppers. Contact these buyers to find out if they have further interests in purchasing property and, if so, what their interests are. It isn't hard to find the active players in a market. Many of these buyers will welcome an additional pair of eyes, ears, and legs working for them. Keep in mind that these people can be prospects for both listing and selling.

Lenders. Check with local lenders about their **real estate owned (REO)** properties. Find out how to get a key to show the property, as well as what commission will be paid, if any.

Some brokers offer full service for lenders. They offer cleanup service and full maintenance services to protect the property until it can be sold. These services give them an advantage over other brokers as to exclusive listings besides creating another profit center.

Besides local lenders, contact the Department of Housing and Urban Development (HUD) and the Federal Deposit Insurance Corporation (FDIC), as well as the Federal Housing Administration (FHA) and the Department of Veterans Affairs (VA) for foreclosure lists. Many agents specialize in selling lender-owned property.

Chambers of commerce. Check with your local chamber of commerce. Ask to be notified of inquiries made by people or companies planning to relocate to your area. If you can reach them first by letter or email, you may be in a preferred position as a possible selling agent.

Membership in a chamber of commerce will help you obtain inquiry information in a timely fashion. Membership can also provide networking opportunities that can bring business. Many networking groups are limited to one representative from each industry. You don't want to end up in a group dominated by other real estate agents.

Open houses.   Open houses can be a good source of both buyer and seller leads. Many people who stop at an open house can't be buyers until they sell their present homes. Some agents will hold open houses on homes listed by other agents within their firm if the property has an attractive exterior (curb appeal) and is on a high-traffic street. Each open house can build a pool of potential buyers with some similarity of interests. If you intend to specialize in an area, price range or type of property, conducting open houses that fall into the category you are interested in can help build a huge pool of new listings to contact. (Open houses are covered in detail in Unit 7.)

> The endless chain method is the process of using prospects to recommend other prospects ad infinitum.

Endless chain.   The basis of the **endless chain**, or referral, method of prospecting is to ask every prospect to recommend other prospects. The use of an endless chain can result in an amazing number of referral prospects. For example, if you secure the names of two prospects from every person you interview, you would get two names from your first prospect; these two should yield four; these four should provide eight; and so on. This can continue, eventually resulting in thousands who are at least potential clients, people whose needs have not yet been determined.

Your friends.   One of the first things you should do on entering the real estate business is to make a list of all the acquaintances and friends you have made over the years. Your list should contain a minimum of 50 names. A good place to start is your holiday card list. Send these people an announcement that you are in the real estate business and indicate how proud you are that your work may give you an opportunity to help them in the future. Be sure to send announcements to the professional people who serve you and who over the years have had your faith and confidence—your doctor, dentist, attorney, and any other professional people you deal with. Because you do business with them, it is likely they will be willing to do business with you.

Another community resource that should not be overlooked is the people with whom you do non–real estate business. You have to buy food, clothing, gas, personal services, and so on. Tell the people who sell things or services to you that you are in the real estate business. These people come in contact with other people every day, and from time to time they hear of someone who is thinking of listing and selling a home or buying a new home. Such communication is commonly called **networking**.

Your sellers.   A sale normally is part of a chain reaction. Sellers of property generally become buyers of other properties, and those sellers, in turn, buy again. Even before a property is sold, find out the intention of the owners. If they will be buyers within the area, you want to be the agent who will sell to them. If they are leaving the area, consider that a referral fee could be possible from an agent in their new community.

Your buyers.   Most people are glad they purchased their homes. If you sold houses to some of these satisfied buyers, you can turn this positive feeling buyers have about their purchases to your benefit. Stopping by with a small housewarming gift several weeks after they take occupancy will give you an opportunity to talk about their relatives and friends who have real estate needs. Whenever you get a listing in the area, contact former buyers by phone or email to see if they have friends who might be interested.

You can also use the approach of asking them to help another:

> I could use your help. I'm trying to find a home for [a retired couple] who wish to live in your area because [they want to be close to their grandchildren]. Do you know anyone in the area who might consider selling or anyone who has had a change in family size because of marriage, divorce, birth, or graduation?

Note: Always use a real prospect, but never give out personal information without

Your neighbors.   Another broker's sign on a neighbor's home shows that you have failed to make your neighbors realize that you are a real estate professional who is available to meet their needs. When you enter the real estate profession, consider a mailing to your neighbors. Figure 4.4 is a broker letter to neighbors of a new sales associate.

Take a walk around your neighborhood with your child or your dog to give you an opportunity to talk to neighbors. Let them know you are in real estate and where you live. Hand out business cards. By asking questions you can find leads. In most neighborhoods, there are a few people who seem to know everything that is happening. These people should be developed as your extra pairs of eyes and ears.

In condominium complexes and mobile home parks, spend time around the recreational facilities. You will seldom have any trouble finding someone to talk to. By knowing what to ask, you can quickly discover what is happening in the area.

Centers of Influence

Another successful prospecting method is to cultivate the friendship of influential persons in the community or territory. These **centers of influence** can help you obtain prospects by referring people who can use your services. These influential people can tell others about you and tell you about people they know who might require professional real estate services. Centers of influence serve to bring you together with potential sellers and buyers.

The objective of cultivating relationships with centers of influence is to establish genuine friendships, whenever possible. It is important that they know their help will be appreciated in your search for contacts. Let your centers of influence know the results of their efforts. This will come naturally if the friendship is genuine, and it will encourage the person to keep helping you.

Some agents refer to these helpers as **bird dogs**. This term is not derogatory. It merely indicates that they point the way. Keep in mind that help won't come to you unless you ask for it.

> **Centers of influence** are people who are influential in your community.

You must explain what you are looking for, such as a friend or acquaintance who has had a change in family size. Having several dozen extra pairs of eyes and ears working for you can provide a great many leads. The best bird dogs are people who help you because they like you and want to see you succeed. However, for continued effort on your behalf, these helpers must feel they are appreciated. Your appreciation can be verbal; better yet, take them to dinner or give a small personal gift to show your appreciation. While it is a violation of the real estate law to reimburse an unlicensed party for acts requiring a real estate license, compensation may be provided to an individual whose involvement is limited to putting two parties together. Prohibited acts would be paying fees to persons soliciting buyers or sellers, showing property, giving property information, or engaging in any form of negotiation.

FIGURE 4.4: **New Associate Announcement Letter**

Note: Don't give out personal information about anyone, even your own salespeople, without permission. Many people don't want information about their children given out.

Good Centers of Influence

- Prominent club members
- Friends
- Relatives
- Attorneys
- Doctors
- Accountants
- Physical therapists
- Dog groomers
- Hair dressers
- Prominent members of civic and charitable organizations

- Golf and tennis professionals
- Ministers, priests, and rabbis
- Bankers
- Public officials
- Teachers
- Health club employees
- Business executives
- People with whom you share a mutual interest, such as a hobby or recreational activity

Community Service

Closely akin to the centers-of-influence method is prospecting through local community service groups. Making contacts by participating in community activities can not only bring in more business but also provide personal satisfaction from working for the benefit of others.

Community service organizations recommended for involvement include the following:

- Churches and other houses of worship
- PTAs
- Educational groups
- College associations
- Chambers of commerce
- Civic organizations
- Service groups
- Boys and girls clubs
- Boy Scouts and Girl Scouts
- Recreational clubs (ski, travel, biking, boating, etc.)
- YMCAs and YWCAs
- Political organizations
- Senior centers

Community activities can also provide these benefits:

- Opportunities to counsel fellow members in such areas as investments, property management, and commercial realty
- Constant exposure to referral sources
- Constant exposure to other property owners
- Personal development, by learning and growing through participation
- Development of a more professional image as a real estate licensee

Your peers will have greater respect for a colleague who participates in community activities. The key is to get involved with people and help fulfill their needs. In seeking contacts through community service groups, however, beware of overcommitment. It is important to develop the ability to say no gracefully. Overcommitting yourself can upset your timetable and also may jeopardize your health. Follow these guidelines:

- Work in only one or two organizations at one time; strive for quality, not quantity

- Anticipate time-consuming assignments before becoming involved

- Do not play personalities for an advantage

- Do not play politics

To stay aware of what is going on, participate where possible in carefully selected committees. Membership on the following committees has proved to be most helpful to licensees:

- Greeting committee (new members)

- Membership committee

- Social or party committee

- "Sunshine" (visit the sick, etc.) committee

Be cautious in using membership as a prospecting technique, because it is easy to turn off fellow members by being overly aggressive. Obtain help from others, but do not abuse them. When you first join a club or association, keep a low profile. It is advisable to do something for the organization and strengthen your relationships before you ask members for referrals.

Fundraising for a worthwhile charity is an excellent way to meet people. While there may be a negative reaction to having to open their wallets, you will have shown that you are a person with a positive community interest.

Build a Referral List

Agents must bring some sort of order to their prospect lists to avoid getting stuck with a briefcase full of names and little else. To build a list and successfully use referrals, the licensee should follow these guidelines:

Develop a systematic plan. This includes studying prospects as you talk to them. Ask for leads as soon after contact as feasible, and ask the prospects how you can improve your services.

Keep track of the results of your methods.

Utilize all sources of information. This includes friends, neighbors, professionals, people in businesses of all kinds, and social contacts.

Make them all aware that you are in the real estate business and would appreciate all referrals.

Follow up referrals by reporting back to the referrer. Also important is to use a computer contact management system to record referrals for future calls. A person giving a negative response now may still be in the market in the future.

There are a number of software programs for contact management. Sage Software has *Act! Premium Software*, a specific program for real estate professionals.

FARMING

Farming is working or prospecting an area or area of interest for sellers as well as buyers. The area chosen for farming can be geographic or non-geographic (a special interest area). Your farm should be chosen based on your personal goals, interests, and your specific market area. The longer you work a farm, the more productive it becomes. Farming requires constant attention and regular contacts.

Geographic Farms

A **geographic farm** is a specific area with definite boundaries that is worked by an agent. Within the specific area, the agent seeks a dominant share of the marketplace.

The best geographic farms tend to be homogeneous areas having similarly priced homes, or they share other characteristics such as age, attitude toward recreational activity, family type, and so forth. Areas of common identity, such as a particular subdivision, or mobile home park generally make good farming areas. By farming an area they already live in, agents will have existing contacts and exposure within the farm area.

Farming yields a crop of listings.

In choosing a farm area, consider how you relate to the people in the area or group. If you are comfortable with and have a special interest in the area or group, you are likely to put forth the effort required for success.

If someone already is actively farming an area with great success, you might consider an area with less active competition. Although you should not mind competition, there might be equally desirable areas with little or no competition, which would mean less resistance to overcome. Just one day of knocking on doors could reveal whether an area is being actively farmed by another professional.

Some experts claim that a farm area should not exceed about 500 homes. We believe the size should be based on the size of the area, considering reasonable, identifiable boundaries as well as the agent's available time and techniques used to devote to farming activities. The fact that there are no hard and fast rules governing farm size can be shown by **megafarming**. Some agents farm areas of several thousand homes. Some of these agents use salaried assistants to help them. The internet is an easy and almost cost-free method of farming and allows for larger farms. Still other agents are able to handle larger than normal farms by specializing in listing activities rather than sales.

A farm takes time to produce a crop of sellers and buyers. Like an agricultural farm, it must be constantly worked to be productive. Generally, agents working geographic farms strive for a minimum of one contact per month with every owner within their farm area. The contact might be direct mail, the internet, a phone conversation that does not violate do-not-call rules, or a face-to-face meeting. Besides letters and personal contacts, email newsletters are very effective at minimal cost. Many agents blog on neighborhood group websites and/or have their own blog website. Getting to know owners and, more important, letting them get to know you places you in an excellent position to work with owners as buyers or sellers when a sale or purchase is needed or desired.

Nongeographic Farms/ Social Farm

A **nongeographic farm** is a particular segment of the marketplace defined according to property differentiation or buyer/seller differentiation. For example, an agent could choose to work a particular ethnic group. If an agent works a particular ethnic or nationality segment of the population, it would be a significant plus if the agent were a member of the group and had the necessary language skills of the group.

An agent might work only a type of property for small investors, such as duplexes. There are a number of agents who specialize in horse properties (properties zoned for horses).

A number of agents farm expired listings, providing owners with updates on listings and sales, as well as seeking personal contact. If your broker has an internet address (URL) tied to your farm area, it will show broker commitment to your area. The site could be both a personal site and one that is connected to properties and blogs. It can also be a marketing tool. Brokers who specialize in auction sales often vigorously farm expired listings for their auction sales.

In a nongeographic farm, door-to-door canvassing will seldom be effective. Acquiring membership lists of organizations and even religious groups, as well as buying specialized mailing lists, will allow you to work this type of farm by direct mail.

The internet can be a valuable source for leads when working a nongeographic farm. Using one of the search engines, you should be able to zero in on your area of specialty within your marketing area. You will find organizations, companies, or groups that can provide leads as to buyers, sellers, lessors, or lessees. You will also find organizations, companies, or groups outside your marketing area that have access to information within your marketing area.

Whatever type or area of farm you choose, keep in mind that farming must be continuous. If you slow down your efforts, you will begin to lose market share from your farm at a fairly rapid pace. Although every successful agent does not farm, either by geographic areas or by special interest, every successful agent does prospect for buyers and sellers.

Niche Marketing

Specializing in a narrow segment of the market is known as **niche marketing**. As you gain exposure to the many possibilities of niche marketing, you may decide to choose a niche that you feel best meets your personality, experience, and needs.

In choosing a niche that serves a particular group of buyers or sellers, you must be cognizant of both your moral and your legal responsibilities concerning discrimination. (See Unit 2.)

Niche marketing is specialization in a narrow segment of the marketplace.

An excellent way to find a niche category of buyers is to go through your old files to see if you have been serving a certain group more than other groups. When you have identified a customer segment, draw a profile of its demographic and psychological characteristics. Prospecting and after-sale surveys are two avenues for accumulating this kind of information. When you analyze past customers, try to determine why they came to you, how effectively you helped them, and the areas in which you feel you may have been weak. This will help you put together a plan to draw more people like them to your customer segment. You also will gain more from your advertising and marketing strategies if these strategies are coordinated around those surveys. Customer segment specialization helps you build a known area of expertise that will enhance your reputation, result in referrals, and keep your customers coming to you, instead of going somewhere else.

Customer segmentation could be flippers who buy, fix and sell, investment property owners, no-down-payment buyers, et cetera. Your niche could be the property type, such as foreclosures, mobile homes, homes with acreage, et cetera.

DEVELOP A PROSPECTING PLAN

Without a definite prospecting plan, prospecting becomes more of a "when you think about it" activity. The results will be far less than optimum. Figure 4.5 shows a sample prospecting plan.

You can evaluate the effectiveness of your prospecting plan by keeping track of the sources of new prospects as well as the results of working with the prospects. Quality of leads is really more important than quantity of leads.

By considering the time spent on your prospecting activities, you may discover that your interests would be better served by a reallocation of time, a change in your plan, or both. Your initial prospecting plan should not be cast in stone. It is a guide that may change, based on your interests and effectiveness in working with different types of situations.

FIGURE 4.5: **Sample Prospecting Plan**

1. Each Monday morning call on the weekend FSBO ads as well as FSBO signs you have observed so you can view for your buyer clients.
2. Contact owners within a one-block radius of every new listing taken within three days of listing.
3. Send letters or make personal contact each Friday morning on foreclosures and evictions listed in a legal newspaper.
4. Contact at least one former buyer each week to ask about friends and/or relatives interested in your area or neighbors who might be relocating.
5. Have lunch at least once each week with a person who has provided or can provide referrals.
6. Make a minimum of 30 contacts each week to locate a home for prospective buyers with whom you are working.
7. For new investment property listings, contact owners of similar property within the neighborhood of the listing. (You need not be limited to your office listings.)
8. Conduct at least one open house each week.
9. Ask at least three people each week for referrals and buyer-seller leads.
10. Contact people whom you have previously asked for help at least once each month.
11. Send weekly e-mails about new listings to previous buyers and sellers, as well as any new contacts you are working with.
12. Give out at least five business cards each day.

SUMMARY

Prospecting is a process used to locate prospective buyers and sellers of real property. There are many methods of prospecting, including door-to-door canvassing, direct mail canvassing, emails, expired listings, newspaper leads (For Sale by Owner ads; rental ads; trades; engagement, marriage, and birth announcements; and death notices), legal notices (foreclosures, probate, evictions, building permits, code violations, bankruptcy, tax delinquency), advertising, looking for problems, the internet, property neighbors, investors and speculators, lenders, chambers of commerce, open houses, endless chain referrals, your sellers, your buyers, your neighbors, centers of influence, and community services.

Telephone solicitation has been significantly limited by the do-not-call regulations. Emails must comply with CAN-SPAM regulations, and fax solicitations are limited to recipients who have given written permission for the fax.

The use of the internet has grown in significance, allowing buyers to visualize properties before the first contact.

Farming is working a particular segment of the market intensively. It can be a geographic area or a nongeographic area, which could consist of a certain type of property or an ethnic group.

A prospecting plan forces agents to evaluate how they will prospect and to evaluate results. It is important to have a contact management system so that contacts don't slip away.

CLASS DISCUSSION TOPICS

1. Be prepared to role-play a door-to-door canvassing situation with another student.

2. Identify what you feel would be logical geographic farms in your area, as well as nongeographic farming opportunities.

3. Prepare a prospecting plan for yourself. Include goals and time to be spent executing the plan.

4. List what you expect will be your five best sources of listings in order of effectiveness.

5. Identify three centers of influence that should be useful to you in prospecting.

6. Bring to class one current-events article dealing with some aspect of real estate practice for class discussion.

UNIT 4 QUIZ

1.   The CAN-SPAM Act puts controls on unsolicited
     a.   fax messages.
     b.   misleading emails.
     c.   residential phone calls.
     d.   real estate assistants.

2.   You may legally pay a referral fee to an unlicensed person who
     a.   shows listings to prospective buyers.
     b.   assists in sale negotiations.
     c.   introduces a prospective buyer to the broker.
     d.   tells buyers about the beneficial property features.

3.   Direct mail solicitation for listings is more effective if you
     a.   use window envelopes.
     b.   use a mailing machine and bulk rate.
     c.   use mailing labels.
     d.   indicate you will be contacting them.

4.   Under do-not-call regulations, which call would be improper?
     a.   Calling for survey purposes
     b.   A call to a business phone
     c.   A call within three months of an inquiry
     d.   A call on a For Sale by Owner ad to solicit a sale listing

5.   Which classified ad category is likely to provide listing leads?
     a.   Homes for rent
     b.   Leases/options to purchase
     c.   Mobile homes for rent
     d.   All of these

6.   Legal notices provide good leads for listings. Which is *NOT* a legal notice?
     a.   Eviction
     b.   Foreclosure
     c.   Probate
     d.   Vacancy

7. Which would be an indication that an owner might be interested in selling an income property?
   a. A high vacancy rate
   b. Tenant evictions
   c. Code violations
   d. All of these

8. Endless chain refers to
   a. the long-term effects of advertising.
   b. obtaining additional prospects from every lead.
   c. the fact that your buyer will eventually become a seller.
   d. the fact that most buyers are sellers and sellers are buyers.

9. The term *farming* as used in real estate refers to
   a. determining what your market area will be.
   b. operation by season, such as a listing season, open house season, selling season, and so forth.
   c. specialization in a particular field of real estate activity.
   d. working or prospecting a geographic area or special interest area for buyers and sellers.

10. An example of a nongeographic farm would be specialization in
    a. mobile homes.
    b. income property.
    c. lots.
    d. any of these.

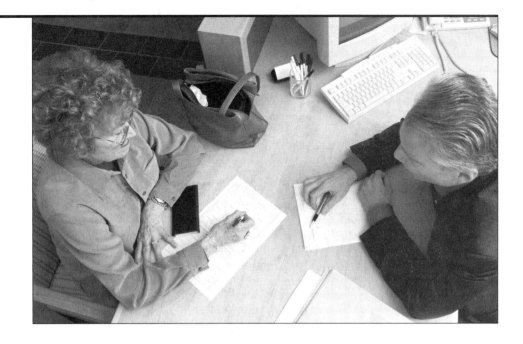

LISTING PRESENTATION PACKAGE

LEARNING OBJECTIVES

When you have completed this unit, you will be able to

- describe a comparative market analysis,

- explain how to estimate seller process,

- list what should be included in a listing presentation, and

- describe the information to be included in buyer listing material.

KEY TERMS

adjusted selling price
buyer listings
comparable properties

comparative market
  analysis
estimated seller's
  proceeds

for sale by owner
listing presentation
  manual

PREPARATION

Getting to the point of an effective face-to-face presentation takes a great deal of effort. An attempt to "wing it" and come in unprepared is more likely to result in failure than success. You should have the material to justify the offering price of the property, to be able to convince the owners that agency representation is in their best interests, and to promote yourself as a professional who understands their needs and is able to meet them.

If your appointment was based on an offer of a **comparative market analysis** (CMA), then we recommend you start at this point. However, if the owners have indicated an interest in listing their property, you might want to start with the listing presentation material.

COMPARATIVE MARKET ANALYSIS

The CMA is really a comparison analysis used by real estate agents to aid in determining a proper list price for a property. Often owners believe their home is worth far more than the CMA would indicate as a fair market value. Your comparables must be presented in an honest, logical, and convincing manner so that the owner realizes that if the property is to sell, it must be priced based on the market. The CMA provides information on **comparable properties** that have been placed in the marketplace, so that they can be compared with the property to be evaluated to determine an offering price. (Comparables are often called *comps*.) Similar property currently on the market is the competition the property owners must go against.

The CMA is not an appraisal. Only certified or licensed appraisers can appraise property. The CMA should be used for single-family residences and for multifamily residential properties of up to four units. In some cases, the CMA can be used for lots. However, it is not an effective tool for larger residential income properties or for commercial or industrial properties.

When relevant property data are selected, the CMA reflects the realities of the marketplace. It should include the following three separate areas:

1. On market now

2. Reported sold prior six months

3. Reported expired prior six months

It is important to have information about all sales in the immediate area over approximately the past six months. If there have been relatively few sales, you might have to go back to expand the analysis to include similarly desirable areas. Similarly, if there were a great many similar sales, the time period could be shortened or the sales area compressed, or both.

An agent could conceivably be liable for damages if a CMA negligently omitted recent similar sales or used unrealistic comparables that resulted in the owner selling a property for less than fair market value. If a court determines that a CMA was prepared to intentionally mislead an owner as to value, then a court might award the owner punitive damages in addition to compensatory damages. For lender-owned properties, you should label them as lender owned and indicate they are offered "as is." Short sales and foreclosure sales should also be indicated as such.

The *on-market-now list* (current listings) merely indicates to an owner the prices that competitors (other owners) are asking for their products (homes). Other owners are competitors because they are seeking to attract the same buyers. The on-market-now list shows an owner what a prospective buyer will see and how the owner's pricing will compare with that of the competition. It does not indicate what an owner can expect to receive from a sale.

> By using comparable properties, the comparative market analysis reflects the reality of the marketplace.

The *reported-sold-prior-six-months list* is more valuable than the list of current properties on the market because it shows actual sales prices. In a market undergoing change, the older the data, the less reliable they are. Prices paid six months ago could be significantly higher than a seller might expect to receive today if the market is falling. On the other hand, prices paid six months ago could be lower than might be anticipated today if the market is rising. Therefore, strive to obtain data covering a period of about the past three months. Use older data only when more current data are not available; even then, older data should be adjusted for market changes.

Adjustments
+ Add for inferior
– Subtract for superior

No two properties are identical. Properties differ by size, age, condition, design, area, view, orientation, and amenities. Adjustments to comparable properties should be made based on the property that is the subject of the CMA. For example, if the comparable property had a better view than the subject property, then the sale price of the comparable would be reduced. If the comparable had two baths and the subject property had 2½ baths, the adjustment would be a higher price for the comparable. The adjusted price is known as the **adjusted selling price**.

Subject Property	Comparable Property	Adjustment to Comparable
2-car garage	3-car garage	–
2½ baths	2 baths	+
9,000 sq. ft. lot	12,000 sq. ft. lot	–
Excellent condition	Needs work	+

There may be sales prices that seem unusual. These too-high or too-low prices are often the result of market imperfections, as covered in Unit 1. Short sales, auctions, and lender "as is" sales could require adjustments. It is also possible that the price paid reflects particular problems or benefits of a property that are not evident from the listing data provided. While prices of sold comparables can be expected to vary within a 10% range of what you consider the value to be (mean point), a variation of 20%, not reflected by the property itself, might be an aberration and not reflect a true market picture. Before you use figures, pull out the old listings and make certain you are not comparing apples and oranges. Information about a property that is significantly different in terms of utility and desirability will give an owner a false sense of value.

The *expired listings* (reported-expired-prior-six-months) *group* is the list of losers. These properties are losers because they failed to sell. Like properties that sold, the more current the expiration of a listing, the more valuable it is for comparison purposes. Often, a property fails to sell because it is overpriced in relation to its competition. From your data, you will likely find that the average list price of homes that failed to sell will be higher than the average list price of homes that sold. Listing prices might be significantly higher than the actual selling prices of the homes that sold. This information can inform owners in a powerful manner that you will not be doing them a favor if you overprice their property. In fact, you could be doing the owners a disservice because the likelihood of selling the property will be decreased. Even when an owner merely hopes for a higher price but will take less, overpricing will keep buyers away. The reported-expired-prior-six-months group also should reinforce your own knowledge that an overpriced listing is not an asset. Instead, it is a liability because it will steal the time and money you spend promoting it with little likelihood of success.

Obtaining Comparables

Comparables are easy to come by. After becoming a member of the local association of REALTORS®, you can log on to the multiple listing service and pull comps from the computer, input the area desired, the square footage, and other amenities to give you a list of comparable homes that have sold recently in the area. You can also perform a radius search. The advantage is speed—the computer produces comps within seconds. You can use the computer to check the current listings as well as the expired listings in the area. There are also services that will prepare comparables for you.

Personalized CMA

If you treat the CMA you have prepared as a valuable document, it will increase the owners' feeling of value. When you give owners a CMA, you want them to feel that you did some hard work on their behalf. A feeling of indebtedness or obligation goes a long way toward the signing of a listing agreement.

Some offices bind a CMA with a plastic ring binder and prepare a nice cover, using their computer printer. The cover indicates that the CMA was prepared for the named owners by the agent and also indicates the basis of the information enclosed. Rather than use a paper presentation, many offices use a laptop computer for their visual presentation. For comparables, they can show virtual tours. The computer presentation allows a more realistic comparison.

The personalized CMA starts with a sheet on the owners' property. It shows owners that you appreciate their home. Be certain that the narrative includes features that owners particularly pointed out to you when they showed you their home. Owners must feel that you have carefully evaluated the property.

Include a view of their home, as well as of the comparables. You should be able to download them from MLS information on the internet. If you don't have a good photo but the comparable has good eye appeal, take the time to get a photograph. A photograph of a house that looks as nice as or better than the home you are attempting to list for sale, coupled with a list price or sale price less than owners have indicated they desire, can go a long way toward putting owners in a realistic frame of mind. It's trite but true: "A picture is worth a thousand words."

If a comparable has features that the home you want to list lacks, Make certain it is covered in your visuals. It emphasizes the strength of the competition.

Your CMA data always should be as accurate and as current as possible. It should lead to your estimate of the price range in which the owners' home could be sold. This estimate should consider the owners' property, comparable sales, and market changes. A range is more realistic than a single price because it allows for minor variations in the marketplace. Be scrupulous in preparing your CMA. Again, using only the comparables that support your own position can be considered fraudulent.

Although an owner might want to list at a price toward the top edge of the range, by using the range, you have prepared the owner to consider any offer within the range as being a reasonable reflection of value. In a sellers' market, with many buyers and few sellers, the range is likely to be far narrower than it would be in a buyers' market, with many more prospective properties available than there are buyers. So, although you show the range, you might want to recommend a listing at the midpoint or even near the low limit of the range, depending on market conditions and the owners' need for a quick sale.. The reasoning for your recommendation should be made clear by the attachments to the CMA.

CMA Software Programs

There are a number of software programs that will make CMA preparation relatively easy and provide a professional-appearing document. These programs use photographs and property details to help you arrive at a recommended list price. We have included CMA material from ToolkitCMA™, a web-based software program of Realty Tools, Inc. (www.realtytools.com) as Figure 5.1A through Figure 5.1H.

WEB LINK

@

Computer people use the term *GIGO*, which stands for *garbage in, garbage out*. If your comps were not realistic, you would have a hard time developing a trend. A sale far outside your anticipated range is an aberration, but it should be considered in determining averages. (See Figures 5.1A and Figures 5.3 through 5.6I.)

This material can be a help not only in listing at the price indicated by your CMA but also in listing below the price your CMA recommends as a list price when the seller is strongly motivated to sell. Often a sale at a below-market price is in an owner's best interest, when compared with the alternative of not procuring a buyer during the listing period or even facing foreclosure. By using your laptop computer to present your CMA, you can use listing photos, including virtual tours, which will give owners a realistic understanding of the marketplace.

Let Owners See the Competition

Often owners want a price that cannot be justified by market conditions as revealed by your CMA. They need a harsh dose of reality. Some agents will conduct a short excursion with the owners to several comparable properties on the market. The agent asks the owners to compare the features of their home and the homes viewed. The owners are then requested to guess the price asked of the various properties. When the agent tells the owners what the list price is, it can serve as an aid to helping owners understand the reality of the current market.

For comparables, use vacant properties. You do not want to intrude on owners when the benefit is other than a sale of that property.

It is an unethical and unfair practice to take an overpriced listing with the secret intent of then trying to influence the owner to reduce the price or to take the listing to sell other properties. Some agents will show an overpriced property to make another property appear to be bargain priced.

Owners who insist on a price above what you consider to be a fair market value range should realize the following:

1. The higher the price, the longer it will take to sell the property.

2. The higher the price, the lower the chance of sales success .

3. Even if the sale is successful, it is likely to fall in the fair-market range or less.

FIGURES 5.1A – 5.1H: **CMA Material from ToolkitCMA™**

Determining the Value of Your Home

A Comparative Market Analysis (CMA) is essential to determine the value of residential property. Location and characteristics of the property are the key elements in determining value. Therefore, the basis for valuation is similar properties in your area. The market analysis takes into account the amount received from recent sales of comparable properties and the quantity and quality of comparable properties currently on the market. The desired end result is to find a price that will attract a willing and able buyer in a reasonable time.

Once the value of your home has been determined, you can decide on an offering price that will achieve your goals. Generally, the price should not exceed the value by more than 5% or potential buyers may not even make offers. Naturally, if you want to sell quickly your asking price should be very near the value.

The following are a few things to keep in mind about pricing:

- Realistic pricing will achieve maximum price in a reasonable time.
- Your cost or profit desire is irrelevant; the market determines the price.
- The cost of improvements are almost always more than the added value.
- Houses that remain on the market for a long time do not get shown.
- A house that is priced right from the beginning achieves the highest proceeds.

 Angela McKendrick, CRS, GRI
Office: 410-555-1234
Home Office: 410-432-7890
Fax: 410-555-5607
Web Site: www.demorealty.com/angela
Email: angela.mckendrick@demorealty.com

 Green Leaf Realty
www.greenleafrealty.com

A.

The Importance of Intelligent Pricing

Determining the best asking price for a home can be one of the most challenging aspects of selling a home. It is also one of the most important. If your home is listed at a price that is above market value, you will miss out on prospective buyers who would otherwise be prime candidates to purchase your home. If you list at a price that is below market value, you will ultimately sell for a price that is not the optimum value for your home. As *Figure 1* illustrates, more buyers purchase their properties at market value than above market value. The percentage increases as the price falls even further below market value. Therefore, by pricing your home at market value, you expose it to a much greater percentage of prospective buyers. This increases your chances for a sale while ensuring a final sale price that properly reflects the market value of your home.

Figure 1 - Percentage of Buyers by Asking Price

Another critical factor to keep in mind when pricing your home is timing. A property attracts the most attention, excitement and interest from the real estate community and potential buyers when it is first listed on the market *(see Figure 2)*. Improper pricing at the initial listing misses out on this peak interest period and may result in your property languishing on the market. This may lead to a below market value sale price *(see Figure 3)*, or, even worse, no sale at all. Therefore, your home has the highest chances for a fruitful sale when it is new on the market and the price is reasonably established.

Figure 2 - Activity Versus Timing

We can give you up-to-date information on what is happening in the marketplace and the price, financing, terms, and condition of competing properties. These are key factors in getting your property sold at the best price, quickly and with minimum hassle.

Figure 3 - The Effect of Overpricing

 Angela McKendrick, CRS, GRI
Office: 410-555-1234
Home Office: 410-432-7890
Fax: 410-555-5607
Web Site: www.demorealty.com/angela
Email: angela.mckendrick@demorealty.com

 Green Leaf Realty
www.greenleafrealty.com

B.

Why use a REALTOR®?

When selling your home, your REALTOR® can give you up-to-date information on what is happening in the marketplace including price, financing and terms of competing properties. These are key factors in a successful sale of your property at the best price in the least amount of time.

Only real estate licensees who are members of the NATIONAL ASSOCIATION OF REALTORS® are properly called REALTORS®. REALTORS® subscribe to a strict code of ethics and are expected to maintain a higher level of knowledge of the process of buying and selling real estate. They are committed to treat all parties to a transaction honestly. REALTOR® business practices are monitored at local board levels. Arbitration and disciplinary systems are in place to address complaints from the public or other board members.

Your REALTOR® can help you objectively evaluate every buyer's proposal and then help write an appropriate legally binding sale agreement. Between the initial sales agreement and settlement, questions may arise. For example, unexpected repairs may be required to obtain financing or a problem with the title is discovered. Your REALTOR® is the best person to help you resolve those issues and move the transaction to settlement.

 Angela McKendrick, CRS, GRI
Office: 410-555-1234
Home Office: 410-432-7890
Fax: 410-555-5607
Web Site: www.demorealty.com/angela
Email: angela.mckendrick@demorealty.com

 Green Leaf Realty
www.greenleafrealty.com

C.

Important Factors In Choosing A Real Estate Agent

A variety of factors influence a seller's decision to list with a particular real estate agent.

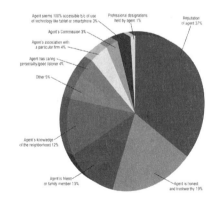

Source: National Association of Realtors®
Profile of Home Buyers and Sellers.

 Angela McKendrick, CRS, GRI
Office: 410-555-1234
Home Office: 410-432-7890
Fax: 410-555-5607
Web Site: www.demorealty.com/angela
Email: angela.mckendrick@demorealty.com

 Green Leaf Realty
www.greenleafrealty.com

D.

FIGURES 5.1A – 5.1H (continued): CMA Material from ToolkitCMA™

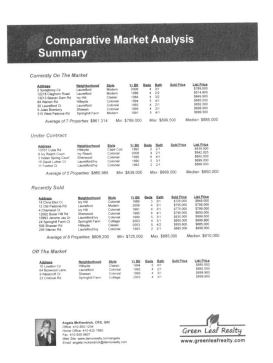

Comparative Market Analysis Summary

E.

Comparative Market Analysis Graphed by Status

F.

Comparative Market Analysis Statistics

Graphic Analysis of Currently On The Market Properties

Summary Statistics of 7 Properties:

Average Price: $861,314
High Price: $899,500
Low Price: $789,000
Median Price: $885,000
Average Year Built: 1992

G.

Pricing Your Property to Sell

Pricing your property correctly is crucial. You want to sell your property in a timely manner at the highest price possible. Current market conditions determine the value.

Pricing too high or too low can cost you time and money. Realistic pricing will achieve a maximum sale price in a reasonable amount of time.

Analysis of the comparable properties suggests a list price range of:

$783,954 to $832,446

H.

Used with permission of Realty Tools, Inc.

ESTIMATED SELLER'S PROCEEDS

The **estimated seller's proceeds** (also called the net sheet), what an owner actually receives in cash and/or paper from a sale, are of vital importance to owners. Owners who receive less than what they anticipated are going to be disappointed. They are going to be unhappy with you and your firm. When owners are unhappy, the chances that problems will arise during escrow tend to escalate. From the standpoints of good business, agency duty, and basic fairness, you want the owners to understand what they will net from a sale if sold at list price. The owners should know what costs they will incur.

> The estimated seller's proceeds should show what the seller would net, based on a particular sale price.

While there are computer programs that will give you printouts of seller costs based on data you supply to the computer, the completeness of the form increases the likelihood that actual figures will vary only slightly from the estimate. Make sure that you will know the amounts the seller will likely incur. For example, all counties in California charge a documentary transfer tax, but some cities charge an additional tax. The seller should be made aware of these small but important charges. Many agents like to estimate seller costs just a little on the high side, so any surprises are more likely to be pleasant ones. You would prepare a new Estimated Seller's Proceeds form if the price were adjusted or if an offer were received at a price other than the one set forth in the listing.

THE LISTING PRESENTATION MANUAL

The listing presentation manual is a valuable visual tool for obtaining listings. It can be a paper presentation using a three-ring binder with plastic protector sheets for each page, but agents are more likely to use a laptop display. You want a visual tool that works hand in hand with your dialogue to make a structured and effective presentation. The listing presentation material sells the owner on benefits—the benefit of using an exclusive agent and the benefit of your firm as that agent. It should not be used in place of the verbal presentation. Basically, as the agent turns the pages or changes the images, the visual message reinforces the agent's verbal message. Separate listing presentation visuals should be prepared for sale listings and buyer listings, although some of the pages will be identical.

Using the laptop presentation forces the owners to sit close to you to view the monitor. While prospects are likely to get defensive if you invade their space, with a laptop presentation, they are the ones getting close to you. The advantage of physical proximity is that it is easier to gain trust and acceptance than it is from across a room.

Listing presentation manuals should be divided into two areas:

1. *Why* list?

2. *Why* us? (Your firm and you)

FIGURE 5.2:   **Good Faith Estimate of Seller's Net Sales Proceeds**

GOOD FAITH ESTIMATE OF SELLER'S NET SALES PROCEEDS
On Sale of Property

Prepared by: Agent _____   Phone _____

Broker _____   Email _____

NOTE: This net sheet is prepared to assist the Seller by providing an estimate of the amount of net sales proceeds the Seller is likely to receive on closing, based on the price set in the agreement, the estimated amount for expenses likely to be incurred to market the property and close a sale, and any adjustments and pro rates necessitated by the sale.

The figures estimated in the net sheet may vary at the time each is incurred due to periodic changes in charges for professional services, administration fees and work enforcement made necessary by later inspections, and thus constitute an opinion, not a guarantee by the preparer.

If the property disposed of is IRC §1031 property and the seller plans to acquire replacement property, use a §1031 Profit and Basis Recap Sheet to compute the tax consequences of the Seller's §1031 Reinvestment Plan. [See **ft** Form 354]

DATE: _____, 20_____, at _____, California.

1. This is an estimate of the fix-up, marketing and transaction expenses Seller is likely to incur on a sale, and the likely amount of net sales proceeds Seller may anticipate receiving on the close of a sale under the following agreement:

☐ Seller's listing agreement   ☐ Purchase agreement   ☐ Counteroffer
☐ Escrow instructions   ☐ Exchange agreement   ☐ Option to buy

1.1   dated _____, 20_____, at _____, California,

1.2   entered into by _____, as the Seller, and

1.3   _____, as the Buyer,

1.4   regarding real estate referred to as _____.

1.5   The day of the month anticipated for closing is _____.

2. **SALES PRICE:**

2.1   Price Received. . . . .   (+)$_____

3. **ENCUMBRANCES:**

3.1   First Trust Deed Note . . . . $_____

3.2   Second Trust Deed Note . . . . $_____

3.3   Other Liens/Bonds/UCC-1 . . . . $_____

3.4   TOTAL ENCUMBRANCES: [Lines 3.1 to 3.3] . . . .   (–)$0.00_____

4. **SALES EXPENSES AND CHARGES:**

4.1   Fix-up Cost . . . . $_____

4.2   Structural Pest Control Report . . . . $_____

4.3   Structural Pest Control Clearance . . . . $_____

4.4   Property/Home Inspection Report. . . . . $_____

4.5   Elimination of Property Defects . . . . $_____

4.6   Local Ordinance Compliance Report . . . . $_____

4.7   Compliance with Local Ordinances. . . . . $_____

4.8   Natural Hazard Disclosure Report . . . . $_____

4.9   Smoke Detector/Water Heater Safety Compliance . . . . $_____

4.10   Homeowners' (HOA) Association Document Charge . . . . . . $_____

4.11   Mello-Roos Assessment Statement Charge . . . . $_____

4.12   Well Water Reports . . . . $_____

4.13   Septic/Sewer Reports . . . . $_____

4.14   Lead-Based Paint Report . . . . $_____

4.15   Marketing Budget. . . . . $_____

4.16   Home Warranty Insurance. . . . . $_____

4.17   Buyer's Escrow Closing Costs . . . . $_____

4.18   Loan Appraisal Fee . . . . $_____

4.19   Buyer's Loan Charges. . . . . $_____

4.20   Escrow Fee. . . . . $_____

4.21   Document Preparation Fee . . . . $_____

– – – – – – – – – – – – – – – *PAGE ONE OF TWO — FORM 310* – – – – – – – – – – – – – – – – – –

FIGURE 5.2 (continued): **Good Faith Estimate of Seller's Net Sales Proceeds**

— *PAGE TWO OF TWO — FORM 310* —

4.22	Notary Fees	$_____
4.23	Recording Fees/Documentary Transfer Tax	$_____
4.24	Title Insurance Premium.	$_____
4.25	Beneficiary Statement/Demand	$_____
4.26	Prepayment Penalty (first).	$_____
4.27	Prepayment Penalty (second).	$_____
4.28	Reconveyance Fees	$_____
4.29	Brokerage Fees	$_____
4.30	Transaction Coordinator Fee	$_____
4.31	Attorney/Accountant Fees	$_____
4.32	Other _____	$_____
4.33	Other _____	$_____
4.34	TOTAL EXPENSES AND CHARGES [Lines 4.1 to 4.33]	(–)$0.00_____

5. ESTIMATED NET EQUITY: . . . . (=)$0.00_____

6. PRO RATES DUE BUYER:

6.1	Unpaid Taxes/Assessments	$_____
6.2	Interest Accrued and Unpaid	$_____
6.3	Unearned Rental Income	$_____
6.4	Tenant Security Deposits	$_____
6.5	TOTAL PRO RATES DUE BUYER [Lines 6.1 to 6.4]	(–)$0.00_____

7. PRO RATES DUE SELLER:

7.1	Prepaid Taxes/Assessments	$_____
7.2	Impound Account Balances	$_____
7.3	Prepaid Association Assessment	$_____
7.4	Prepaid Ground Lease	$_____
7.5	Unpaid Rent Assigned to Buyer	$_____
7.6	Other _____	$_____
7.7	TOTAL PRO RATES DUE SELLER [Lines 7.1 to 7.6].	(+)$0.00_____

8. ESTIMATED PROCEEDS OF SALE: . . . . (=)$0.00_____

8.1 The estimated net proceeds at line 8 from the sale or exchange
analyzed in this net sheet will be received in the form of:

a. Cash	$_____
b. Note secured by a Trust Deed.	$_____
c. Equity in Replacement Real Estate.	$_____
d. Other _____	$_____

I have prepared this estimate based on my knowledge and readily available data.	I have read and received a copy of this estimate.
Date: _____, 20_____	Date: _____, 20_____
Broker: _____	Seller's Name: _____
DRE #: _____	
Agent: _____	
Signature: _____	Signature: _____

FORM 310   08-11   2011 **first tuesday**, P.O. BOX 20069, RIVERSIDE, CA 92516 (800) 794-0494

©2015 RPI — Realty Publications, Inc.

You must convince the owner or the buyer about the concept of a listing as your first step and then show that you should have the listing.

SALE LISTINGS

Owners feel that a listing will cost them money. They are likely to initially view the idea of a listing as negative rather than look at the benefits you can offer. Therefore, you must overcome the negative thoughts and help owners realize the benefits offered.

Why List?

When you deal with a **for sale by owner** (FSBO), realize that a significant reason the owners want to sell the home themselves is to save the commission. They feel if they can sell their property without an agent, the agent's fee will be additional money for them. Therefore, begin your presentation with a discussion of who actually saves when an agent is not involved.

Even when you are not dealing with an FSBO, you could be in competition with the owners, as well as with other agents, for a listing. While not stated or even denied, the owners could be considering selling without an agent as one of their options. Therefore, we believe that all listing presentation material should begin with a discussion of the false savings of FSBO offerings.

Consider starting your presentation with the following visual question and answer:

> The primary reason owners want to sell without an agent is to avoid paying a commission.

Question:

Who saves when an owner sells without an agent?

Answer:

The buyer

Note: This question-and-answer technique is very effective and easy to prepare. Put only one question and answer on a page or screen. For a book, pages should be read on the right side of your book. We show suggested verbal presentations following each question and answer. You can use appropriate ideas to tailor your own presentation materials to your needs.

> I understand why you would want to sell [might consider selling] your home without an agent. You would like to save the agent's fee. Owners who do succeed in selling without an agent—and there aren't that many of them—find that they're not the ones who save. If there are any savings to be had, the buyer enjoys them.

Buyers who approach owners who advertise their homes for sale or put signs in their front yards will want to reduce any offer they might make by at least the amount of the agent's fee, even though the price might have been set to reflect all or part of this savings.

Buyers will not even settle for half because they realize it is buyers, not sellers, who really pay the commission. The price the buyer pays includes a commission, and although the seller may pay it, it is paid for with dollars that come from the buyer's savings and not the seller's pockets. When an owner sells direct, losing the commission is just for starters. Buyers often view for-sale-by-owner situations as opportunities to make a profit for themselves. They believe that for sale by owner indicates a distress sale, and that belief explains some of the ridiculous offers that owners receive.

Question:

> Why are most For Sale by Owner signs replaced by agent signs?

Answer:

> Because owners are seldom successful in selling their homes, most owners who try to sell without an agent end up listing their property with a licensed agent. They wasted time and money on their futile effort.

Few buyers seek out For Sale by Owner ads and signs, and when they do give an offer it is usually at a price the owner will not consider. Many times, buyers who are considering making an offer on a for-sale-by-owner property will make an opening offer of at least 5% less than they would otherwise offer because they figure that the seller is not paying a commission. Many buyers use this as a negotiating tool.

Question:

Whom does this sign attract?

Answer:

Bargain hunters

"Lookie Lous"

Unqualified buyers

With a For Sale by Owner sign on your front lawn, you will attract bargain hunters of all types.

Your home will be on the Sunday entertainment tour of "Lookie Lous," who might be interested only in how you have decorated your home or are simply using you as a way to fill an otherwise vacant day.

Your For Sale by Owner ads and signs will attract people who might truly love your home but don't have a prayer of getting necessary financing. These people can waste a great deal of your time. Even if they give you an offer, the sale will never be closed.

A For Sale sign says "come on in" to the whole world. When you show people your home and belongings, you are really allowing strangers in. You let them see into closets and places that your best friend will never see, and you have no idea why they are there. While talking to one prospective buyer, another could be going through your jewelry box or medicine cabinet. I wish it weren't a problem, but safety is a problem today. People put in expensive alarm systems and then invite strangers into their homes, allowing them to see who lives there and what is there. Is this wise?

Question:

What does this sign mean?

Answer:

Wasted time

Wasted effort

Likelihood of legal problems

Failure/discouragement

Owners who try to sell without an agent are prisoners in their own homes, waiting for a phone call on the ad or a passerby to ring their doorbell.

When they accept an offer, they might find that the other party views the agreement differently from what the owners thought was agreed to. The likelihood of a lawsuit is increased many times when an agent is not part of the transaction.

Actually, a lawsuit is seldom a problem, because most owners who try to sell without an agent never even get an offer.

Question:

Why do most serious buyers employ real estate agents?

Answer:

Because agents have the inventory, understand the market, know how to qualify buyers, and can negotiate a sale with all the paperwork.

[Mr. and Mrs.], when you were looking for a home to purchase, I bet you visited real estate agents, am I right? The reason you went to at least one agent is because agents knew what was on the market and were able to quickly locate properties that met your needs. Without agents, buyers would have to contact dozens of individual property owners to check out properties, even though inspection might reveal that a property did not come close to meeting their needs. Buyers today are no different than you were when you purchased this home. Buyers who are serious about buying contact agents. Buyers dealing with agents understand they will have to pay a price dictated by the market and that they are not going to get anything for nothing.

We suggest you take a positive approach regarding the benefits of agency representation. Owners who understand the benefits of professional representation are less likely to resist paying a reasonable fee for these services.

Note: The word *fee* denotes a professional charge for benefits, whereas *commission* has a negative connotation to some people.

> The word *commission* has a negative connotation, but *fee* is positive in that it is a charge for benefits received.

Question:

What do you get for your fee?

Answer:

These important benefits:

Help and advice on making your home more salable

Promotion and advertising (paid by the agent)

Exposure on seven websites

Multiple-listing benefits

Qualifying of all prospects

Freedom to enjoy your time

Advice on offers and counteroffers

Problem solving during escrow

We work with you to make your house salable at the highest possible price. We promote your home with advertising and open houses. We prepare advertising flyers on your home for other agents, for responses to inquiries, and for those visiting your home. We also feature your home on our own website, as well as seven other websites. Of course, we bear all of these costs.

Information on your home is made available through our multiple listing service to [137] offices and more than [1,814] agents and through the website that has [more than 3,000] hits per day. This is the kind of exposure that is possible for your home.

An effective visual tool is to have a computer print-out listing every agent who is a member of your MLS service. The size of the printout helps impress upon the owners the number of people who will be able to work to sell their home.

We properly qualify anyone we bring to your home. We know who they are, where they live and work, and who can afford to buy your home before they cross your threshold.

You receive our advice on all offers received. We will work with you and the buyer in turning an unacceptable offer into an advantageous sale.

We work with buyers in obtaining financing to ensure that the purchase will close.

We monitor escrow to make certain there are no hang-ups. If a problem arises, we inform you and work to overcome it so the sale can progress.

This question-and-answer approach is just one of many approaches that can be used for your listing presentation material. Whatever material you use should flow toward the desired goal of overcoming any resistance by the owners to signing an agency agreement. You must be comfortable with the approach you use. If you are not comfortable with the material, chances are your effort will reflect your attitude, which will translate into few successful listings.

WEB LINK

Figures 5.3 and 5.4 were provided by Realty Tools, Inc. (www.realtytools.com) and show the benefits of listing and having agency representation.

FIGURE 5.3:   Why Use a REALTOR®?

Why use a REALTOR®?

When selling your home, your REALTOR® can give you up-to-date information on what is happening in the marketplace including price, financing and terms of competing properties. These are key factors in a successful sale of your property at the best price in the least amount of time.

Only real estate licensees who are members of the NATIONAL ASSOCIATION OF REALTORS® are properly called REALTORS®. REALTORS® subscribe to a strict code of ethics and are expected to maintain a higher level of knowledge of the process of buying and selling real estate. They are committed to treat all parties to a transaction honestly. REALTOR® business practices are monitored at local board levels. Arbitration and disciplinary systems are in place to address complaints from the public or other board members.

Your REALTOR® can help you objectively evaluate every buyer's proposal and then help write an appropriate legally binding sale agreement. Between the initial sales agreement and settlement, questions may arise. For example, unexpected repairs may be required to obtain financing or a problem with the title is discovered. Your REALTOR® is the best person to help you resolve those issues and move the transaction to settlement.

Angela McKendrick, CRS, GRI
Office: 410-555-1234
Home Office: 410-432-7890
Fax: 410-555-5607
Web Site: www.demorealty.com/angela
Email: angela.mckendrick@demorealty.com

Green Leaf Realty
www.greenleafrealty.com

Used with permission of Realty Tools, Inc.

FIGURE 5.4: **Services You Will Receive**

Services You Will Receive

- We will help you determine the best selling price for your home.

- We will suggest what you can do to get your home in top selling condition.

- We will develop a strategy to show your home.

- We will enter your home in the Multiple Listing System.

- We will implement the enclosed marketing plan.

- We will talk with you to review progress periodically.

- We will advise you of changes in the market climate.

- We will present all offers to you promptly and assist in evaluating them.

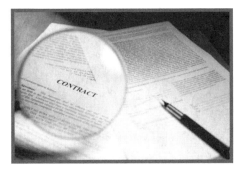

- We will monitor progress toward closing when a contract is accepted.

- We will monitor the appraisal and buyers loan approval.

- We will immediately advise you of events that may threaten closing.

- We will coordinate and monitor the settlement process.

Angela McKendrick, CRS, GRI
Office: 410-555-1234
Home Office: 410-432-7890
Fax: 410-555-5607
Web Site: www.demorealty.com/angela
Email: angela.mckendrick@demorealty.com

www.greenleafrealty.com

Used with permission of Realty Tools, Inc.

Why Us?

To obtain a listing, you have to convince owners that you and your firm deserve their trust. This is particularly important when owners are hesitant about listing their property because of a previous unsatisfactory experience with another agent.

You must build rapport with property owners. The owners must not only want to list their property, they also must want to list with you because they feel you are a capable, truthful person representing a reputable firm.

Sell yourself to the owners as a caring person who understands their problems and wants to help produce solutions. If you are unsuccessful, you could end up doing all the groundwork for an easy listing by another agent who has been able to develop greater empathy with the owners.

Listen to what the owners say during and after your presentation. Address them by their last names (Mr. Owner, Mrs. Seller). Answer questions slowly and fully. Ask questions to determine if you are communicating fully with the owners.

Don't *tell* the owners, *ask* them. Don't talk down to them or dismiss questions with flippant remarks. Don't use technical terms or acronyms. They may not understand what this "girl" Fannie Mae has to do with their property. In the initial phase of the presentation, keep in mind that the product you are selling is really yourself.

> You must sell yourself as worthy of an owner's trust.

The *Why Us?* portion of your listing material should cover you personally, as well as your firm. You might want to start with a one-page résumé titled "Want to Know About [Lester Jones]?"

Keep your résumé simple. You should have printed copies of this résumé so you can give the owners a copy. You are asking them to entrust you with the sale of their home, so they deserve to know something about you. When you give the owners your résumé, take no more than one minute to tell them about yourself. You should emphasize knowledge of the community, success in sales, special training, professional designations, and so forth.

A photo of your office or, if more than one office, a collage of photos can be effective. If your office has been in business a long time, a caption such as "Servicing [Midvale] since [1953]" is appropriate. If you are with a large firm or franchise, the caption could read "[8] offices and [146] professionals ready to serve you." If you have a large office, a group photo of your sales force with the name of your firm is effective.

Your narrative could simply be the following:

> We offer the advantage of 8 offices and 146 salespeople. Isn't this the kind of sales force you want for success?

For a franchise, consider this presentation:

> [Franchise Name] [Logo]
> [1,823] Offices
> [36,000] Salespeople
> Our Name Means: Instant Recognition
> National Referrals

Your possible narrative could be this:

> The name [VIP Realty] means instant recognition even to those who are new to our community. Because we are a [VIP] office, you can benefit from our national referral system.

| You must sell the benefits that your firm has to offer. |

If your firm is small, use a photo of your office and turn your small size into a positive with a narrative such as the following:

> Because we specialize in a small number of select properties, our owners receive maximum service. Your home will not be competing with 400 other office listings. We can provide the individual attention your home deserves in order to have a successful sale.

As an alternative, you might use a caption to illustrate your small firm as part of a large organization:

> [Loring Realty] is part of a multiple listing service offering you [237] offices and more than [2,000] salespeople, all working for your success.

Your narrative might be as follows:

> With [Loring Realty] representing you, you can take advantage of this huge sales force working together for your success.

Perhaps you want a separate sheet providing information on your multiple listing service. Your possible narrative might be this:

> By appointing [Loring Realty] as your agent, [in less than one hour] the information on your home will be available to these [237] offices and more than [2,000] salespeople. This sales force can be working for you.

An alternative narrative for a multiple listing service would be the following:

> Assume every agent in our multiple listing service is working with just two buyers for a home in your home's general price range. Now that may seem to be a very low figure, but consider that tomorrow morning your home can be exposed to those two buyers by [2,000] agents. That's [4,000] potential buyers for your home.

If you are a REALTOR®, consider a sheet with just the REALTOR® trademark. Your narrative could be this one:

> Every broker is not a REALTOR®. Only REALTORS® can use this symbol. [Loring Realty] is a member of the California Association of REALTORS® and the National Association of REALTORS®. As REALTORS® we are pledged to a Code of Professional Conduct.

If your firm is a member of the National Association of Real Estate Brokers, a similar approach could be used.

A collage of press releases can be effective as follows:

> The fact that [Loring Realty] has played a dominant role in [community activities] and [development] brings us instant name recognition as a professional leader.

Tell owners how your firm advertises to attract potential buyers. For a larger firm, you could have a sheet stating this:

2013

[$2 Million] + Advertising Budget

Your narrative could be this one:

> Our advertising budget of [$] means [$] per week spent to bring in buyers. This budget has given us name recognition and dominance in the marketplace. Our dominance is reflected in our sales record.

FIGURES 5.5A – 5.5E: **Presentation Samples**

Determining the Value of Your Home

A Comparative Market Analysis (CMA) is essential to determine the value of residential property. Location and characteristics of the property are the key elements in determining value. Therefore, the basis for valuation is similar properties in your area. The market analysis takes into account the amount received from recent sales of comparable properties and the quantity and quality of comparable properties currently on the market. The desired end result is to find a price that will attract a willing and able buyer in a reasonable time.

Once the value of your home has been determined, you can decide on an offering price that will achieve your goals. Generally, the price should not exceed the value by more than 5% or potential buyers may not even make offers. Naturally, if you want to sell quickly your asking price should be very near the value.

The following are a few things to keep in mind about pricing:

- Realistic pricing will achieve maximum price in a reasonable time.
- Your cost or profit desire is irrelevant; the market determines the price.
- The cost of improvements are almost always more than the added value.
- Houses that remain on the market for a long time do not get shown.
- A house that is priced right from the beginning achieves the highest proceeds.

Angela McKendrick, CRS, GRI
Office 410-555-1234
Home Office 410-432-7890
Fax 410-555-5607
Web Site www.demorealty.com/angela
Email angela.mckendrick@demorealty.com

A.

In Conclusion

When you choose Angela McKendrick **you will receive:**

- Excellent service and support.
- A market analysis of your home.
- A winning marketing plan.
- Every effort to sell your home promptly.
- The resources of Green Leaf Realty.

***List Your Home Now
with Angela McKendrick!***

Angela McKendrick, CRS, GRI
Office 410-555-1234
Home Office 410-432-7890
Fax 410-555-5607
Web Site www.demorealty.com/angela
Email angela.mckendrick@demorealty.com

B.

Customer References

Sellers...

Fred & Susan Fredericks	23 Elm Street	822-4554
Joe & Lisa Johnson	1400 N. Timonium Road	922-2222
Ron & Dawn Larkin	2311 E. Roundtop Circle	444-3948
Debra Jones	433 Forest Drive	231-6932
Don & Julia Smith	32 E. Running Road	211-4599
Len & Hanna Leonard	443 Forest Drive	343-6798

Buyers...

Mark & Joan Dawson	2300 S. Timonium Road	666-3033
Suzanne Swift	22 Forrest Avenue	667-9888
Ron & Joan Burns	55 W. Running Road	333-9843
Joe & Ann Reese	321 Pine Forest Lane	222-4563
Robert Johnson	324 82nd Terrace	342-6879
Jay & Sarah Volkers	75 Winding Way	234-1098

Angela McKendrick, CRS, GRI
Office 410-555-1234
Home Office 410-432-7890
Fax 410-555-5607
Web Site www.demorealty.com/angela
Email angela.mckendrick@demorealty.com

C.

Resume

Angela McKendrick

Experience:
1998-Present: Real Estate Agent specializing in single family, multi-family, condominiums, and land sales.
1994-2002: Marketing Director for McCormick Company.

Affiliations:
Greater Baltimore Board of Realtors.
Maryland Association of Realtors.
National Association of Realtors.
Residential Sales Council.

Education:
Columbia University
North Carroll High School
Professional Courses sponsored by the National Association of Realtors.

Community:
Former American Cancer Society "Person of the Year."
Hunt Valley Community Association.
Greater Baltimore Association.
Scoutmaster Troop 211.

Personal:
Married to Jason McKendrick.
Children: David (31) and Anna (26).
Hobbies: Golf and Tennis.

D.

FIGURES 5.5A – 5.5E (continued): Presentation Samples

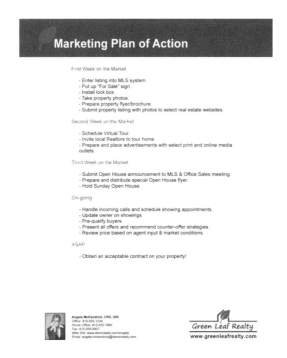

E.

Used with permission of Realty Tools, Inc.

For a small firm, consider a collage of your ads, web listings, or both. You could say: You can see we publicize our listings.

If your office advertises in a foreign paper places listings on foreign websites or has relationships with brokerage offices in other countries, this should be emphasized. Many owners feel that foreign buyers pay top price, so that access to them is important.

The Only Office in [Sacramento] Advertising in

Nihon Keizai Shimbun
Japan's Largest Business Daily Newspaper

We market our properties to the largest possible market. We go to the buyers. Besides our area advertising, our international advertising has built up a referral network of agents who work with us to locate buyers.

FIGURES 5.6A –5.6I: Presentation Samples

A.

Real Estate Services Proposal

Prepared Especially for:
Tom & Mary White
7 Deep Run Court
Hunt Valley, MD 21030

For marketing the property located at:
7 Deep Run Court

Prepared by:
Angela McKendrick, CRS, GRI
Agent
Green Leaf Realty
123 Main Street
Hunt Valley, MD 21030

Office: 410-555-1234
Home Office: 410-432-7890
Fax: 410-555-5607
Web Site: www.demorealty.com/angela
Email: angela.mckendrick@demorealty.com

Date: August 20, 2015

This analysis is not an appraisal. It is intended only for the purpose of assisting buyers or sellers or prospective buyers or sellers in deciding the listing, offering, or sale price of the real property.

Green Leaf Realty
www.greenleafrealty.com

B.

Real Estate Services Proposal

Prepared Especially for:
Tom & Mary White
7 Deep Run Court
Hunt Valley, MD 21030

For marketing the property located at:
7 Deep Run Court

Prepared by:
Angela McKendrick, CRS, GRI
Agent
Green Leaf Realty
123 Main Street
Hunt Valley, MD 21030

Office: 410-555-1234
Home Office: 410-432-7890
Fax: 410-555-5607
Web Site: www.demorealty.com/angela
Email: angela.mckendrick@demorealty.com

Date: August 20, 2015

This analysis is not an appraisal. It is intended only for the purpose of assisting buyers or sellers or prospective buyers or sellers in deciding the listing, offering, or sale price of the real property.

Green Leaf Realty
www.greenleafrealty.com

C.

Subject Property Profile for

7 Deep Run Court

The following features have been identified to aid in the search for properties that are comparable to yours. This will help in determining proper pricing for your home.

City: Hunt Valley	Neighborhood: Orchard Valley	Year Built: 1988
Fin SqFt: 2160	Lot Desc: Backs To Trees	Lot Size: 1.04
Style: Colonial	Levels: 3	Bedrooms: 3
Bathrooms: 2/1	Const: Cedar Siding	Roofing: Cedar/Shake
Basement: Fully Finished	Basement: Walkout Level	Heat: Heat Pump
Fuel: Electric	Cool: Central A/C	Parking: Garage
Garage Spaces: 2	Exter Feat: Deck	Water: Well
Sewer: Septic	# Fireplaces: 2	Amenities: Auto Gar Dr Opn
Amenities: Built-In Bookcases	Amenities: Mba/Sep Shwr	Other Rms: Den/Stdy/Lib
Other Rms: Family Room		

Angela McKendrick, CRS, GRI
Office: 410-555-1234
Home Office: 410-432-7890
Fax: 410-555-5607
Web Site: www.demorealty.com/angela
Email: angela.mckendrick@demorealty.com

Green Leaf Realty
www.greenleafrealty.com

D.

Marketing Plan of Action

First Week on the Market
- Enter listing into MLS system.
- Put up "For Sale" sign.
- Install lock box.
- Take property photos.
- Prepare property flyer/brochure.
- Submit property listing with photos to select real estate websites.

Second Week on the Market
- Schedule Virtual Tour.
- Invite local Realtors to tour home.
- Prepare and place advertisements with select print and online media outlets.

Third Week on the Market
- Submit Open House announcement to MLS & Office Sales meeting.
- Prepare and distribute special Open House flyer.
- Hold Sunday Open House.

On-going
- Handle incoming calls and schedule showing appointments.
- Update owner on showings.
- Pre-qualify buyers.
- Present all offers and recommend counter-offer strategies.
- Review price based on agent input & market conditions.

ASAP
- Obtain an acceptable contract on your property!

Angela McKendrick, CRS, GRI
Office: 410-555-1234
Home Office: 410-432-7890
Fax: 410-555-5607
Web Site: www.demorealty.com/angela
Email: angela.mckendrick@demorealty.com

Green Leaf Realty
www.greenleafrealty.com

FIGURES 5.6A –5.6I (continued):   Presentation Samples

Subject Property Profile for

7 Deep Run Court

The following features have been identified to aid in the search for properties that are comparable to yours. This will help in determining proper pricing for your home.

City	Hunt Valley	Neighborhood	Orchard Valley	Year Built	1988
Fin SqFt	2160	Lot Desc.	Backs To Trees	Lot Size	1.04
Style	Colonial	Levels	3	Bedrooms	3
Bathrooms	2/1	Const.	Cedar Siding	Roofing	Cedar/Shake
Basement	Fully Finished	Basement	Walkout Level	Heat	Heat Pump
Fuel	Electric	Cool	Central A/C	Parking	Garage
Garage Spaces	2	Exter Feat.	Deck	Water	Well
Sewer	Septic	# Fireplaces	2	Amenities	Auto Gar Dr Opn
Amenities	Built-In Bookcases	Amenities	Mba/Sep Shwr	Other Rms	Den/Stdy/Lib
Other Rms	Family Room				

 Angela McKendrick, CRS, GRI
Office: 410-555-1234
Home Office: 410-432-7890
Fax: 410-555-5607
Web Site: www.demorealty.com/angela
Email: angela.mckendrick@demorealty.com

 Green Leaf Realty
www.greenleafrealty.com

E.

Services You Will Receive

- We will help you determine the best selling price for your home.
- We will suggest what you can do to get your home in top selling condition.
- We will develop a strategy to show your home.
- We will enter your home in the Multiple Listing System.
- We will implement the enclosed marketing plan.
- We will talk with you to review progress periodically.
- We will advise you of changes in the market climate.
- We will present all offers to you promptly and assist in evaluating them.

- We will monitor progress toward closing when a contract is accepted.
- We will monitor the appraisal and buyers loan approval.
- We will immediately advise you of events that may threaten closing.
- We will coordinate and monitor the settlement process.

 Angela McKendrick, CRS, GRI
Office: 410-555-1234
Home Office: 410-432-7890
Fax: 410-555-5607
Web Site: www.demorealty.com/angela
Email: angela.mckendrick@demorealty.com

 Green Leaf Realty
www.greenleafrealty.com

F.

Resume

 Angela McKendrick

Experience:
1998-Present: Real Estate Agent specializing in single family, multi-family, condominiums, and land sales.
1994-2002: Marketing Director for McCormick Company.

Affiliations:
Greater Baltimore Board of Realtors.
Maryland Association of Realtors.
National Association of Realtors.
Residential Sales Council.

Education:
Columbia University
North Carroll High School
Professional Courses sponsored by the National Association of Realtors.

Community:
Former American Cancer Society "Person of the Year."
Hunt Valley Community Association.
Greater Baltimore Association.
Scoutmaster Troop 211.

Personal:
Married to Jason McKendrick.
Children: David (31) and Anna (26).
Hobbies: Golf and Tennis.

 Green Leaf Realty
www.greenleafrealty.com

G.

Customer References

Sellers...

Fred & Susan Fredericks	23 Elm Street	822-4554
Joe & Lisa Johnson	1400 N. Timonium Road	922-2222
Ron & Dawn Larkin	2311 E. Roundtop Circle	444-3948
Debra Jones	433 Forest Drive	231-6932
Don & Julia Smith	32 E. Running Road	211-4599
Len & Hanna Leonard	443 Forest Drive	343-6798

Buyers...

Mark & Joan Dawson	2300 S. Timonium Road	666-3033
Suzanne Swift	22 Forest Avenue	667-9888
Ron & Joan Burns	55 W. Running Road	333-9843
Joe & Ann Reese	321 Pine Forest Lane	222-4563
Robert Johnson	324 82nd Terrace	342-6879
Jay & Sarah Volkers	75 Winding Way	234-1098

 Angela McKendrick, CRS, GRI
Office: 410-555-1234
Home Office: 410-432-7890
Fax: 410-555-5607
Web Site: www.demorealty.com/angela
Email: angela.mckendrick@demorealty.com

 Green Leaf Realty
www.greenleafrealty.com

H.

FIGURES 5.6A –5.6I (continued):   Presentation Samples

I.

Used with permission of Realty Tools, Inc.

If your office has a home protection plan, consider this:

[Loring Realty] Offers Buyers
Home Protection Plan
That Makes Your Home More Desirable to Buyers

Our home protection plan protects buyers against structural problems and system breakdowns for [one] year after purchase. This protection has given us a word-of-mouth reputation to the extent that many buyers would not consider using another agent to purchase a home.

If your office belongs to a national referral network but is not a franchise office, consider a sheet or computer screen that reads as follows:

Member
[Home Relocators]
A National Relocation Referral Service
[1,838] Cooperating Member Firms in 50 States

Your possible narrative might be as follows:

Would you like to take advantage of referrals from every corner of the nation? We constantly receive calls about people relocating to our area because of our [Home Relocators] membership. We want our owners to have every sales advantage possible. I'm sure that's the kind of representation you want.

Emphasize your internet site:

I'm sure you realize that the internet is of prime importance in selling real estate. These are a few pictures of our internet site.

Show a home presentation from the site, as well as your office home site. If your site features virtual tours, explain what they are and the benefits they offer (with a high-speed wireless connection, you can access the sites on your laptop for a very effective presentation):

[Loring Realty] takes second place to no one in using technology to market our homes.

Emphasize your internet presence:

"We will be placing your home (photos, video, virtual tour) on nine websites visited by [over 85,000] viewers each day."

If you purchase enhanced coverage on websites, you should point out how their property will stand out from other listings. If your firm specializes in the area where you are seeking a listing, a sheet should show this specialization:

[Palm Desert Greens]
Housing Specialists

Your narrative could be something like this:

We specialize in [Palm Desert Greens]. We have built up a reputation of being the [Palm Desert Greens] broker. Prospective buyers come to us because we have the inventory and make the sales. When other agents get a buyer who is interested in [Palm Desert Greens], they frequently call us. Our cooperation with others and our knowledge of the market have resulted in a record of success in [Palm Desert Greens] that is second to none.

By using computer information from your local multiple listing service, you should be able to find statistics that show your firm is outstanding in several areas. Sheets should be prepared to showcase these distinctions. But be careful when you use statistics. If you emphasize that 50% of your listings are sold, it also points out a 50% failure rate. Approaches that are more positive would be these:

[Loring Realty]
[42%] Better Record of Success

According to the records of the [Tri-County Multiple Listing Service], listings with [Loring Realty] had a [42%] greater chance of success than the board average for [20XX].

[Loring Realty]
We Get More for Your Home

According to the records of the [Tri-County Multiple Listing Service], the average home in [20XX] sold at [84%] of its listed price. In [20XX], [Loring Realty] home sales averaged [94%] of list price. That's [10%] more money in the pockets of our sellers than our competition. Is getting the most money from your home important to you?

Another approach could be this:

For all practical purposes, you get our services free. Let me tell you why. The average sale as reported by the [Tri-County Multiple Listing Service] for [20XX] was at [84%] of list price. In [20XX], [Loring Realty] sales averaged [94%] of list price. Therefore, we were able to get our owners an increase over the average sale in excess of our fees received.

The percentage of your own listings that are sold by your office can be a positive statement about your firm:

[20XX] Multiple Listing Figures
Sales Made by Listing Office
Average [26%]
[Loring Realty] [51%]

At [Loring Realty] we don't just list and hope one of the cooperating offices finds a buyer. From these figures, you can see that we feel obligated to work hard for our owners. When we represent you, you come first.

Would you like to know how we will sell your home?

You should have a visual marketing plan (see Figure 5.5E, page 200). Your plan should indicate the following as applicable:

Signs, talking signs

Property flyers

MLS distribution

Office website

Other websites used (domestic and foreign)

Enhanced websites

Electronic lockboxes

Virtual tours

Agent caravan

Open houses

Papers, magazines, and other media

Owner suggestions

Staging

Owner communications

Communications with other agents

Constant evaluation of efforts, property, and results

The last page or screen of your presentation should really be a trial closing:

[Mr. and Mrs. Garczynski], don't you want [Loring Realty] to represent you?

Your narrative would simply be the question asked.

Additional Listing Tools

Another tool to bring to a listing presentation is a completed property flyer of the owner's home with a good color photograph of the home and known information (other information left blank, as well as price). This should be left with the owner even if the listing is not obtained.

Some agents also prepare a website presentation that can be viewed on a laptop computer. An attractive visual such as this can help convince the owners they should have you as their agent.

If you use talking signs, a rider strip showing the radio frequency, the base unit, and a radio to listen to a prepared voice message could put you a step above much of the competition.

Bring an electronic lockbox the owners can handle. People like to feel things. It is in our human nature. Let owners hold the lockbox while you explain the security aspects and the information it provides.

BUYER LISTINGS

To obtain listings from buyers, you should explain the normal agency where the agent represents the seller or has dual agency duties. An understanding of seller agency will make the need for buyer agency representation very apparent.

Owners must also understand what you will do for them and how you will be paid your fee. You can use a variation of the question-and-answer technique with just questions where the answers are obvious:

Whom does the property listing agent represent?

Will the property listing agent try to find the home that is best for you, or will the agent try to sell his clients' property?

Some lenders selling foreclosed properties pay brokers a selling fee less than is usually charged. Will a seller's agent want to show you these homes when they have listings that offer them higher fees?

Will the property listing agent try to sell you the property at the lowest possible price?

Does the property listing agent get greater compensation when the price is greater?

The sellers have an agent looking out for their best interests. Should you be similarly protected?

You should explain that your services will generally be paid for by the seller because you will accept the multiple listing service commission split as compensation, which is paid by the seller.

For your presentation, consider the similar material developed by Realty Tools, Inc., or by other software suppliers. In addition, some of the same material you developed for sales listings would be applicable to buyer listings.

Note: Buyer presentation material can also be used as an enclosure when responding to an inquiry, as well as presented to prospective buyers where a buyer listing is not being sought.

COMMERCIAL AND INVESTMENT PROPERTY

WEB LINK

While you can modify residential listing presentations for commercial and investment property, a better approach would be to use software designed for the purpose. Some examples of providers of such software are www.realdata.com, www.costart.com, and www.realhound.com.

SUMMARY

The comparative market analysis is an excellent tool for arriving at a recommended list price, as well as for convincing owners that it is in their best interests to initially list their home at a realistic price. The attachments you provide clearly illustrate the effect of pricing on the time to sell, as well as on the likelihood of success.

The Estimated Seller's Proceeds form is really a disclosure form to fully inform the owners of what they will net from a sale at list price. By receiving this information at the time of listing, the owners are prepared for what they will actually receive. Unpleasant surprises can mean sales that fail to close.

The listing presentation manual is a paper or computer visual tool to be used along with the agent's narrative to provide a structured, effective listing presentation.

The presentation manual is broken down into two sections. One is *Why List?* and the other is *Why Us? The Why List?* presentation shows owners why it is in their best interests to employ an exclusive selling agent. The *Why Us?* presentation tells the owners about you and your firm. It shows the owners the advantages your firm offers. It is a positive approach because it sells benefits and leads to a trial closing.

A separate listing presentation manual should be prepared for buyer listings.

CLASS DISCUSSION TOPICS

1. Comparative market analysis

Prepare a comparative market analysis on a property (use real or fictitious comparables). Present the analysis to an owner (use another student) and explain how you arrived at your recommendations.

2. Estimated Seller's Proceeds form

Prepare an Estimated Seller's Proceeds form, based on costs in your area, for a home that has a $181,000 first trust deed. The seller will be paying 6% commission on the $300,000 sale. (Do not prorate taxes, insurance, or consider impound accounts.)

3. Listing presentation manual

Prepare either the *Why List?* or *Why Us?* portion of the listing presentation manual. Be prepared to make a presentation in class on your portion of the listing presentation manual to another student as though you were addressing an owner.

4. A prospective seller will be interviewing other agents.

Prepare, in writing, the reasons the prospective seller should choose you or your firm rather than your competitors.

5. Bring to class one current-events article dealing with some aspect of real estate practice for class discussion.

UNIT 5 QUIZ

1. A CMA is *BEST* described as
    a. a formal appraisal.
    b. the cooperative marketing approach of multiple listings.
    c. a reflection of the reality of the marketplace.
    d. the comparative mortgage analysis performed by agents in advising buyers as to lender and loan type.

2. In making your recommendation of list price for a single-family home, the *MOST* important portion of the analysis deals with
    a. list prices of homes on the market now.
    b. list prices of homes where the listings expired.
    c. prices of comparable properties that sold.
    d. possible rental income.

3. You should realize that for data used on a CMA,
    a. the older the data, the less reliable they are.
    b. sales prices that seem unusually high or low are often the result of market imperfections.
    c. both of these are true.
    d. both of these are false.

4. Owners must be made to realize that
    a. the higher they price their home over fair market value, the longer it will take to sell.
    b. the higher they price their home over fair market value, the lower the likelihood of a sale during the listing period.
    c. both of these are true.
    d. both of these are false.

5. A recommended list price below what the CMA indicates as the likely sale range is in an owner's best interest when
    a. a sellers' market exists.
    b. the seller must get the highest net.
    c. the seller must sell quickly.
    d. the seller is not strongly motivated to sell.

6. What a seller receives in hand from a sale is the
   a. gross sale price.
   b. net sale price.
   c. net profit.
   d. seller's net proceeds.

7. The principal reason owners try to sell their homes without an agent is
   a. to have a quick sale.
   b. to save the commission.
   c. to be able to pick the buyer.
   d. none of these.

8. Your listing presentation material should
   a. be organized to follow your listing presentation.
   b. not be used in lieu of a verbal presentation.
   c. be helpful in selling an owner on the concept of listing in general and listing with your firm in particular.
   d. be all of these.

9. Which statement is the *BEST* approach to take when selling the benefits of listing with a small office?
   a. "We try harder because of the competition."
   b. "All we need to find is one buyer, and even we can do that."
   c. "We need the business more than the large firms do."
   d. "We specialize in a small number of select properties."

10. Which would be the MOST effective statement to make during a listing presentation?
    a. Last year we sold 26% of the listings we took during the listing period.
    b. Our office has six full-time and nine part-time salespeople.
    c. Last year our average sale was at 86% of the list price.
    d. Our average time to sell was 32 days last year compared with a MLS average time to sell of 54 days.

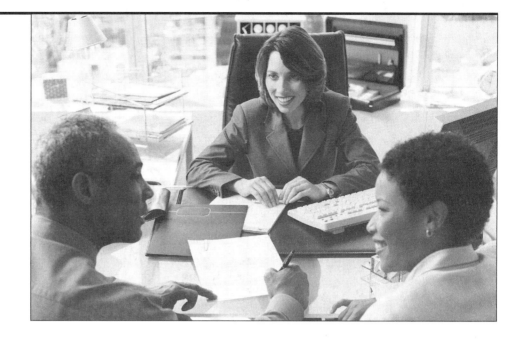

LISTING PRESENTATIONS AND LISTING CONTRACTS

LEARNING OBJECTIVES

When you have completed this unit, you will be able to

- define listing agreement and explain its elements,

- analyze the exclusive-authorization-and-right-to-sell listing and the exclusive-right-to-represent agreement (buyer's listing), and

- describe the listing transaction.

KEY TERMS

bilateral agreement	exclusive-right-to-	safety clause
clincher	represent agreement	short sale
exclusive-agency	net listing	trial closing
listing	open listing	Uniform Electronic
exclusive-	option combined with	Transaction Act
authorization-and-	a listing	unilateral contract
right-to-sell listing	procuring cause	

THE LISTING AGREEMENT

Of all the documents used in the real estate business, none is more important than the listing agreement. This is the instrument that defines a broker's rights and duties. It is the broker's employment contract and gives the broker the right to compensation.

Definition

A *listing agreement*, when executed (signed) by the parties, becomes a legally binding *contract* that authorizes a broker to serve as agent for a principal in a real estate activity. Listing contracts may be entered into for the purpose of securing qualified persons to buy, sell, lease, or rent property or to locate property for lease or purchase. Agents are authorized to find a purchaser or a lessee for a particular property at a specified price and terms, within a certain time limit, or to locate a property for a prospective buyer or a lessee, commonly known as a *buyer agency listing*. The agreement spells out the rights to and obligations of the broker and the seller or the broker and the buyer.

The agreement creates an agency relationship. Brokers who fulfills their part of such contracts are entitled, both legally and morally, to be paid for these efforts. Just a few years ago, buyer agency listings were practically unknown. Now they are quite common because they make sense to buyers who want an agent who represents their interests.

Elements

Because the listing is a contract, it must include all the essential elements of a contract, including competency of parties, lawful object, proper offer and acceptance (mutual consent), and consideration.

California has adopted a modified version of the Uniform Electronic Transaction Act. Parties can agree to conduct a transaction by electronic means. This could apply to listing agreements.

To be enforceable, listing contracts must be in writing [Civil Code 1624(5)]. Oral listings provide the broker with no legal protection whatsoever, because without a written contract, the broker cannot enforce payment of compensation if the principal refuses to pay it. "My word is my bond" is no bond at all in a court of law.

The *consideration* in a listing contract is the broker's promise to "use diligence in locating a ready, willing, and able buyer" in exchange for the seller's promise to pay a commission or the agent's promise to locate a property for a buyer with compensation paid by the buyer or the seller. The promise (seller or buyer to pay commission) given for a promise (broker to use diligence in finding a buyer/property) is a **bilateral agreement**, which is a promise made in exchange for another promise.

The consideration that passes between parties in a real estate contract can be anything of value.

FIGURE 6.1: **Who May Sell a Property and Receive a Commission under Three Types of Listing Agreements**

Open Listing   Exclusive-Agency Listing   Exclusive-Right-to-Sell Listing

Types of Listing Agreements

There are many variations of the basic listing agreement from various publishers, as well as computer program forms and special forms used by real estate franchises. Some are for general residential property; others are for special types of property, such as industrial, income, farm, or unimproved property. Despite the variations, there are three basic kinds of listings: open listings, exclusive-authorization-and-right-to-sell listings, and exclusive-agency listings. Net listings and option listings are additions to the three aforementioned listing contracts. A buyer's listing can also be an open listing. The purpose of a listing agreement generally is to define the relationship between the seller (or buyer, in the case of a buyer's listing) and the broker. You may find it useful to group listings into two kinds of agreements, exclusive and nonexclusive. Figure 6.1 classifies listings according to the relationship between seller and broker.

Open listing. An **open listing** is a nonexclusive written memorandum that when signed by the seller or buyer, authorizes the broker to serve as an agent for the sale or purchase of property. Under an open listing, the owner agrees to pay a commission if the broker procures a buyer or property that is purchased. Because the broker is not obligated to use diligence to locate a buyer or property, an open listing is considered to be a **unilateral contract**. It is a promise that is accepted by the agent's action in procuring a buyer or a property.

The seller or buyer may give this type of listing to as many brokers as he or she sees fit. If the owner has given agents permission to erect signs, there could be multiple For Sale signs on a property. The first agent who finds, according to the listing terms, a ready, willing, and able buyer acceptable to the seller or an acceptable property for the buyer gets the commission. This cancels all other open listings and negates the payment of any other commission. An open listing allows the owner to sell the property herself or the buyer to buy the property himself without being liable to the broker(s) for any compensation.

From the seller's or the buyer's point of view, open listings may appear to provide a wider market than exclusive agreements. However, more sophisticated sellers and buyers often conclude that brokers receiving this type of listing are unlikely to give them preferred attention. Sellers and buyers soon discover that "what is everybody's business is nobody's business" and that carefully selecting a single competent broker is almost always to their advantage.

Most real estate offices will not take an open sale listing because they know that the likelihood of a sale is slight and that allowing the owner to feel the office is using diligence could be a disservice to the owner. With an open listing, there can be owner/agent competition for the same buyer. Owners will often try to make the sale themselves to avoid paying a commission. In order to be protected as the **"procuring cause"** of a sale, the broker must register a buyer with the owner. The agent who is the procuring cause must have initiated an uninterrupted series of events that led to the sale. Experienced agents will hold out for an exclusive-right-to-sell listing and, if they are unable to obtain one, will walk away. The fact that others might agree to an open listing can actually help them. After the owner and the open listing agents have tried unsuccessfully to market the property for several months, the owner should be more receptive to a prepared marketing plan under an exclusive-right-to-sell listing.

Exclusive-authorization-and-right-to-sell listing. An **exclusive-authorization-and-right-to-sell listing** gives a broker the sole right to procure a purchaser for a property. With this type of listing, the broker is the sole agent and has the right to a commission if a buyer is found for the property by anyone—even the owner—during the term of the listing. The listing broker has earned a commission when a bona fide offer from a ready, willing, and able buyer at a specified or accepted price and terms is produced, whether or not escrow closes. (The listing is to produce a buyer.)

An exclusive-authorization-and-right-to-sell listing entitles the listing agent to the compensation, no matter who sells the property.

All exclusive listings, by law, must have a definite termination date. Listings should be dated when they are taken, and the effective term should be set forth so clearly and definitely that there can be no mistake. An exclusive listing may not contain such wording as "effective until date of sale" or "until canceled in writing." California Real Estate Law Section 10176(f) states that a licensee is subject to disciplinary action for

claiming, demanding, or receiving a fee, compensation, or commission under any *exclusive* agreement authorizing or employing a licensee to sell, buy, or exchange real estate for compensation or commission where such agreement does not contain a *definite, specified date* of final and complete termination. [emphasis added]

The agent must give the owner a copy of any exclusive listing at the time it is signed. Because open listings are frequently just letters from an owner and need not be signed by the agent, an agent is not required to give the owner copies of these open listings, although it is strongly recommended that the owner receive copies of all listings. Figure 6.2 is a residential listing agreement, an exclusive-authorization-and-right-to-sell listing form.

FIGURE 6.2:   Residential Listing Agreement (Exclusive Authorization and Right to Sell)

(The following form is copyrighted by the California Association of REAL-
TORS®, © 2014, and is reprinted under a limited license with permission.
Photocopying or any other reproduction, whether electronic or otherwise,
is strictly prohibited.)

CALIFORNIA
ASSOCIATION
OF REALTORS®

RESIDENTIAL LISTING AGREEMENT
(Exclusive Authorization and Right to Sell)
(C.A.R. Form RLA, Revised 11/13)

1. **EXCLUSIVE RIGHT TO SELL:** _____ ("Seller")
   hereby employs and grants _____ ("Broker")
   beginning (date) _____ and ending at 11:59 P.M. on (date) _____ ("Listing Period")
   the exclusive and irrevocable right to sell or exchange the real property in the City of _____,
   County of_____, Assessor's Parcel No. _____,
   California, described as: _____ ("Property").

2. **ITEMS EXCLUDED AND INCLUDED:** Unless otherwise specified in a real estate purchase agreement, all fixtures and fittings that
   are attached to the Property are included, and personal property items are excluded, from the purchase price.
   ADDITIONAL ITEMS EXCLUDED: _____.
   ADDITIONAL ITEMS INCLUDED: _____.
   Seller intends that the above items be excluded or included in offering the Property for sale, but understands that: (i) the purchase agreement
   supersedes any intention expressed above and will ultimately determine which items are excluded and included in the sale; and (ii) Broker
   is not responsible for and does not guarantee that the above exclusions and/or inclusions will be in the purchase agreement.

3. **LISTING PRICE AND TERMS:**
   A. The listing price shall be: _____
   _____ Dollars ($ _____).
   B. Additional Terms: _____
   _____.

4. **COMPENSATION TO BROKER:**
   **Notice: The amount or rate of real estate commissions is not fixed by law. They are set by each Broker
   individually and may be negotiable between Seller and Broker (real estate commissions include all
   compensation and fees to Broker).**
   A. Seller agrees to pay to Broker as compensation for services irrespective of agency relationship(s), either ☐ _____ percent
   of the listing price (or if a purchase agreement is entered into, of the purchase price), or ☐ $ _____,
   AND _____, as follows:
     (1) If during the Listing Period, or any extension, Broker, cooperating broker, Seller or any other person procures a ready, willing, and
     able buyer(s) whose offer to purchase the Property on any price and terms is accepted by Seller, provided the Buyer completes the
     transaction or is prevented from doing so by Seller. (Broker is entitled to compensation whether any escrow resulting from such offer
     closes during or after the expiration of the Listing Period, or any extension.)
   OR (2) If within _____ calendar days (a) after the end of the Listing Period or any extension; or (b) after any cancellation of this
     Agreement, unless otherwise agreed, Seller enters into a contract to sell, convey, lease or otherwise transfer the Property to
     anyone ("Prospective Buyer") or that person's related entity: (i) who physically entered and was shown the Property during
     the Listing Period or any extension by Broker or a cooperating broker; or (ii) for whom Broker or any cooperating broker
     submitted to Seller a signed, written offer to acquire, lease, exchange or obtain an option on the Property. Seller, however,
     shall have no obligation to Broker under paragraph 4A(2) unless, not later than 3 calendar days after the end of the Listing
     Period or any extension or cancellation, Broker has given Seller a written notice of the names of such Prospective Buyers.
   OR (3) If, without Broker's prior written consent, the Property is withdrawn from sale, conveyed, leased, rented, otherwise transferred,
     or made unmarketable by a voluntary act of Seller during the Listing Period, or any extension.
   B. If completion of the sale is prevented by a party to the transaction other than Seller, then compensation due under paragraph
   4A shall be payable only if and when Seller collects damages by suit, arbitration, settlement or otherwise, and then in an
   amount equal to the lesser of one-half of the damages recovered or the above compensation, after first deducting title and
   escrow expenses and the expenses of collection, if any.
   C. In addition, Seller agrees to pay Broker: _____.
   D. Seller has been advised of Broker's policy regarding cooperation with, and the amount of compensation offered to, other brokers.
     (1) Broker is authorized to cooperate with and compensate brokers participating through the multiple listing service(s)
     ("MLS") by offering to MLS brokers out of Broker's compensation specified in 4A, either ☐ _____ percent of the
     purchase price, or ☐ $_____.
     (2) Broker is authorized to cooperate with and compensate brokers operating outside the MLS as per Broker's policy.
   E. Seller hereby irrevocably assigns to Broker the above compensation from Seller's funds and proceeds in escrow. Broker may
   submit this Agreement, as instructions to compensate Broker pursuant to paragraph 4A, to any escrow regarding the Property
   involving Seller and a buyer, Prospective Buyer or other transferee.
   F. **(1)** Seller represents that Seller has not previously entered into a listing agreement with another broker regarding the Property,
     unless specified as follows: _____.
     (2) Seller warrants that Seller has no obligation to pay compensation to any other broker regarding the Property unless the
     Property is transferred to any of the following individuals or entities: _____
     _____.
     (3) If the Property is sold to anyone listed above during the time Seller is obligated to compensate another broker: (i) Broker is

Seller's Initials (_____)(_____)

EQUAL HOUSING
OPPORTUNITY

FIGURE 6.2 (continued):   **Residential Listing Agreement (Exclusive Authorization and Right to Sell)**

Property Address:_____ Date:_____

not entitled to compensation under this Agreement; and (ii) Broker is not obligated to represent Seller in such transaction.

5.   MULTIPLE LISTING SERVICE:

A. Broker is a participant/subscriber to _____ Multiple Listing Service (MLS) and possibly others. Unless otherwise instructed in writing the Property will be listed with the MLS(s) specified above. That MLS is (or if checked ☐ is not) the primary MLS for the geographic area of the Property. All terms of the transaction, including sales price and financing, if applicable, (i) will be provided to the MLS in which the property is listed for publication, dissemination and use by persons and entities on terms approved by the MLS and (ii) may be provided to the MLS even if the Property is not listed with the MLS.

BENEFITS OF USING THE MLS; IMPACT OF OPTING OUT OF THE MLS; PRESENTING ALL OFFERS

WHAT IS AN MLS? The MLS is a database of properties for sale that is available and disseminated to and accessible by all other real estate agents who are participants or subscribers to the MLS. Property information submitted to the MLS describes the price, terms and conditions under which the Seller's property is offered for sale (including but not limited to the listing broker's offer of compensation to other brokers). It is likely that a significant number of real estate practitioners in any given area are participants or subscribers to the MLS. The MLS may also be part of a reciprocal agreement to which other multiple listing services belong. Real estate agents belonging to other multiple listing services that have reciprocal agreements with the MLS also have access to the information submitted to the MLS. The MLS may further transmit the MLS database to Internet sites that post property listings online.

EXPOSURE TO BUYERS THROUGH MLS: Listing property with an MLS exposes a seller's property to all real estate agents and brokers (and their potential buyer clients) who are participants or subscribers to the MLS or a reciprocating MLS.

CLOSED/PRIVATE LISTING CLUBS OR GROUPS: Closed or private listing clubs or groups are not the same as the MLS. The MLS referred to above is accessible to all eligible real estate licensees and provides broad exposure for a listed property. Private or closed listing clubs or groups of licensees may have been formed outside the MLS. Private or closed listing clubs or groups are accessible to a more limited number of licensees and generally offer less exposure for listed property. Whether listing property through a closed, private network - and excluding it from the MLS - is advantageous or disadvantageous to a seller, and why, should be discussed with the agent taking the Seller's listing.

NOT LISTING PROPERTY IN A LOCAL MLS: If the Property is listed in an MLS which does not cover the geographic area where the Property is located then real estate agents and brokers working that territory, and Buyers they represent looking for property in the neighborhood, may not be aware the Property is for sale.

OPTING OUT OF MLS: If Seller elects to exclude the Property from the MLS, Seller understands and acknowledges that: (a) real estate agents and brokers from other real estate offices, and their buyer clients, who have access to that MLS may not be aware that Seller's Property is offered for sale; (b) Information about Seller's Property will not be transmitted to various real estate Internet sites that are used by the public to search for property listings; (c) real estate agents, brokers and members of the public may be unaware of the terms and conditions under which Seller is marketing the Property.

REDUCTION IN EXPOSURE: Any reduction in exposure of the Property may lower the number of offers and negatively impact the sales price.

PRESENTING ALL OFFERS: Seller understands that Broker must present all offers received for Seller's Property unless Seller gives Broker written instructions to the contrary.

Seller's Initials ( ) ( )	Broker's Initials ( ) ( )

B. MLS rules generally provide that residential real property and vacant lot listings be submitted to the MLS within 2 days or some other period of time after all necessary signatures have been obtained on the listing agreement. Broker will not have to submit this listing to the MLS if, within that time, Broker submits to the MLS a form signed by Seller (C.A.R. Form SELM or the local equivalent form).

C. MLS rules allow MLS data to be made available by the MLS to additional Internet sites unless Broker gives the MLS instructions to the contrary. Seller acknowledges that for any of the below opt-out instructions to be effective, Seller must make them on a separate instruction to Broker signed by Seller (C.A.R. Form SELI or the local equivalent form). Specific information that can be excluded from the Internet as permitted by (or in accordance with) the MLS is as follows:
(1) Property Availability: Seller can instruct Broker to have the MLS not display the Property on the Internet.
(2) Property Address: Seller can instruct Broker to have the MLS not display the Property address on the Internet.
Seller understands that the above opt-outs would mean consumers searching for listings on the Internet may not see the Property or Property's address in response to their search.
(3) Feature Opt-Outs: Seller can instruct Broker to advise the MLS that Seller does not want visitors to MLS Participant or Subscriber Websites or Electronic Displays that display the Property listing to have the features below. Seller understands (i) that these opt-outs apply only to Websites or Electronic Displays of MLS Participants and Subscribers who are real estate broker and agent members of the MLS; (ii) that other Internet sites may or may not have the features set forth herein; and (iii) that neither Broker nor the MLS may have the ability to control or block such features on other Internet sites.
(a) Comments And Reviews: The ability to write comments or reviews about the Property on those sites; or the ability to link to another site containing such comments or reviews if the link is in immediate conjunction with the Property.

Seller's Initials (_____)(_____)

RLA REVISED 11/13 (PAGE 2 OF 5)

RESIDENTIAL LISTING AGREEMENT - EXCLUSIVE (RLA PAGE 2 OF 5)

FIGURE 6.2 (continued):   **Residential Listing Agreement (Exclusive Authorization and Right to Sell)**

Property Address:_____ Date:_____

    (b) Automated Estimate Of Value: The ability to create an automated estimate of value or to link to another site containing such an estimate of value if the link is in immediate conjunction with the Property.

6.   **SELLER REPRESENTATIONS:** Seller represents that, unless otherwise specified in writing, Seller is unaware of: (i) any Notice of Default recorded against the Property; (ii) any delinquent amounts due under any loan secured by, or other obligation affecting, the Property; (iii) any bankruptcy, insolvency or similar proceeding affecting the Property; (iv) any litigation, arbitration, administrative action, government investigation or other pending or threatened action that affects or may affect the Property or Seller's ability to transfer it; and (v) any current, pending or proposed special assessments affecting the Property. Seller shall promptly notify Broker in writing if Seller becomes aware of any of these items during the Listing Period or any extension thereof.

7.   **BROKER'S AND SELLER'S DUTIES:** (a) Broker agrees to exercise reasonable effort and due diligence to achieve the purposes of this Agreement. Unless Seller gives Broker written instructions to the contrary, Broker is authorized to (i) order reports and disclosures as necessary, (ii) advertise and market the Property by any method and in any medium selected by Broker, including MLS and the Internet, and, to the extent permitted by these media, control the dissemination of the information submitted to any medium; and (iii) disclose to any real estate licensee making an inquiry the receipt of any offers on the Property and the offering price of such offers. (b) Seller agrees to consider offers presented by Broker, and to act in good faith to accomplish the sale of the Property by, among other things, making the Property available for showing at reasonable times and, subject to paragraph 4F, referring to Broker all inquiries of any party interested in the Property. Seller is responsible for determining at what price to list and sell the Property. Seller further agrees to indemnify, defend and hold Broker harmless from all claims, disputes, litigation, judgments attorney fees and costs arising from any incorrect information supplied by Seller, or from any material facts that Seller knows but fails to disclose.

8.   **DEPOSIT:** Broker is authorized to accept and hold on Seller's behalf any deposits to be applied toward the purchase price.

9.   **AGENCY RELATIONSHIPS:**
    A. Disclosure: If the Property includes residential property with one-to-four dwelling units, Seller shall receive a "Disclosure Regarding Agency Relationships" (C.A.R. Form AD) prior to entering into this Agreement.
    B. Seller Representation: Broker shall represent Seller in any resulting transaction, except as specified in paragraph 4F.
    C. Possible Dual Agency With Buyer: Depending upon the circumstances, it may be necessary or appropriate for Broker to act as an agent for both Seller and buyer, exchange party, or one or more additional parties ("Buyer"). Broker shall, as soon as practicable, disclose to Seller any election to act as a dual agent representing both Seller and Buyer. If a Buyer is procured directly by Broker or an associate-licensee in Broker's firm, Seller hereby consents to Broker acting as a dual agent for Seller and Buyer. In the event of an exchange, Seller hereby consents to Broker collecting compensation from additional parties for services rendered, provided there is disclosure to all parties of such agency and compensation. Seller understands and agrees that: (i) Broker, without the prior written consent of Seller, will not disclose to Buyer that Seller is willing to sell the Property at a price less than the listing price; (ii) Broker, without the prior written consent of Buyer, will not disclose to Seller that Buyer is willing to pay a price greater than the offered price; and (iii) except for (i) and (ii) above, a dual agent is obligated to disclose known facts materially affecting the value or desirability of the Property to both parties.
    D. Other Sellers: Seller understands that Broker may have or obtain listings on other properties, and that potential buyers may consider, make offers on, or purchase through Broker, property the same as or similar to Seller's Property. Seller consents to Broker's representation of sellers and buyers of other properties before, during and after the end of this Agreement.
    E. Confirmation: If the Property includes residential property with one-to-four dwelling units, Broker shall confirm the agency relationship described above, or as modified, in writing, prior to or concurrent with Seller's execution of a purchase agreement.

10. **SECURITY AND INSURANCE:** Broker is not responsible for loss of or damage to personal or real property, or person, whether attributable to use of a keysafe/lockbox, a showing of the Property, or otherwise. Third parties, including, but not limited to, appraisers, inspectors, brokers and prospective buyers, may have access to, and take videos and photographs of, the interior of the Property. Seller agrees: (i) to take reasonable precautions to safeguard and protect valuables that might be accessible during showings of the Property; and (ii) to obtain insurance to protect against these risks. Broker does not maintain insurance to protect Seller.

11. **PHOTOGRAPHS AND INTERNET ADVERTISING:**
    A. In order to effectively market the Property for sale it is often necessary to provide photographs, virtual tours and other media to buyers. Seller agrees (or ☐ if checked, does not agree) that Broker may photograph or otherwise electronically capture images of the exterior and interior of the Property ("Images") for static and/or virtual tours of the Property by buyers and others on Broker's website, the MLS, and other marketing sites. Seller acknowledges that once Images are placed on the Internet neither Broker nor Seller has control over who can view such Images and what use viewers may make of the Images, or how long such Images may remain available on the Internet. Seller further agrees that such Images are the property of Broker and that Broker may use such Images for advertisement of Broker's business in the future.
    B. Seller acknowledges that prospective buyers and/or other persons coming onto the property may take photographs, videos or other images of the property. Seller understands that Broker does not have the ability to control or block the taking and use of Images by any such persons. (If checked) ☐ Seller instructs Broker to publish in the MLS that taking of Images is limited to those persons preparing Appraisal or Inspection reports. Seller acknowledges that unauthorized persons may take images who do not have access to or have not read any limiting instruction in the MLS or who take images regardless of any limiting instruction in the MLS. Once Images are taken and/or put into electronic display on the Internet or otherwise, neither Broker nor Seller has control over who views such Images nor what use viewers may make of the Images.

12. **KEYSAFE/LOCKBOX:** A keysafe/lockbox is designed to hold a key to the Property to permit access to the Property by Broker, cooperating brokers, MLS participants, their authorized licensees and representatives, authorized inspectors, and accompanied prospective buyers. Broker, cooperating brokers, MLS and Associations/Boards of REALTORS® are not insurers against injury, theft, loss, vandalism or damage attributed to the use of a keysafe/lockbox. Seller does (or if checked ☐ does not) authorize Broker to install a keysafe/lockbox. If Seller does not occupy the Property, Seller shall be responsible for obtaining occupant(s)' written permission for use of a keysafe/lockbox (C.A.R. Form KLA).

RLA REVISED 11/13 (PAGE 3 OF 5)   Seller's Initials (_____)(_____)
                                                                                 EQUAL HOUSING OPPORTUNITY

RESIDENTIAL LISTING AGREEMENT - EXCLUSIVE (RLA PAGE 3 OF 5)

FIGURE 6.2 (continued):   **Residential Listing Agreement (Exclusive Authorization and Right to Sell)**

Property Address: _____ Date:_____

13. **SIGN:** Seller does (or if checked ☐ does not) authorize Broker to install a FOR SALE/SOLD sign on the Property.

14. **EQUAL HOUSING OPPORTUNITY:** The Property is offered in compliance with federal, state and local anti-discrimination laws.

15. **ATTORNEY FEES:** In any action, proceeding or arbitration between Seller and Broker regarding the obligation to pay compensation under this Agreement, the prevailing Seller or Broker shall be entitled to reasonable attorney fees and costs from the non-prevailing Seller or Broker, except as provided in paragraph 19A.

16. **ADDITIONAL TERMS:** ☐ REO Advisory Listing (C.A.R. Form REOL) ☐ Short Sale Information and Advisory (C.A.R. Form SSIA)

_____

_____

_____

_____

_____

17. **MANAGEMENT APPROVAL:** If an associate-licensee in Broker's office (salesperson or broker-associate) enters into this Agreement on Broker's behalf, and Broker or Manager does not approve of its terms, Broker or Manager has the right to cancel this Agreement, in writing, within **5 Days** After its execution.

18. **SUCCESSORS AND ASSIGNS:** This Agreement shall be binding upon Seller and Seller's successors and assigns.

19. **DISPUTE RESOLUTION:**
    A. **MEDIATION:** Seller and Broker agree to mediate any dispute or claim arising between them regarding the obligation to pay compensation under this Agreement, before resorting to arbitration or court action. Mediation fees, if any, shall be divided equally among the parties involved. If, for any dispute or claim to which this paragraph applies, any party (i) commences an action without first attempting to resolve the matter through mediation, or (ii) before commencement of an action, refuses to mediate after a request has been made, then that party shall not be entitled to recover attorney fees, even if they would otherwise be available to that party in any such action. THIS MEDIATION PROVISION APPLIES WHETHER OR NOT THE ARBITRATION PROVISION IS INITIALED. **Exclusions from this mediation agreement are specified in paragraph 19C.**
    B. **ARBITRATION OF DISPUTES:**
    Seller and Broker agree that any dispute or claim in Law or equity arising between them regarding the obligation to pay compensation under this Agreement, which is not settled through mediation, shall be decided by neutral, binding arbitration. The arbitrator shall be a retired judge or justice, or an attorney with at least 5 years of residential real estate Law experience, unless the parties mutually agree to a different arbitrator. The parties shall have the right to discovery in accordance with Code of Civil Procedure §1283.05. In all other respects, the arbitration shall be conducted in accordance with Title 9 of Part 3 of the Code of Civil Procedure. Judgment upon the award of the arbitrator(s) may be entered into any court having jurisdiction. Enforcement of this agreement to arbitrate shall be governed by the Federal Arbitration Act. Exclusions from this arbitration agreement are specified in paragraph 19C.
    "NOTICE: BY INITIALING IN THE SPACE BELOW YOU ARE AGREEING TO HAVE ANY DISPUTE ARISING OUT OF THE MATTERS INCLUDED IN THE 'ARBITRATION OF DISPUTES' PROVISION DECIDED BY NEUTRAL ARBITRATION AS PROVIDED BY CALIFORNIA LAW AND YOU ARE GIVING UP ANY RIGHTS YOU MIGHT POSSESS TO HAVE THE DISPUTE LITIGATED IN A COURT OR JURY TRIAL. BY INITIALING IN THE SPACE BELOW YOU ARE GIVING UP YOUR JUDICIAL RIGHTS TO DISCOVERY AND APPEAL, UNLESS THOSE RIGHTS ARE SPECIFICALLY INCLUDED IN THE 'ARBITRATION OF DISPUTES' PROVISION. IF YOU REFUSE TO SUBMIT TO ARBITRATION AFTER AGREEING TO THIS PROVISION, YOU MAY BE COMPELLED TO ARBITRATE UNDER THE AUTHORITY OF THE CALIFORNIA CODE OF CIVIL PROCEDURE. YOUR AGREEMENT TO THIS ARBITRATION PROVISION IS VOLUNTARY."
    "WE HAVE READ AND UNDERSTAND THE FOREGOING AND AGREE TO SUBMIT DISPUTES ARISING OUT OF THE MATTERS INCLUDED IN THE 'ARBITRATION OF DISPUTES' PROVISION TO NEUTRAL ARBITRATION."

    | Seller's Initials _____ / _____ | Broker's Initials _____ / _____ |

    C. **ADDITIONAL MEDIATION AND ARBITRATION TERMS:** The following matters shall be excluded from mediation and arbitration: (i) a judicial or non-judicial foreclosure or other action or proceeding to enforce a deed of trust, mortgage or installment land sale contract as defined in Civil Code §2985; (ii) an unlawful detainer action; (iii) the filing or enforcement of a mechanic's lien; and (iv) any matter that is within the jurisdiction of a probate, small claims or bankruptcy court. The filing of a court action to enable the recording of a notice of pending action, for order of attachment, receivership, injunction, or other provisional remedies, shall not constitute a waiver or violation of the mediation and arbitration provisions.

RLA REVISED 11/13 (PAGE 4 OF 5)   Seller's Initials (_____)(_____)

RESIDENTIAL LISTING AGREEMENT - EXCLUSIVE (RLA PAGE 4 OF 5)

FIGURE 6.2 (continued):   **Residential Listing Agreement (Exclusive Authorization and Right to Sell)**

Property Address:_____ Date:_____

20. **ENTIRE AGREEMENT:** All prior discussions, negotiations and agreements between the parties concerning the subject matter of this Agreement are superseded by this Agreement, which constitutes the entire contract and a complete and exclusive expression of their agreement, and may not be contradicted by evidence of any prior agreement or contemporaneous oral agreement. If any provision of this Agreement is held to be ineffective or invalid, the remaining provisions will nevertheless be given full force and effect. This Agreement and any supplement, addendum or modification, including any photocopy or facsimile, may be executed in counterparts.

21. **OWNERSHIP, TITLE AND AUTHORITY:** Seller warrants that: (i) Seller is the owner of the Property; (ii) no other persons or entities have title to the Property; and (iii) Seller has the authority to both execute this Agreement and sell the Property. Exceptions to ownership, title and authority are as follows: _____
_____.

☐ REPRESENTATIVE CAPACITY: This addendum is being signed for Seller by an individual acting in a Representative Capacity as specified in the attached Representative Capacity Signature Disclosure (C.A.R. Form RCSD). Wherever the signature or initials of the representative identified in the RCSD appear on this Agreement or any related documents, it shall be deemed to be in a representative capacity for the entity described and not in an individual capacity, unless otherwise indicated. Seller (i) represents that the entity for which the individual is signing already exists and (ii) shall Deliver to Broker, within 3 Days After Execution of this Agreement, evidence of authority to act (such as but not limited to: applicable trust document, or portion thereof, letters testamentary, court order, power of attorney, resolution, or formation documents of the business entity).

By signing below, Seller acknowledges that Seller has read, understands, received a copy of and agrees to the terms of this Agreement.

Seller_____ Date _____
Address _____City _____State _____ Zip _____
Telephone _____ Fax _____ Email _____

Seller_____ Date _____
Address _____City _____State _____ Zip _____
Telephone _____ Fax _____ Email _____

Real Estate Broker (Firm) _____ Cal BRE Lic.# _____
By (Agent) _____Cal BRE Lic.# _____ Date _____
Address _____City _____State _____ Zip _____
Telephone _____ Fax _____ Email _____

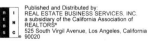

Published and Distributed by:
REAL ESTATE BUSINESS SERVICES, INC.
a subsidiary of the California Association of
REALTORS®
525 South Virgil Avenue, Los Angeles, California
90020

Reviewed by _____ Date _____

RLA REVISED 11/13 (PAGE 5 OF 5)

RESIDENTIAL LISTING AGREEMENT - EXCLUSIVE (RLA PAGE 5 OF 5)

With an exclusive-agency listing, the broker is not entitled to a commission if the owner sells without an agent's assistance.

Exclusive-agency listing.   An **exclusive-agency listing** differs from the exclusive-authorization-and-right-to-sell listing in one major respect: the seller will pay a commission to the listing broker regardless of which agency makes the sale, but it does not prevent owners from selling their own property and paying no commission.

Owners will often want an exclusive-agency listing because they have one or more parties who have expressed interest in the property and don't want to have to pay a fee for the agent selling to "their" prospect. In order to avoid competition with the owner, the agent should suggest an exclusive authorization-and-right-to-sell listing with exceptions for named parties for a period of time, such as seven days. If the buyer's prospects are seriously interested, they will have to decide quickly or they will realize that the owner will be paying a fee, which reduces any advantage they may feel they have in buying direct from the owner. Such an agreement helps the owner because it could mean a quick sale or saving wasted time with a party who is not a serious buyer. After the stated time, which in this case was seven days, the broker has an exclusive-authorization-and-right-to-sell listing without exceptions. The broker might also gain prospects for the purchase of other properties.

It is important to keep in mind that whenever there is an excluded party from an exclusive-right-to-sell listing, the listing agent should disclose the exclusion to other agents. Failure to do so could make the listing agent responsible for paying a commission to another agent, even though the listing agent did not receive compensation for the transaction.

Net listing.   A **net listing** is not truly a type of listing. Net listings could be open, exclusive-right-to-sell, or exclusive-agency listings. Net refers to commission. A clause in the agreement states that the owner is asking a certain sum of money from the sale of property. All expenses, including the broker's commission, are to be covered by any sum the broker is able to obtain in excess of the selling price (net) specified by the seller.

Net listings provide that the commission shall be the excess over a net price set by the seller.

Net listings are seldom used. They make agents vulnerable to charges of fraud, misrepresentation, and other abuses against which the real estate law offers sellers protection. For example, a broker might fail to tell an owner that the price the owner wants is too low or be tempted to persuade the seller to ask for the lowest possible amount so that the broker can sell the property at a much higher price to collect a large commission. These types of actions go against the broker's duties as an agent. In fact, net listings are illegal in a number of states because of the inherent conflicts of interest. Even though they are legal in California, they are generally avoided.

Nevertheless, if a broker takes a net listing, California law requires that the broker disclose, in writing, the selling price and the broker's compensation before acceptance of any offer.

Note: An agent's failure to disclose the selling price under a net listing is cause for license revocation or suspension.

Option combined with a listing. An option is an irrevocable right to buy a property at an agreed price. An **option combined with a listing** entitles the broker to compensation under the listing if the property is sold to a third person, as well as the agent's right to buy the property herself. Law forbids a listing broker who has an option combined with a listing to profit at the expense of the owner. If the broker finds a buyer willing to pay more than the option price, and if the broker then exercises an option to buy to make a greater profit from resale of the property, the broker must make a full disclosure to the owner. California law covering this is stated as follows:

> *If a broker employed to sell property is also given an option to purchase the property himself, he occupies the dual status of agent and purchaser and is not entitled to exercise his option except by divesting himself of his obligation as agent by making a full disclosure of any information in his possession as to the prospect of making a sale to another.*

Even though an option listing may be legal if the proper disclosures are made, an agent who makes an extraordinary profit might nevertheless become involved in a lawsuit. This action could negatively reflect on his or her reputation. It is strongly recommended that both net listings and option listings be avoided.

Buyer broker agreement—exclusive right to represent. Buyers want to be shown the property that best meets the their needs, regardless of the fact it is listed for sale or for sale by owner or lender. They also want to purchase at the lowest possible price. To accomplish these goals, buyers want their own agents. New contract forms were developed for buyer representation. See Figure 6.3. Although this form is for an exclusive representation, buyer listings (like seller listings) could be exclusive agency, under which a buyer could buy without an agent and not be obligated to pay a fee, or could even be an open listing.

The form is similar in many respects to the exclusive-authorization-and-right-to-sell listing. It gives authority to the broker to act as the agent of the buyer rather than the seller. The buyer's broker looks at the entire transaction from the buyer's standpoint, without a shared loyalty. The new contract form allows the buyer to tailor the broker's services to meet the buyer's needs and adjust the compensation accordingly.

The buyer's broker is held to the same standard of performance in serving the buyer as the listing broker owes to the seller. The commission is negotiable, and the contract must contain a definite termination date.

FIGURE 6.3: **Buyer's Listing Agreement**

BUYER'S LISTING AGREEMENT
Exclusive Right to Buy, Exchange or Option

Prepared by: Agent _____   Phone _____
Broker _____   Email _____

NOTE: This form is by a buyer's agent when employed by a buyer as their sole agent to locate and acquire property for a fixed period of time.

DATE: _____, 20_____, at _____, California.
Items left blank or unchecked are not applicable.

1. RETAINER PERIOD:
    1.1   Buyer hereby retains and grants to Broker the exclusive right to locate real property of the type described below and to negotiate the terms and conditions for its purchase, lease or option, acceptable to Buyer, for the period beginning on _____, 20_____ and terminating on _____, 20_____.

2. BROKER'S OBLIGATIONS:
    2.1   Broker to use diligence in the performance of this employment.

3. GENERAL PROVISIONS:
    3.1   Buyer acknowledges receipt of the Agency Law Disclosure. [See **ft** Form 305]
    3.2   Buyer authorizes Broker to cooperate with other brokers and divide with them any compensation due.
    3.3   Before any party to this agreement files an action on a dispute arising out of this agreement which remains unresolved after 30 days of informal negotiations, the parties agree to enter into non-binding mediation administered by a neutral dispute resolution organization and undertake a good faith effort during mediation to settle the dispute.
    3.4   The prevailing party in any action on a dispute will be entitled to attorney fees and costs, unless they file an action without first offering to enter into mediation to resolve the dispute.
    3.5   This agreement will be governed by California law.

4. BROKERAGE FEE:
    NOTICE: The amount or rate of real estate fees is not fixed by law. They are set by each Broker individually and may be negotiable between Client and Broker.
    4.1   Buyer agrees to pay Broker ☐ _____% of the purchase price, or ☐ _____, IF:
        a.   Buyer, or any person acting on Buyer's behalf, purchases, leases, exchanges for or obtains a purchase option on real property sought under this agreement during the retainer period.
        b.   Buyer terminates this employment of Broker during the listing period.
        c.   Within one year after termination of this agreement, Buyer enters into negotiations which result in Buyer's acquisition of an interest in any property Broker has solicited information on or negotiated with its owner, directly or indirectly, on behalf of Buyer prior to this agreement's termination. Broker to identify prospective properties by written notice to Buyer within 21 days after termination. [See **ft** Form 123]
    4.2   Buyer's obligation to pay Broker a brokerage fee is extinguished on Broker's acceptance of a fee from Seller or Seller's Broker of property acquired by Buyer.
    4.3   In the event this agreement terminates without Broker receiving a fee under §4.1 or §4.2, Buyer to pay Broker the sum of $_____ per hour of time accounted for by Broker, not to exceed $_____.

TYPE OF PROPERTY SOUGHT:
GENERAL DESCRIPTION _____
LOCATION _____ SIZE _____
RENTAL AMOUNT/TERM _____

I agree to render services on the terms stated above.	I agree to employ Broker on the terms stated above.
Date: _____, 20_____	☐ See attached Signature Page Addendum. [ft Form 251]
Buyer's Broker: _____	Date: _____, 20_____
Broker's CalBRE #: _____	Buyer's Name: _____
Buyer's Agent: _____	
Agent's CalBRE #: _____	Signature: _____
	Buyer's Name: _____
Signature: _____	Signature: _____
Address: _____	Address: _____
Phone: _____ Cell: _____	Phone: _____ Cell: _____
Email: _____	Email: _____

FORM 103   12-14   ©2014 **first tuesday**, P.O. BOX 5707, RIVERSIDE, CA 92517 (951) 781-7300

The buyer's broker, who is entitled to be compensated by the buyer, is motivated to show the buyer all known applicable properties, including:

- For-sale-by-owner properties

- Foreclosure and probate sales

- Unlisted properties

- Open listings

- Any other available properties

Figure 6.3 is a written contract between the broker and a buyer. Therefore, it must be filled out correctly and signed by the necessary parties. (**Note:** Specific clauses and organization will vary in forms prepared by different publishers.)

ANALYSIS OF RESIDENTIAL LISTING AGREEMENT EXCLUSIVE AUTHORIZATION-AND-RIGHT-TO-SELL LISTING FORM

Because the listing agreement is a written contract between the broker and the seller, it must be filled out correctly and signed by the necessary parties. The exact wording on each listing form will vary, depending on the details of the transaction. However, certain basic provisions are part of each listing contract. Figure 6.2 is a form for an exclusive-authorization-and-right-to-sell listing. The following paragraphs analyze this sample form.

Paragraph 1: Exclusive-Right-to-Sell

Enter here the name of the owner and the real estate office or broker receiving the listing. If a salesperson rather than a broker takes the listing, the salesperson should write his or her employing broker's name. The salesperson completing the form signs his or her name at the bottom of the form. Note that the words *exclusive and irrevocable* make this listing an exclusive authorization and right to sell.

After the broker's name, enter the time period, including the beginning and the termination dates. Three-month to six-month periods are common; however, if the broker thinks the property will take longer to sell, he or she may ask for more time.

Next, enter the location of the property by city and county as well as by an unmistakable address within the city. Occasionally, in addition to the street address, the location by lot, block, and tract or a metes-and-bounds legal description may be given. It may be necessary to add a legal description as a signed attachment to the listing.

Paragraph 2: Items Included and Excluded

Items of personal property that may be included in the purchase are listed, as are items of real or personal property excluded from the sale. Misunderstandings can arise as to what property the seller intends to include, and listing the items will help alleviate such a problem. Examples of personal property often sold with a residence are major appliances and drapes.

Paragraph 3: Listing Price and Terms

The terms of sale include the price at which the property is being offered. Additional space is provided for stipulating the exact terms the owner requires to sell the property. This includes financial arrangements, such as cash, second trust deeds, or loan assumptions. Unless terms are specified, the owner is not obligated to pay a commission when he or she refuses a full-price offer unless the offer is for cash.

Paragraph 4: Compensation to Broker

Bold face type points out that commission is negotiable and not set by law. This statement is required for listings of 1–4-unit residential properties.

Subparagraph A indicates the rate or amount of commission that will be paid if the property is sold.

Subparagraph A-1 stipulates that commission is due regardless of who actually produces a potential buyer. All that is required is that the purchase offer either meets the price and terms of the agreement (as stated in Paragraph 2) or includes a different price and terms that are acceptable to the seller. The offer also must be made during the listing period stated in Paragraph 1.

The safety clause protects you from attempts to evade paying your fee even after the listing expires.

Subparagraph A-2 is the **safety clause**. It provides that the listing agent shall be entitled to a commission if the property is sold within a specified number of days after expiration of the listing to a prospective buyer whose name was furnished by the agent to the owner within three calendar days of expiration of the listing or was sold to a buyer who was shown and physically entered the property during the listing period.

Subparagraph A-3 states that the seller agrees to pay a commission if the seller sells, leases, or rents the property; withdraws it from the market without the consent of the broker; or otherwise renders the property unavailable for sale before the expiration date.

Subparagraph B provides that if completion of the sale is prevented by a party other than the seller and the seller collects damages, then the total commission is to be the lesser of the commission due under Paragraph 4A or one-half of the damages recovered after deducting expenses.

Subparagraph C provides for any additional seller compensation, such as MLS fees or other broker expenses.

Note: Several brokerage firms have been charging sellers a transaction fee or document preparation fee in the $200 range in addition to the commission. If any additional charges are to be made to the seller, they should be clearly set forth in the listing contract. If the fee is in conjunction with a federally related loan, then the fee may violate the Real Estate Settlement Procedures Act, which requires an actual service provided for every fee. Agents may not charge duplicate fees.

Subparagraph D provides that the broker may cooperate with other brokers and divide the commission in any manner acceptable to them or an agreed percentage.

Subparagraph E states that the seller irrevocably assigns to the broker the broker's compensation from the seller's proceeds. In the past, some sellers have notified an escrow not to pay the broker but to turn the funds over to the sellers. Because the escrow is not the agent of the broker, the escrows complied. An assignment agreement protects the broker's fee.

Subparagraph F is the owner's warranty that the owner is not obligated to pay a commission to any other broker if the property is sold during the listing period, with the exception of listed prospective buyers. If such a listed buyer purchases the property during the listing, the broker is not obligated to pay the listing broker and the listing broker is not obligated to represent the owner in the sale.

Paragraph 5: Multiple Listing Service

The parties agree that listing information is to be provided to an MLS. Without authorization from the owner, the agent would not have the right to cooperate with subagents or give the listing or sale information to an MLS or to third parties.

The seller has the right to exclude property information from websites, as well as website features such as viewer comments.

Paragraph 6: Seller Representations

Seller represents that he or she is unaware of a notice of default recorded against the property; delinquencies due under loans; bankruptcy, insolvency, or other proceedings affecting the property as well as any litigation pending or threatened that could affect the seller's ability to sell and any current or proposed special assessments. If the seller becomes aware of any of the above during the listing, the seller agrees to promptly notify the agent.

Paragraph 7: Broker's and Seller's Duties

The broker agrees to use diligence in achieving the purpose of the listing agreement. The seller agrees to consider offers received in good faith and to hold the broker harmless for claims resulting from incorrect information supplied or the failure to disclose information to the broker.

Paragraph 8: Deposit

This section authorizes the listing agent to accept the deposit. Without this authorization, an agent taking a deposit could be doing so as the agent of the buyer.

Paragraph 9: Agency Relationships

This paragraph explains that the broker represents the seller and will not be the agent of the buyer; however, if a buyer is procured by the listing agent, it may be necessary for the broker to act in a dual agency capacity. The seller is informed that the broker also represents other sellers. The agency is to be confirmed prior to or concurrent with the execution of a purchase agreement.

Paragraph 10: Security and Insurance

This section explains that the broker is not responsible for loss or damage to personal property, regardless of the presence of a lockbox, and that the owner must take precautions to protect valuables and obtain insurance for risks involved.

Paragraph 11: Photographs and internet Advertising

Owner can agree or refuse to allow photographs to be used for MLS listings and advertising. The owner acknowledges that visitors may take photos but owner has the option of having MLS listing indicate photos are not to be taken.

Paragraph 12: Key Safe/Lockbox

This provides authorization to install a lockbox. The lockbox makes the property more available for showing by other agents in the MLS. The agent is not liable to the owner for loss or damage resulting from access via the lockbox. If the seller wants the property shown by appointment only, then the listing agent may not want to use a lockbox, and the seller can elect whether or not to use it.

Owners should realize that by refusing to allow a lockbox, the number of showings by other offices will likely be reduced. Showings by other offices would likely require the listing agent to accompany selling agents to view the property.

Paragraph 13: Sign

Putting a For Sale sign on the property makes the property more recognizable. However, the agent must obtain authorization from the seller to do so.

Paragraph 14: Equal Housing Opportunity

The property is offered in compliance with antidiscrimination laws. Members of a protected class cannot be denied the right to purchase property due to their protected class

Paragraph 15: Attorney's Fees

If there is any disagreement between the seller and broker and they go either to court or to arbitration, the loser in either incident must pay the costs. This paragraph tends to reduce frivolous lawsuits.

Paragraph 16: Additional Terms

Space is provided for any other owner-broker agreements or terms.

Paragraph 17: Management Approval

If an associate licensee enters into this agreement, the broker or manager has the right to cancel this agreement within five days.

Paragraph 18: Successors and Assigns

This agreement shall be binding upon the seller and seller's successors and assigns.

Paragraph 19: Dispute Resolution

Subparagraph A provides that the broker and seller agree to mediate any disputes arising from this agreement prior to any other action that is available. They are not, however, required to resolve the dispute through mediation.

Subparagraph B provides that by initialing, the parties agree to neutral binding arbitration of any dispute, thus giving up rights to have the dispute litigated in the courts.

Subparagraph C also provides that matters excluded from mediation and arbitration include foreclosure proceedings, unlawful detainer action, mechanics' liens, matters within court jurisdiction, and tort injuries from latent or patent defects to the property.

Paragraph 20: Entire Contract

It is agreed that this agreement is the entire agreement and may not be contradicted by prior agreements or verbal statements.

Paragraph 21: Ownership Title and Authority

This paragraph warrants that the sellers are the only persons who have title to the property unless indicated otherwise, and that the seller has the authority to execute this agreement and sell the property

Signatures

The seller acknowledges that he or she has read, understands, and accepts the agreement and has received a copy of it.

ANALYSIS OF THE BUYER LISTING AGREEMENT—EXCLUSIVE RIGHT TO REPRESENT BUYER

Compare this buyer's listing with the seller listing (exclusive-authorization-and-right-to-sell agreement) in Figure 6.2. You will notice similarities and differences.

The **exclusive-right-to-represent buyer agreement** sets forth the type of property that the buyer wishes to purchase, its size location, and the price. The specific obligations of the broker are set forth.

The general provisions include acknowledgment of agency disclosure, an authorization to cooperate with other brokers, dispute resolution and an attorney fee provision.

The buyer agrees to pay broker agreed compensation if a purchase is made or owner terminates agreement. A safety provision includes entitlement to compensation for one year after termination if a purchase is made of a property the broker introduced the buyer to and identified said property to the buyer within 21 days of termination of the agreement.

The buyer's obligation to pay a brokerage fee is extinguished if broker accepts a fee from seller or seller's agent.

THE LISTING PROCESS

Real estate brokers must pay careful attention to listing details to ensure a smooth transaction.

Preparing for the Listing

An old adage about the listing process is that it is "80% preparation and 20% selling." The time spent on research before the first appointment with a prospective seller is critical in obtaining the listing.

Step 1: Obtain information about the property.   Ownership records, as well as public information about a property, is available online from public as well as private websites. Sites such as *www.propertyshark.com* can provide ownership records, information or recent building permits, taxes, assessor data, etc.

Generally, real estate firms use their title company to obtain property information. A property profile can generally be obtained instantaneously using public records searches available within any local MLS. Besides title and liens, you should ask for a search of federal tax liens. In addition to the public data available through the MLS, your title company also can give you comparable sales by neighborhood, or even by street, and provide copies of deeds if desired.

Step 2: Prepare your comparative market analysis (CMA).   (See Unit 5.)

Step 3: Drive by the current and expired listings and by the property that has sold.   Drive by the prospective property and then by the comparables to get a feeling for the amenities of the property you are going to list as well as to compare it visually with other existing and expired listings in the marketplace. Take photos, if none are available, so the owners can see the types of property their home will be competing with for buyers.

Keep an open mind as to value until you have analyzed the available data. Just like owners, agents will sometimes have preconceived notions about value, based on a single sale or misinformation.

Check comparable properties before you go for your listing presentation. Often what appears as a comparable on your printout is not even close to being a comparable property when utility and desirability are considered. If an owner knows the property you are using as a comparable and knows of problems it has that should have excluded it as a comparable, you will have lost credibility as an expert. Your chances of obtaining a listing could be significantly reduced.

The Sales Listing Interview

With your preparation and research taken care of, you are ready to call on your listing prospect.

On the first visit, you should ascertain the owners' motivation for selling and view the property to prepare your comparative market analysis and your listing presentation. Normally, you will make your listing presentation on your second visit to the property; however, if the owners appear receptive and you have a good feel for the value, you should go into your listing presentation during your first visit to the property.

After arriving for your second visit, ask the owners if it is all right if you go through their home once again. This relieves tension and shows your interest. If you haven't yet determined the owners' reason for selling, ask them. They will generally give you an honest response. Ask what the owners have done to the home. Owners will be more receptive to agents who they feel appreciate their home.

An excellent place to present your material to owners is the kitchen table. It presents a nonthreatening informal setting, and you are able to sit close to the owners.

(It is easier to be argumentative from a distance.) You also want them to be able to easily view your visual material.

The comparative market analysis (CMA).   In presenting your comparative market analysis, don't rush. You must show you appreciate their house, but present the comparables fairly to lead up to your recommendations. Watch owners for reactions. If they show little reaction, ask questions such as "Are there any recent area sales that I missed?"

Sometimes owners have an inflated idea of what their property is worth. It may be based on a sale under different conditions or on what they heard someone say a house sold for. Often owners have a value in mind based simply on what they want. Consider the following:

[Mrs. Jones], buyers, not sellers or brokers, determine market value. I have shown you what homes similar to yours are for sale at as well as what similar homes have sold for. Is there any information you know of that I have not considered?

If the owners say that another agent told them they could get more for their house, ask to see the comparative market analysis that the price was based on. Chances are there won't be one. Then consider the following rebuttal:

I don't know how that agent was able to arrive at a value so quickly and without a detailed analysis. A value off the top of one's head is a hunch at best. If it is too high, a listing at that price simply means a lot of time wasted and no sale. I showed you the effect of overpricing a home on the likelihood of a sale. If a hunch is too low, someone will get a bargain at your expense. I won't price your home on a hunch, and I'm sure you wouldn't want me to do that.

There are many approaches, but all have the same goal: to convince the owners that your value has validity and that offering the property at a competitive price would be in the owners' best interests.

You want to get the owners to agree on an offering price at this time. If you can't obtain an agreement, your further efforts will be futile. However, if the owners agree on an offering price, you are more than halfway along to a listing:

Do you agree with my recommendation that your home should be placed on the market for ($___)?

Accepting a listing at an unreasonably high price could be a violation of your fiduciary duty to your client.

If an owner is adamant about to what you consider an unrealistically high price, a short drive to some neighboring properties for sale might bring the buyers back to earth. Choose unoccupied homes with lockboxes to show without disturbing owners.

If the owners have been very receptive to your presentation with the comparative market analysis or if the owners contacted you to list the property, it should not be necessary for you to go through the listing presentation. You can cut right to the listing. Start by obtaining the owners' signatures on the Estimated Seller's Proceeds form. (See Unit 5.) Never delay when parties are receptive because delay can lead to indecision.

The listing presentation.   After you have finished presenting your comparative market analysis, ask the owners if they can spare a few minutes for you to present some information they will want to hear. Because you have gone to a great deal of effort on behalf of the owners, you can expect a positive response.

Go through the listing presentation book or computer presentation, using narratives such as those developed in Unit 5. Of course, use your narratives with your visuals as you turn the pages of your book. When you have finished, you should be ready for a closing.

PowerPoint, a Microsoft developed program, is an excellent program to use for preparation of a computer presentation. It can combine text with graphics, slides, movies, and audio for a professional and effective presentation. Additionally, if you are making your presentation using an iPad or other tablet device, consider preparing your presentation in Keynote or another third-party application.

> ### Be Positive
> Use positive terms in your presentation. An agency representation indicates you will be doing something for an owner, whereas listing may have a negative connotation. In the same manner, a fee is something that they can understand is due a professional, but commission is a word that can have a negative connotation.

Make certain the owners understand what they will actually net from an offer. Be up front with them. When you use the Estimated Seller's Proceeds form, be realistic in your figures. As previously stated, it is better to be on the low side than to estimate a net significantly higher than the owner will actually receive. Disappointed owners lead to loss of goodwill toward your firm and could result in a failure to close the sale. After the sellers sign the statement, give them a copy.

You should explain agency relationships and have the owners sign that they have received a copy of the agency disclosure (Unit 3). While the signing of the Seller's Estimated Proceeds form and the Disclosure Regarding Real Estate Agency Relationships form do not obligate the owners, it should now be a natural act to sign the listing when it is presented. A **trial closing** tries for an agreement to sign the listing. The choice should not be to list or not to list. As an example, the question "Would you want me to serve as your marketing agent for 90 days or should we make it 120 days?" gives owners a choice between two positives, not between a positive and a negative.

If the owners respond positively to your trial closing, give each of the owners a copy of the listing. It could be prepared in advance so you need to insert only minor items. Go through the listing slowly. Answer any owner questions. When you get to items calling for initials, give each owner a pen and ask each to initial where recommended. Make certain they understand that the option is theirs.

Every presentation you give will not necessarily run smoothly. There will be objections that must be overcome in a straightforward, logical manner. You might consider starting with the following:

I'm glad you mentioned that because...

That's an excellent point. You're absolutely right but...

Owners who hesitate to sign the agreement are signaling that they have a problem. You must find out what the problem is if you are to overcome it. Most of the objections should be readily overcome by material covered in Unit 5 and included in your listing presentation.

A common objection is, "I want to sell, in fact I need to sell. That's why I can't be tied up with a listing." Your response could be:

That's exactly why I suggest an exclusive-right-to-sell agency agreement at the price I have indicated. We know from experience that it takes longer for an owner not represented by an agent to sell a home than it takes with an agent. In addition, in working on your own, you more than double your chance of running into time-consuming and costly problems when you do find a buyer. You are not tying up your property with an exclusive-right-to-sell agency agreement; instead, you are taking the first step toward a sale.

Many objections center on paying compensation. As previously stated, you should always refer to it as a *fee*. Consider the following approaches:

The fee is paid out of money the buyer puts up. The buyer's price includes the fee so they feel they are the ones paying it. When buyers know that an agent isn't involved, they typically reduce any offer that they're willing to make by an amount to cover the fee involved with an agent even if the price was reduced to reflect this. Buyers may not be willing to split it because they may feel that it comes out of their money.

If an owner asks you to reduce your fee, one approach to use would be:

A reduced fee would not be fair to you. Studies have shown that a reduced fee increases the length of time it takes for a sale as well as reduces the likelihood of a sale.

If there are varying commission rates in your area, check the records of your listing service before making the listing presentation. You may discover that listings taken by firms offering a significantly lower fee have a lower sales record than listings taken by your firm at a more normal fee. If so, you could present this information visually with a bar graph and use a narrative such as:

Based on the computer records of [Cedar Creek Brokers Association], listings taken by [Champion Realty] at a [6%] fee have a [46%] greater likelihood of being sold during the listing period than listings taken by other firms at a [4%] fee. This points out that you get what you pay for. A lower fee simply reduces the likelihood of a sale. A lower fee may mean no fee at all and an unsold house. Is that a bargain?

Another objection concerns *listing price*. Some owners want to add your fee to what they want for the home to determine an offering price. Owners may be unrealistic for many reasons, but it isn't enough just to get a listing; you want a listing that is likely to sell. While you have a duty to an owner to get the maximum possible from a property, you also have a duty to advise the owner as to what would be in the owner's best interests.

Several approaches you can use include:

Let's assume that we offer the property at the price you suggest [$]. Assume further that we find a buyer at that price. The sale would be unlikely to be made because lenders make loans based on appraisals of market value, not what a buyer is willing to pay. From my comparables, I have shown you data on market value. Appraisers have access to this same data. What do you suppose will happen when the buyer is notified that the loan is not approved because the property is worth less than the buyer has offered?

> Too high a list price does not help the owner.

Assume you are a buyer and you are looking at homes and you see these comparable properties I have shown you at lower prices than your home is listed at. What do you suppose a buyer's reaction will be? Pricing that is not reflective of the market would not be fair to you, because you would be eliminating many potential buyers.

An overpriced listing is unlikely to sell. Your failure will help another agent in obtaining a listing at a realistic price. By taking an overpriced listing, you will get a reputation both of failure and of having an inventory of overpriced properties.

If the owners indicate that they want to list at their price to see what happens and perhaps reduce the price later, an approach to use would be:

When a property is realistically listed, agents are enthusiastic and will spend their best efforts on selling that property. If they regard a listing as a "hard sell," they will show the property only if more attractively priced properties are not available.

When you finally reduce your price, that price adjustment is not greeted with the enthusiasm of a new listing. In addition, when buyers know a price was reduced and the property has been on the market for a long time, they will sense desperation. Any offer will then likely be significantly less than the reduced price. If you really want to sell your home at the best possible price, I suggest we list it at [$]. Doesn't this make sense?

Sometimes it takes a **clincher**. Final persuasion for an owner who has been trying to sell without an agent could be:

[Mr. and Mrs. Jones], do you realize that this house is holding you captive? With your sign and your ads, you likely feel that you have to be here every weekend waiting for the telephone or doorbell to ring. Even people who say they will be here seldom show up. I'm offering to relieve you of these obligations.

Whenever you make a closing that implies a signature, offer the owner a pen. The owner who puts it down still has questions that must be eliminated. Don't be afraid to try again and again for a closing. A closing is not a one-time win-or-lose proposition.

Prepare yourself so answers to objections and closings come naturally. If you can't close a listing, you won't be able to close a sale. If you can't close a sale, you become an order taker who shows merchandise and waits for a buyer to decide, not a problem solver—and certainly not a professional salesperson.

Follow through.   After you obtain the listing, thank the owners. Be certain you leave the following items:

- A copy of the signed listing with your card attached

- A copy of your comparative market analysis

- The Estimated Seller's Proceeds form

- A copy of the signed agency disclosure form if not covered in the listing

Let the owners know what will be happening (your marketing plan) when the for sale sign will be installed and when you will be contacting them again.

The Buyer Agency Presentation

It is difficult to get buyers to agree that you should be their exclusive agent to find them property to buy unless they feel that you fully understand their needs, that you are competent and able to locate a property for them, and that it would be in their best interests to have you as their exclusive agent. Similarly, you don't want to take an agency responsibility and expend your best efforts for prospective buyers until you realize they are motivated to buy, have the resources and/or credit to consummate a purchase, and have needs you can reasonably fulfill.

A good time to make a presentation for exclusive-agency representation to buyers would be after you have interviewed them about their needs, shown them several properties, and questioned them further about property impressions. By then, you will have understood fairly well the buyers and sold yourself as a professional.

A good approach would be to tell your prospective buyer(s) that you would like to have them obtain preapproval for a loan so that they'll have the financing when they find a property. By handling an internet loan application and printing out a loan preapproval letter, you will show your professionalism and make the prospects feel they are a step closer to a new home. A loan preapproval will also enhance the likelihood of an offer being accepted by an owner.

A number of internet sites are available where your client can get preapproved for a loan in as little as 15 minutes. You should explain to your clients that being preapproved, subject to verification, does not obligate the buyers to deal with that specific lender. The preapproval letter can be attached to any offers made.

You could now conduct a presentation using buyer-listing presentation material, or you could use a narrative such as the following:

> *I would like to help you in finding the best home for you. I imagine we will spend a good deal of time together in accomplishing this goal. Do you feel comfortable working with me?*

You can, of course, expect a positive response and people are unlikely to say they are uncomfortable working with you.

> *Most agents are really agents of the owners and have a duty to get the highest price possible for a property. However, I would like to represent you alone rather than an owner. As your agent, my duty would be to fulfill your needs with the best property for you at the lowest price. Is that what you want?*

Prospective buyers can be expected to give a positive response, as they of course want the best property at the lowest price.

> *I'll be using my best efforts to work for you and to meet your needs. However, my services will likely be paid, not by you, but by sellers who have listed properties with other agents. While I'll share in the fee paid by a seller, my sole obligation will be to you. Does that type of arrangement sound reasonable to you?*

Note: You are asking if it sounds reasonable and the response will likely be positive. It is implied that they are agreeing to an agency relationship.

> *I want you to be partners with me in meeting your needs. If you see a house that is for sale, a house you're interested in, or an internet listing that perks your interest, contact me and I'll get more information for you. If it seems promising, I'll arrange for you to see the property.*

> *I would like to go over the agency representation that I think would best meet your needs.*

You can then give your prospective buyer(s) copies of the exclusive-right-to-represent agreement and go through the agreement with them explaining the meaning of each paragraph. You should explain to the prospective buyers that by signing the agreement, they are not obligated to make any purchase and that in cases where the property is listed for sale with a broker, the seller would be the one paying your fee. By having them initial each page as you complete the agreement, signing it will be a natural act.

Listing a Short Sale

There may be listing situations that at first glance appear hopeless because the owner owes more than can be netted from a sale.

A saleable listing is still possible if you can convince a lender that it is in their best interest to agree to a **short sale** where the lender agrees to accept sale proceeds as settlement of the loan obligation. See Unit 7 for how to handle short-sale situations.

Before a lender will agree to this the lender has to be convinced that the borrower will otherwise default on the loan and that the listing price you are proposing is as good as they can expect in the market. If a lender gives approval for a short sale of 1-4 residential units, a deficiency judgement is not possible.

SUMMARY

A listing contract is an agency contract to sell or locate property.

A valid listing must be in writing and must meet the four requirements of any contract:

1. Competent parties

2. Lawful object

3. Proper offer and acceptance (mutual consent)

4. Consideration

There are six basic types of listings:

1. Open listing (nonexclusive)

2. Exclusive-authorization-and-right-to-sell listing

3. Exclusive-agency listing

4. Net listing

5. Option listing

6. Exclusive-right-to-represent listing

The real estate agent must understand every paragraph used in both the sale and buyer-listing forms to answer owners' and buyers' questions and properly meet owners' and buyers' needs.

The agent must prepare for the listing transaction. The first step is to obtain information about the property; the second step is to prepare the comparative market analysis; the third step is to drive by comparables to make certain that your comparables are truly comparable and that you have a good sense of value.

The listing presentation normally starts with going through the comparative market analysis. The seller should understand the validity of your information before you proceed further.

If the owners are not ready to list their property, go through your listing presentation material, using a narrative with your visuals. This material should answer two owners' questions, why list? and why you? This should lead you to a trial closing that is intended to gain an agreement to sign the listing. After a listing is signed, be certain to leave a copy along with copies of the Estimated Seller's Proceeds form and your comparative market analysis and agency disclosure information if not included in the listing form. Be certain the owners know when you will contact them again.

To obtain a buyer's agency agreement you must prove your competency to locate property and the buyers must feel you fully understand their needs and are willing to work for them.

If a home is encumbered with a trust deed greater than the fair market value of the property, a listing is still possible if the lender will agree to a short sale. In a short sale the lender accepts the net sale proceeds as full settlement for their lien.

CLASS DISCUSSION TOPICS

1. Prepare a list of ten possible objections that an owner might raise to signing a listing.

2. Be prepared to enact a classroom role-playing situation in which objections are raised by the owner. (You might be called on to take the part of either the agent or the owner.)

3. Prepare a five-minute (maximum) presentation to a prospective buyer, showing why he or she should be represented under a signed buyer-listing agreement.

4. Role-play closing a listing with your instructor as the owner. Be prepared with more than one closing.

5. Special assignments (if indicated by instructor):

    a. Using a form supplied by your instructor or one used in your area, complete an exclusive-authorization-and-right-to-sell agreement for the following:

Property:	Single-family residence, 217 W. Clark Lane, Fillmore, California, Ventura County
Owners:	Sam and Loretta Smyth
Broker:	(Name Yourself)
Listing Period:	Four months commencing this date
Price:	$548,000
Personal Property:	Refrigerator, pool equipment, and fireplace accessories go with property
Special Conditions:	No lockbox or sign. Two-hour notice of all showings limited to 3–5 pm daily and 8 am until noon on weekends and holidays.
Broker's Compensation:	Six percent of sale price. 90-day safety period for commissions to parties whom agent(s) negotiated with prior to expiration of listing and whose names were furnished to owner.

b. Using a form supplied by your instructor, complete an exclusive-right-to-represent agreement for the following:

Buyer:	Henry and Sally Corleone
Broker:	(Name Yourself)
Period of Authorization:	Three months from this date
Property:	Single-story 3–4 BR home with 2½ baths, 3-car garage, fireplace, and golf course views in gated community
Price:	$650,000 to $800,000
General Location:	Palm Desert, Rancho Mirage, or Indian Wells, California
Other:	Spanish architecture preferred
Compensation:	3½% of acquiring price. If compensation is paid by another party, any excess shall be paid to broker. If within 60 days of termination buyer buys a property that broker introduced buyer to during life of this agreement, then buyer shall pay broker the compensation.
Agency:	This shall be a single agency only.

6. Explain either a sales listing or buyer agency form, paragraph by paragraph, as if you were explaining it to a prospective seller or buyer.

7. Bring to class one current-events article dealing with some aspect of real estate practice for class discussion.

UNIT 6 QUIZ

1. A valid exclusive listing requires
   a. a lawful purpose.
   b. mutual consent.
   c. consideration.
   d. all of the above.

2. An agent sold a property where the owner had verbally agreed to pay a commission. The agent would be legally entitled to a commission from the owner for the sale if the agent had
   a. relied on the verbal promise.
   b. made a written memorandum of the agreement signed by the agent.
   c. obtained a valid buyer listing agreement.
   d. none of the above.

3. Which listing would you be *LEAST* likely to advertise?
   a. Nonresidential property
   b. An open listing
   c. An exclusive-agency listing
   d. An exclusive-right-to-sell listing

4. A listing under which the owner can sell the listed property without payment of a commission but the agent is nevertheless an exclusive agent is a(n)
   a. open listing.
   b. exclusive-right-to-sell listing.
   c. exclusive-agency listing.
   d. net listing.

5. An agent who did not obtain a purchase offer but who initiated an uninterrupted chain of events that led to a sale would be considered the
   a. agent of record.
   b. procuring cause
   c. exclusive agent.
   d. cooperating broker.

6.   An exclusive-right-to-sell listing likely includes
     a.   an agency relationship disclosure.
     b.   an attorney fee provision.
     c.   an arbitration agreement.
     d.   all of the above.

7.   All of the following statements regarding an exclusive-right-to-sell listing are true *EXCEPT*
     a.   escrow does have to close for an agent to be entitled to a commission.
     b.   it must have a termination date for the agent to be able to collect a commission.
     c.   the agent must give the owner a copy of the listing when the owner signs.
     d.   the agent is precluded from working with

8.   The type of listing that has the greatest likelihood of resulting in a sale would be a(n)
     a.   open listing.
     b.   exclusive-agency listing.
     c.   exclusive-right-to-sell listing.
     d.   reduced-fee listing.

9.   An owner tells you that Agent Jones told her she could get far more for her home than your CMA indicates. What is your *BEST* response?
     a.   "Many unethical agents will promise the moon to get listings and then fail to perform."
     b.   "I am willing to take the listing at that price, but if we don't attract buyers we will reevaluate the price."
     c.   "I don't believe it. No agent who knows the market would set a price that high."
     d.   "I think my comparative market analysis covers all recent comparables and clearly shows the market value. May I please look at the comparative market analysis that Agent Jones prepared for you?"

10. By taking a listing at a low fee that will result in a less than normal fee for any cooperating brokers, you are benefiting
     a.   your office.
     b.   a selling office.
     c.   the owner.
     d.   none of the above.

7

SERVICING THE LISTING

LEARNING OBJECTIVES

When you have completed this unit, you will be able to

- explain owner/agent communication,

- describe how to prepare a property for a sale,

- describe seller disclosures and explain how to modify or extend a listing,

- list the components of a marketing plan, and

- explain how to handle a short sale listing.

KEY TERMS

agent property
  evaluation
broker open house
caravan
communication
Equator Platform

homeowner
  instructions
information boxes
neighborhood
  information request
open house

pocket listing
property brief
staging
talking sign
virtual tour
weekly activity report

OWNER-AGENT COMMUNICATION

The reason most often cited by owners who have been unhappy with the agent who took the listing on their property is not the failure of the agent to secure a buyer; it is the failure of the agent to communicate with them after the listing is signed.

It's easy for owners to feel abandoned by their agents. There is a For Sale sign on the lawn and a listing on the internet. Occasionally, someone calls for an appointment, and people rush through the home in silence.

Owners want to know what is happening. Some agents even become hard to reach when owners want to know what is happening. The agent paved the way so smoothly in the presentation to get the listing, but now there seems to be a communication breakdown.

> Owner discontent is usually based on the agent's failure to communicate with the client.

The problem in these cases may be that the agent failed to explain what would be happening in advance and doesn't want to tell an owner that very little is happening now. Sometimes, unprofessional agents make unrealistic promises to get listings and want to avoid the unpleasant task of telling the owners that they have not located buyers for their properties. When a listing expires, some agents don't even want to face the owners again to try for an extension.

What Will Be Happening

Owner-agent **communication** should start with the listing. Agents should inform owners what will be happening in the few days immediately following. Agents should make definite appointments to meet soon after a listing to discuss their marketing approaches.

Broker Introduction

Chances are the owners have never met your broker. Your broker should send a letter to the owners thanking them for entrusting the sale of their home to his or her firm. The letter should state that the listing agent is the owners' contact person with the firm but that if any problems arise, they should feel free to contact the broker.

Postlisting Meeting

You should consider a post-listing meeting with the owners soon after the listing was obtained. At the post-listing meeting, go through the house again and make recommendations to the owners of things they should do to help with marketing, called "staging," their home. Impress on the owners that marketing is really a team effort.

> The owner's cooperation can increase the likelihood of a sale.

Homeowner instructions.   Give the owners **homeowner instructions** to follow. (See Figure 7.1.) When you recognize that work needs to be done, advise the owners to do it or have it done. Show that it is in the owners' interest and not yours that the house appears at its best.

FIGURE 7.1:   Instructions for Sellers

Homeowner Hints for a Successful Sale

I. Exterior
  A. Grass and shrubs: Keep trimmed. Consider a fast-greening fertilizer such as ammonium sulfate (inexpensive) for a deep green lawn.
  B. Pets: If you have a dog, clean up any dog dirt on a daily basis. If you have a cat, change your litter box daily. Secure pets when the house is being shown.
  C. Fences: Make any needed repairs. A neat, well-painted fence gives a positive impression.
  D. Flowers: Plant seasonal blooming flowers, especially near the front door and in any patio area. A profusion of color can have your home half-sold before the door is even opened.
  E. Bird feeders: Hummingbird feeders and birdhouses create a pleasant mood, especially when they are close to any patio area.
  F. Paint:
    1. Front door should be refinished or painted if it shows excessive wear.
    2. Check exterior paint. Often only the trim or, depending on sun exposure, only one or two sides of the house need painting. Keep in mind the fact that paint is cheap compared to the extra dollars a home with a clean fresh appearance will bring.
  G. Lawn furniture: Place lawn furniture in an attractive, leisurely manner. A badminton net; croquet set-up or barbeque gives a positive image as well.
  H. Roof: If the roof needs to be repaired or replaced, it's best to have the work done. Otherwise, buyers will want to deduct the cost even if your price already reflects the required work. Delaying repairs can actually cost you twice as much.
II. Interior
  A. Housekeeping: You are competing against model homes, so your home must look as much like a model as possible. Floors, bath fixtures, and appliances must be sparkling. Make beds early in the day. Unmade beds and late sleepers create a very negative image.
  B. Odors and aromas: Avoid using vinegar or frying or cooking strong-smelling foods such as cabbage just before showing. The odors last and work against the image you are trying to create. On the other hand, some smells have a positive effect on people: Baked bread, apple pie, chocolate chip cookies, and cinnamon rolls are examples of foods that can help sell your home. Consider keeping packaged cookie or bread dough in the refrigerator. Just before a scheduled showing, the smell of these baking foods can be a great help to us. Garbage containers should be emptied regularly and cleaned. For exterior garbage cans, seal daily garbage in plastic bags to avoid odor.
  C. Paint: If you have leftover paint, you can accomplish a great deal by touching up paint where needed. If the paint is dark, repaint with light colors such as off-white, oyster, light beige, or pale yellow. Light colors make rooms appear fresh as well as larger.

FIGURE 7.1 (continued):   **Instructions for Sellers**

D. Plumbing: Repair any leaky faucets. Make certain you don't have a gurgling toilet or cracked toilet seat.

E. Shades and blinds: Replace any torn shades or broken blinds.

F. Drapes: If drapes need cleaning, have it done. If they are old and worn, stained or dark, consider replacing them with light colors. (Large department stores or catalog houses will have products that can solve the problem.) Vertical blinds might be considered as an alternative to drapes. They are less expensive than all but the cheapest drapes and have a clean, appearance.

G. Carpets: Dirty carpets should be either professionally steam cleaned (preferred), or you should rent a heavy-duty cleaner to do it yourself.

H. Lighting: If any room appears dark, increase the wattage of your light bulbs. Before a showing, open the blinds and drapes and turn on the lights, even during the day. You want the house as light as possible. Make certain your light fixtures and windows are clean.

I. Closets: If closets appear crowded, remove items not needed and put them in boxes. The boxes can then be stacked neatly in a corner of the basement, attic, or garage.

J. Too much furniture: Many houses appear crowded, with too many pieces of large furniture as well as bric-a-brac. Consider putting excess furniture in a rental storage unit.

K. Family photos and mementos: Put very personal items in drawers. While they are important to you, visitors must be able to visualize it as their house, not your house. Many prospects feel intrusive when they are among personal items of others.

L. Garage and basement: Spruce up your work area. Consider a garage sale to get rid of the excess items too good to throw away but of no use to you. Put excess items in boxes and stack them neatly in a corner. Consider using a commercial garage floor cleaner to remove excess oil and grease marks on the garage floor and driveway. You might consider a commercial steam cleaner (not carpet cleaner).

   A. Temperature: On cold days, a natural fire in the fireplace will help us sell your home. Start the fire before the showing is scheduled. On hot days, consider turning the air conditioner several degrees cooler than normal. The contrast will seem phenomenal, giving a very positive reaction. In moderate weather, open windows for fresh air.

III. You

When your home is shown, it's best that you disappear for a while. Buyers feel restrained with an owner present. If buyers will not voice their concerns, then their questions cannot be answered and their problems cannot be solved. Many buyers will feel they are intruding if you are present. Buyers then tend to spend less time in the property, which can reduce salability.

If you must remain in the house, try to stay in one area. Excellent places to be are working in the garden, on the lawn, or in the workshop. These activities create a positive image. While soft music is fine, do not have a TV on. Never, never follow the agent around the house during the showing, volunteer any information, or answer questions the buyers may have. You have engaged professional real estate salespersons. We will ask you questions if necessary.

[Clyde Realty]   [555-8200]   [www.CRE.com]

Besides cleaning and performing needed repairs, there could be a situation in which an improvement might increase property value in excess of the cost of the improvement. Should this be the case, inform the owners of this possibility. In the event they improve the property after it is listed, an adjustment in the list price should be considered.

It is not enough that owners understand what is expected of them, they should understand why. Owners must understand that their house is in competition with other homes for the same buyers. Therefore, they must do everything feasible to make their home a winner.

Some owners may want to meet prospective buyers and follow you around and volunteer information; after all, it is their home. While they have the right to do so, they should understand that being there could inhibit prospective buyers from freely voicing concerns. If a concern of a prospective buyer is not known to you, you can't overcome it. You must explain that like most people, buyers may not want to criticize because it could be taken personally by the owners. On the other hand, voicing a problem to you is really a sign of interest with a "but" attached. Getting rid of the "but" can turn that interest into a sale.

Explain to the owners that at times prospective buyers may come to their door. Owners should ask for the name of the prospect and call your office at once, so an agent can come to show them the home.

Figure 7.2, "Preparing Your Home for Showing and Sale," and Figure 7.3, "When an Appointment Is Made to See Your Home," are taken from the Toolkit for Presentations and are reproduced with the permission of Realty Tools, Inc.

Security.   You should advise owners to secure small expensive items when the home will be available to unsupervised visits by other agents. If the property has a security system, do not make the code readily available to all other agents. Listing agents often arrange to meet buyer agents and disarm the system. Many security systems allow remote monitoring where you can turn off and reset the system when an agent calls your office.

Do not turn off security systems without the owner's permission. While it makes showings easier, it creates great risks. In La Habra, California, an unoccupied furnished home listed on the market was trashed and looted by hundreds of teenagers led to the property by internet party invitations. The security system had been turned off.

Staging.   As the sales market tightens, the need to have properties outshine competing properties is apparent. Owners are competing against other homeowners and even lenders and flippers. The advantage your owner can have is the ability to make their house look move-in ready.

FIGURE 7.2: **Preparing Your Home for Showing and Sale**

Preparing Your Home

Your home has just one chance to make a great impression with each potential buyer. And it can! The following "tricks of the trade" will help you keep track of what needs to be done. The whole idea is to present a clean, spacious clutter-free home--the kind of place you'd like to buy. Accomplish a little everyday, and before long your home will be ready to make the impression that can make the sale.

Your Home's Curb Appeal

- ❏ Mow lawn
- ❏ Trim shrubs
- ❏ Edge gardens and walkways
- ❏ Weed and mulch
- ❏ Sweep walkways and driveway, remove branches, litter or toys
- ❏ Add color and fill in bare spots with plantings
- ❏ Remove mildew or moss from walls or walks with bleach and water or other cleaner
- ❏ Take stains off your driveway with cleanser or kitty litter
- ❏ Stack woodpile neatly
- ❏ Clean and repair patio and deck area
- ❏ Remove any outdoor furniture which is not in good repair
- ❏ Make sure pool or spa sparkles
- ❏ Replace old storm doors
- ❏ Check for flat-fitting roof shingles
- ❏ Repair broken windows and shutters, replace torn screens, make sure frames and seams have solid caulking
- ❏ Hose off exterior wood and trim, replace damaged bricks or wood
- ❏ Touch up exterior paint, repair gutters and eaves
- ❏ Clean and remove rust from any window air conditioning units
- ❏ Paint the front door and mailbox
- ❏ Add a new front door mat and consider a seasonal door decoration
- ❏ Shine brass hardware on front door, outside lighting fixtures, etc.
- ❏ Make sure doorbell is in good working order

General Interior Tips

- ❏ Add a fresh coat of interior paint in light, neutral colors
- ❏ Shampoo carpeting, replace if necessary
- ❏ Clean and wax hardwood floors, refinish if necessary
- ❏ Clean and wash kitchen and bathroom floors
- ❏ Wash all windows, vacuum blinds, wash window sills
- ❏ Clean the fireplace
- ❏ Clean out and organize closets, add extra space by packing clothes and items you won't need again until after you've moved

- ❏ Remove extra furniture, worn rugs, and items you don't use; keep papers, toys, etc. picked up--especially on stairways
- ❏ Repair problems such as loose door knobs, cracked molding, leaking taps and toilets, squeaky doors, closets or screen doors which are off their tracks
- ❏ Add dishes of potpourri, or drop of vanilla or bath oil on light bulbs for scent
- ❏ Secure jewelry, cash and other valuables

The Living Room

- ❏ Make it cozy and inviting, discard chipped or worn furniture and frayed or worn rugs

The Dining Room

- ❏ Polish any visible silver and crystal
- ❏ Set the table for a formal dinner to help viewers imagine entertaining here

The Kitchen

- ❏ Make sure appliances are spotless inside and out (try baking soda for cleaning Formica stains)
- ❏ Make sure all appliances are in perfect working order
- ❏ Clean often forgotten spots on top of refrigerator and under sink
- ❏ Wax or sponge floor to brilliant shine, clean baseboards
- ❏ Unclutter all counter space, remove countertop appliances
- ❏ Organize items inside cabinets, pre-pack anything you won't be using before you move

The Bathrooms

- ❏ Remove all rust and mildew
- ❏ Make sure tile, fixtures, shower doors, etc. are immaculate and shining
- ❏ Make sure all fixtures are in good repair
- ❏ Replace loose caulking or grout
- ❏ Make sure lighting is bright, but soft

The Master Bedroom

- ❏ Organize furnishings to create a spacious look with well-defined sitting, sleeping, and dressing areas

The Garage

- ❏ Sell, give away, or throw out unnecessary items
- ❏ Clean oily cement floor
- ❏ Provide strong overhead light
- ❏ Tidy storage or work areas

The Basement

- ❏ Sell, give away, or throw out unnecessary items
- ❏ Organize and create more floor space by hanging tools and placing items on shelves
- ❏ Clean water heater and drain sediment
- ❏ Change furnace filter
- ❏ Make inspection access easy
- ❏ Clean and paint concrete floor and walls
- ❏ Provide strong overhead light

The Attic

- ❏ Tidy up by discarding or pre-packing
- ❏ Make sure energy-saving insulation is apparent
- ❏ Make sure air vent is in working order
- ❏ Provide strong overhead lighting

When It's Time To Show

- ❏ Make sure your property profile folder, utility bills, MLS profile, house location survey, etc. are available
- ❏ Open all draperies and shades, turn on all lights
- ❏ Pick up toys and other clutter, check to make sure beds are made and clothes are put away
- ❏ Give the carpets a quick vacuuming
- ❏ Add some strategically placed fresh flowers
- ❏ Open bathroom windows for fresh air
- ❏ Pop a spicy dessert or just a pan of cinnamon in the oven for aroma
- ❏ Turn off the television and turn on the radio music at a low volume
- ❏ Make a fire in the fireplace if appropriate
- ❏ Put pets in the backyard or arrange for a friend to keep them
- ❏ Make sure pet areas are clean and odor-free
- ❏ Make sure all trash is disposed of in neatly covered bins

Angela McKendrick, CRS, GRI
Office: 410-555-1234
Home Office: 410-432-7890
Fax: 410-555-5607
Web Site: www.demorealty.com/angela
Email: angela.mckendrick@demorealty.com

Green Leaf Realty
www.greenleafrealty.com

Used with permission of Realty Tools, Inc.

Some agents give advice to owners as to repainting, landscape work, rearranging furniture, storing excess belongings, etc., however many agents lack the training and experience to be really effective.

There are professional stagers who will make a property look as if Martha Stewart lived there. Some will instruct the owner what to do for a few hundred dollars while others will do the entire job. They may just add accessories, remove clutter and use much of what the owner has. In some case they will repaint, refinish floors, change cabinets, paint, re-landscape and completely furnish and accessorize the home with new rental furniture. The property, the market, as well as the owner's willingness to cooperate will determine the extent of the staging. Flippers have found that professionally staged homes sell more quickly than vacant homes and can mean greater profit because of both shorter holding times and higher sale prices. Coldwell Banker tracked 2772 home sales and found that based on list prices, staged homes sold for almost 5% higher price than unstaged homes and took half as long to sell. California does not require licensure to act as a stager.

WEB LINK

@

There are several organizations of home stagers: International Association of Home Staging Professionals at www.iahsp.com and Real Estate Staging Association at www.realestatestagingassociation.com.

Professional Property Inspection

You should inform your owners that your property inspection only covered defects that a reasonable visual inspection would reveal and that most sale contracts provide for the buyer being able to have access for a professional inspection.

Many sales agreements fall apart when defects are found. If corrections are necessary, usually it is the seller who agrees to the cost.

Explain that a better approach would be for the owner to have a professional inspection now so that there will be no surprises and any problems could be solved now. In addition, the professional inspection report could be a sales tool to help convince a buyer.

You could give the owner the names of several inspectors you have had good relations with and consider competent.

FIGURE 7.3:   When an Appointment Is Made to See Your Home

When An Appointment Is Made

Agents from many real estate firms will want to show your home. Please allow any agent who calls to show your home at the suggested time. If you are not frequently available, it is suggested that you allow a lockbox to be installed on your door. You will increase your odds for a sale by allowing more qualified buyers to see your home. You do not want to miss an out-of-town transferee because your home was not able to be shown.

During a showing:

- Open all draperies and window shades during daylight hours.

- The kitchen & bathroom should sparkle.

- Open windows one half hour before showing to circulate fresh air.

- Open all the doors between rooms to give an inviting feeling.

- Place fresh flowers on kitchen table and/or in the living room.

- If possible, bake cookies or bread to add an inviting aroma.

- Turn on all lights and replace bulbs with high wattage bulbs where needed.

- Pets should be confined or restricted from view. Eliminate pet odors. Not everyone may share your love of animals. Some people may be allergic to them.

- All jewelry and small valuables should be stored in a safety deposit box or in a locked closet.

- Replace any items not included in the sale, or tag them appropriately with "to be replaced with..." or "not included" signs.

- Beds should be made & clothes picked up. Bathrooms should be clean, with towels folded and toilet lid down.

- When you leave the house, please leave it as if you know it is going to be shown. You never know when the right person is going to look at it!

 Angela McKendrick, CRS, GRI
Office: 410-555-1234
Home Office: 410-432-7890
Fax: 410-555-5607
Web Site: www.demorealty.com/angela
Email: angela.mckendrick@demorealty.com

www.greenleafrealty.com

Used with permission of Realty Tools, Inc.

Weekly activity report.   Tell the owners what you have already done, what you are doing, and what you will be doing. Owners should understand that you will be sending them a **weekly activity report**, and that if they have any questions at any time they should call you. (See Figure 7.4.)

While some agents would rather make monthly reports simply because they show more activity, owners don't want to wait that long. Prepare reports on all of your listings every week so they become a part of your routine. Weekly reports also will force you to review your own sales activity and to consider what can or should be done to bring about a sale.

FIGURE 7.4:   Weekly Activity Report Form

[Jones Realty]
Weekly Progress Report   Week Ending _____
Property: _____
Owners: _____
Number of Inquiries: _____
Number of Showings: _____
Advertising: _____
Open House Date(s): _____
Number of Visitors: _____
Comments of Agents and Prospective Buyers: _____
_____
_____
_____

As an attachment to weekly activity reports, you can include any ads for the property, a printout of the property, copies of property postings on internet sites, and even emails sent promoting the property (don't include the addressees or you might find that the seller will contact the prospective buyers directly, posing a problem for the listing agent).

Showings.   Owners must understand that although agents try to give them notice well in advance of a showing, this may not always be practical. Explain that in showing another property, an agent might realize that the owners' property better fits the needs of a certain buyer than properties that originally were selected for viewing. At times, prospective buyers may ask agents about certain houses while looking at other properties. If a property fits a buyer's needs, the prospective buyer could well turn into an actual buyer. The fact that they, not the agent, found the property can influence a sale.

Also explain that the reverse can happen: owners might be prepared for a visit by an agent who fails to show. While you generally will notify owners of canceled appointments, there will be times when such notification is difficult.

During hot weather, suggest that the owner leave soft drinks in the refrigerator for agents from your office and their prospective buyers. Explain that offering prospects cold bottled water or a soda and getting them to sit down can help them view the home from a more relaxed point of view. If the owners agree to do this, and they generally will, make certain the agents within your office know about it. Some agents display their company label on bottled water. Besides stocking owners' refrigerators, they use the bottled water at their office and at open houses as a refreshing advertisement. Incidentally, a good place to sit is close to a pool or garden, if available. Otherwise, pick the room that has the best ambiance.

Your office advertising policy.   You should explain that internet advertising has become the media of choice for most buyers. Classified ads for homes have all but vanished in most newspapers. While you may still spend a significant portion of your advertising dollar in print media, what you do on the internet is of prime importance. Help your owners fully understand your print advertising policy and the media used. Explain that every home is not advertised every day because this isn't necessary to successfully market a property. Explain that buyers often buy a different house from the one in the advertisement that attracted their attention. Explain that many people who answer ads are hoping for a bargain and tend to inquire about homes priced at less than they expect to spend.

A property doesn't need to be advertised every day.

In the same vein, other homes priced in the same or even a higher or a lower price range create inquiries. When qualifying these prospective buyers, the agent may discover that the owners' house is likely to meet the buyers' needs. Thus, advertising for other houses creates prospects for their home. Explain that by endeavoring to cover a range of both price and special features, you can in effect advertise every home in your inventory each day with just a handful of ads.

The owner can be a source of valuable information.

Neighborhood information request. Another way in which you can make the owners feel they are part of your marketing effort is to ask them to complete a **neighborhood information request**. (See Figure 7.5.) This information can be extremely valuable, and filled-out copies should be readily available to all salespersons in your office. Agents who know what buyers want will have special ammunition to sell particular houses. Although other homes might have area activities or neighbors that would make them equally desirable, the agent who does not have the information cannot use it to make the sale. As an example:

Johnny, do you like baseball? Well, you're in luck, there is a Little League here, and they play just two blocks away at McKinley Park.

Knowing the architect. For distinctive homes, you should ask the owner if they know the name of the architect, being sure to verify this information before using it. Mentioning the architect's name to prospects can add a panache to the property. If the architect is well known, it can reflect in both the sales price and the time required to sell. You can Google the name of the architect and find important buildings/homes that the architect designed. This can be additional sales information. If the owner does not know the architect, you can check with city planning. The building permit records and/or plans on file should reveal the name of the architect.

FIGURE 7.5: **Neighborhood Information Request**

Neighborhood Information Request

Owner: _____   Address: _____

Having an in-depth knowledge of your neighborhood and neighbors can give us a competitive advantage over less informed sales agents who represent other properties.

We would therefore appreciate your completion of this form to the best of your ability.

1. Neighborhood features you feel a buyer would likely be most pleased with: _____
   _____
   _____

2. School districts are:
   _____

3. School bus stops at:
   _____

4. Youth activities in the area (Little League, junior hockey, soccer league, etc.):
   _____

5. Public recreational facilities in area (parks, pools, playgrounds, tennis courts, golf courses, etc.): _____
   _____

6. Hike and/or bike paths:
   _____
   _____

7. Nearest public transportation route:
   _____

8. Nearest medical facilities:
   _____

9. Nearest community center (for children, seniors, etc.):
   _____

10. Nearest churches and synagogues (and denominations):
    _____

11. Nearest shopping area:
    _____

12. Any pet-friendly facilities (dog park):
    _____

Please send your completed form to my attention in the enclosed postage paid envelope.

Your help in providing this data is greatly appreciated.

Appreciatively yours,

_____

Change in Agents

If an agent who took a listing leaves the office, the broker should assign another salesperson to serve as listing agent and liaison with the owners. This agent should meet with the owners and go over their work to that point in time as well as to discuss ways the property can be made more readily salable (if applicable).

Preparing the owners for an offer.   Give owners a blank copy of a purchase contract and explain to them that the form is the one that will be used by a buyer. By explaining the clauses and leaving a copy with the owners, you will reduce the chance that they will get upset about any clause when they receive an offer.

Also prepare owners for quick offers. Explain that the first few weeks after a listing is taken can be very productive because other agents as well as prospective buyers tend to get excited over new listings. You can point out that when some owners get a quick offer, they feel that it indicates they set their price too low when it actually means they priced their property right. They reject good offers, and they later regret the rejection. In pointing out this fact, you reduce the likelihood of a negative reaction to a quick offer.

NECESSARY INFORMATION AND DISCLOSURES

You want the sellers to complete the Real Estate Transfer Disclosure Statement (see Unit 3) as soon as possible so it can be given to a prospective buyer. If the owners reveal problems that you feel should be corrected before a sale, you should advise them to take corrective action.

Have the owners complete a FIRPTA/California Withholding form (Unit 14). If the property is leased, obtain copies of lease(s). You should also obtain estoppel certificates from tenant(s) that they have no defenses or offsets against the landlord.

If the property is a common interest development, you should obtain copies of the bylaws, CC&Rs, current financial statement, minutes of meetings, and any information about changes in assessments or pending legal actions. The CAR purchase contract is going to require that this information be provided to the buyers during their contingency periods. It's important to ensure that this information is current and available to buyers.

You should have the sellers sign the Water Heater Statement of Compliance that the water heater will be properly braced as of close of escrow, as well as the Smoke Detector Statement of Compliance that operable smoke detectors shall be in place at close of escrow as required by law.

The Lead-based Paint and Lead-based Hazards Disclosure Acknowledgment and Addendum should also be signed by owners indicating knowledge of any lead-based paint.

You will want a property profile from a title company or through the public records module of the MLS. This could reveal problems that might make a sale difficult or even impossible if not corrected, such as judgments, silent owners, liens, and so forth.

You will also want to know the lot size that may be available from plat maps. You should also obtain the Natural Hazards Disclosure report as soon as practical.

LISTING MODIFICATION (ADJUSTMENT)

If it becomes apparent that you made an error in your assessment of the property value, let the owners know at once. If you suggest a different price, be able to defend your position. When you suggest lowering the price, you are, in effect, asking the owners to give up something they think they have. *Modification* or *adjustment* does not have the immediate negative connotation of *lowering*.

Changes in the market can turn a proper original listing price into a price that is either too high or too low. After taking the listing, for example, several comparable properties are put on the market at significantly lower prices that will affect the ability to attract interest in your property. Taking the owners to visit one or more recently listed, competitively priced, comparable properties, as covered in Unit 5, will help the owners realize that a price adjustment on their property is needed to be competitive.

If owners refuse to adjust their price when you feel such an action is necessary to find a buyer, consider the ultimate in persuasion: offer to return the listing. Ask the owners to sign a release relieving you of all agency obligations under the listing. Ask to be let out of your agreement to exercise diligence on their behalf. Although owners might not really be sold on your representing them, no one likes to be the one rejected. A release offer often convinces owners to adjust their price to the level recommended.

The worst-case scenario is that you will give up an overpriced listing that had less than a good chance of attracting buyers. From a rational point of view, of course, giving up a poor listing makes sense, but you may feel that if you don't succeed, you are a loser. You actually will be a winner, because you will be able to devote your time to probabilities rather than remote possibilities. You do not have to take or retain overpriced listings.

Don't look at this approach as a bluff, because you shouldn't be bluffing. To be sure, it's an either/or approach, but it's unfair to the owners to continue to offer their home at a price that will fail to attract prospective buyers.

Don't change the original listing when making a listing adjustment. Use a modification form or separate signed and dated letter that will enable you to later determine what was done should a problem arise.

A significant downward price adjustment on a listing should be communicated to local area cooperating brokers and salespersons by email. It will get more attention than an MLS computer update by itself. You should update all internet presentations.

LISTING EXTENSION

Several weeks before your listing expires, schedule a meeting with the owners to go over the listing and what you have been doing on their behalf. If the owners feel that you have been diligent in working for them and have kept them informed, you have an excellent chance of obtaining a listing extension. However, if you fail to keep the owners informed and they have to call you to find out what is happening, your chances of obtaining an extension to the listing are materially diminished.

If you obtain an extension, a thank-you letter from your broker is appropriate. Also, don't forget to immediately communicate the extension to your MLS.

If the owners do not wish to extend the listing, supply the names of people who viewed the property. This must be in writing to protect your firm from the owner making a sale to one of these prospects during the safety period.

YOUR MARKETING PLAN

You should have a marketing plan. By following the suggestions in this section, you will see a marketing plan develop. A copy should be provided to the owners as soon as it is prepared. See Figure 5.5E for a sample plan.

Signs

When you obtain the listing, put up a For Sale sign immediately after leaving the house. If you do not, you should tell the owner when one will be installed. If your office uses huge wooden holders for metal signs, you should have smaller lawn signs that can be used in the interim. Tell the owners when your large sign will be installed.

Besides the broker's name and telephone number, some brokers include their website addresses so that prospective buyers can obtain more information right away on their own.

FIGURE 7.6:   **Rider Strip Example**

Rider strips.   A rider strip can emphasize a desirable feature not evident from the exterior, such as "Pool and Spa," "5 Bedrooms," "Home Theater," etc. See Figure 7.6.

QR codes.   Real estate agents can order signs or create fliers with quick response (QR) codes on them. These codes allow users to scan them quickly using an application on their smartphones or other devices to obtain immediate information on the property in question. These can be just as effective as other advertising media and allow for a call to action to visit a website or call the listing agent from the property itself. The ability to rapidly transmit information through QR codes has made this a popular choice for real estate agents.

Information Boxes

All of the real estate supply houses as well as some REALTOR® board or association office stores carry **information boxes** or tubes that can be attached to your yard signs. These boxes are a low-cost, effective way to interest buyers. Inside the box, insert a supply of property information sheets (briefs) that describe the listed property in a manner that is likely to interest the prospective buyer and encourage them to contact your office. Information boxes can also include information on similar properties and the broker's internet address where more information is available, as well as an email address.

Photos

Photographs of the home should be taken as soon as possible after the listing is taken. You want interior photos emphasizing desirable aspects of the home as well as exterior photos. You want the photos for property magazines, property briefs, ads, mailings, and displays as well as for internet sites. Photos also have to be taken for virtual tours if your internet site includes them.

Lockbox

If possible, install a *lockbox*, or *keybox*, used by your MLS right after taking the listing. If there is going to be a delay, inform the owners when a lockbox will be installed. Lockboxes are simply large boxes that have a separately locked compartment to hold the house keys. They may be locked to door handles, electric meters, metal railings, etc.

The latest lockbox models are electronic marvels. Besides containing the key, they tell you by a simple phone call who has used the lockbox, including date and time. Lockboxes are now available where the agent can access the data online. This information is valuable for security reasons. Electronic lockboxes can even monitor the status of the lockbox battery and restrict access to preselected agents or grant access to agents from other real estate organizations. It also lets you tell the owner in your weekly activity report who entered the property by using the lockbox. You can also call agents who viewed the property for their comments. This is the type of information an owner should be made aware of. Like the talking sign, these electronic lockboxes are a superb marketing tool that can be effectively used in your listing presentation.

There is a REALTOR®-approved lockbox from SentriLock, LLC. You insert a credit-card-sized card in the slot. The card has a microprocessor chip. You then punch in your number on the box's keypad. A green light tells you to remove your card and the box opens. The system logs the last 70 people who entered the property. The lockboxes are sold through REALTOR® Associations and MLS services. The California Association of REALTORS® requires the use of approved lockboxes for security reasons, as well as to have uniform access to properties.

Owners should understand that allowing other people access to their homes when they or you are not present does create a security risk. You should suggest that they make certain that their insurance will adequately cover theft or mysterious disappearances of furnishings. You might also suggest that expensive objects be locked up or removed from the premises.

The Multiple Listing Service

To provide greater market coverage for their listings, a group of brokers often conducts a cooperative listing service, or MLS. The group often consists of members of a local real estate board or association; however, membership in the board or association is not a prerequisite to membership in the service. The MLS is used most often with an exclusive-authorization-and-right-to-sell listing, but it may be used with other listings as well. A member of the group who takes any listing turns it in to a central bureau that distributes it to all participants in the service, usually on the internet. All members have the right to sell the property; however, they must have the listing broker's permission to advertise or promote it. When a sale is made on an MLS listing, the listing broker and the broker who found the buyer share the commission.

Suppose, for example, an MLS commission split was 50/50. The listing broker would get 50% of the commission, and the broker who found the buyer would get the other 50%. Within each agency the broker would, according to the contractual agreement between the broker and the salesperson, also split his or her share of the commission with the salesperson who had actual contact with the seller or buyer. (Only brokers can receive commissions, but they may share them with the salespeople who work with them.) Figure 7.7 illustrates a possible split of the 6% commission on a property that sold for $440,000.

Commission splits will vary among offices, often based upon broker services as well as the market. As an example, when there are many buyers and few sellers the listing commission could be greater than the sales commission.

FIGURE 7.7:   Splitting a Commission on an MLS Listing

It is important that owners fully understand the role of an MLS service and the agency implications.

If, for any reason, a broker does not submit a listing to the MLS service and precludes other agents from showing the property, it would be considered a *pocket listing*. Refusing cooperation would generally not be in the best interests of the principal and could be a breach of the agent's fiduciary duty as well as MLS rules.

A new listing should be placed on your office website, as well as the other Internet sites that you use, as soon as possible. A printout of the material included on the site should be provided to the owner(s). (For information about what your website should include, see Unit 8.)

Your Website

While other websites might have restrictions, you are not under constraint as to your own office website. You can offer your own format and more data with multiple photos, virtual tours and even videos. A drone's birds-eye view can be an effective means to show the house in its environment as well as focus on area amenities. Drones can produce exceptional videos. Cost for these professionally produced videos has decreased so that they are not limited to the upper end of the price spectrum. Be aware that the use of drones for commercial purposes requires FAA approval.

Property Brief (Information Sheet)

As soon as you have your photographs, prepare a property brief. A **property brief** is simply a one-page flyer about the property pointing out attractive features. It must have a photograph or drawing of the home. If the owners purchased the property from a developer, there is a good chance they have kept the original sales material; check it over if they do have it. There could be an attractive pen-and-ink drawing of the house that would reproduce well for your property brief. If there is a floor plan, it may be possible to reproduce this on the back of the property brief along with some information on special features.

A professional-quality property brief can be prepared in a few minutes with a laser printer and any number of available desktop publishing software programs. Owners will be impressed with a quality flyer featuring their home so soon after you have taken the listing. (See Figure 7.8.)

The backside of this particular property brief provides additional photos.

| A property brief is an advertising flyer about a particular property. |

The property briefs should include an internet address where the prospect can obtain further information including additional photos on the property as well as other properties.

For your listings, you want the property brief to indicate your name, license, identification number, cellphone number, email address, fax number, personal website, etc. You want to be contacted.

Copies of the property brief should be left at the home to be given to prospects as well as agents who will view the property. Therefore, deliver the property briefs to the home before any visits take place. They should be placed close to the front door, preferably on a table, so that a visitor will not miss them. A small "Take One" sign can be used. If the For Sale sign has an information box, a good supply should be placed inside it. Give a supply of property briefs to every agent in your office. You might also give them to agents from other offices who are particularly active in the area or in the type of property you are offering. Be sure to check the information box on your For Sale sign whenever you visit the property to see whether the property briefs need to be replenished.

Property briefs also are given out at open houses. It is a good idea to have a supply of property briefs on similar homes as well as briefs on the home that is open. Briefs may also be sent in response to mail, phone or internet inquiries.

Other Internet Sites

WEB LINK

The National Association of REALTORS® has a website, www.realtor.com, where a prospective buyer or tenant can find properties in all areas of the country. The site allows a broker to post a picture of the property as well as a great deal of information to interest prospective buyers. The viewer can obtain further information and a blowup picture of the property on request. In addition, a number of boards of REALTORS® and groups of boards have area websites. The appendix includes a list of some of the many internet sites that are available.

You will be limited to what you place on sites that you don't control. You want a good exterior photo as you will likely be allowed to place only one on the website. The information you provide will likely have to be in a specific format. While you should carefully choose descriptive wording on your own website, multiple-broker sites generally limit your descriptions.

If you prepare a video of a listing, it could be used on YouTube and other sites featuring videos.

FIGURE 7.8: **Example of a Property Brief**

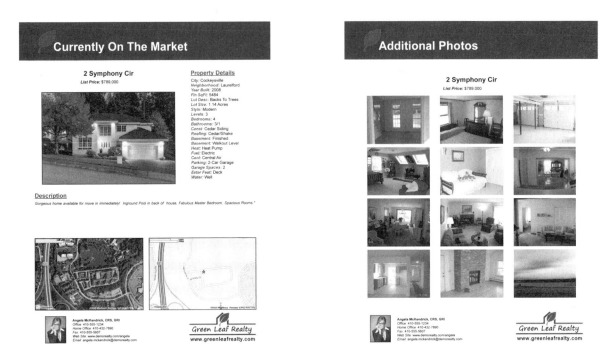

Used with permission of Realty Tools, Inc.

For an additional fee you can get special enhanced coverage for your property on many of the property websites. Realtor.com offers Showcase treatment that can include an agent's photograph and contact information, a yellow banner of search results page, ability to add up to 25 jumbo photos, full motion video and virtual tours, open house alerts, custom headings and descriptions and exposure for up to three additional listings. Your use of showcase treatment will be well received by the owners. It can also be an excellent listing tool.

Virtual Home Tours

Technology has evolved so that it is possible to offer virtual home tours while seated before a personal computer. Providing virtual home tours on the internet impresses owners of listed properties and saves buyers' and agents' time. A viewer can move from side to side, backward and forward, and from room to room when viewing the site. A specially trained photographer usually takes 360-degree photographs of the interior, exterior, and even the neighborhood. Today, software programs are available that allow an agent to prepare a virtual tour using a plain digital camera; such a software program costs around $300. If you are interested in creating your own virtual home tour, two of the sources you might wish to consider are www.paradym.com and Photo Vista Virtual Tour available through www.z-law.com. This program can produce film or digital photographs. Homes & Land will prepare a virtual tour for you from six or more photos; however, you must advertise in its home magazine. Its website is www.homesandland.com.

While at present, it is estimated that less than 30% of listings can be seen as a virtual tour, having virtual tours on your website is an excellent marketing tool for both selling properties and obtaining listings.

Before you prepare a virtual tour for the internet, obtain the owner's permission in writing to do so. There is a danger that the virtual tour will provide access information to persons interested in what is in the house and not the house itself. A virtual tour could be a home shopping site for a burglar. Visitors to the home are usually prequalified or register. This is not true of a person who can view the contents on a computer. Owners should be advised to review their insurance coverage, especially if the home contains valuable art objects and/or antiques.

Brokers find that with virtual tours, they can show a home when it is not available for a physical showing. It is believed by many brokers that virtual tours will replace the flat photographs currently used on most websites. Most house hunter sites now offer virtual tours. While virtual tours consist of a number of shots taken from the same point to provide an unbroken panorama, a video tour is a movie using a video camera that provides images as though touring the property. The terms are often used interchangeably.

YouTube sites are now being used for video home tours by many agents. A number of programs are available to make professional quality real estate video tours designed to excite buyers to want more information. If prospective buyers are offered a choice between still photographs and a video of a property, they will usually choose the video. Video tours may also be used on your firm's website. Other real estate websites generally have restrictions.

Advertising

After you have given the listing to your MLS, prepared a property brief, and posted the property information and photograph on the internet, prepare at least three classified advertisements on the property, as well as one open-house ad. Take your time because you want your presentation to have maximum effectiveness. If you are preparing print ads, a number of excellent books can help you produce superior ads. Using different approaches, your ad can be tailored to appeal to various groups of readers, based on features advertised and the form of your appeal. By preparing at least three ads, you are less likely to repeat an ad, which generally results in reduced response. You won't be caught with an ad deadline and six other tasks that need immediate attention, which usually means a mediocre ad at best.

If your firm uses one of the home magazines, prepare an ad for it as well, even though a decision may not yet have been made to advertise the listing there. By having the ad ready, the likelihood of its being used has measurably increased.

Be sure to send owners copies of the ads on their property when it is advertised. Keep in mind that advertising does not sell property—salespersons sell. What advertising does is to create responses that professional agents can convert into sales.

Office Caravans

The owners should be told in advance about the office caravan and the MLS caravan. Many offices **caravan** their office listings. The name *caravan* comes from the long lines of cars that agents drive from home to home to view properties. Have all the salespeople fill out an agent questionnaire after they walk through the property. (See Figure 7.9.) The information from this **agent property evaluation** questionnaire should be supplied to the owners with your suggestions. If the agent property evaluation indicates a serious problem, meet with the owners as soon as possible to decide how to resolve it.

MLS Caravan

Large real estate MLSs have many more listings than the agents could possibly visit in one morning or even in one day. However, the listings are broken down into areas. Most agents want to see only the homes at the price and in the area where they feel they are most likely to have prospective buyers. Again, the effective agent concentrates more on probabilities than on possibilities.

Give the owners as much advance notice as you can about the caravan. The owners should have the property "standing tall (in show condition) for inspection." The following are some general rules for caravans:

- Owners should not be at home. Agents tend to spend more time in a home when owners are not present.

- Offer agents hot coffee or lemonade, depending on the weather. Fill the cups or glasses about two-thirds full, so the agents can carry them while they view the home. This will tend to slow the viewing process.

- Give each agent a property brief. The agents see so many homes that most will not remember which features went with which house.

- Consider mood setting. Have the stereo playing soft music. If the weather is cold, have the fireplace going; if it is hot, set the air-conditioning between 68° and 70° so it feels like a cold blast when agents enter the house.

- Ask the owner to bake some chocolate chip cookies, cinnamon rolls, or fresh bread. The aroma will be pleasant, and agents will like something to eat.

- Be at the house or have an assistant present during the caravan.

Concentrate your viewing time on properties you're most likely to sell.

FIGURE 7.9:   Agent Property Evaluation

Agent Property Evaluation

Property Address _____

1. Features of this house that will be most appealing to buyers: _____
    _____
    _____

2. Features or lack of features that buyers are likely to view as a negative:
    _____

3. I feel that the price is:
    ☐ Too high   ☐ Too low   ☐ Realistic
    By how much? $ _____
    Why? _____
    _____

4. To increase salability, the owner should consider:
    _____
    _____
    _____

During slow markets, some agents put out a buffet lunch for caravan members. In a large MLS, instead of having only 15% of the agents visit the property, you may increase it to 60% or more of the agents on caravan by providing them food. An agent open house is different in that it is designed to attract agents who did not view the property on the MLS caravan. Providing refreshments during the caravan increases caravan viewing, and agents remain in the property for a longer time. An expenditure such as this makes sense for a property that shows well, is priced right and needs a quick sale.

Some agents use the internet to view properties rather than go on caravans. It is likely that at some time in the future, caravans will no longer be necessary.

Area Canvass Letter

Within one week of taking a new listing, you should send a letter to residents living within at least one block of the listed property. This letter informs the neighbors of the listing and asks their help in locating a buyer. (See Figure 7.10.)

Check the Files

As soon as you get a new listing in an office, all salespersons in the office should go through their prospect files to try to match their current prospects with the new listing. This activity has two major advantages:

1. Prospective buyers tend to get excited over brand-new listings. They might treat property on the market for a long period of time as shopworn merchandise, but a new listing elicits interest and can also have a sense of urgency. They are seeing this property before it is being visited by perhaps hundreds of agents, all of whom have prospective buyers. Right now the property can be theirs if they wish. This is one of the reasons that the most productive period for sales tends to be the first 20 days after the listing is taken.

FIGURE 7.10:   Canvass Letter

[Date]

_____

_____

_____

Dear [   ]:

Our office has recently listed the home of a neighbor at [322 Maple Lane] for sale. You have probably noticed our For Sale sign.

I am writing to ask for your help in locating a buyer for this fine home.

I have enclosed a descriptive sheet on the property. We think it is a lot of house for the money, and the neighborhood is great so you would be helping anyone you suggest. If you can come up with any suggestions about your friends who might also want to be your neighbors, I would appreciate hearing from you.

Sincerely,

_____

_____

[Note: Be certain to include a property flier and follow through.]

2. The second advantage of immediately calling prospects is that it creates traffic within a few days of taking the listing. The owners' impression of you as a professional and of your firm is likely to be set within the first few weeks of the agency. After that period, it will be difficult to change the owners' perception.

Some brokers make the consideration of new listings part of their weekly meetings. The broker asks agents to think about their prospects and who likely would be interested in the property. By directing thoughts toward solving a problem, agents frequently generate ideas they would not have had otherwise.

Broker Open House

If you have an unusual property, a property that must be sold or several identical properties close to each other, consider a **broker open house**. In large associations, agents can't physically visit every new listing. They have to pick and choose. Therefore, a great many agents could miss your home on a caravan because they only visited, say, 12 of 35 new listings. Even listings that were visited were only viewed for a few minutes, and if you asked an agent a week later which home had which feature, most agents would give you a wrong answer.

Because of the longer period of time spent at a property, an agent open house impresses on agents the details of that property. The offer to stop by for food and drink can bring in many agents. It also serves a dual purpose because owners like these events; it shows extraordinary marketing.

Broker open houses provide maximum exposure of new listings to agents, whereas the MLS caravan only allows quick viewing of a small portion.

Although you may have balloons, flags, and other accoutrements outside, you don't have to host an elaborate party to attract agents. Cheese, crackers, and nuts will do. Wine or champagne should be served in plastic glasses. One way to encourage agents to linger awhile is a drawing using agents' business cards. The prize could be anything from a book of 10 free car washes to a weekend vacation package.

If you have the cards of the agents who were there, you can get them to complete a questionnaire giving their views on the property location and price, as well as letting you know whether they are working with any potential buyers.

While taking an overpriced listing might be a violation of the agent's fiduciary duty, many agents continue to do so.

Open House

Having an open house on an overpriced property will generally be a waste of both time and money. In addition, it will leave viewers with a negative feeling toward you and your firm. Therefore, you want open houses that are priced competitively. Best results can be expected from fresh property (recently listed).

Owners must be encouraged to have the house as presentable as possible for a standard **open house**. Treat the buyer open house as you treated homes for caravans and broker open houses. You want the home to appear light, bright, and as fresh as possible. There is one exception to having the house as close to perfect as is possible. That is an open house for a property advertised as a fixer-upper. If this is the case, the home will need more than minor repairs or touch-ups, although it should be clean.

If you are able to, greet the parties at the door and introduce yourself as you extend your hand. The normal reaction will be to give you their name. Use the prospects' names when answering or asking questions. Use the sales skills of Unit 10; don't be passive.

By asking each visitor to fill out a registration card or guest book, you can find out why they came and if they are buyers or sellers. Instead of registration cards, some agents give visitors clipboards with attached pencils, asking them to rate the house as to how it fits their needs. Figure 7.11 is an example of such a form. Of course, the comments from visitors should be relayed to your owners in their weekly activity report.

Many real estate agents today are relying on iPad or other tablet sign-in sheets for their open houses instead of traditional paper sign in sheets. Some visitors might be hesitant to sign in on a physical sign in sheet but today's consumer is quite accustomed to entering electronic information.

Various apps designed to manage open house leads are available. Many agents are reporting that the consumers are not pushing back at all on these electronic sign-in sheets.

Also, having the consumer information already in a database allows the agent to easily follow up on these leads with emails and phone calls without having to manually move the data into another system.

By offering the viewer notification of new listings, you can obtain email addresses, as well as permission to make phone calls even if they are on the do-not-call registry.

Draw Attention to the Property

Besides ads, you should have signs and arrows directing traffic from major streets. Always ask other property owners if you can put a directional sign on their lawns. They will generally allow you to do so, but if you do not ask, the sign likely will be removed.

Some agents tie a group of balloons to a mailbox or tree to attract attention. This is fine, as are flags, banners, helium balloons, and so forth. Feather flags are particularly effective in gaining attention. A feather flag is a relatively narrow cloth flag on a vertical pole. Sizes range from 8 inches to around 15 feet in height and from 2 to 4 feet wide. This vertical flag is read from top to bottom. Keep it simple with just Open House in large print. The thin material vibrates with just the slightest breeze and is readily readable. A number of flag companies keep Open House feather flags in stock. One Los Angeles–area broker uses a machine to spew out thousands of large soap bubbles. Another agent flies a 20-foot helium-filled blimp lettered "Open House." Some developments prohibit open house signs and limit For Sale signs as to size and color. By parking an "Open House mobile" or car parked in the driveway with Open House magnetic signs on the sides, you can generally get around these restrictions. Anything to make the house stand out can be used. You don't want to keep an open house a secret. Invite neighbors, as well as prospective buyers you are working with who have not seen the house. You want to generate traffic.

Give every open-house visitor a copy of your property brief and your business card. Property briefs of other homes you have in the same and lower-price brackets also should be available. By questioning visitors, you can find their interests and needs, and you may excite their interest in a property better suited to them. For this reason, it is absolutely critical to be fully aware of any properties that might better suit a prospective buyer's needs.

Open houses are a time to make contacts and gather information, so ask questions. You can use general qualifying questions and determine specific interests. If visitors seem enthusiastic, use a trial closing. Don't think the sole function of an open house is only to show; it is to sell as well. Open houses tend to please owners because they show positive action on your part. They are often a source of listings because many visitors must sell before they can buy. They are a source of prospective buyers for other properties as well as the property shown. Therefore, you should look at the whole picture. With every visitor, ask yourself, "How can I fulfill this person's real estate needs?"

| Open houses provide a variety of benefits. |

When you have or your office has several open houses in the same general area and price range, each open house should have a property brief of the other open house(s) and maps showing how to get to each property.

Some brokers advertise an open-house "Lotto," where a visitor to one house gets a card and a sticker. Another sticker is given at each additional home visited. If all the homes are visited, the visitor is awarded a gift, such as a baseball cap (with the firm's name).

It is possible for a single agent to conduct several open houses in a single day. For optimum effect, the homes should be in close proximity and should likely appeal to the same house hunters. The open houses should have staggered times such as 12 to 2 pm and 2:15 to 4 pm.

A variation of the above is an open house caravan where visiting time is relatively short, such as 15 minutes, and the caravan proceeds to the next home. Viewers should also be given clear directions to each home. Again, the homes should all appeal to the same potential buyers.

When a property has been extensively remodeled, neighbors will want to see what has been accomplished. An open house where neighbors have been specially invited can be beneficial not for a sale to the neighbors but for friends of the neighbors who might be interested in a home in the area.

FIGURE 7.11:   Visitor Rating Form

Visitor Rating

Property _____

Your name _____   Phone _____

Address _____   E-mail _____

Date _____

I am visiting this open house because of   ☐ Advertising   ☐ Signs

☐ Other (specify): _____

_____

Features I particularly like: _____

_____

_____

Features I do not like: _____

_____

_____

I believe the price quoted is: ☐ Low   ☐ About right   ☐ High

My reason for visiting is: _____

_____

Do you presently own your home? _____ Is it currently for sale? _____

General comments: _____

_____

_____

☐   I would like to receive e-mails, with pictures, or new listings and other open houses.

☐   You may call me about future new listings.

_____ (Signature)

Facebook Marketing

In this unit, we talk about the marketing plan associated with taking a new listing. Once a listing is taken most real estate agents will do the standard marketing plan consisting of placing a sign on the property, putting it in the MLS and doing some light direct mail. However, the real estate licensee should also have a Facebook strategy in place.

The unique aspect of Facebook advertising is that Facebook has a database of unique information on users. We self-populate what our interests are, where we are at any given time, and who our friends are. This allows marketing to be extremely targeted.

For example, imagine that you have a listing in a given city on a home that has a wine cellar. You could take a picture of the wine cellar and create a Facebook ad around this image. Facebook allows you to target your audience based on interests, gender, age, and other demographic criteria. An agent could target users who live within 15 miles of the listing, are 35 and older, and have indicated interests in "wine," "chardonnay," or other relevant search terms relating to wine.

The thought behind this isn't so much that you are going to find a buyer immediately but that the picture of the wine cellar and your listing will get "liked" and "shared" across the internet and may end up ultimately catching the eye of an interested buyer.

Servicing Buyer Agency Agreements

While keeping in touch with buyers is usually not a problem, prospective buyers you were unsuccessful in helping should not be forgotten, even if you don't have an agency agreement with them. It is a good idea to send emails or letters at least once a week on new listings. Provide website information for viewing or send property briefs. At least every two weeks you should contact the prospects by phone and ask for their comments about properties presented. If positive, set up a showing. It is not uncommon for some buyers to spend months looking for a home. While this is often the fault of the salespersons, some people are just procrastinators when it comes to a final decision. When you have determined that the buyers are ready, willing, and able to buy, keep working and help them decide.

SHORT SALE LISTINGS

A great many homes in America are underwater in that their loan indebtedness exceeds market value. In such cases, sellers would actually have to come up with cash to sell their homes. Most of the time, they are unable to do so. A solution is a short sale in which the lender agrees to accept the net receipts of the sale as a discharge of borrowers' obligations. The advantage to lenders is that they save the time and money a foreclosure would require, do not have to secure the property, and would not be subject to holding costs or the expense of repair and sales expenses. In most cases, a short sale would be an advantage to the lender over foreclosure.

In some instances where there is private mortgage insurance, the lender may want to foreclose and go against the insurer for their loss. Most major lenders use Equator Platform as a standardized short sale system. Agents log in at www.equator.com/ home and click on "Initiate Short Sale." They indicate the lender or the loan servicer and provide the loan number. The agent then completes the short sale application by following the lender's instructions.

Where the Equator Platform is not used, your first step in a short sale should be to contact the lender's loan mitigation officer. Different lenders have different titles. It may take a number of calls to contact the right party. You should tell the officer what you plan to do and indicate you will be sending a package explaining that a short sale is planned. Your package will include the following:

- Comparative market analysis showing all recent comparable sales in the area for three months

- A hardship letter from the owners (letter should show why a sale is needed and why the loan terms cannot be honored [e.g., physical problems and expenses, loss of job, reduced income, job relocation, etc.]) If the homeowner is not in default and there is not a genuine hardship, short sale approval is unlikely.

- Financial statement showing assets and liabilities of the owners

- Copies of bank statements (checking and savings) for past three months

- Credit card statements for past three months

- Estimated lender's net based on list price

- Copy of sale listing

You should ask the loan mitigation officer if there is anything else you should send.

The same package should be sent to the lender when an offer is received, along with the purchase offer and the borrower's prequalification for a loan. While some lenders claim a *fast track* on short sale approvals, a wait of two to four months, and sometimes much longer, is not unusual.

A shorter approval is more likely if the offer is void of contingencies and the earnest money is substantial. If subject to inspection, the period for inspection should be very short.

Some buyer's agents recommend a statement in bold print in their offer that says, "Buyer will pay all closing costs and fees." They believe such a statement will increase the likelihood of a fast approval.

Buyers will sometimes offer several thousand dollars above the broker's advertised price to protect against another agent's submitting a full price offer on the property.

Normally, when a debt is forgiven, the debtor's forgiven obligation is taxed as income. The Mortgage Forgiveness Debt Relief Act removes federal tax liability on such debts. The act was extended through 2015 and further extension is likely. California has a similar act that expired but may be extended.

THE OFFER AND BEYOND

Servicing the listing actually includes your communication and efforts from the time you obtain an offer to purchase until close of escrow. This aspect of servicing the listing is included in Unit 11, "From Offer to Closing."

SUMMARY

In this unit, you learned that honest and complete agent-owner communication, even when the communication is not good news, is better than a breakdown in communication. Owners want and deserve to know what is happening.

Owner-agent communications start with the listing. Owners should know when they will be seeing you again and why. The purpose of your next visit probably will be a postlisting meeting, when you will inform owners what you will be doing, including your marketing plan, and what you expect of them.

The owners should understand the instructions given them and the reasons for those instructions. Owners who do not understand why an instruction is given and that it is given for their best interests are not likely to follow the instruction.

The owners should understand that they will be receiving weekly activity reports about what is happening. Let owners know that if they have any questions or suggestions, they can contact you.

Owners who understand the showing procedure will realize the need to be prepared for showings at short notice.

Owners should realize that when print ads are used to advertise other houses as well, agents are bringing in calls about a wide range of properties. After buyers are qualified, it often is the case that another house better meets their needs than the one they inquired about.

Obtaining neighborhood information from the owners furnishes your office with the special ammunition necessary to give prospective buyers that last little nudge that results in a sale. Knowledge about the neighbors, similar interests, ages of children, and even employment can make a home more desirable to buyers.

Should an agent leave an office, the broker should immediately notify the owners of the departed agent's listings and establish a new contact person to meet with the owners as soon as possible.

The owner should complete the Transfer Disclosure Statement as soon as possible. All owner certificates and disclosures should be signed.

If a listing needs to be modified for any reason, let the owners know and meet with them. If you made a mistake in pricing, admit it and show the owners what it should be. If conditions have changed since the owners gave their listing, show them the changes along with your recommendations.

If you feel a modification is necessary in order to find buyers, and the owners will not accept the modification, ask to be relieved of the listing. This powerful approach will often serve to convince owners to accept your recommendations. If you do give back the listing, chances are you got rid of a liability, not an asset.

Go to owners for an extension before a listing expires. Review what you have done for them. If you have used diligent effort on behalf of the owners and have communicated with them, you will have a good chance of obtaining an extension.

The owners should understand your marketing plan, a plan that likely begins with a For Sale sign. A rider strip showing your evening phone number can give you additional calls. A rider strip for a particularly desirable feature, such as four bedrooms, will increase the sign's effectiveness.

Talking signs are radio transmitters. The sign outside directs people to tune to an AM or FM station number. The signs, usually the property of the listing agent, are an excellent listing tool.

A number of information boxes are available that can be attached to For Sale signs. They are used to hold brochures or property briefs on the property being sold. They are an effective tool to interest prospective buyers.

The lockbox, if appropriate, should be attached as soon as possible after the listing is taken. New electronic lockboxes can provide you with information about all persons who used the lockbox.

Take photographs of the property listed as soon as the proper light is available. They will be needed for the MLS, property briefs, office display boards, window displays, and internet presentations.

Post the property on your internet site, as well as on other sites, as soon as possible. If you prepare a virtual tour, take proper pictures of the property.

Get the listing information to your MLS as soon as possible. Prepare a property brief within a day or two of taking a listing. Also prepare advertisements for placement.

Prepare owners for the office caravan, showing the property to agents from your office. Ask agents to complete an agent property evaluation so you can provide the owners with the reactions of other professionals. The owners should also be prepared for an MLS caravan of agents from other offices. If possible, the listing agent should be at the property during the caravan period.

Immediate interest in the listing can be obtained by direct mail or direct contact with neighbors, asking them for help in finding a buyer, and by all agents going through their files for likely buyers.

An agent open house is another way to bring agents into the property. If you offer food and drinks at the end of the day, many agents will come to these open houses.

Regular open houses must be prepared for in the same manner as a caravan showing. The open house can serve as a source of listings and a source of buyers for other properties, as well as for the open-house property.

If the mortgage amount exceeds fair market value, notify the loan mitigation officer as to a short sale.

Servicing the listing extends all the way until close of escrow. It is a process whereby you make a plan, work your plan, and communicate.

CLASS DISCUSSION TOPICS

1. Prepare a marketing plan with dates from the listing for a single-family home. (Use the following assumptions: The owner is highly motivated to sell, and the property is listed at a price below those of most comparable properties; however, there have been few recent sales in the area.)

2. Prepare a property brief for a specific property.

3. Visit one open house held by another office. Discuss how it was held and what suggestions you would make for the agent (if any).

4. Discuss any property you know of that you feel is not being properly marketed. Be prepared to justify your recommendations.

5. Bring to class one current-events article dealing with some aspect of real estate practice for class discussion.

UNIT 7 QUIZ

1. The reason that an expired listing was not extended with the original listing office MOST likely is dissatisfaction with
    a. the commission percentage.
    b. communications.
    c. price.
    d. the length of listing.

2. Agent advice to owners on showing their home would NOT include
    a. instructions to be present so they can volunteer information.
    b. cleaning instructions.
    c. landscaping instructions.
    d. repair instructions.

3. When there has been little, if any, interest in a property, the listing salesperson should
    a. convey this information.
    b. tell the owner the property is priced 10% too high.
    c. wait until there is something good to report.
    d. tell the owner that you are expecting an offer.

4. The Equator Platform is a system for
    a. locating property.
    b. loan approval..
    c. short-sale approval
    d. a title search.

5. You want owners to give you neighborhood information
    a. to keep the owners busy.
    b. to give your listings a competitive advantage.
    c. to use it to get more listings.
    d. for none of these.

6. An owner should understand that reducing a list price to the CMA value
   a. increases the likelihood of a sale.
   b. does not mean that an owner is giving up anything.
   c. results in both of these.
   d. results in neither of these.

7. If possible, you should place a rider strip on your listing signs that shows
   a. your fax number.
   b. all your professional designations.
   c. a desirable feature.
   d. all of these.

8. A property brief should *NOT* be used as a
   a. handout at open houses.
   b. substitute for internet advertising.
   c. handout at caravans.
   d. mailing piece to answer inquiries.

9. A broker open house is of greatest value when the property
   a. is in a large market with hundreds of listings.
   b. is overpriced.
   c. has a very limited use.
   d. has been reduced in price.

10. Advantages of open houses include
    a. pleasing owners because they indicate activity.
    b. locating buyers for other property.
    c. obtaining leads for listings.
    d. all of these.

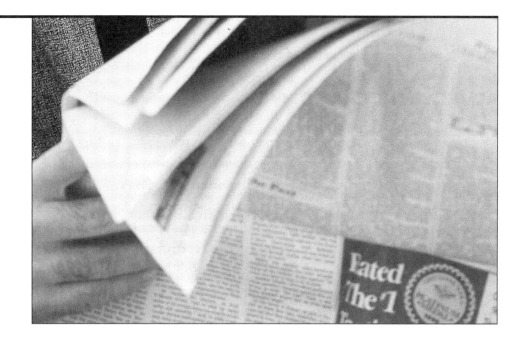

UNIT EIGHT 8

ADVERTISING

LEARNING OBJECTIVES

When you have completed this unit, you will be able to

- explain the objective of advertising and describe the AIDA approach to advertising;

- describe basic advertising guidelines, including media choices;

- evaluate advertising effectiveness;

- explain the legal implications of advertising; and

- describe an advertising budget.

KEY TERMS

AIDA approach	company dollar	operational advertising
annual percentage rate	direct mail advertising	outdoor advertising
bait-and-switch	display advertising	press releases
advertising	institutional	specialty gifts
blind ads	advertising	specific advertising
business card	media choice	Truth in Lending Act
car sign	name tag	
classified advertising	newsletters	

ADVERTISING OBJECTIVES

Advertising is the process of calling people's attention to something to arouse a desire to buy or to obtain more information about the product or service being promoted. The real estate industry could not exist without advertising. In addition to advertising products for lease or sale, the real estate industry also advertises for sellers and for salespeople. You will see that real estate advertising takes many forms.

Real estate advertising may be divided into two major types: institutional advertising and specific advertising. These two categories describe the two goals of real estate advertising.

Institutional advertising attempts to create a favorable image of the real estate company, the broker, and the salesperson. It keeps the company's name in the public eye and aims to inspire trust, confidence, and goodwill. Institutional advertising, often done by organized groups having similar interests, manifests pride in and respect for the real estate business. Individual brokers may be required to share some of the costs incurred in this type of advertising.

Specific advertising, also called **operational advertising**, is concerned with immediate results. It describes a particular piece of property and stimulates activity in a specific property or an entire tract of homes. In specific advertising, a broker's advertisements are in direct competition with the advertisements of other brokers.

THE AIDA APPROACH TO ADVERTISING

The most common, and probably most important, reason for advertising is to find ready, willing, and able buyers for sale listings. All the listings in the world will do you no good unless someone finds a ready, willing, and able buyer and makes that elusive sale.

Why do people buy? Prospective purchasers buy a particular piece of property for the benefits it offers. The most fundamental benefit is shelter, but the property also might provide other things that are important—security, good schools, convenience, recreation, prestige, and a lot more. The purpose of advertising is to communicate these benefits through the property's features—its price, size, location, and so on. People do not buy for the physical features of a property, but rather for the benefits those features offer, such as a relaxing life style, a feeling of security or love of family. Some people buy based upon how others will react.

If an ad is to be read and thus attract buyers, it usually must be designed to grab the reader's Attention, stimulate his or her Interest, generate a Desire, and lead the reader to Action. This is commonly referred to as the **AIDA approach,** from an acronym made up of the first letter of each step involved.

- **Attention**—The first step in any type of advertising is to gain attention. *Attention getters* include headlines that use words and word combinations, as well as typefaces and layouts that attract prospective buyers and encourage them to read further. You might gain attention with color, movement, message, sound, or even something odd or out of place, such as a misspelled word or an outrageous statement. It could even be humor. Whatever is used, you cannot get a message across until you have gained the attention of the intended recipient of the message.

- **Interest**—The ad should arouse interest in the specific product or service offered. Probably one of the best ways to arouse interest is through curiosity. Curiosity can be stimulated by ensuring that the ad allows the reader to imagine using and enjoying the benefits of the product or service.

- **Desire**—Once the person's attention is attracted and her interest is aroused, the ad can create desire by appealing to the senses and emotions. At this stage, language must be clear and concise and inspire the reader's confidence. Wherever possible, the advertising should try to build mental images and picture the reader as the final recipient of the product or service.

| The **AIDA** approach: Attention, Interest, Desire, Action |

- **Action**—Finally, the ad should move potential buyers to take action. The advertisement should be directed toward helping them make a decision, to convince them that they want to know more. The action desired by a real estate advertisement is either a phone call, email, or fax to you or your office; an actual visit to your office, an open house, or a project; or a visit to your website for pictures and more information. If an ad fails to evoke action from a recipient of the message, then, to that person, the ad is really institutional in nature. It helps in name identification and general goodwill but has failed to bring in a prospective buyer.

ADVERTISING GUIDELINES

There are five basic tenets of advertising:

1. Advertise the right property

2. Know when to advertise

3. Choose the right market

4. Use the proper media

5. Use effective advertising techniques

By use of the internet, it is now possible for a real estate office to advertise all listings at the same time. This is not possible with print advertising. If you are trying to generate a great number of prospects, consider placing the listings that have the greatest general appeal in a predominant position on your website. We know that buyers responding to a real estate advertisement are likely to buy a property other than the property advertised. For this reason, we strive to advertise properties in areas and/or price ranges where we also have other available properties. This tactic increases the likelihood that prospects who respond to advertisements will become buyers.

Knowing when and where to advertise, whom you want to reach, and the features to emphasize is extremely important. You probably would not feature a swimming pool in an advertisement for a home in northern California at the beginning of a cold winter; a fireplace would be a more appropriate feature. Likewise, you would probably avoid advertising an elegant, expensive home in a local shoppers guide that is distributed primarily to low-income families.

ADVERTISING MEDIA

Choosing Advertising Media

In determining media choice, the advertiser must begin with three basic considerations:

1. The target audience to be reached

2. The message to be conveyed

3. The money available for media purchases

This means that in addition to determining what to say, the broker must evaluate which medium or combination of media will deliver the maximum number of potential customers for the expenditure the broker can afford.

Because the message cannot contribute to sales until prospective buyers are exposed to it, the message must be delivered within sight or earshot of such prospects. The various advertising media perform the delivery function.

Media choices available include the following:

- Personal advertising

- Internet property sites

- Office and personal internet sites

- Social media

- General circulation daily

- General circulation weekly

- Weekly throwaway

- Foreign language and ethnic papers

- Special-interest papers (such as mobile home news)

- Special-interest publications

- Homebuyer magazines

- Radio

- Television

- Outdoor advertising

- Signs

- Direct mail

- Newsletters

- Telephone directories

- Press releases

- Specialty gifts

When choosing the medium, keep in mind that the objective is not necessarily to reach the largest number of people but to reach the greatest number of potential prospects at the least possible cost.

In determining the media to be used, ask yourself the following two questions:

1. What are my marketing goals?

   — To get more sale listings?

   — To get more buyer listings?

   — To attract more potential buyers?

   — To increase market share?

   — To enhance recognition of name?

   — To enhance recognition of professionalism?

   — To sell listed properties?

2. Which specific media will reach my target audience?

Personal Advertising

Personal advertising should start with a **name tag** identifying you as a real estate professional. The tag should be readable from at least 6 feet away. Preferably, it should use the same color as your office signs and business cards. If you are a REALTOR®, "REALTOR®" should be on your name tag. If you have achieved a significant professional designation, such as GRI, this also should be on your name tag.

| Personal advertising concentrates on you, rather than on your firm. |

Your personal advertising should include your **business card**. You want people to be able to identify your card among a group of cards. The easiest way to accomplish this is with your photograph on the card. As stated in Unit 1, your card should include your email address, fax number, and cell phone number. If you have foreign language skills and feel they are important in your work, your card should indicate those skills. Your real estate license number must be on your business card. It is required on cards because they are a first point of contact.

Some agents are now using personal logos on their business cards, personal websites, mailings, property briefs and advertising. While firm information is also provided, the logo helps to distinguish the agent from other agents and sells the individual.

Because of the amount of information that you may require, you might consider a foldout card.

Smartphones can read QR (quick response) codes. A smartphone can scan and capture a business card with a QR code. The code can contain business card data, as well as access to websites, resumes, et cetera. Data can be transferred from one smartphone to another by a simple scanning process.

A magnetic **car sign** is a good low-cost advertising tool. Include your name, the name of your firm, REALTOR® (if applicable), and firm logo (a firm-identifying design). The logo should appear on all advertisements, signs, cards, and so forth. Magnetic signs that proclaim "Open House," as well as your name, can turn your vehicle parked in a driveway into an invitation to visit.

It is a good idea to print out copies of your résumé with your photograph. You can give them to prospective buyers and sellers, as well as use them as an enclosure with mailings (both snail mail and email).

Your own column.   In smaller-circulation local papers, it may be possible to write a weekly real estate column. Being an author of a column will increase your name recognition, as well as show your knowledge and professionalism.

Personal business sites. Many agents now have their own websites that include personal information, as well as information on properties they are offering, frequently with links to other sites. Because salespeople in 100% commission offices act much like independent brokers, it makes sense for such agents to have their own websites.

The salesperson's own website can include many of the links from the office site, but it must include the broker's name and the salesperson's license number.

Blogs. A blog is a website maintained by an individual with emphasis on a particular subject with regularly updated news and comments. Many blogs allow viewers to leave comments. It should be separate from your personal business website. A blog could be centered on an activity or a particular geographical area such as "Sun City Happenings." It might include community events, information on residents, as well as real estate data on listings, sales, rentals and valuation trends. By including valuable information, you promote yourself in a positive manner. There are many sports blogs about particular local teams. There are even blogs as to social activities, such as line dancing or bridge.

A blog should not look like a commercial home page. It should be loaded with information for the targeted audience.

A problem with blogs is that they can take much of your time. Some agents use personal assistants to keep the blogs current after they have been established.

Social networking sites. Social networking is not just for teenagers with agile thumbs. A vast array of social networking sites is now available to help companies and/or an individuals in their business endeavors. Social networking allows a dialog with followers. New ways of using these sites are being discovered almost daily. A growing number of companies on the internet offer tutorials about the business use of social networking and offer to handle your page on a site.

Avoid religion and politics on your websites unless you want to eliminate a great number of potential clients. Don't use social media to make yourself seem important. Use it to show yourself as caring, helpful and community-minded individual. Don't overload your websites with garbage information. Keep in mind that real estate is local, so what is happening in your community will be of greatest interest.

A number of books and videos are available on how to use social networking sites. In addition, a number of firms and organizations offer seminars on social media marketing.

- Twitter is a service that enables users to send and read text messages up to 140 characters. An estimated 500 million tweets are sent daily. While unregistered individuals can read tweets, registered members can post them. Business tweets often talk about non-business items to gain the interest of readers. They can target interest groups.

  Tweets can be inspirational to agents and informative as to offers, price reduction, et cetera. They can be sent to prospective buyers, sellers, and clients. Tweets can be used to invite specific individuals or people in general to an open house or to promote a new listing. They can announce a sale or be used for a welcome to a new neighbor. Tweets are also used to promote blog postings and websites. There is a great deal of free help, as well as a subscription service, about using Twitter for business. The website www.chrisbrogan.com offers free ideas to real estate professionals for using Twitter.

  A hashtag # can be used on Twitter, as well as on other social media. The hashtag is used for key words so the tweet can be found on a tweet search. As an example, #Brentwood Foreclosure or #Yucaipa Horse Ranch.

- Facebook connects people. The largest social networking system available requires participants to register before creating a personal profile. Many firms are now including Facebook link information on their press releases. Some Facebook pages are community oriented with news to garner followers. A Facebook page can include simple sign-ups for emails and newsletters with software such as Mail Chimp (www.mailchimp.com).

- Instagram, owned by Facebook, is a photo and video sharing website. Forty million photos are posted each day. A filter system allows photos to be manipulated in ways similar to Adobe Photoshop. Instagram is available for smartphones and iPads. Hashtags can be used to get attention and listings. Videos are limited to 15 seconds. You can adapt other videos with your voice to describe a property as though you were showing it. One technique is a neighborhood map showing locations of listings giving the user the ability to view each listing with photos or video.

■ LinkedIn is a business networking website that can reach developers, investors, and others who can help your business. You can tell your story on your company page.

■ The above noted sites are just a few of the many available.

YouTube.   Youtube.com is a video-sharing website. Content is uploaded by registered individual users. Unregulated users can view the videos. Many real estate agents post virtual tours of their properties on YouTube. Some agents host their own shows to highlight their knowledge and inform buyers and sellers. YouTube allows for a video blog.

Photo sharing.   Photo sharing is the publishing or transfer of digital images online. Photo blogs allow you to classify photos and add captions and comments.

The internet offers amazing opportunities and is the future of real estate communication.

Newspaper Advertising

Newspapers are the oldest advertising medium in the nation and in the past have been the keystone of the real estate business. Although the first advertisement appeared in the *Boston Newsletter* in 1704, newspapers were rather scarce until 1790. After many decades of phenomenal growth, newspaper sales and readership are now in sharp decline. The high cost of advertising and growth of the internet has resulted in less reliance on real estate classified advertising. The classified ad sections of large circulation newspapers have declined from several pages to a few columns. However, there is still a place for print advertising.

Newspapers have a degree of audience selectivity. Because of their wide circulation, they may be considered to have extensive coverage. They also have time-and-place flexibility and are especially important for local advertising. Because of their tremendous circulation, newspapers reach all classes of consumers. A drawback of newspaper advertising is that its effective life span is short.

Since the 1990s, a third of household growth and about 12% of first-time buyers have been immigrants. Foreign language papers should be considered if an office wishes to tap into this market. Real estate agents must avoid advertising exclusively in minority publications because it might be construed as steering, a violation of the real estate law.

Weekly newspapers in smaller communities are still an effective media for real estate ads because the percentage of readers remains high due to their local news content. The cost of advertising in local weeklies is manageable. Generally, newspaper readers are graying. The average age of readers is increasing. The product advertised can be targeted to the older reader.

Newspaper advertising is divided into classified and display advertisements. Any newspaper ad should provide a broker name, phone number, and internet address. Advertisements that do not identify the advertiser as a broker are called **blind ads** and are illegal in California. A blind ad is deceptive because readers are induced to contact the advertiser in the belief that they are dealing directly with an owner rather than an agent.

Classified advertisements. All forms of newspaper advertising are important, but the most common form used in the real estate business is still **classified advertising**.

While not as productive as internet sites, print advertising still produces sales. People interested in buying or leasing real estate still check the classifieds where available, although they will likely spend more time on the internet. People older than 60 are more likely than those younger than 50 to seek out classified ads before they use the internet.

Keep in mind that your classified advertisements have a very short lifespan and will be in direct competition with many other ads, including those on the internet. A mediocre ad generally means a mediocre response. Strive for ads that achieve maximum effectiveness by analyzing likely buyers for a property and appealing to those buyers' needs.

Your classified ad should indicate an internet address that offers more information and additional properties: Examples are "More information and properties, www.seeahome.com" or "Property Tour, www.seeahome.com." People who find attractive properties on the internet feel that they played an active role in a home search rather than passively letting a salesperson decide which homes they were going to see. When a prospective buyer "discovers" a property, the chances of an actual offer are enhanced.

Classified ads are read by willing readers looking for properties. Therefore, the best heading would be the most desirable feature of the property: "4 Bedrooms," "Beverly Hills," or even price, "$397,500." However, you would not waste an ad heading such as "Beverly Hills" if the newspaper classification was for "Beverly Hills Property." Avoid redundancy. Figure 8.1 includes examples of ads with headings that cover one or more of a home's prime attractions.

When you don't have a super feature to advertise or there are many competing ads, consider an attention-grabbing heading to make your ad stand out from the others. Figure 8.2 includes examples of such ads.

Advertisements normally tell us how good a product is. If an ad listed the faults of a product, no one would normally be expected to buy it. Real estate, however, is different. Ads for fixer-upper properties often result in an exceptional response. A likely reason is that a property with problems spells opportunity to a great many buyers. The worse you make a property appear, the greater the response. Figure 8.3 includes sample fixer-upper ads. Before you use ads of this type, obtain the owners' permission in writing. Many owners will become upset if you degrade or make fun of their home, even if it brings in a buyer.

FIGURE 8.1:   Sample Feature Ads

Westlake

You can own a like-new, 3BR, 2½ bath Tennessee Colonial with all the fine detailing and craftsmanship you thought had been forgotten. A 2½-car garage, central air, a family room and a prestigious

WESTLAKE

address are yours for just $487,500

UR

HOME REALTY

Call Amber at 760-555-8200
View at www.ur-home.net

You can call attention to location by using a split heading, which is effective for a highly desirable area.

Spanish Omelet

Arches, tile and huge beams combine to make this 3-bedroom, 2-bath, West Side masterpiece a very tasty dish at

$579,500

Special features include family room, 3-car garage, central air, delightful fenced yard and giant Norway pine. One look and we will put up the "sold" sign. For a virtual tour, check #82 at www.ur-home.net.

UR

HOME REALTY

Call Amber at 760-555-8200
Tour at www.ur-homenet

The split heading features architectural style and price. The reader is invited to view the property on the Internet.

> Adjectives add desirability to ads.

Adjectives.   The use of adjectives to paint word pictures of features can spark readers' interest. It generally is false economy to write bare-bones ads in a competitive market. Often an ad that is 20% longer because of the use of adjectives earns a response rate that far outweighs the 20% higher ad cost. A response increase exceeding 100% is not uncommon.

As an example of how descriptive words can paint an image, consider how you might describe a bathroom to paint a picture for the reader:

> Sumptuous master bath, sensuous master bath, sinfully sensuous master bath, deliciously sumptuous bath, Roman bath, opulent Phoenician bath, Grecian bath, garden tub, antique claw-footed tub, sky-lit bath, enchanting garden bath

FIGURE 8.2: Sample Attention-Grabbing Ads

Maxine and Marvin Slept Here

for 10 years, but Marvin was transferred to Phoenix, so they must regretfully take their bed and leave this 3BR, 2-bath, red brick Georgian Colonial in the nicest area in all of Woodland Glen. The home features a tantalizing Jacuzzi tub in the master bath, which is why the shower is practically new; walk-in closets; music room for little Ralph, who is learning to play the drums; and a kitchen any chef would fry for. Priced to get Maxine and Marvin on their way at $437,500.

UR

HOME REALTY

760-555-8200
View at www.ur-home.net

Who Used the Tub?

We suspect Mr. Buckley of our office has been bathing in the Italian marble tub in the sumptuous master bath of this 3BR, 2½-bath Italian Renaissance estate in Westhaven. Every afternoon he visits the house and takes along a towel. When he returns, he's singing Italian arias. When you see the tantalizing Roman baths, you'll understand why. The estate has an aura of elegance that makes you want to pamper yourself. With more than 3,500 sq. ft. of sheer luxury and almost a half-acre of grounds, this is your chance to be good to yourself for $849,500. After all, who deserves it more?

UR

HOME REALTY

760-555-8200
View at www.ur-home.net

The above heading is a real attention getter.

Lady Saxophone Player

must sell her 3BR, cedarshake, Westfield Cape Cod in order to seek fame and fortune. There is a garage, several magnificent hickory trees, a family of squirrels, a somewhat neglected garden and a kitchen big enough to seat an 8-piece band. The price hits a pleasant note at $529,500.

UR

HOME REALTY

760-555-8200
www.ur-home.net

Before you feature an owner in your ad, obtain the owner's permission to run the ad.

FIGURE 8.3: Sample Fixer-Upper Ads

A Monument to Bad Taste

If you have more money than taste, you'll love this gaudy French Provincial with Italianate influence, finished to excess in a sort of baroque style. There are 11 huge rooms, all equally ugly. It does command a premier West Hills location, offering every conceivable amenity; but while you might like to visit, you wouldn't want to live here. Mr. Clements of our office, a former Edsel owner, thinks it's beautiful—just the way he imagines a movie star's home to be. It's priced far below reproduction costs at $689,000, but then who would want to reproduce it?

UR

HOME REALTY

760-555-8200
www.ur-home.net

As strange as it may seem, this ad will bring in calls from qualified buyers.

Decorator's Nightmare

Leprous yellow walls, jarring purple accents, and blood-red tile are just a few of the features in this 3-bedroom Dutch Colonial that prove money and good taste aren't synonymous. This appears structurally sound, and it does offer an excellent West Side location as well as an attractive exterior and landscaping. The price reflects the poor taste of the decorator—$369,500.

UR

HOME REALTY

760-555-8200
www.ur-home.net

This ad is a variation on the fixer-upper ad. Be certain you have the owner's permission before you comment negatively on the decorating.

It Could Be Worse

The roof doesn't appear to leak, but just about everything else in this 3BR, 2-bath, brick English Tudor in Westwood is in need of mending. While it has expansive lawns, hedges and flower beds, you'll have to imagine how it will look trimmed without the weeds and bare spots and with flowers blooming. If you love to tinker, you have enough work for a lifetime. The only redeeming feature is the price, $339,500.

UR

HOME REALTY

760-555-8200
www.ur-home.net

Yuk! This Place Is Unbelievable

This 3-bedroom, West Side American Traditional appears to have been neglected from the day it was built. It will take a semi to haul away the junk in the backyard. Perhaps under all that dirt you may find shining spendor, but don't count on it. But then for $189,500, what do you expect?

UR

HOME REALTY

760-555-8200
www.ur-home.net

This was adapted from an ad by Ian Price, Surfer's Paradise, Australia.

You can see that adjectives can bring a desired image to the reader, so use them. The use of adjectives is also important for your internet ads. While you are not limited on your office websites, many websites limit the space allowed for property descriptions.

Large circulation papers.   The greater a paper's circulation, the higher the cost of advertising. It doesn't take many large classified ads in the *Los Angeles Times* to use up the advertising budget of many firms. You can use a relatively short ad to perk a reader's interest to check further on the internet. Here are examples:

Many single-office real estate brokers avoid large newspapers, such as the *Los Angeles Times*, because so much of the circulation is beyond the brokers' market area. They attempt to target their areas by advertising in smaller-circulation papers that are local in scope.

Display advertisements.   Display advertising may be either institutional or operational in nature. It may combine the two, so that it is used primarily to build goodwill and prestige and keep the name before the public, while at the same time advertising specific properties. Be sure to include an internet address that can offer additional information.

Because of costs, display ads are primarily used for selling developments rather than single homes. An exception would be newspapers in smaller communities offering lower advertising costs. Consider obtaining professional help for display advertisements.

General Rules for Display Advertising

- Most people read from the upper left corner to the lower right corner.

- Therefore, the ad should be composed with the heading on top, illustration and copy in the center, and firm name, phone number, and Web address in the lower right quarter. One large picture is generally more effective than several small pictures.

- If reproduced well, photographs may be more effective than drawings, but most photographs require professional retouching to increase contrast, remove distracting features, and blur backgrounds.

- Include white space. White space emphasizes the message.

- Don't use more than two typefaces in an ad.

- Ads in the outside columns will generate more interest than ads in the inside columns.

- Typefaces with serifs (the fine lines at the end of letter strokes) are generally more readable than sans-serif typefaces (without the lines).

- Lowercase letters are easier to read than capital letters.

- Short sentences are more readable than long sentences.

- Short words are more readable than long words.

- If you pull readers through the first three lines, they are likely to read the entire ad.

- Use words that are readily understood.

- Don't be too subtle or sophisticated.

- Always tell the reader what to do (call, come in, or check the internet).

- Always use the same logo in your ads.

Magazine Advertising

The cost of advertising in a magazine having mass appeal generally is prohibitive. However, magazines appealing to special-interest groups could be productive for the right property. As an example, if you had 40 acres zoned for a salvage yard with railroad siding access, you might consider advertising it in a trade magazine for salvage yard operators.

Special city or area magazines are usually slick paper magazines with very limited circulation. They are likely to be most effective for very impressive homes.

Area homebuyer magazines are found in most areas of California. These magazines are particularly effective for newcomers to the area. There are variations of these magazines that cover just new home developments and rentals. It is believed that the prevalence of websites will diminish the effectiveness of these magazines.

Similar to homebuyer magazines, e-brochures are for the internet. They can be sent as emails or included on a CD business card. Software to prepare e-brochures can also be used to prepare printed brochures. You might want to check www.imprev.com for more information.

Radio and TV Advertising

Compared with print media, radio broadcasting is a relatively new advertising medium. The first paid advertisement on radio appeared in 1922. Today radio can reach, at one time or another, nearly 99% of the households in the United States. Customers can be reached traveling to and from work, to and from the market, at the beach, or in their own homes. Radio is effective because the audience can listen while doing something else.

In using radio advertising, match the property with the demographics of those who listen to the station. Unless you hope to sell a multimillion-dollar estate to a rock star, don't advertise it on a hard-rock station. Foreign language stations are being used effectively for brokers who are trying to tap into immigrant groups.

Television delivers advertising messages to both the eye and the ear. What's more, it permits the use of motion and color and usually delivers the message in the home. Television advertising, however, is expensive, and it is used sparingly for general real estate advertising. It is used most often by large real estate firms, franchisers, and developers.

Home showcase programs are becoming popular on television, particularly in smaller markets. They allow photos, as well as a verbal descriptions of property benefits. There are cable stations that have 24-hour bulletin boards of things for sale. Some brokers have reported excellent responses to these bulletin-board stations for low-cost and low-down-payment homes as well as rentals.

Outdoor Advertising

Outdoor advertising is used less frequently than other media, depending largely on the size of the town and the availability of advertising billboards. Usually, billboards are used by larger brokerage offices or chain operations.

However, signs may be painted on buildings, fences, bus-stop benches, or other display places by individual real estate offices as well.

Because of their cost, which can be several thousand dollars per month depending on features and location, the real estate use of billboards has been primarily for large new developments.

For Sale Signs

While relatively inexpensive, For Sale signs are effective and they work seven days a week, 24 hours per day. The design of a licensee's For Sale signs should be unique, original, quickly informative, and as attractive as possible. The attention-getting value of the signs will be enhanced through the use of color, unique design, an identifiable logo, and design and size of print. Rather than plain paint for your For Sale signs, consider reflective paint that stands out when light hits the sign. A new twist is a glow-in-the-dark paint that remains bright for several hours after dusk. (Your sign firm should be able to offer this product.) Solar-powered light fixtures are also available that allow signs to stand out at night.

> Your sign should be distinguishable from that of your competition.

Colors used should provide a high degree of contrast for readability (the best color contrast is yellow and black). To distinguish their signs from those of competitors, some brokers have changed the shape of their signs. A simple change is a vertical rectangle rather than a horizontal one. Others have gone to oversized signs or odd-shaped signs. Whatever their makeup, signs should be coordinated with any printed material being created for the office. Riders for special features or for listing a salesperson's name and phone number and even an Web address should be considered. (Talking signs and sign information boxes were covered in Unit 7.)

Direct Mail

Although **direct mail advertising** is rather expensive per contact, it can be an effective way to reach a selected audience. It may be institutional in nature or be designed to promote a new subdivision, an area, or even a specific piece of property. Various vehicles are used in this method of advertising, including pamphlets, brochures, letters, postcards, booklets, pictures, and maps. You can spread the word about new listings with regularly scheduled targeted mail using readily available merge software.

This medium may encourage the reader to seek more information by returning a response device that may result in additional material and inclusion in mailing lists and other sales promotions. An excellent approach is to offer prospective customers free email updates of new listings, including photos, by simply sending you an email. Of course, every direct mail piece should reference your firm's website. Direct mail approaches were more fully discussed in Unit 4.

Direct Email

We have shown you one way to obtain email addresses of prospects with the visitor rating form in Unit 7. We will be showing you more ways to have prospects willingly provide their email addresses. The beauty of a direct approach with email is that, except for preparation time, it is a no-cost approach. Direct approach emails can include colored pictures, movement (motion), and even sound. You can email a zip code by utilizing mailing list firms that also have email addresses. Like any other advertising, you want your direct mail and email ads to stand out from the commonplace. An unsolicited email must clearly indicate that it is an advertisement piece and comply with the CAN-SPAM regulations.

Newsletters

Many offices, as well as individual agents, successfully use **newsletters**. They include information that would be of interest to the recipient, as well as information about the firm or agent. They are particularly valuable in niche marketing. As an example, one agent who has established her niche in marketing mobile homes in a particular park has a monthly newsletter that includes personal information about residents and information on new residents and club schedules and special events. Computer programs and numerous services are available that will allow you to quickly publish a quality newsletter. You can also subscribe to services that print and distribute newsletters with your photo and contact information. Paper newsletters have been diminishing in importance because of the growth of email newsletters and agent blog websites.

Telephone Directories

Although real estate firms have yellow-page listings, often in bold type, display ads in telephone directories are not likely to be as cost-effective as those in other advertising media. The effectiveness of your yellow-page ad can be increased significantly by use of your internet address; for example, "View Available Homes at www.seeahome.com."

Press Releases

Press releases are really free advertisements. If you look in the real estate section or supplement of any newspaper, you will find that most of the articles are taken from press releases. Your local newspaper will publish press releases that are well written and have a newsworthy message. Some examples of such messages are the grand opening of an office, the groundbreaking for a development, the listing of a historic building, any sale where the buyers or sellers are newsworthy, special awards or designations received by agents, and office promotions.

Press releases are free advertisements.

Whenever possible, include a high-quality digital photo. Include a caption, and if people are shown, be sure to identify them in the caption.

Specialty Gifts

Most offices include **specialty gifts**, or promotional giveaway items, in their advertising budget. These may include notepads, maps, magnetic holders, calendars, pencils, directories, and pens with a salesperson's and the firm's identification. Such items promote you or your company continually and can be dispensed through the office, at business and social gatherings, at open houses, and during door-to-door canvassing. They are excellent door openers and can be used effectively to get acquainted in a neighborhood.

The Internet

The internet has become the predominant marketing tool. Just a few years ago, it was rare to have a transaction where the buyer or the seller contact resulted from information contained on a website. Today, many offices are reporting that most of their contacts result from internet postings. Surveys of property buyers reveal that in many areas over 90% of buyers indicated that they used the internet for their property search. Some 63% of buyers say they viewed homes they first found on the internet. While there are a great many sites where you can post your listings, it is extremely important that you have your own office website if you are going to be competitive.

Websites have been getting more elaborate, frequently with multiple pictures of each property and with sound and motion. Virtual tours allow a viewer to "walk through" the property; this virtual "walk-through" can either half-sell the property or eliminate it for a prospective buyer. By paying an extra fee, many home search websites offer enhanced property coverage, which increases the effectiveness of your property presentation.

One advantage of the internet is its relatively low cost once your website has been established. Be sure to include your web address in all your advertising in other media.

A decreasing portion of the advertising pie goes to print advertising. The internet is now considered more productive. Corzen, Inc., a New York–based provider of advertising data, claims that the internet is over twice as effective as print for real estate firms. Because the internet is the best bargain in town, print ads are dwindling in most papers and magazines. The internet allows a small firm to have a large presence within a market area. Some companies are now going 100% internet in their marketing efforts. Other firms claim to be using newspapers sparingly and then primarily to placate owners.

Before you prepare a website, we recommend you view the websites of a number of large brokerage offices in major metropolitan areas across the country. Note the differences in quality of the sites and in site features. Make a note of the features you want in your site, as well as why you feel some sites are outstanding. Now you are ready for your webpage preparation.

Features that you want to include on your website are as follows:

- **About us**—This feature allows a viewer to obtain information about your firm and its personnel; includes résumé and testimonial letters.

- **Inventory**—Here you provide photos and descriptions of your listings. If there are a great many listings, the viewer should be able to enter parameters such as price, size, and location to narrow the search for properties. If a property is advertised by number, the viewer should be able to go directly to that property. The inventory should also include the ability to increase size of photos, as well as view additional photos. Virtual tours should be considered for all listings.

■ **Area map**—This can show the locations of properties, as well as the broker's office.

■ **Email offer**—Each page of your site should offer the viewer an opportunity to receive emails of new listings before they are advertised.

■ **Motion and/or sound**—These features hold the viewer's attention and will distinguish your site from others.

■ **Loan qualifying opportunity**—This viewer option will provide information on the prospect and allow further direct contact.

■ **800 number**—By providing this number, you encourage calls from outside your immediate area.

■ **Back to home page**—This feature should be on every page of your website.

■ **Contact us**—This will allow the viewer to send an email to you. Agents can also include a link that says, "Search MLS here," an, through the use of a system known as IDX, pull MLS data to display on the agent's website.

While agents can prepare their own webpages using one of the inexpensive webpage programs, these are often boilerplate sites and fail to provide maximum viewer impact. As previously stated, we strongly suggest that a professional `webpage designer create your site. Before you hire a designer, be certain to view other sites created by the designer. A correctly designed website can ensure long-term use and will attract prospective buyers, sellers, lessors, and lessees, as well as enhance the image of your firm.

Besides your personal and office websites, it is important that your property information be distributed to MLS and other area and national websites.

Many agents have reported success with internet classified sites such as www.craigslist.org/about/sites and www.wantedwants.com.

Pay-per-click ads.   Many firms have reported success with pay-per-click ads on websites other than real estate sites. Sites that sell the benefit of a community are logical sites for pay-per-click ads. Every time a website viewer clicks on your ad, you pay a small fee. A click on the ad could lead to your website's homepage, which could then lead to information about you and the available inventory.

Other Forms of Advertising

There are many other ways to advertise: movie screens, videotapes, window displays, transit ads, bus shelter and bench ads, electric message boards, marquee ads, supermarket carts, and so on. You will find that your advertising is limited only by the limits of your imagination and the thickness of your pocketbook.

ADVERTISING EFFECTIVENESS

Is your advertising program producing the results you want? There is an old saying in advertising: "Half of my advertising is worth the money. The problem is that I don't know *which* half!" If you don't set up an evaluation system, you will never know. Identifying the part of your advertising dollar that is producing your sales can be critical to success. You must be able to determine which types of advertising are most effective for you and which produce the most income. You can do that by tracking ads and determining their cost compared with the amount of business they generate. You can even pinpoint which approach and/or medium is most effective for a particular type of property.

The key to a good measurement system is simplicity. One method to use when you run a newspaper ad or send out a letter or direct mail piece is to put a code on the bottom of the piece. A simple technique is to use a designated telephone number. Thus, respondents who contact you by a call to that number indicate that they are responding to a particular ad. If possible, try to identify separately for each ad the number of prospects and sales that result, so you will know the quality as well as the quantity of leads you obtain. Then determine the cost of each advertisement. Many offices require that the receptionist who handles incoming calls keep telephone logs. The receptionist can ascertain the type of ad seen by the caller and the ad medium and can enter this information into the log.

You should evaluate ads for effectiveness.

Just because one medium is not as effective as another in terms of number of responses does not mean the medium is ineffective.

EXAMPLE   Jane Freyman placed two ads in different newspapers for the same period. The ads were identical. She knew that this was important because she wanted to test which publication worked best. If she used different-quality ads, one would naturally pull better because it was a better ad, not because the publication was better. She ran the ads at the same time for the same reason. The only difference was that the ad in paper A directed people to ask for department X, whereas the ad in paper B told people to ask for department Y.

There was a difference in the cost of running the ads. A had a circulation of 20,000 and charged $200 for the ad. B had a circulation of 100,000 and charged $1,000. The following are the results that Freyman tabulated:

Paper A	Paper B
15 prospects	27 prospects
5 eventual sales	9 eventual sales

Which paper is a more attractive advertising medium? Does Freyman simply want greater numbers of sales, or does she want to get more sales more cost-effectively?

Assuming that the amounts of the individual sales were comparable, B probably would be more attractive to Freyman if she wanted more sales. The ad in B generated more eventual sales. However, if Freyman was more interested in cost-effectiveness, she probably would prefer A. The sales numbers were smaller, but so were the costs—not only the cost of the ad but also the cost per sale:

$$\$200 \div 5 \text{ sales} = \$40 \text{ per sale}$$

$$\$1,000 \div 9 \text{ sales} = \$110 \text{ per sale}$$

LEGAL IMPLICATIONS OF ADVERTISING

Advertising of real property is regulated by California real estate law, the regulations of the real estate commissioner, and the federal Consumer Credit Protection Act (Truth in Lending Act). The following sections from the California Business and Professions Code and the Regulations of the Real Estate Commissioner are merely condensations of the actual statues and regulations.

California Real Estate Law

Section 10139—"Penalties for Unlicensed Person." This law stipulates that any unlicensed person acting as a licensee who advertises using words indicating that she is a broker is subject to a fine not to exceed $20,000 and/or imprisonment in the county jail for a term not to exceed six months. If the violator is a corporation, it is subject to a fine of $60,000.

Section 10140—"False Advertising." This section states that every officer or employee who knowingly advertises a false statement concerning any land or subdivision is subject to a fine of $1,000 and/or one year's imprisonment. In addition, the licensee may have his license suspended or revoked.

Section 10140.5—"Disclosure of Name." Each advertisement published by a licensee that offers to assist in filing applications for the purchase or lease of government land must indicate the name of the broker and the state in which she is licensed.

Section 10140.6—"False Advertising." Licensees may not publish in any newspaper or periodical or by mail an ad for any activity for which a real estate license is required that does not contain a designation disclosure that they are performing acts for which a license is required.

While the law requires licensees to include their license number in contact material, newspaper and periodical advertising are exempt, as are For Sale signs and television ads.

Section 10235—"Misleading Advertisement." A licensee may not advertise, print, display, publish, distribute, televise, or broadcast false or misleading statements regarding rates and terms or conditions for making, purchasing, or negotiating loans or real property sales contracts, nor may a licensee permit others to do so.

Section 10236.1—"Inducements." A licensee may not advertise to offer a prospective purchaser, borrower, or lender any gift as an inducement for making a loan or purchasing a promissory note secured directly by a lien on real property or a real property sales contract.

Section 10131.7—"Mobile Home Advertising."   A licensee is prohibited from engaging in the following activities:

- Advertising a mobile home that is not in an established mobile home park or is being sold with the land

- Failing to withdraw an advertisement of a mobile home within 48 hours of removal from the market

- Advertising or representing a used mobile home as a new one

- Making a false statement that a mobile home is capable of traveling on California highways

- Falsely advertising that no down payment is required on the sale of a mobile home when in fact one is required

Regulations of the Real Estate Commissioner

The real estate commissioner can adopt regulations that have the same force and intent as law. Two of these regulations follow.

Article 9, Section 2770.1—"Advertising License Designation."   Use of the terms *broker, agent, REALTOR®, loan correspondent*, or the abbreviations *bro., agt.*, or other terms or abbreviations, is deemed sufficient identification to fulfill the designation requirements of Section 10140.6 of the Business and Professions Code.

Article 9, Section 22773—"Disclosure of License Identification Number on Solicitation Materials."   All first point-of-contact solicitation material must disclose the licensee's eight-digit real estate license number. This includes business cards, stationary, websites, flyers, et cetera.

Code of Ethics of the National Association of REALTORS®

Even though the Code of Ethics of the National Association of REALTORS® is a moral code and as such is not enforceable by law, its guidelines are observed by most real estate licensees in California. Professional courtesy and ethics should not end with those acts that have been sanctioned by law. The individual who tries only to stay on the border of the law may at some time step across that border.

Regarding advertising, Article 12 of the 2015 Code of Ethics states that

> REALTORS® shall be honest and truthful in their real estate communications and shall present a true picture in their advertising, marketing, and other representations. REALTORS® shall ensure that their status as real estate professionals is readily apparent in their advertising, marketing, and other representations, and that the recipients of all real estate communications are, or have been, notified that those communications are from a real estate professional.

> 12-4　REALTORS® shall not offer for sale/lease or advertise property without authority.

> 12-5　REALTORS® shall not advertise nor permit any person employed by or affiliated with them to advertise real estate services or listed property in any medium (e.g., electronically, print, radio, television, etc.) without disclosing the name of that REALTOR®'s firm in a reasonable and readily apparent manner.

> 12-6　REALTORS®, when advertising unlisted real property for sale/lease in which they have an ownership interest, shall disclose their status as both owners/landlords and REALTORS® or real estate licensees.

Truth in Lending Act

The **Truth in Lending Act**, or Regulation Z, a part of the federal Consumer Credit Protection Act of 1968, requires disclosure of credit costs as a percentage, as well as total finance charges. It is enforced by the Federal Trade Commission.

Truth-in-lending applies to credit extended with a finance charge or credit payable in more than four installments. If the amount or percentage of down payment, the number of payments or period of repayment, or the amount of payment or amount of finance charges (trigger terms) is included in any advertisement, then the ad must include three elements:

1. Amount or percentage of down payment

2. Terms of repayment

3. **Annual percentage rate** (APR) (the true interest rate considering points and other loan costs; the nominal rate is the rate stated on the note)

Advertising the APR alone will not trigger the these disclosures.

If creditors extend credit secured by a dwelling more than five times per year, they must furnish the purchaser a truth-in-lending disclosure showing all loan facts. However, the total amount of finance charges for the term of the loan need not be shown for first mortgages or loans used to purchase real property. (Because escrow impounds for taxes and insurance are not considered loan costs, they need not be listed.)

Truth-in-lending makes **bait-and-switch advertising** (advertising property that agents don't intend to sell or that is not available in order to attract buyers for other property) a federal offense.

Rescission right.   If the loan is for consumer credit secured by the borrower's residence, the borrower has the right to reconsider and cancel. This right is valid until midnight on the third business day following loan completion. (Rescission right does not apply to home purchase loans but does apply to home equity loans and home refinancing.)

Exemptions.   Loans exempt from all truth-in-lending disclosure requirements are business loans, agricultural loans, construction loans, personal property loans over $25,000, and interest-free loans with four or fewer installments. Non-owner-occupied housing is considered a business and thus exempt from disclosure. Carryback financing for most sellers (not more than five times per year) also is exempt.

CIVIL RIGHTS ACT OF 1968

The Civil Rights Act of 1968 prohibits discriminatory advertising (see Unit 2). Discriminatory advertising includes advertising that indicates any preference, limitation, or discrimination because of race, color, religion, sex, handicap, familial status, or national origin.

There are some discriminatory words and phrases that are not readily recognized by many as being discriminatory. In addition, some words carry different connotations among different social, ethnic, and economic groups. Words also have different meanings based upon geographic location.

A number of groups have tried to clarify what was and was not acceptable wording for advertising by publishing lists. These lists varied greatly. Some lists went so far as to indicate that advertising the "view" was discriminatory to the blind. Prudent agents will follow the BRE guidelines for advertising (see Figure 8.4).

While the Department of Housing and Urban Development (HUD) enforces the Fair Housing Act, the federal agency was reluctant to provide guidance. There was a partial clarification on January 9, 1995, when HUD sent a memo to its staff as to guidelines for investigation of discrimination allegations. The memo addressed the following five points:

1. **Race, color, national origin.** Complaints should not be filed for use of "master bedroom," "rare find," or "desirable neighborhood." Some groups felt that "master" indicated slavery, and "rare find" and "desirable neighborhood" indicated areas without minorities.

2. **Religion.** Phrases such as "apartment complex with chapel" or "kosher meals available" do not, on their face, state a preference for persons who might use such facilities. Prior to HUD's memo, groups were advising that any reference in an ad to religion would violate the federal Fair Housing Act.

3. **Sex.** Use of the terms "master bedroom," "mother-in-law suite," and "bachelor apartment" does not violate the act because they are commonly used physical descriptions.

4. **Handicap.** Descriptions of properties such as "great view," "fourth-floor walk-up," and "walk-in closets" do not violate the act. Services or facilities such as "jogging trails" or references to neighborhoods such as "walk to bus stop" do not violate the act. Because many handicapped individuals cannot perform these activities, it was formerly thought that references to walking, biking, jogging, and so on would violate the law. It also is acceptable to describe the conduct required of residents, such as "nonsmoking" or "sober." You can't, however, say "nonsmokers" or "no alcoholics" because these describe persons, not barred activities. You can advertise accessibility features such as "wheelchair ramp."

5. **Familial status.** While advertisements may not contain a limitation on the number or ages of children or state a preference for adults, couples, or singles, you are not "facially discriminatory" by advertising properties as "2-BR, cozy, family room," services and facilities with "no bicycles allowed," or neighborhoods with "quiet streets."

The HUD memo still leaves a great deal unanswered; however, HUD seems to indicate that the rule is one of reasonableness. If an ordinary person would feel an ad favored or disfavored a protected group, it would be discriminatory. Organizations have come up with updated lists that tend to reflect this thinking.

FIGURE 8.4: Advertising Guidelines

STATE OF CALIFORNIA
BUREAU OF REAL ESTATE

LICENSE DISCLOSURE REQUIREMENTS FOR MORTGAGE ADVERTISING

RE 858 (REV. 3/16)

The following chart shows the required disclosures of licensure based on the purpose of the mortgage loan advertisement. In addition to the information in the chart, the requirements of Business and Professions Code (B&P) Section 10140.6(b) apply to all first point-of-contact materials designed to solicit the creation of a professional relationship between the licensee and consumer.
Please note: All disclosure requirements of licensure can be located in B&P Sections 10140.6, 10235.5, 10236.4, and Title 10, beginning with Section 2770, of the Regulations of the Real Estate Commissioner. (See below.)

Advertising Media

The disclosures are required in all advertising including, but not limited to, flyers, mailers, TV, radio, newspapers, magazines, yellow pages, and the Internet.

Questions?

If you have questions, please call the Mortgage Loan Activities section at (916) 263-8941 or write to: Bureau of Real Estate, Attn: Mortgage Loan Activities, P.O. Box 137000, Sacramento, CA 95813-7000.

Required Disclosures	Advertising Purposes		First Point of Contact Only (Business cards, email, etc.)
	Soliciting for Borrowers	Soliciting for Investors/Lenders and/or Note Purchasers	
Phrasing	CA Bur of Real Estate – Real Estate Broker; or Real Estate Broker – CA Bur of Real Estate - AND - Broker, agent, Realtor, loan correspondent or abbreviations bro., agt., or other similar terms or abbreviations	Broker, agent, Realtor, loan correspondent or abbreviations bro., agt., or other similar terms or abbreviations	Broker, agent, Realtor, loan correspondent or abbreviations bro., agt., or other similar terms or abbreviations
CalBRE License Number	8-digit license number of each licensee in the advertisement - AND - 8-digit license number of the broker	8-digit license number of each licensee in the advertisement - AND - 8-digit license number of the broker	8-digit license number of each licensee in the advertisement
NMLS Unique Identifier*	Unique identifier of each licensee in the advertisement* - AND - Unique identifier of the broker*	N/A	Unique identifier of each licensee disseminating the materials* (Unique identifier of the employing broker or corporation *not* required)
Font Size Requirement	No less than the smallest font used in the advertisement	No less than the smallest font used in the advertisement	No less than the smallest font used in the advertisement

*Only applies to residential mortgage loan originators, as defined in Section 10166.01 of the Business and Professions Code.

PERTINENT CODES & REGULATIONS

Business and Professions Code

Disclosure of Licensed Status in Advertising
10140.6. (a) A real estate licensee shall not publish, circulate, distribute, or cause to be published, circulated, or distributed in any newspaper or periodical, or by mail, any matter pertaining to any activity for which a real estate license is required that does not contain a designation disclosing that he or she is performing acts for which a real estate license is required.

(b) (1) A real estate licensee shall disclose his or her license identification number and, if that licensee is a mortgage loan originator, the unique identifier assigned to that licensee by the Nationwide Mortgage Licensing System and Registry, on all solicitation materials intended to be the first point of contact with consumers and on real property purchase agreements when acting as an agent in those transactions.

The commissioner may adopt regulations identifying the materials in which a licensee must disclose a license identification number and, if that licensee is a mortgage loan originator, the unique identifier assigned to that licensee by the Nationwide Mortgage Licensing System and Registry.

(2) For purposes of this section, "solicitation materials intended to be the first point of contact with consumers" includes business cards, stationery, advertising fliers, and other materials designed to solicit the creation of a professional relationship between the licensee and a consumer, and excludes an advertisement in print or electronic media and "for sale" signs.

(3) Nothing in this section shall be construed to limit or change the requirement described in Section 10236.4 as applicable to real estate brokers.

FIGURE 8.4 (continued):   Advertising Guidelines

RE 858 – Reverse

(c) The provisions of this section shall not apply to classified rental advertisements reciting the telephone number at the premises of the property offered for rent or the address of the property offered for rent.

(d) "Mortgage loan originator," "unique identifier," and "Nationwide Mortgage Licensing System and Registry" have the meanings set forth in Section 10166.01.

Advertising of Loan – License Disclosure

10235.5. (a) No real estate licensee or mortgage loan originator shall place an advertisement disseminated primarily in this state for a loan unless there is disclosed within the printed text of that advertisement, or the oral text in the case of a radio or television advertisement, the Bureau of Real Estate license number and the unique identifier assigned to that licensee by the Nationwide Mortgage Licensing System and Registry under which the loan would be made or arranged.

(b) "Mortgage loan originator," "unique identifier," and "Nationwide Mortgage Licensing System and Registry" have the meanings set forth in Section 10166.01.

Disclosure of License Number in Advertisement; License Number and CalBRE License Information Telephone Number in Disclosure Statements

10236.4. (a) In compliance with Section 10235.5, every licensed real estate broker shall also display his or her license number on all advertisements where there is a solicitation for borrowers or potential investors. Every mortgage loan originator, as defined in Section 10166.01, shall also display the unique identifier assigned to that individual by the Nationwide Mortgage Licensing System and Registry on all advertisements where there is a solicitation for borrowers.

(b) The disclosures required by Sections 10232.4 and 10240 shall include the licensee's license number, the mortgage loan originator's unique identifier, if applicable, and the department's license information telephone number. *

(c) "Mortgage loan originator," "unique identifier," and "Nationwide Mortgage Licensing System and Registry" have the meanings set forth in Section 10166.01.

[*The CalBRE's licensing information telephone number is not required on advertisements for loan activities. The number is required to be on the Lender/Purchaser Disclosure Statement and the Mortgage Loan Disclosure Statement.]

Commissioner's Regulations

2770.1. Advertising - License Designation.
Use of the terms broker, agent, Realtor, loan correspondent or the abbreviations bro., agt., or other similar terms or abbreviations, is deemed sufficient identification to fulfill the designation requirements of Section 10140.6(a) and (c) of the Business and Professions Code.

Use of the terms and abbreviations set forth above does not satisfy the requirements of Sections 10235.5 and 17539.4 of the Code.

2773. Disclosure of License Identification Number on Solicitation Materials – First Point of Contact with Consumers.

(a) A real estate broker or salesperson, when engaging in acts for which a license is required, shall disclose its, his or her eight (8) digit real estate license identification number on all solicitation materials intended to be the first point of contact with consumers. If the name of more than one licensee appears in the solicitation, the license identification number of each licensee shall be disclosed. The license numbers of employing brokers or corporate brokers whose names or logos or trademarks appear on solicitation materials along with the names and license numbers of licensed employees or broker associates do not need to appear on those materials.

Solicitation materials intended to be the first point of contact with consumers, and in which a licensee must disclose a license identification number, include the following:

(1) Business cards;

(2) Stationery;

(3) Websites owned, controlled, and/or maintained by the soliciting real estate licensee; and

(4) Promotional and advertising fliers, brochures, email and regular mail, leaflets, and any marketing or promotional materials designed to solicit the creation of a professional relationship between the licensee and a consumer, or which is intended to incentivize, induce or entice a consumer to contact the licensee about any service for which a license is required.

The type size of the license identification number shall be no smaller than the smallest size type used in the solicitation material.

(b) For the purposes of Business and Professions Code Section 10140.6, solicitation materials do not include the following:

(1) Advertisements in electronic media (including, without limitation, radio, cinema and television ads, and the opening section of streaming video and audio);

(2) Print advertising in any newspaper or periodical; and

(3) "For Sale" signs placed on or around a property intended to alert the public the property is available for lease, purchase or trade.

2847.3. Disclosure of License and Issuing Department.
(a) Use of either of the following statements shall satisfy the requirements of Sections 10235.5 and 17539.4 of the Code.

(1) Real estate broker, California Bureau of Real Estate.

(2) California Bureau of Real Estate, real estate broker. The words "California" and "Bureau" may be abbreviated only as "CA" or "CAL" or "Calif" and "Bur". A dash (-) may be used in lieu of the comma appearing in the statements set forth above in paragraphs (1) and (2).

(b) The type size of the statement as set forth in subdivision (a) will also satisfy the designation requirements of Section 10140.6 of the Code.

(c) Use of either statement as set forth in subdivision (a) will also satisfy the designation requirements of Section 10140.6(a) and (c) of the Code.

Supervising social media advertising

Real estate licensees should take care to ensure that the names on Instagram, Facebook, and other social media accounts don't give the impression that the salesperson is acting without being under the supervision of a licensed broker.

For example salesperson Betty Thomas at XYZ Brokerage, Inc., should not have an Instagram account that gives the impression that she is operating on her own. One could argue that www.instagram.com/bettythomasrealestatebroker or www.instagram.com/bettythomasrealty could be deemed deceptive and against the rules of the real estate commissioner if obtained by a salesperson.

Ideas of what to post on social media.   As you start your career in real estate, it is important to make a decision as to how your accounts on social media are going to be set up.

- Are your social media accounts going to be separated into personal and business, or are you going to use one account for both?

- If they are going to be split, how often are you going to post to your business account? If you are going to use the same accounts for both, what percentage do you see being devoted to each aspect of your life?

Most social media experts agree that your business posts don't always have to consist of hard-selling content. You can mix lighter material with the fact that you are in business and want more customers.

Here's one idea for posting:

- Photos of houses or properties that you have just sold or listed. As a new real estate licensee, you might not have properties that you have sold or listed yet. In that case, consider posting pictures of properties that your company has listed or sold recently and the caption could be, "Our team just listed 123 Any Street! Message me for details!"

This lets your follower base know that you are active and in the real estate business.

It is a common marketing strategy among real estate agents to send just listed/sold postcards to a given database upon obtaining signatures on a contract. In the world of digital marketing, it should also be standard that a real estate agent post on all social media of their recent success completing a transaction. This means an Instagram, Facebook, and Twitter message announcing your recent transaction.

ADVERTISING BUDGET

Every successful real estate office has developed a system for budgeting its expenses. One of the expenses that must be accounted for is advertising. Advertising is one of the most important steps in the marketing of real property, but it does cost money. Soon after starting in the business, a broker learns that a certain amount of the firm's income dollar must be allocated to this item to maximize returns.

WEB LINK

@

An advertising budget involves more than just the number of dollars to be spent in advertising; it should determine how the dollars should be allocated. According to HomeGain (www.homegain.com), in September 2005 the typical real estate advertising budget was allocated in the following manner:

- Newspapers   39%
- Other print   20%
- Direct mail   17%
- Online   11%
- Yard signs   8%
- Yellow Pages   4%
- Telemarketing   1%

HomeGain believed that a more appropriate budget should be as follows:

- Newspapers   10%
- Other print   5%
- Direct mail   10%

- Online   52%

- Yard signs   20%

- Yellow Pages   3%

- Telemarketing   0%

HomeGains' projections of how a real estate advertising budget should be allocated have been largely realized. According to Borrell Associates, by 2015, real estate agents and brokers had spent nearly 75% of their advertising budget online.

The advertising dollar budget of an office is influenced by the advertising costs within a community, as well as by market conditions. As a rule, the time to increase advertising is when market sales are increasing. It is rare for expansion of advertising in a declining market to make economic sense, although reallocation of expenses should be an ongoing consideration.

Many offices plan their advertising budget as a percentage of their anticipated income dollar. As an example, a firm might plan to use 20% of the office share of commissions (the **company dollar**) for advertising. Because economic changes can be rapid, a budget should be adjusted to reflect market change. In a down market, while total advertising dollars will decrease, the percentage of the company dollar spent on advertising will increase. Similarly, in an active market where total ad dollars will likely increase, the percentage of advertising costs to the company dollar will decrease.

A number of agents who charge reduced fees make up for some of their fee reduction by charging owners advanced advertising expenses. Expenditures are then made with the owner's funds.

SUMMARY

Advertising is the process of calling people's attention to a product or service. The real estate industry could not exist without the ability to disseminate information.

Advertising falls into two broad categories: institutional, which is basically advertising to promote the goodwill of the firm, and specific or operational advertising, which is to sell or lease a particular property.

The AIDA approach to advertising is basically that an effective ad should gain **A**ttention, **I**nterest the party intended, create **D**esire, and result in **A**ction. The five basic tenets or guidelines for advertising are as follows:

1. Advertise the right property

2. Know when to advertise

3. Choose the right market

4. Use the proper media

5. Use effective advertising techniques

Advertising really begins with the salesperson's personal advertising that includes a name tag, business cards, and magnetic car signs.

While a broad array of media choices are available, most of a firm's advertising budget was formerly devoted to classified advertising. To be effective, a classified ad must have a highly desirable feature in the heading or else have an attention-getting heading. While negative ads are generally not successful, in real estate they may be very effective. Fixer-upper ads that emphasize what is wrong with a property often receive an exceptional rate of response. Internet advertising is considered more effective than print ads at a fraction of the cost and has replaced print ads in budget emphasis.

Display advertising, because of cost, is more appropriate for expensive properties or large developments. Specialty magazine ads can also be effective.

The For Sale sign is effective at relatively low cost. Direct mail can be effective, but there is a high cost per contact.

Other advertising includes telephone directories, press releases, newsletters, and specialty gifts.

The internet is the most effective media today including personal and company websites, property websites, classified ad websites, blogs, and social networking sites.

It is essential that a firm understand the effectiveness of its advertising. By keeping track of responses, we can learn which medium or approach is most effective for which type of property. This knowledge will allow advertising planning based on past results, not just by intuition.

As a licensee, you are responsible for knowing the legal implications of real estate advertising. Licensees are prohibited from false, misleading, and discriminatory advertising. Of particular interest is the Truth in Lending Act. Besides prohibiting bait-and-switch advertising, advertising the amount or percentage of down payment, the number of payments or period of repayment, or the amount of payment or finance charge all will trigger the full-disclosure provision of this law. Certain words may have discriminatory connotations, so care must be taken in describing properties.

Today, the largest portion of the advertising budget is related to the internet. The advertising budget of an office will vary based on advertising costs within the market area. Many offices plan advertising based on a percentage of anticipated office income.

CLASS DISCUSSION TOPICS

1. In addition to a photograph, what other ways can agents make their business card stand out?

2. Prepare two classified ads, one with a feature heading and the other with an attention-getting heading, to sell the home in which you live.

3. Discuss all the ways a typical real estate office in your area advertises (include both institutional advertising and specific advertising).

4. Check the websites of local brokers. Evaluate the sites as to quality, giving your reasons for your evaluation.

5. From the cautionary words shown on the Miami Valley word and phrase list, pick out a word that could be used in both a discriminatory and a nondiscriminatory manner and be prepared to give examples.

6. Bring to class one current-events article dealing with some aspect of real estate practice for class discussion.

UNIT 8 QUIZ

1. The AIDA approach does *NOT* include
   a. attention.
   b. demand.
   c. interest.
   d. action.

2. Personal advertising includes
   a. name tags.
   b. blog websites.
   c. car signs.
   d. all of these.

3. What does the term *logo* refer to?
   a. Your firm name
   b. An identifying design or symbol
   c. Length of gross opportunity, which refers to the time span of attention generated by an ad
   d. None of these

4. Blind ads are ads that fail to include
   a. a price.
   b. the address of property.
   c. broker identification.
   d. property specifics.

5. The MOST cost-effective advertising medium for selling a home likely would be
   a. television.
   b. the internet.
   c. classified newspaper ads.
   d. billboards.

6. Classified ads are different from most other forms of real estate advertising because they are
    a. actually sought out by the reader.
    b. ineffective for expensive homes.
    c. less reader-selective than other printed ads.
    d. unemotional.

7. Real estate professionals know that ads that tell about the problems of a property are
    a. a waste of advertising dollars.
    b. likely to give a firm a bad name.
    c. unlikely to attract any calls.
    d. none of these.

8. An advertiser with an extremely low advertising budget would most likely avoid
    a. press releases.
    b. For Sale signs.
    c. billboards.
    d. the internet.

9. Which statement is *FALSE* about display ads?
    a. Readers' eyes tend to move from upper left to lower right.
    b. One large picture is generally more effective than several smaller ones.
    c. Short words are easier to read than long words.
    d. Capital letters are easier to read than lowercase letters.

10. In preparing display ads, a good advertiser should
    a. eliminate as much white space in the ad as possible for maximum effect.
    b. use different logos in different ads to avoid repetition.
    c. use no more than two typefaces in an ad.
    d. avoid using a serif typeface in the text.

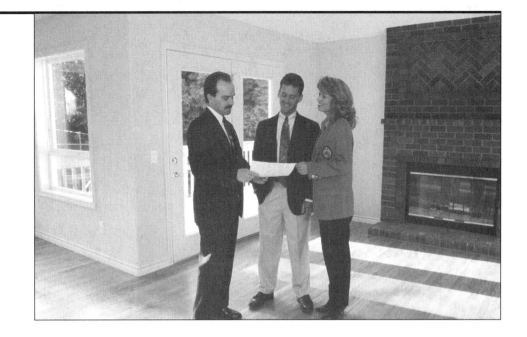

THE BUYER AND THE PROPERTY SHOWING

LEARNING OBJECTIVES

When you have completed this unit, you will be able to

- explain why a call from a prospective buyer resulting from a sign differs from an inquiry resulting from an ad or website;

- describe how to turn inquiries into firm appointments;

- explain how to prepare for your first meeting with prospective buyers and how to qualify these prospective buyers regarding needs, motivation, and financial ability;

- describe how to reduce security risks; and

- describe how to use qualifying information in selecting homes to view and understand that qualifying is an ongoing process.

KEY TERMS

back-end ratio	front-end ratio	open-end questions
closed-end questions	LTV	prequalify
floor time	negative motivation	

THE APPOINTMENT

Your initial buyer contact from advertising generally takes the form of a telephone call. Prospective buyers generally call about ads, For Sale signs, or your website picture and description, rather than coming to your office for general information. Your goal regarding the call is not to sell the property—no one *buys* property over the telephone. Your goal is to turn that call into an appointment so you can be in a position in which a sale is possible.

A call is a valuable commodity. A telephone inquiry from which you fail to obtain an appointment or, at the very least, the caller's name and telephone number is a total loss of overhead dollars. If you were to compute all office overhead, including advertising, and divide that monthly figure by the number of telephone inquiries your office receives in the month, you would understand how much it really costs to bring in each inquiry. Wasting a telephone inquiry might well be equivalent to throwing $100 or $200 into the wind. Good telephone technique reduces the percentage of wasted calls.

Many offices have designated periods of **floor time**, or *opportunity time*, where agents are given inquiries in rotation. If you have floor time, be prepared to turn telephone inquiries into appointments.

Telephone inquiries are not limited to office hours and floor time. Calls can be at all hours and on home phones and personal cell phones. In addition, you will receive inquiries by email and fax messages.

Prepare to Receive Telephone Calls

You should be prepared to field inquiries at all times. Have copies of both your own current ads and your office ads from the prior weekend, as well as all office listings, so that they are readily accessible. Make notations on ads so you know what property each ad refers to. Review the listings so the information is fresh in your mind. Also, consider likely **switch property** priced up to 20% more or less than advertised properties. In the event you reveal some feature that "turns off" the person inquiring, you need something at hand to switch to.

Have a map of your community readily available with numbered adhesive markers referencing all your office listings. If you have wall space near your desk, this is an excellent place for this map, but you also want one to carry with you. This map is essential because callers on For Sale signs often have the wrong street but usually the right general area. Consider switch property for sign inquiries. As a general rule, you know that callers on For Sale signs

- like or would be satisfied with the area, and

- like or would be satisfied with the appearance of a home with a similar exterior.

Handling the Inquiry

Switch properties are other properties that a caller about a particular property is likely to be interested in.

People calling about ads usually buy property other than the property they initially inquired about. The same is true for calls prompted by For Sale signs. This is why it is important to know your inventory. You will be able to readily switch your discussion to appropriate properties as necessary. For this reason, as you begin your real estate career, it would be wise to spend time each day physically visiting properties for sale and studying the available inventory.

People who call in reference to a sign might not tell you that a price you have quoted is beyond their means. In fact, they might even ask for more information. However, you won't know this unless you mention a switch property priced significantly less than the property called about. If the callers show interest in the switch property, the original property that they called about may be too expensive. As to switch properties, keep in mind that while callers on For Sale signs are often looking beyond their means, callers on priced ads are often hoping to buy a property that is less than they can afford to pay.

If a caller has viewed the property on the internet, you know that the caller likes the appearance of the property and the description seems to "fit" her needs. You also know that the property is priced within the range the caller expects to pay and that the property's location and address are satisfactory. Prospects who call about an internet posting are more likely to buy the property they are interested in than are prospects calling from other advertising. An internet inquiry is, therefore, a valuable inquiry because the callers have half-sold themselves on the property.

The following are some general rules about dealing with telephone inquiries from prospective buyers:

- Obtain the caller's name and telephone number

- Ask questions about family size and needs

- Find out what interested them about the ad

- Find out what the prospective buyer is interested in and why

- Find out if the caller has been prequalified or approved for a loan and for how much

- Hold the details—give a little more information than was in the ad. The less information given, the greater the chance of ending the telephone call with an appointment.

- Answer home elimination questions with a question. For example, if a caller asks, "Does that house have three bedrooms plus a den?" your answer should be "[Mrs. Jones], do you need three bedrooms plus a den?" If the caller asks the price, you should ask, "What price range were you interested in?" If the questioning reveals complete unsuitability of the property, you should be able to switch to a similar property that has the required features.

- Close on an appointment. The choice given should be what time, not whether the caller wants to see the property.

- Set the place for the meeting. There are only two places for an initial meeting with a potential buyer:

  1. At your office (preferred)

  2. At the buyer's home

(You may meet a prospective buyer at a property that the buyer wishes to purchase after having successfully preapproved them with a lender.)

- Include mention of other property that may interest the prospects. This will help reduce the likelihood of a no-show.

- Keep the call short and end the call after the appointment is set.

For an internet inquiry, because the caller generally wants to see the property, there should be no difficulty setting up the appointment.

Lovely 3BR, 2-bath ranch home
in Willow Springs.
Reduced to $389,500.
Owner financing available.

Oasis Realty   760-976-4132

www.oasispropertytour.com

A suggested approach to calls on the ad shown is as follows:

My name is Howard Young. What is your name, please?

Note: If the ad indicated a web address, you want to know if the caller viewed the property on the internet. If the caller has, treat the call like gold because the caller is already half-sold on the property.

Yes, that is a lovely three-bedroom home, Mrs. Jones. How large is your family, [Mr./Mrs.] Jones?

That home is in one of the nicer areas of Willow Springs. Is that the area you are interested in?

Are there any other areas that you are considering?

That home is priced at $389,500. Is that the general price range you are interested in?

I can arrange to show this lovely home as well as another home that I think will interest you 5:00 pm today, or would 6:00 pm be more convenient for you?

Notice that the choice is the time, not whether they want to see the property. If your prospective caller indicates neither time is convenient, ask when it would be convenient to show the property.

If the caller indicates he is not free at all that day, say:

Let's set it up for tomorrow at 5:00 pm. I'll meet you and your spouse at my office. Our office is on the corner of Third Street and Lake Boulevard. You can't miss our orange sign.

Have you been prequalified for a loan? (If yes, "For how much?")

(If not), If you could come 15 minutes early, I can get you prequalified so in the event you wish to buy a home, the seller will be more likely to accept any offer you make. Can you come a little early?

If the caller doesn't object, you have a definite appointment. Whenever you have an appointment for the next day, call the prospects in the morning of that day to remind them of the appointment. When you call, be enthusiastic and tell them you have another property you feel they also will be interested in. This will reduce the no-shows. Never indicate you have another property if you don't have one.

| Get more information from the caller than you give. |

As you see, asking questions gives you control of the conversation. You get an appointment without giving out too much information and without undue delay and you have set the mood for buying not just looking.

By mentioning another house to Mr. or Mrs. Jones, you probably aroused some interest and set the stage for alternative properties, if necessary. Now say:

I will see you and [Mr./Mrs.] Jones at my office at 6:00 pm. Do you have a pencil and paper handy? Our office is at [1911 Elm Street across from the Security Bank]. Are you familiar with the area? [If not, give specific directions.] Again, my name is Howard Young. I look forward to seeing you.

Your question is about the caller's knowledge of your office location, not where you will meet the caller. You are telling, not asking for, the place of the meeting.

You can see from this sample script that the agent didn't really give information beyond what was in the ad. Instead, the agent asked for information. The call was kept very short and was ended as soon as an appointment had been set.

As we have stated, there are only two places to meet a prospective buyer for the first time. These are at the buyer's home or in the agent's office. Some agents like to visit the buyer's home to get a better insight into the buyer's lifestyle and needs, but the agent's office allows for an uninterrupted qualifying process controlled by the agent. If you are to meet the prospects at their residence, you should let someone in your office know where you are going and whom you are to meet. For safety reasons, you can also check if that person is a resident at that address. You can go to www.msn.intelius.com and click on "Reverse Lookup." Enter the address to get the occupants' names. If you must meet prospective buyers at their homes, you should complete the buyer financial qualifying process before you discuss properties. With wireless access to your MLS, you can go directly from the prospect's home to properties.

Getting a Caller's Name

In some offices, telephone calls are answered by a receptionist, who usually will get a caller's name for you. At times callers will, for one reason or another, resist giving their names. You will also encounter calls where caller ID is blocked. If there is resistance to giving a name, don't make an issue of it because there are a number of simple techniques you can use to get callers' names.

> Let me put you on hold while I get some information that should interest you. In case we get disconnected, what is your telephone number so I can call you back?

If you get the telephone number, there should be no caller hesitancy in proving a name.

If the call results in an appointment, try the following:

> In the unlikely event I get tied up for some reason, what is your home number so I can call you to reset the appointment?

Even though you may have the caller's name and number with your caller ID, you want the caller to give you the number. Callers who give you their number will probably also give their name if asked.

Another effective way to get callers' names owes its effectiveness to the fact that it is nonthreatening:

> I have a flyer with a photo of that property, as well as information on several other properties, one in particular that I feel you will be interested in. Would it be all right if I prepared a packet of information and put it in the mail or emailed it to you?

If you offer sincere, knowledgeable assistance, this nonthreatening approach of mailing the information will result in a positive response in 90% of cases in which prospects initially hesitate to give a name. Callers must now give you a name and an address or email address. Also ask if they would like to receive email alerts as to new listings as soon as they come on the market. Once you have prospects' names, they will provide the other information you need.

If you have not been able to obtain an appointment, the following approach can be very effective in keeping communications open:

> I email pictures and details of new listings to prospective buyers who request them. These are sent out before the property is advertised. Are you interested in being alerted to new listings and having first chance?

Not every contact is a good contact. Reluctance to give a name is often a signal that the caller is not a serious buyer, but it could also mean that the caller is afraid of being harassed by overzealous salespeople. The call could be for information not related to buying, such as a call from a curious neighbor. Your greatest efforts should be directed toward callers who are open as to identity and needs rather than those who are secretive. Your maximum efforts should be directed toward probabilities rather than remote possibilities.

"I Just Want the Address"

You will have callers who haven't used the internet and want the address of the property so they can drive by for a quick look. Generally, the caller wants an exterior look to either eliminate the property from consideration or make a decision to view it. Unfortunately, a drive-by might eliminate you as well as the property from the caller's consideration. As a response to such a request, consider:

> Let me send you some interior photos of the house and back garden. The street view alone doesn't do it justice. What is your email address?

If you are unable to get an appointment with callers and they still want the property address, it is good policy to get the callers' name and telephone number before giving out the address. This is very important because should prospective buyers not be particularly interested in the property from a drive-by look, they would be lost to you for future contact. However, if you have a name and telephone number, you can encourage prospects to drive by the property and also note any other properties nearby with For Sale signs that appear interesting. Let the callers know you will call them back for their impressions of the property and to obtain information for them on other properties that appeared desirable.

Technology and Caller Data

Technology has gone beyond caller ID where you only have the name and number of a caller. It is now possible to know where the caller lives, family size, and even financial data. This information is now available, not just for the calls you answer but also for calls that were unanswered because your line was busy or prospects called and failed to leave a message. If you desire information on such services, one service provider is *www.callsource.com*.

Locking In the Caller

When callers are motivated buyers, there is a good likelihood that they will continue looking through ads, as well as websites, and will contact other agents. You can't do anything about calls made before prospective buyers called you, but it is relatively easy for you to keep them off the phone.

> [Mrs. Smith], if you have the time, I would appreciate it if you could check our website at www.palmspringshomes.com and the classified ads and note any other properties that interest you. Bring the website information and the paper with you when we meet at [4 pm today], and I'll be able to give you information on other properties. Perhaps you might want to see one or more of them. By having you check what interests you, I can also learn a great deal about what you desire and will be able to find the home you will want to own.

This keeps the possible buyer off the phone. It might possibly give you other property to show and provide information on the buyer's desires.

Email Contacts

If you receive an email contact about a property on the web, you will likely also get a name, which allows you to call rather than email your response. It is easier to set up an appointment when in direct phone contact than it is by email. Contacts about a particular property shown on your website should be treated like gold. Be prepared to close on an appointment to show the property.

Can't Get an Appointment

If you can't turn a call into an appointment, use it to set the stage for further contact.

> Would it be all right if I called you should a property be listed that [has five bedrooms and is priced under $300,000]?

This approach will generally result in a positive response and a name and telephone number if you have otherwise been unable to obtain this information.

After the appointment—keep the prospect off the phone.

Similarly, you could ask:

> Would it be all right if I emailed you some information on other properties that I think might interest you?

This nonthreatening approach is likely to receive a positive response.

You should also ask the caller if it would be all right to add them to an email alert system through the MLS that will send them automated information of any new listings that you feel might interest the caller. It's a nonthreatening approach, and you now have a reason to call to discuss any email property you presented. Of course, you should again try to set up an appointment.

Internet Leads

When the buyers' inquiry is from an ad they saw online, they may or may not be serious about purchasing the given property. Previously many real estate brokers and agents would believe that internet leads were worthless, because they didn't take the time to pick up the phone and make an actual call. However, perspective has now shifted as most buyers start their home search online and it is quite common practice for an interested party to make initial contact electronically rather than with a phone call. Therefore, these leads should be taken seriously as well.

The same rules apply with regard to internet leads as they apply to other leads. Here are some best practices with regard to handling internet inquiries:

1. Responsiveness is mandatory. In the age of instantaneous information, your prospects are used to getting fast responses to their inquiries. The buyer is probably surfing around many different websites, and often the most responsive agent is the one that will win.

2. Continuous follow-up is critical with web inquiries. Your prospects are not only on your website. They are visiting the sites of all your competitors too. Couple this with the fact that web inquiries are often long sales cycles, follow-up is mandatory.

3. These buyers should be set up through an automatic drip system in the MLS. Most MLS systems are going to have a mechanism wherein the agent can input the criteria of the buyers and the system will automatically email them listings that match their search. This allows the agent to leverage the technology in the MLS without actually having to pull manual searches each day.

THE MEETING

Your Safety

Unfortunately, personal safety has become an issue in recent years. Agents have been attacked by people posing as "buyers." To reduce jeopardizing your personal safety, meet prospective buyers at your office whenever possible. People who have anything on their minds other than a purchase will generally not want to show themselves to other people. After they come to your office and undergo a qualifying process, the likelihood of a safety problem will be significantly reduced.

Some agents ask to see photo identification to make certain the person is who he claims to be.

Some agents like to introduce prospects to other agents or their broker, as potential troublemakers won't risk being exposed. Other safety precautions include notifying your office or voice mail of a change in a showing schedule, always leaving the front door of a dwelling unlocked during the showing, and having the prospect walk ahead of you. If you must meet a prospect for the first time at a property, you want to make certain an owner, tenant, or another agent from your office will be present.

Always let someone know where you are going. Some offices have a code. As an example, an agent could call an office and say, "Could you check the red file on 1250 North Main Street? I'm there now." The words "red file" could be an alert for agents who feel they are in trouble.

Consider making yourself less attractive as a victim. Avoid ostentatious jewelry; a Gucci bag and/or Rolex watch may be signs of success, but they could also make you a target of opportunity. Stiletto heels or cowboy boots may be fashionable, but they inhibit your ability to move quickly when required.

Many agents now carry pepper spray or electronic devices that emit a loud piercing noise. A loud whistle can also be used.

Avoid parking in the driveway of the property you are showing. Besides showing disrespect for the property, you place yourself in a position where your car can be blocked in case of an emergency.

Never drive to a property in a client's vehicle. If the client insists on driving, take two vehicles.

Some agents take photos of clients and vehicles showing license plate numbers and email the photos to their office.

You lessen your personal danger by telling the prospect that someone else from your office will be arriving shortly.

Safety Issues

Many times, the excitement of getting new clients and meeting them overshadows thoughts of individual safety.

Best practices surrounding safety.   Salespeople should be encouraged to do the following:

1. Require 100% of all potential buyers to be preapproved by a lender before scheduling a tour. Remind your buyer that in the vast majority of cases, the preapproval process is done at no cost or obligation.

2. Always keep your customer in sight while on tour.

3. Let your office manager, receptionist, or another agent know where you are going to be and who you are going to show property to.

4. Have a plan of exit if you feel unsafe in any way.

Brokers should be able to add to the above based on local custom to tailor their own safety program for their sales staff.

Prepare to Meet the Prospective Buyer

Before you meet your prospective buyers for the first time, think through the qualifying process. You also might want to make some tentative appointments to show specific properties.

Schedule your first meeting with a prospective buyer at your office.

Because the qualifying process often reveals that properties inquired about do not really meet the needs, resources, or both of the prospective buyers, you want the owners to understand that the appointments are only tentative at this time and may need to be canceled or postponed.

Make certain you have a "qualifying room," free and clean, with fresh coffee or soft drinks available. We suggest you qualify prospective buyers in a separate office or closing room. This reduces distractions and provides a chance to learn about the prospects without interruption.

First Impressions

When you meet with prospective buyers, make a mental point of remembering their names. By repeating their last name several times to yourself and thinking of people you know with the same first names, you won't have to ask the buyers their names when writing an offer to purchase.

Make certain you are pronouncing names correctly. If you are uncertain, ask. Because people like to be addressed by their names, use them frequently during the discussions. Explain that you will be able to save the prospective buyers a great deal of time by spending just a few minutes to decide what they really need in a home. Serve bottles of water or large cups of hot or iced coffee (or tea). Seat the clients close to you during your qualifying session because it gives you more control.

Needs and Interests

Keep in mind that the primary purpose of this meeting is for you to gain information. When you are talking, it should usually involve asking a question. People like people who are interested in them, and chances are they're not really interested in you. Their interest is in what you can do for them. To communicate effectively, you must ask **open-end questions** that require explanations and reasons rather than **closed-end questions** that can be answered with a simple "yes" or "no" but fail to inform you as to why. Ask about hobbies, special interests and pets. You could be wasting time in showing a house with a small backyard if the prospects own two Great Danes. Keep in mind that the only dumb question is the one you failed to ask.

Some agents use the FORD acronym as a guide to learning about their prospects:

- Family

- Occupation

- Recreation

- Dreams

Many agents use a qualification form so they won't forget the information prospective buyers give them. The use of a form also reduces the chances of forgetting to obtain some needed information. Figure 9.1 is an example of a form you might consider using. You can also put the information directly into your contact management system.

FIGURE 9.1: **Prospective Buyer Confidential Information Sheet**

Prospective Buyer Confidential Information Sheet

Name(s) _____ Phone no. _____

Fax no. _____ E-mail _____

Address _____

Size of family _____

Names and ages of children or other dependents living with you: _____
_____
_____

Pets _____

Initial contact with the firm was because of (advertisement, Web sites, sign, referral, etc.)
_____

Present address _____

How long at above address? _____

Do you presently own your own home? _____

If yes, must you sell before you buy? _____

If yes, is your present home currently listed for sale? _____

With _____

How long has it been on the market? _____

Your reason for seeking to buy a new home _____

What features do you like about your present home? _____

What features don't you like about your present home? _____

Why? _____

What feature(s) do you consider to be most important for your new home? _____
_____

Why? _____
_____
_____

What are your hobbies or special interests? _____
_____
_____
_____

Have you qualified for or been turned down for a home loan within the past year? _____
_____

If you qualified for a loan, what was the name of the firm and loan amount? _____
_____

How soon would you like to be in your new home? _____

Buyer Qualifying Process

The qualifying process is really a three-part process involving the following:

1. Needs and interests of the buyers
2. Buyers' motivation
3. Preapproval by an institutional lender

The form tells you the needs of buyers, as well as why they are buyers. Keep in mind that qualifying buyers is a continuing process leading right up to receiving an offer. By asking for reactions to homes shown, you gain insight into what prospective buyers really want. The reality could be far different from what a buyer claims to want. Your contact management systems should not only include the information you obtain about prospect needs and interests but also indicate the properties they have seen and their reactions to the showings.

A simple buyers-needs evaluation can be made by just having the buyers list the 10 most important features they want in their new home. Then have them rate the features in order of importance. This rating will help you in choosing homes to show, as well as in obtaining a purchase offer.

Financial qualifying.   You should know FHA and VA loan limits and down payment requirements if your prospective buyers are likely to be eligible for these types of financing. You also should know down payment requirements for various types of loans.

> You should have an in-depth understanding of current qualifying ratios being used by lenders in your area. You should also understand how the FHA and VA qualify purchasers.

Lenders use the terms *front-end* and *back-end ratios*. **Front-end ratio** customarily refers to the ratio of a buyer's housing costs to income. Generally, gross income is used for front-end qualifying. For many institutional lenders, the front-end ratio is 28%, which means the *buyers' total monthly housing costs (principal, interest, taxes, and insurance [PITI]) cannot exceed 28% of their gross income.*

total monthly payment ÷ gross monthly income = 28% or less

A person's total housing expense plus long-term debt obligations cannot exceed 36% of gross income (**back-end ratio**).

PITI + total monthly credit obligations ÷ gross monthly income
= 36% or less

Qualifying ratios will be covered in more detail in Unit 12.

Down payment requirements vary by the lender and type of loan. Lenders express the loan-to-value ratio by the acronym **LTV**. If the borrower pays for private mortgage insurance, the down payments requirement may be reduced.

Self-employed individuals frequently have difficulty qualifying for loans. Lenders often require that self-employed buyers furnish two years of tax returns with their loan applications. Although buyers may indicate to you or the lender that they make X dollars a year, the tax returns may reveal a very different financial profile. Self-employed buyers may have to consider homes for which seller financing is available, make a larger down payment, or be willing to pay a higher interest rate from a subprime lender.

The maximum loan for which they can qualify plus their down payment sets the maximum limit on housing that prospective buyers can purchase. Further details on financial qualification of buyers are included in Unit 12. Keep in mind that qualification ratios are not rigid. Lenders will make loans to individuals failing to meet qualification tactics when the type of loan, down payment, or interest rate is considered more favorable to the lender.

We recommend that you **prequalify** buyers or obtain lender preapproval whenever possible before you show properties. Failure to prequalify prospective buyers could result in showing the prospects homes they cannot afford. Besides resulting in wasted effort, it becomes difficult to sell the prospects less costly housing later.

By completing a prequalification online, you can get approval for a loan amount based on verification of given information.

You should be sending prequalification lending information to a lender you recommend before you leave your office to show a property. If you don't get an immediate answer, this is a reason for the prospective buyers to come back to your office after the showing. Also, by prequalifying a buyer, you have changed the buyers' attitude from looking to buying. Prequalifying buyers also reduces the likelihood that they will seek out other agents. Prequalifying buyers can make them your customers.

Start the lender financial qualification process before you leave to show homes to customers.

Should prospective buyers be reluctant to give financial information to you, have the prospects complete the computer loan qualification process themselves. They will be less reticent when providing the information directly to the lender.

Actual lender approval is based on more than income and expenses. Their credit score (FICO score) will determine if they will be given a loan, as well as the interest rate and down payment requirements.

Because of the mortgage crisis and its great many defaults, lenders are reluctant to lend to persons with any blemishes on their credit. You might have to consider lower-price homes so that the down payment available will be a larger percentage of the purchase price. Another possibility would be a lease option in which the buyers are lessees until they have enough equity to obtain financing.

If you handle the qualifying process in a professional manner, you will be setting the stage for the buyers to regard you as a professional and a person they can relate to. (Another advantage of financial qualifying is that you tend to eliminate "Lookie Lous.")

After the buyers' financial qualifying, it might become apparent that what the buyers indicate they need may not be possible based upon financial restrictions. Keep in mind what a buyer expresses as a need may be only a "want." The agent must not mislead buyers into believing they can fulfil a wish list when it is clearly not possible because of financial restrictions. Referring to property as a "starter home" allows buyers to keep their perfect dream home alive but postpone it for the future.

As an alternative, you can point out that you will show property with the potential of fulfilling the buyers' wishes through repair, renovation, or future expansion. Explain that their aspirations are within reach if they are able to visualize what a property can become.

Preparing the Buyer

During the financial qualification process, you discussed the down payment. Before you show property, you should discuss earnest money. Earnest money deposits are made with offers. Prospective buyers should understand that their check will be held uncashed until their offer is accepted. Ask a question that makes the prospective buyers visualize writing a check, such as the following:

> If we are fortunate and find the perfect home for you today, would you be able to make a deposit of [$] with your offer? Should we find the home that meets your needs, is there anything that would stop you from making a decision today?"

It is better to know about possible problems as soon as possible so that you can prepare to deal with them. It also lets the prospects anticipate buying rather than just looking.

Give prospective buyers a copy of the purchase contract your office uses before you leave the office. Ask them to look the form over at their convenience and explain that when you succeed in finding them a home they wish to purchase, this will be the form used. Buyers who receive the form up front are less likely to object to the form later, and signing it will be an easier task.

What Happens to the Buyers' Offer?

Buyers should understand that three things can happen when they make an offer:

1. Acceptance means that they have purchased a home.
2. A counteroffer from the owners gives the buyers the opportunity to accept it (and have the house), make their own counter to the counteroffer, or reject it.
3. Rejection of the offer means the entire earnest money deposit is returned to the offerors.

If you approach the qualifying process in an organized fashion, you should be able to start looking at homes less than an hour from the time prospective buyers arrive at your office.

Be certain to explain agencies and have your prospective buyers sign the agency form. (See Unit 3.) You should explain your disclosure obligations, as well as disclosures of the owner when buyers find a home that meets their needs.

You may decide that you can best serve your prospective buyer as a buyer's agent. If this is the case, you should discuss the benefits of exclusive buyer representation with your prospective buyers and obtain a buyer listing.

Planning Your Efforts

From your qualifying questions, you will have determined why the prospective buyers want to buy and if they can buy now. If they must sell a home first to become buyers, discuss an offer contingent on the sale of their own home should they find a house that meets their needs. If your prospects want to sell before they place an offer, you should still spend some time with them to whet their appetites for a new home. An advisable approach would be one showing session plus frequent phone calls about the progress of their own home sale and emails on new listings that you feel would be of interest.

If you know about a person's special interests, you can use this information in selecting homes for showing. As an example, if a prospective buyer has indicates a strong interest in physical fitness, showing a house with a room that is used or could be used as a workout room would be a wise choice.

When the author first began in real estate sales, he showed a listing sight unseen. The prospective buyers, a well-dressed couple with a young daughter, stopped at the office after seeing an ad that indicated the home was located on a large wooded lot, and that it had seven rooms and a large garage-workshop. Because it was located in an excellent area, the potential buyers wanted to know if the listed price of the property, which was low, was a mistake. This untrained agent did everything wrong. He failed to get any qualifying information from the prospective buyers and was off to show a property he knew nothing about other than by reading a few lines on the office listing. Before he showed the property, one of the other agents told him, "It's a dog. You'll never sell it!"

However, he discovered that the home was an old farmhouse with imitation brick, roll-asphalt siding, and the garage was a large machine shed/barn with a dirt floor. The pine floors in the house were covered with linoleum. There were no closets in the bedrooms, and because the house had been vacant for a long time, there was a very unpleasant odor throughout the place.

He asked the prospective buyers what they thought of the home. The response was, "It definitely has possibilities." Fifteen minutes later they signed an offer and within a month had moved into their new home. Because the father was a disabled veteran, this was the only home they could afford in this desirable school district. It was the answer to their dreams, but to other agents it was a dog. If this agent had previously viewed the property and understood the needs and abilities of the buyers, he would have realized the perfect match. There was nothing wrong with the property; it simply needed to be matched with the right buyers. You should not substitute what *you* want for what *others* might want.

In selling, the ability to be a good listener is even more important than the ability to be a good talker. Unfortunately, many people have poor listening skills and pretend to listen, but do not hear. To add to the problem, the human mind can take in and process around 500 words a minute, yet we speak at a rate of only about 100 to 150 words a minute. The difference makes it easy to be distracted and allow your mind to wander. Practice active listening so you will be sure to hear words that are relevant to the customer's needs, problems, and solutions.

A good listener listens actively by reinforcing the speaker with words of understanding, repeating what was said (especially when objections arise), and nodding or making some show of approval.

Silence also is an excellent tool; when in doubt, the best solution is to keep silent. Discreet silence at the right time often shows an excellent command of the language. Also, active listeners do not interrupt or formulate a response when the speaker is talking.

Remember to Listen

Remember, you will not make sales by winning arguments. Speakers need the opportunity to make known their points and voice their feelings of doubt or displeasure. Listen with your eyes, as well as with your ears. Keep a relaxed tone while speaking, and mean what you say. When you are finished, stop.

In selecting property for showing, first consider properties from the internet that the prospective buyers have shown interest in. These properties can be half sold. If the buyers feel they discovered a property, the likelihood of a purchase is enhanced.

Agents must be careful to listen to buyers and choose properties for showing according to wishes and interests shown and not to substitute what the agent likes for what buyers express interest in.

Showing property priced significantly higher than the limits set by buyers when you don't fully realize their financial situation could be a disaster. You could sell buyers on a property or features they cannot obtain.

California is a more mobile society, so neighborhood is less important than in many Eastern communities where family and friends have been located within a small area for generations. When buyers insist on a designated area and their "want" list cannot be met based on their financial ability, consider first showing property within the area and then what a move outside the designated perimeter can achieve as to what they want in a home.

Chinese Buyers

There has been a significant influx of buyers from China. These buyers have been purchasing upscale homes, usually for cash, in prestigious locations.

There are an estimated 2.5 million Chinese millionaires. Many are now seeking a safe place for their wealth, as well as a place for family safety and educational opportunities. A U.S. visa program (EB-5) allows wealthy aliens to obtain permanent residency in the United States if they invest $500,000 to $1 million in a U.S. investment that will create at least 10 jobs. The visa covers the investor's spouse as well as children under age 21. Some 80% of the EB-5 visas have been going to mainland China. China has topped Canada in home purchase dollars. According to the National Association of Realtors®, Chinese buyers purchased $28.6 billion in U.S. real estate in the 12 months preceding March 2015. It is believed that approximately half of this investment has been in California, primarily in the greater Los Angeles area, San Francisco, and San Diego. Buyers have been seeking areas with substantial Chinese populations. Irvine, California, in Orange County has become a mecca for many Chinese buyers. Some subdivisions have reported over 50% of sales to Chinese nationals.

Real estate agents should strive to understand the culture of diverse groups. Chinse buyers often rely heavily on opinions of friends and family members and may wish to consult with them before making a decision. A great many Chinese pay attention to feng shui in home purchase decisions. What you may consider the perfect home for a Chines family could be rejected because of bad feng shui.

Feng Shui

Feng shui (pronounced fung shway) translates as "wind-water" in English. It is an ancient Chinese practice to orient the energy of a dwelling. It positions objects and structure design for the favorable flow of chi, which is life force for good fortune.

Where a sale to a Chinese national is likely, some agents bring in a feng shui practitioner for an evaluation and hopeful approval. Fees for this service range from under $200 to around $400 depending on area and home size.

Feng shui consultants will offer solutions to correct problems with energy flow. Sometimes a solution can be simple for a property, but at times, the problem can be so severe that many Chinse buyers would not consider the property.

Some problem areas include the following:

- A backyard sloping down, which will take energy away from the house. It can be alleviated with a retaining wall to stop the downward energy flow.

- A T-junction house is considered bad feng shui because the chi coming directly down the road to the house is too aggressive and negatively affects the house.

- A south-facing unit is most preferred and east-facing is considered a bad omen although east-facing windows can create good energy.

- A clean line of sight from the front door to the back door allows good luck to come in and go right out. Minor alterations might solve the problem.

- A front door leading directly to a stairway will allow good energy to flow up or down the stairs to the detriment of the main floor.

- The front door must open inward, not outward which would push away positive energy.

- Trees and shrubs should not block the view of the front door because they would also block energy.

- Sharp corners emit negative energy.

- The bathroom door should not be close to the front door.

- Rooms should be clutter free because clutter resists the flow of positive energy (model homes).

- Work areas (home offices) should be separate from living areas.

- Plants, flowers, and water features are positive energy.

Colors are important to many Chinese buyers. Green is positive because it denotes nature. Yellow equals power, and red and purple are considered lucky.

Numbers are very important to many Chinese. Number 8 is the luckiest of Chinese numbers, while 4 and 14, 5 and 6 are to be avoided. The number 4 is unlucky because it is pronounced similarly to the Chinese word for death (sîwáng).

To avoid the number 4, some agents will set a price, such as $388,888, and a separate price for furnishings, such as $88,888.

Street addresses are also important. Favorable addresses should be emphasized in advertising and in showings.

A basic understanding of feng shui will enable an agent to select homes for showing to Chinese buyers, as well as to consider how to counter possible problem areas.

Prospecting the China Market

China has a number of important home shows that feature foreign property. Beijing luxury property shows brought more than 5,200 wealthy Chinese to view international properties. A number of U.S. brokers have set up elaborate booths at the show. Foreign sellers indicate that setting up a booth at one of many property shows costs from $30,000 to $150,000. Brokers usually represent a new home development or a large condo development with many vacancies. Some brokers travel to China to sell business opportunities to allow Chinese families to obtain a visa. Others enter arrangements with Chinese real estate firms to locate buyers for business opportunities or luxury homes.

There are a number of Chinese real estate websites, some for foreign property. Juwai.com is a global property portal with 2.4 million properties listed in 58 countries.

PROPERTY TOUR PRESENTATION PACKAGE

WEB LINK

Just as presentation material can increase the effectiveness of a listing presentation, presentation material can make showings more effective. Material prepared for a buyer makes it easy for the buyer to evaluate and compare offerings and can lead to a natural closing. When you understand the buyer's needs and have prequalified the buyer, a property presentation package should be considered. Figures 9.2A–9.2J from Realty Tools, Inc. (www.realtytools.com) show a sample buyer tour presentation package. You will note that each property presented includes property details, photographs, a map, and space for viewer's comments. The property comparison sheet shows what the buyers have indicated they are seeking.

THE SHOWING

Preparing to Show

To show property to prospective buyers intelligently, you must make adequate preparation:

- Know all available properties in the area

- Be able to identify school boundaries

- Be cognizant of shopping and recreational facilities in the area

- Be aware of public transportation routes

- Be aware of any other information about the area that might help prospects make a favorable decision

FIGURES 9.2A – 9.2J: **Property Tour Presentation Package**

Property Tour

Prepared Especially for:
Tom & Mary White
7 Deep Run Court
Hunt Valley, MD 21030

Prepared by:
Angela McKendrick, CRS, GRI
Agent
Green Leaf Realty
123 Main Street
Hunt Valley, MD 21030

Office: 410-555-1234
Home Office: 410-432-7890
Fax: 410-555-5607
Web Site: www.demorealty.com/angela
Email: angela.mckendrick@demorealty.com

Date: August 20, 2015

Green Leaf Realty
www.greenleafrealty.com

A.

Home Finders' Profile for

Tom & Mary White

You have identified the following criteria to aid us in the search for your new home. Please review this information and notify Angela McKendrick immediately if there are any changes.

City:	Hunt Valley	*Neighborhood:*	Laurelford
Year Built:	1988	*Fin SqFt:*	5384
Lot Desc:	Backs To Trees	*Lot Size:*	1.04
Style:	Colonial	*Levels:*	3
Bedrooms:	4	*Bathrooms:*	3/1
Const:	Cedar Siding	*Roofing:*	Cedar/Shake
Basement:	Fully Finished	*Basement:*	Walkout Level
Heat:	Heat Pump	*Fuel:*	Electric
Cool:	Central A/C	*Parking:*	Garage
Garage Spaces:	2	*Exter Feat:*	Deck
Water:	Well	*Sewer:*	Septic
# Fireplaces:	2	*Amenities:*	Auto Gar Dr Opn
Amenities:	Built-In Bookcases	*Amenities:*	Mba/Sep Shwr
Other Rms:	Den/Stdy/Lib	*Other Rms:*	Family Room

Angela McKendrick, CRS, GRI
Office: 410-555-1234
Home Office: 410-432-7890
Fax: 410-555-5607
Web Site: www.demorealty.com/angela
Email: angela.mckendrick@demorealty.com

Green Leaf Realty
www.greenleafrealty.com

B.

Presenting

Features Include:

City: Hunt Valley
Neighborhood: Shawan
Year Built: 1995
Fin SqFt: 5684
Lot Desc: Cul-De-Sac
Lot Size: 3.05 Acres
Style: Colonial
Levels: 2
Bedrooms: 4
Bathrooms: 3/1
Const: Brick
Roofing: Shingle-Asphalt
Basement: Full
Basement: Unfinished
Heat: Forced Air
Fuel: Gas Heated
Cool: Zoned
Parking: Garage
Garage Spaces: 2
Exter Feat: Deck
Water: Well

9 Jules Brentony
$898,900

Gorgeous Brick Home with Plenty of Amenities. Great Neighborhood. Short Drive to City.

Comments: _____
_____
_____
_____
_____
_____
_____
_____

Angela McKendrick, CRS, GRI
Office: 410-555-1234
Home Office: 410-432-7890
Fax: 410-555-5607
Web Site: www.demorealty.com/angela
Email: angela.mckendrick@demorealty.com

Green Leaf Realty
www.greenleafrealty.com

C.

Presenting

Features Include:

City: Cockeysville
Neighborhood: Laurelford
Year Built: 2008
Fin SqFt: 5484
Lot Desc: Backs To Trees
Lot Size: 1.14 Acres
Style: Modern
Levels: 3
Bedrooms: 4
Bathrooms: 3/1
Const: Cedar Siding
Roofing: Cedar/Shake
Basement: Finished
Basement: Walkout Level
Heat: Heat Pump
Fuel: Electric
Cool: Central Air
Parking: 2-Car Garage
Garage Spaces: 2
Exter Feat: Deck
Water: Well

2 Symphony Cir
$789,000

Gorgeous home available for move in immediately! Inground Pool in back of house, Fabulous Master Bedroom, Spacious Rooms."

Comments: _____
_____
_____
_____
_____
_____
_____
_____

Angela McKendrick, CRS, GRI
Office: 410-555-1234
Home Office: 410-432-7890
Fax: 410-555-5607
Web Site: www.demorealty.com/angela
Email: angela.mckendrick@demorealty.com

Green Leaf Realty
www.greenleafrealty.com

D.

FIGURES 9.2A – 9.2J (continued):   Property Tour Presentation Package

Presenting

Features Include:

20 Laurelford Ct
$892,000

City: Cockeysville
Neighborhood: Laurelford
Year Built: 1992
Fin SqFt: 5800
Lot Desc: Backs To Trees
Lot Size: 9 Acres
Style: Colonial
Levels: 3
Bedrooms: 4
Bathrooms: 2/1
Const: Vinyl
Roofing: Shingle
Basement: Full
Basement: Finished
Heat: Forced Air
Fuel: Electric
Cool: Central A/C
Parking: Garage
Garage Spaces: 2
Exter Feat: Balcony
Water: Well

FULLY FINISHED WALK-OUT BASEMENT WITH REC ROOM (30X23), GUEST BEDROOM (18X17), FULL BATH & WINDOWS. THIS IS A FULL BASEMENT. 9 ACRES OF BEAUTIFUL GROUNDS, PARK-SETTING. UPPER 2ND LEVEL HAS 2 ROOMS (20X11 & 20X24) FULLY FINISHED. APPROX. 6,000 FINISHED SQUARE FEET. UNIQUE AND DISTINCTIVE."

Comments: _____

Angela McKendrick, CRS, GRI
Office: 410-555-1234
Home Office: 410-432-7890
Fax: 410-555-5607
Web Site: www.demorealty.com/angela
Email: angela.mckendrick@demorealty.com

Green Leaf Realty
www.greenleafrealty.com

E.

Presenting

Features Include:

13213 Beaver Dam Rd
$849,900

City: Cockeysville
Neighborhood: Ivy Hill
Year Built: 1984
Fin SqFt: 4090
Lot Desc: Back To Woods
Lot Size: 1.89 Acres
Style: Classic
Levels: 3
Bedrooms: 4
Bathrooms: 3/2
Const: Cedar Siding
Roofing: Shingle/F-Glass
Basement: Unfinished
Basement: Walkout Level
Heat: Forced Air
Fuel: Bottled Propane
Cool: Ceiling Fan
Parking: Driveway
Garage Spaces: 3
Exter Feat: Patio
Water: Well

HANDCRAFTED OAK FOYER AND STAIRCASE. THE ATTENTION TO ARCHITECTURAL DETAIL IS OUTSTANDING. AMENITIES SUCH AS HARDWOODS, MARBLE, CERAMIC AND BRASS ADD THE FINISHING TOUCHES!"

Comments: _____

Angela McKendrick, CRS, GRI
Office: 410-555-1234
Home Office: 410-432-7890
Fax: 410-555-5607
Web Site: www.demorealty.com/angela
Email: angela.mckendrick@demorealty.com

Green Leaf Realty
www.greenleafrealty.com

F.

Presenting

Features Include:

12218 Cleghorn Road
$814,900

City: Cockeysville
Neighborhood: Laurelford
Year Built: 1986
Fin SqFt: 3862
Lot Desc: Backs To Trees
Lot Size: 1 Acre
Style: Modern
Levels: 3
Bedrooms: 4
Bathrooms: 2/2
Const: Brick
Roofing: Shingle/Asphalt
Basement: Full
Basement: Unfinished
Heat: Heat Pump
Fuel: Electric
Cool: Central A/C
Parking: Driveway
Garage Spaces: 3
Exter Feat: Balcony
Water: Conditioner

PARK-LIKE GROUNDS. MASTER BEDROOM SUITE WITH BALCONY. STAINED GLASS WINDOWS & LARGE FAMILY ROOM. WET BAR AND ATRIUM DOOR TO SIDE PORCH. LIVING ROOM WITH ATRIUM DOOR TO PATIO. LOTS OF WINDOWS. FLOORS HAVE BEEN REFINISHED. VERY CHARMING HOME WITH ELITE AMENITIES."

Comments: _____

Angela McKendrick, CRS, GRI
Office: 410-555-1234
Home Office: 410-432-7890
Fax: 410-555-5607
Web Site: www.demorealty.com/angela
Email: angela.mckendrick@demorealty.com

Green Leaf Realty
www.greenleafrealty.com

G.

Buyer Tour Map

Ref #	Status	Address
1	Currently On The Market	13213 Beaver Dam Rd
2	Currently On The Market	12218 Cleghorn Road
3	Currently On The Market	20 Laurelford Ct
4	Currently On The Market	9 Jules Brentony
5	Currently On The Market	2 Symphony Cir

Angela McKendrick, CRS, GRI
Office: 410-555-1234
Home Office: 410-432-7890
Fax: 410-555-5607
Web Site: www.demorealty.com/angela
Email: angela.mckendrick@demorealty.com

Green Leaf Realty
www.greenleafrealty.com

H.

FIGURES 9.2A – 9.2J (continued): Property Tour Presentation Package

I.

J.

Used with permission of Realty Tools, Inc.

Select previously visited houses for viewing and consider the benefits offered by particular properties to particular buyers.

Don't show a property just to please the owners. Some agents try to show property to impress owners with their work on the owners' behalf rather than to make a sale. This tactic often backfires because prospective buyers will realize that you really aren't listening to them. Instead, you are wasting their time. This tactic materially lessens the likelihood of having a second chance to show properties to these prospects. Don't give preference to your own office listings. What matters is the buyers' needs. By placing buyers' needs first, you are more likely to be successful.

Some agents try to hold back what they consider to be the best property for their prospects. Instead, they show overpriced or unsuitable property first. They believe the property they hope to sell will then appear in a more favorable light. This practice could be considered unethical because the result could be to give prospective buyers a false impression of property values. It is probably best to arrange showings by location to avoid wasting time backtracking.

If the qualifying process indicates that the homes you initially selected for viewing are unsuitable, cancel the appointments and make new ones before leaving your office. Try to show vacant homes on lockboxes first, so that you give owners time to prepare for a showing.

Some agents like to show no more than three or four properties. How many you show should be dictated by the situation. As an example, if buyers have flown into your area to buy a home because of a job transfer, then you want to continue to show them property until a selection can be made. You can keep confusion to a minimum when you show a large number of properties by giving them information sheets with photos of each house. You can break showings into groups of three or four. Take a coffee break after showing each group and discuss the comparative values of the homes. Find out which one of the group buyers liked best. If a clear winner does not appear, consider a second showing of the best home in each group.

Some agents like the idea of showing what they consider the best as their last scheduled showing. They feel that the first homes give the buyers a basis of comparison that allows the benefits of the final home to be fully appreciated. Other agents like to show what they regard as the best first so that other properties, as they are shown, can be compared to the first property.

Successful salespeople will generally show fewer properties per sale than less successful salespeople. Successful salespeople have a better understanding of their buyers and tend to be more selective in properties they show.

Showing Techniques

Sell the neighborhood.   Plan your route to sell the neighborhood. Choose the most scenic route, one that includes schools, public parks, golf courses, and shopping areas. If possible, adapt your route to the interests of the prospective buyers, but do not plan a route to avoid what *you* regard as a negative factor in the area. If you feel there is a negative element that might influence prospective buyers, this must be revealed to them. *However, the presence of a different racial or ethnic group in the area is not considered a negative factor and should not be revealed as if it were.* In fact, if you were to reveal this type of information, it might be regarded as racial steering, that is, directing people based on race. This is a violation of the Civil Rights Act of 1968.

Because people buy a neighborhood as much as they do a specific property, selling the neighborhood cannot be emphasized enough. While driving to the property, endeavor to educate the buyers by discussing only relevant items. If necessary, prepare leading questions. Try to keep the buyers' attention focused on houses of similar price and on the quality of the neighborhood itself. Point out recent sales of comparably priced homes. This should increase the buyers' trust in you and establish a price range in their minds.

A **negative motivation** technique that entails warning buyers about any problem feature often works well. Buyers build these features up in their minds and are relieved when they find a simple solution to a problem or don't perceive the feature as a problem. Also, avoid overenthusiasm on specific points; it may backfire. Instead, permit the buyers' discoveries to be new and exciting experiences.

When you arrive at the property, don't park in the owner's driveway. Park across the street from it if it has good curb appeal. If you pause for a moment when you get out of the car, your buyers will do the same. Ask for their opinion of the house and the area.

Another reason not to park in an owner's driveway is so you don't get blocked in by another vehicle. It also shows respect for the owner's property.

Create a favorable ambiance. It is interesting to note that although some buyers are interested in construction and utility, most are attracted by color, glamour, texture, and style. Don't bore prospects with details unless you are asked. Show a property for the emotional responses. Buyers usually purchase what they want and what they feel good about. Cater to these feelings by creating a favorable ambiance—proper mood and atmosphere. Have the owner provide fresh flowers in vases. Depending on the weather, either prepare the fireplace or have the air-conditioning operating. Encourage the buyer to relax and feel at home.

You want prospective buyers to think like owners. Use language such as "[Jeffrey's school/Longview Middle School] is only three blocks away. Would you like to look at the school after we leave?" You should have ascertained in advance that Jeffrey would indeed be admitted to the school. In some areas, schools have had to limit new students.

If you are unable to answer a prospect's question and you promise to get the information, treat that promise as a priority. It shows you have regard for their concerns and gives you a reason for another contact.

Involve the whole family.   Ask questions of all family members. If you are receiving positive vibrations from prospective buyers, consider "[Jennifer], which bedroom would be yours?" Remember that just because one member of the family is the most vocal does not mean that person is necessarily the decision maker.

Ask, don't tell, if you want to sell.   The following story illustrates what to do and what not to do when you show property:

Mr. and Mrs. Doe are potential real estate buyers. They have decided to go for the traditional afternoon time killer, the Sunday drive. As they tour their town, complaining about the traffic, Mrs. Doe's face lights up when she sees a lovely home with lots of little flags flying. It is crisp, modern, and obviously open for inspection, so she decides that they should stop and look it over. They walk into the house and are greeted by a real estate salesperson, who puts down a comic book and slowly gets up. The salesperson then proceeds to give the demonstration—the cook's tour.

| Ask questions and listen to the answers. |

"This is the living room," the salesperson proclaims with a sweep of the hand. "This is the dining room; notice the roominess. . . . This is the kitchen. These are the kitchen cabinets. This is the oven; it's big and modern." The salesperson continues, "Notice how wide the hall is. Why don't you both look at this bedroom with me? Isn't your husband interested in bedrooms? This is a closet."

By this time, the couple has had enough. They remember how much they wanted a chocolate malt, and off they go. The salesperson returns to the comic book.

Now imagine the same scene with a different character—a professional salesperson who knows how to communicate:

This salesperson rises but waits to let the customers look around the living room for a moment. Then she turns to Mrs. Doe and says, "Where in this living room would you place your sofa?" (Do not sell the space, sell the benefits of the space.)

In the kitchen, the salesperson opens a cabinet and says, "What would you put in here, dry groceries or your kitchen china?" Opening the oven, the salesperson says, "How big a turkey do you think this oven would take?"

True professionals never say, "This is the second bedroom." They always ask, "Whose bedroom will this be?" A professional does not state obvious facts. A professional *sells* by asking who, what, where, or how for every room and every feature:

> There's plenty of room in the bedroom for a king-size bed plus an office area. Would you put the desk in the window alcove?

> Mr. Thomas, how would you use this workroom?

> Would you use this room as a study or as a spare bedroom?

> How do you think your dog will like having her own trees in the fenced yard? Would you use the covered patio for summer entertaining?

The first minutes of entering a home can set the emotional stage for buying or forgetting the property. You want to get prospective buyers involved:

> What do you like about this [house], [room]? What if anything would you change? Why?

Sell benefits, not features. A pool is merely a hole in the ground with chlorinated water in it. The wise real estate salesperson remembers that the pool is, in fact, much more than this.

> Imagine on a hot summer day, Mr. and Mrs. Jones, not having to trek the kids all the way down to the local recreation center to go swimming. You will be able to save gas and time by having the kids play right here in the backyard.

A gourmet kitchen is a place to indulge in one's culinary hobby, not to mention a pleasant atmosphere in which to work out tensions. A fireplace contributes to family togetherness and the kindling of romance. A dishwasher is not a luxury; it is a necessity, given the hectic demands on most people's time. A spa and sun deck promote an image of relaxed enjoyment, as well as being status symbols. Listen carefully to uncover features and benefits that are important to the buyer, as well as probing when appropriate, and then sell those features and benefits.

Ask questions, don't state opinions.

Because the qualifying process is a continual one, after each house shown you must *ask questions, not state opinions.* By asking questions about what prospective buyers liked and what they didn't like and probing for the reasons behind these feelings, you may find that your showing schedule needs modification.

Use tie-downs.   A good communicator uses **tie-downs**, a question that calls for a positive response. They can be used to check out whether a benefit is important or to build a sense of ownership. No professional salesperson ever makes a positive statement without tying it down:

- "This is a spacious room, *isn't it?*"

- "You really need four bedrooms, *don't you?*"

- "Your children should be close to school, *shouldn't they?*"

- "This is the sound investment you've been looking for, *isn't it?*"

These words—*isn't it, can it, won't it, don't you, can't you,* and so on—are powerful selling tools. Little yeses easily lead to the big yes. Sell on minor points.

A series of yes responses can lead to the big YES!

Invite comparisons.   The comparison technique gets buyers involved. Ask such questions as "Did you like the vanity off the bedroom, as it was in the house you just saw, or do you prefer this style?" "Will this dining room set off your antique hutch, or can you see it better in the other house?" These questions get the buyers involved in defining what is important to them. Buyers start selling themselves and get prepared to make the big decision by making a lot of little ones.

By use of comparisons you can discover preferences.

Additional showing tips.   If you know that a property has a feature that the buyers will enjoy, don't point it out to them. Let them discover that pool or large oak tree on their own. Here are other items that may enhance your presentation:

- Occasionally allow the buyers privacy. They may want to feel that they're alone when they discuss personal things.

- Do not assume that just because you like a feature of the property, the buyers will like it as well.

- Do not resent the presence of a friend of the family. Use the friend as an ally.

- Always overcome any objections on the scene. If space is an issue, use a tape measure (let the customer measure). Try to settle any questions on the spot.

- Begin and end the tour of the home in the most beautiful and unique part of the house.

- The buyers will follow your lead. Whenever you enter a room, they will follow.

- Involve children. Wherever possible, direct questions to the children.

- Speak plainly, and avoid technical terms. When people do not understand, your point is lost.

- Call attention to outstanding features, but do not go overboard or you will close the door on the sale of another property.

- Show the rooms in the most productive order. In a home, this is usually front hall, living room, dining room, kitchen, bedrooms, yard or garden, and last of all the most attractive rooms on the first floor. This procedure may be varied to suit special cases.

- If the rooms are small, do not stand in the middle of a room; stand along the side.

When showing furnished property be aware that you have a duty of reasonable care as to the possessions of the occupant. Do not allow prospects to wander about out of your sight. Small expensive items can be a temptation for some people. While the listing agent should have advised owners to secure such objects, they don't always do so and some owners fail to heed warnings.

Establishing a list. A valuable technique to use when showing property is to ask prospective buyers if they would want to include the property on their list for consideration. The list approach prepares the buyer for a purchase choice between several properties they have shown a degree of interest in. The choice you're seeking is which property they will buy, not a to-buy-or-not-to-buy decision.

The list can also be used as a closing technique: "This property meets nine out of 10 of the items on your list; you can't get much better than that."

An alternative showing technique. For vacant property, consider opening the door and telling the prospects to take their time and look around and that you will join them shortly.

When you join them, ask questions as to what they thought about particular features or what they like most about the property. By letting them view the property, they will be relaxed making their own decisions and able to privately discuss their feelings. This "on your own" showing technique is particularly effective when you feel that this is the property your prospective buyers will want. Because of security considerations as to the owners' property, don't use this technique when the property has owner furnishings without specific permission by the owner to do so.

Multiple-prospect home tours. Home tours by bus or caravan are an effective tool to attract prospective buyers and can present competition that can stimulate buying decisions. Buyers do not feel threatened in situations when they are part of a group viewing property. They are more likely to go on a tour of homes than to contact a broker to view particular homes that may interest them.

Most brokers conducting tours require prospects to sign up in advance because space is limited. They also offer to prequalify or even preapprove buyers for loans at no cost or obligation. A call the day before the tour and a little "teaser" information about one property will reduce the number of "no shows." You want a full tour because it can create a feeling of excitement and competition.

Some brokers will offer multiple tours featuring properties based on property type and/or price range. Some tours are limited to new home developments. Others may be limited to properties in foreclosure or short sales. Tours of foreclosed properties, as well as tours of fixer-uppers for flippers, have been very productive. Some brokers advertise the homes they show and the period of time they will be at each property, which allows prospects to go to just one or several of the homes to be viewed.

Providing clipboards with photos and data of each home and places for the prospects to make notes is effective in helping the buyers make their own decisions. With large groups, let the prospects view on their own.

During bus tours, a salesperson will then ask questions of the viewers as to each house after they have seen it. Often a problem raised by one person will be minimized by a solution offered by another viewer.

At the end of the tour, participants are asked to answer a brief questionnaire about the benefits of the tour and their feelings about the properties. Participants are asked if they would like to discuss any particular property or if they would like more information.

While offers are received on the day of the tour, especially when more than one prospect shows interest in the same property, other offers may take a few days. Many participants will sign up for additional tours.

Tours should be followed up with a telephone call.

Rules of Professional Conduct

The following rules help you maintain goodwill and a professional manner as you plan for and conduct showings:

- If you arrive at a property and notice that someone else is showing it, wait inconspicuously until the other salesperson and clients have left.

- When showing a home, leave it as you found it. If drapes were closed, see that they're closed when you leave. If inner doors were closed, close them when you leave. Double-check all outside doors to see that they're locked. Be sure to replace the key in the lockbox where you found it. If dogs, cats, or other animals are confined to a given room, yard, garage, and so forth, see that they do not gain access to other rooms or to the street.

- Notify the listing office immediately if something seems to be amiss at a property you have shown. Treat all listings as you would want to have your own listing treated.

- If a listing specifies "call first," never take a customer to the door and ask to show the home. If, while showing a property, you decide to show another and cannot reach the owner by phone, leave the client in the car while you go to the door and ask the owner for belated permission to show the property. Then abide by the owner's wishes.

- If a listing indicates that the property is to be shown only during certain hours or gives other information regarding particular conditions of showing, do not violate these requests. There must be a reason for them.

- Leave your business card at each property. It is a courtesy to the owner (whether at home or not). It also helps to advertise your own office. It is a good idea to write the date and the time on the back of the card.

- Interoffice courtesy requires that when calling another agency for information, you immediately identify yourself and your company.

- Do not enter a house with a lighted cigarette, pipe, or cigar, and do not light one while in a house. Be certain that prospective buyers also abide by these restrictions.

- Avoid making uncomplimentary remarks about a house, its condition, or its furnishings while in the house. The owner may be in the next room and be embarrassed or hurt by your comments.

KEEP THEM YOURS

After you have completed your first session of showing homes to prospective buyers, it is a good idea to ask them to return to the office to discuss the properties they have seen. If a closing is not going to be possible, consider a way to tie down the prospects so they regard you as their agent. Consider the following approach:

> I prefer to work with just a few buyers. I dedicate my efforts to finding them a property that best meets their needs. Usually, I'm able to meet the needs of my buyers in just a few weeks. I am willing to work for you and concentrate my efforts on your behalf if you are serious buyers. At times, buyers don't really have the down payment they say they have, or for some other reason are not in a position to buy. If I were able to show you a property that has everything you want, would you make an offer?

You want prospective buyers to feel an obligation to work with you.

Your buyers can be expected to assure you that they are serious and willing to make an offer. Continue:

> If you are willing to let me take over the exclusive responsibility of finding the home you want, I will use all my efforts to locate the property that meets all your needs. If you see an ad or internet listing that interests you, if you drive by a home you like, or even if you see an open-house sign, call me about it. If other brokers contact you, tell them to call me and I will cooperate with them. If you are willing to work with me, I am willing to go all out for you. Does this seem fair?

The answer will usually be positive, and many people will live up to the agreement, but it would be better to bring out a buyer-agency agreement at this time. When you find the house that meets their needs, committed buyers will often feel obligated to make an offer when they might otherwise have procrastinated. If you want to act as a buyer's agent rather than a dual agent or seller's agent, now is a good time to obtain a buyer agent listing.

Video Streaming

You can show property to prospective renters or buyers without their being physically present. Using a smartphone, you can provide live-time viewing with apps such as Skype, Facetime, and Periscope. By coordinating viewing time, clients can see a live video feed as the agent uses a camera function to scan rooms and exterior features while talking to the client. The client can ask for close-ups or to return to a particular feature of the property. While some agents have reported receiving purchase offers online from the live feed, it has been particularly valuable as to relocation rentals. Clients are willing to obligate to a one-year lease more readily than a half a million dollar purchase when they have not physically visited the property.

SUMMARY

Contacts generally begin with a phone call. Be prepared for phone inquiries by having current listings, ads, switch property, and location of office listings readily available.

Prospects calling from a For Sale sign usually like the area and exterior; however, the price may not be suitable. Callers from ads are more likely suitable for switch property at a higher price. Callers from the internet like the appearance and price and are more likely to be purchasers of the property inquired about than callers from other sources.

Find out the names and addresses of callers, as well as their needs. Give minimum property information but extract the maximum information on callers' needs and motivations. By giving callers just enough information to keep their interest level high, you can obtain an appointment using a choice of time, not a choice between meeting and not meeting. By asking motivated prospective buyers to mark other ads that interest them, you can lock the prospects in and keep them from calling other agents.

In preparing to meet prospective buyers, you should have some tentative property-showing appointments and a qualifying plan. Before you show any property, you must ascertain prospects' needs, their motivation to buy, and their financial qualifications: the down payment they can afford and the maximum loan they can carry.

Personal security risks will be reduced by meeting prospects at your office and introducing them to your broker and other employees.

The motivation of prospects will affect the level of priority and energy that should be planned for prospective buyers. Based on prospects' needs and financial abilities, your selection of property for showing might need modification. Do not show prospective buyers properties they cannot afford.

Feng shui is the flow of energy and is of importance when dealing with Chinese buyers.

A property tour presentation package can help the buyer keep track of properties and evaluate them. It can lead naturally to a sale.

Plan your showings and ask questions. Don't give opinions during the showing process. Keep in mind that when you conduct a showing, you are selling benefits. Involve the entire family with your questions. The qualifying process should continue right to the point of sale.

Group tours can be effective in showing similar properties. Competitive situations can spark interest and encourage action.

By having buyers select properties for a list for consideration, they can further narrow their choices by property to buy or not buy.

CLASS DISCUSSION TOPICS

1. Role-play an inquiry about your own home with another student. Your goal will be to obtain a name, address, basic needs, and a firm appointment.

2. Role-play a need and motivation buyer-qualification process with another student.

3. Role-play a showing of your classroom with another student cast as a prospective buyer of a classroom.

4. Bring to class one current-events article dealing with some aspect of real estate practice for class discussion.

UNIT 9 QUIZ

1. Callers from a For Sale sign are likely to be
   a. satisfied with the area.
   b. looking for a more expensive home.
   c. satisfied with the general exterior appearance.
   d. both a and c.

2. If we compare callers from classified ads with those from For Sale signs, in general,
   a. callers from signs are more likely to end up buying homes that cost less than the home they called about.
   b. callers from ads are more likely to end up buying homes that cost more than the home they called about.
   c. both of these are true.
   d. both of these are false.

3. Real estate professionals should
   a. limit showing to their own listings.
   b. show overpriced property first to make the one house seem a bargain.
   c. avoid driving through nearby minority areas.
   d. do none of these.

4. In showing property, you should
   a. never show a prospect more than three homes in one day.
   b. show prospects a really nice home they can't afford in order to keep up their interest.
   c. never change your showing plans once you start.
   d. do none of these.

5. The qualifying process includes discovering
   a. the buyers' motivation.
   b. the buyers' needs and interests.
   c. a down payment they can make and the amount they can finance.
   d. all of these.

6. The front-end loan-qualifying ratio is the ratio of
   a. gross housing cost to gross income.
   b. gross income to net income.
   c. net housing cost to net income.
   d. none of these.

7. The back-end qualifying ratio refers to the ratio of
   a. gross housing cost to gross income.
   b. total housing expense plus long-term debt to gross income.
   c. gross income to net income plus housing cost.
   d. none of these.

8. A good policy for a professional real estate salesperson would be to
   a. meet new prospects at the nicest property you think will interest them.
   b. avoid discussing financial matters until an offer is received.
   c. ask open-ended questions of prospective buyers.
   d. limit appointments to the showing of no more than two properties.

9. For personal safety concerns, you should
   a. meet prospects at your office.
   b. avoid ostentatious jewelry or accessories.
   c. leave front doors unlocked at showing.
   d. do all of these.

10. If another agent is showing a home when you arrive for a showing, what should you do?
    a. Bring your prospects in and let them know they are competing with other buyers for the house
    b. Cross the house off your showing list until you are sure it has not been sold
    c. Wait inconspicuously until the other agent completes his or her showing and leaves
    d. Tell your clients that you are certain that the other prospects are buyers so they had better act fast

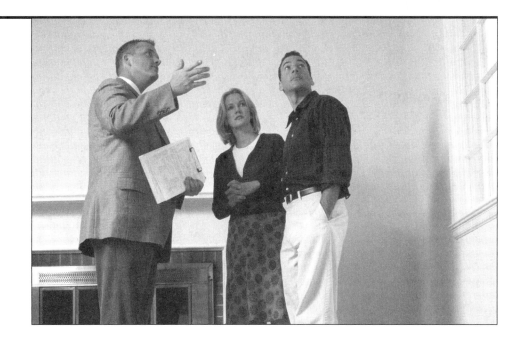

10

OBTAINING THE OFFER AND CREATING THE SALES AGREEMENT

LEARNING OBJECTIVES

When you have completed this unit, you will be able to

■ explain what selling is and how it is accomplished;

■ describe how to obtain an offer to purchase, recognize buying signals, and deal with objections;

■ list various closing techniques;

■ explain and complete the California Residential Purchase Agreement and Joint Escrow Instructions; and

■ estimate buyer costs.

KEY TERMS

assumptive close	estimated buyer's costs	persuasion
buying motives	inducement	positive choice
buying signals	mirroring	trial close
California Residential Purchase Agreement and Joint Escrow Instructions	negative motivation	

WHAT IS SELLING?

If all you accomplished in real estate was to escort people through houses, you would be a tour guide, not a salesperson. Selling is a noble profession because it helps others fulfill their needs and desires. As a salesperson, you influence the outcome of a showing. You influence prospective buyers to become owners by executing a real property purchase contract. Webster defines selling as "to induce others." While in real estate we induce others to buy benefits, selling begins with uncovering client or customer needs and then working for those needs to be satisfied. In other words, salesmanship involves imparting knowledge, amplifying desire and showing how those desires can be fulfilled.

Selling Is Persuading

Persuasion is the central theme in many descriptions of the selling process:

- The personal or impersonal process of persuading prospective customers to buy a commodity or service

- The art of persuading people to accept or to follow certain ideas that lead them to a desired action

- Persuading people to want what you have in terms of products, services, or ideas

Unfortunately, the word *persuasion* reminds many people of someone who convinces them to buy unnecessary products. You can avoid this problem by understanding that people buy benefits that will satisfy their wants and needs, both conscious and unconscious. Your job is to address the needs and show your customers that satisfying *their* needs is most important to *you*.

The good feelings that result will lead to long-term customer satisfaction and future business.

Selling Is Effective Communication

Without effective communication, there is no understanding. Know what you want to say; use listeners' language. Do not use fancy or technical words when simple ones will do. Use the "KISS" method—**K**eep **I**t **S**imple and **S**incere.

A clear idea, sufficient facts, and proper media are of no avail if the communicator uses language that confuses the listener. Words should be chosen with the utmost care, organized, and delivered meaningfully. When you are dealing with parties who have limited English language skills, slow your speech and ask questions so you are certain you are being understood. Avoid using real estate terminology, such as Fannie Mae, or acronyms, such as MLS and FSBO.

Idea.   The most common cause of poor communication is the communicator's own failure to understand the idea he wants to express. You must have something to communicate. As a rule, if you are unsure about what you really mean or are lacking essential facts, it is best not to try to communicate your thoughts to others.

For effective communication, Keep It Simple and Sincere!

Facts.   To make the sales message understood, you must provide sufficient facts. Without facts, the person receiving the message cannot form valid conclusions or take effective action. This is illustrated by the story of a temporary post office employee who was told to take a truck and deliver the New York mail. Six hours later, the department received a telephone call: "I'm out of gas on the New Jersey Turnpike, 11 miles out of New York. Can you wire me some money so I can deliver the mail?" What the boss had forgotten to tell the new employee was, "When we say deliver the New York mail, we mean to drive it two blocks to Union Station and leave it on the train platform."

Receiver.   Words or symbols have different meanings for different people. Assess your listener before attempting to communicate. Recognition of experience, mood, and temperament, as well as knowledge of the product or service, will make or break the communication chain.

Your Voice Personality

Does your selling voice communicate well? If not, the following four guidelines will help you relate to your customer more effectively:

1. Articulate clearly

2. Sound positive and friendly

3. Match your customer's speech in volume, speed, and tone (this is sometimes called mirroring). Remember that just because someone speaks slowly, it doesn't mean that person thinks slowly.

4. Use your customer's descriptive words

Selling Is Discovering

Help your client or customer to discover. For example, ask, "Would it be all right if I ask you a few questions?" Evaluate your inquiry style by asking the following questions:

- Do my questions tell my prospect that I understand the client or customer?

- Do I ask property-oriented (fact-finding) questions?

- Do I follow this with people-oriented (feeling-finding) questions?

- Do I ask open-ended questions to get the other party to "open up"?

> Open-ended questions ask for reasons and feelings. Example: "Why do you want a three-car garage?"

In qualifying prospective buyers, use open-end questions to gain information rather than closed-end questions. Open-end questions ask for reasons and feelings and aid in the communication process, whereas closed-end questions can be answered with a simple "yes" or "no" that does not provide any background about reasoning and motivation. A child's "Why?" is an example of an open-ended question. By asking questions like "Tell me…," you invite the buyer's participation. The buyer will feel more in control.

If you start with fact-finding questions, which appeal to reason, you accomplish the following three things:

1. You relax the prospect.

2. You indicate to the prospect that you have done your homework.

3. You obtain valuable information that helps guide your sales effort.

Then revert to feeling-finding questions, which appeal to emotions. Remember that people are more likely to buy the product or service if they feel that you understand them. By acknowledging the buyer's needs, you can establish a bond of empathy. You must show that you understand both the needs and the concerns of the buyer.

Give buyers a rational reason to fulfill an emotional need.

Customers' reasons for buying traditionally have been divided into two major categories: rational and emotional. *Rational motives* are usually defined as including any considerations that have to do with long-term costs, financing, and benefits from proposed expenditures. In other words, rational motives measure all the costs against all the probable gains. There are probably as many *emotional motives* for buying as there are customers. However, a few that are most frequently seen in real estate are love, fear, convenience, prestige or social approval, and self-improvement. Selling often involves giving a prospective buyer a rational reason for fulfilling an emotional need.

Selling Is Knowing Your Customer

Customers are the heart and soul of your business. Your customers do not have to love you but should like and trust you. It is a good idea for you to love your customers. Always keep in mind how you can best serve them.

Customer types. There have been numerous attempts to pigeonhole prospects and customers. This can be done if you keep in mind the temperamental fluctuations that might occur. Remember, no customer is a single type; each one is a composite of several types. Most experienced licensees have seen an individual display more than one temperament during an interview. Some customers put the salesperson on the defensive; some buyers waver; some are irritable, cynical, or good-humored. Alert salespeople adjust their approaches to the attitudes, temperaments, and buying needs of each customer. Figure 10.1 shows strategies for dealing with various types of prospects.

Selling Is Knowing Your Product

If you are going to satisfy customer needs and wants, you must know what properties are available and their features. Taking a listing, preparing for a showing, going through the multiple listing service listings, and networking with others are all good opportunities for gathering this information. Knowledge and expertise are becoming even more important as consumers become more sophisticated. Several areas of knowledge about your product are discussed in the following paragraphs.

Features of properties include those of the community, as well as those of specific houses. For example, clients may want to know the following:

- Are there good schools nearby? (Private versus public and specialty schools)

- Where is the nearest racquetball court?

- What are the neighborhood amenities?

Because it is difficult to know everything about every community, many salespeople begin by specializing in a specific geographic area. Often, this market area includes the neighborhoods in which you will do the most business. It will serve you well to get involved in these communities, get to know the neighborhood, and keep up with changes.

The brokerage firm, you, and the services you provide also are part of the product. Unanswered questions and objections raised in these areas can kill a sale. Early in your relationship with your clients or prospects, present information that will establish your credibility and show them that you have the resources to work hard for them. Some agents hand out fact sheets or a résumé. An anecdote about a way in which you and the firm have benefited others may help you establish rapport and provide reassurance if the situation seems appropriate:

"There are advantages and disadvantages to this property," said the honest and well-informed real estate agent. "To the north is the gas works, to the east the glue factory, to the south a fish and chips shop, and to the west a sewage farm. These are the disadvantages."

"What are the advantages?" the customer asked.

"You can always tell which way the wind is blowing," was the agent's reply. As this anecdote humorously illustrates, you often can present disadvantages as advantages.

Because it is unlikely that a piece of property will have every feature a client wants, it makes sense to play up the significant features and downplay the ones that are lacking. However, be meticulous about disclosure issues. Do not neglect or change the presentation of negative information just because it is (or may be perceived as) a disadvantage. Both legally and morally, you owe each client a high standard of care—a quality of service that a "reasonably prudent person" would provide. Since the *Easton v. Strassburger* case, awareness of responsibilities has become a prime concern in the real estate profession.

FIGURE 10.1:   Types of Prospects

General Strategies to Use		
Silent Prospect—the "Clam"—Does not indicate whether she is agreeing or disagreeing	=	Ask leading questions; be more personal than usual/
Procrastinator—the "Putter-Offer"—Does not know his own mind; has difficulty making up mind	=	Summarize benefits that prospect will lose if he or she does not act; be positive, self-assured, and dramatic/
Glad-Hander—Talkative or overenthusiastic	=	Lead these prospects back into the sale after letting them talk themselves out!
Argumentative Type—Usually is insincere and tries the salesperson's patience	=	Sincerity and respect on the salesperson's part will create respect. Consider, "You're absolutely right. That's why you'll appreciate . . ."
Slow or Methodical Type—Appears to weigh every word of the salesperson	=	Slow down and simplify details. Adjust your tempo to your prospect's. This approach is often called mirroring and can lead a sales prospect comfortably to a positive decision.
Skeptical or Suspicious Type—Convinced that every salesperson is trying to "pull the wool over her eyes"	=	Stay with the facts, and be conservative in statements. Allay the prospect's fears.
Overcautious or Timid Type—Acts as if he does not trust the salesperson	=	Take it slow and easy. Reassure on every point. Use logic and make it simple.
Impulsive Type—Apt to interrupt presentation before salesperson states all points		Speed up presentation, concentrating only on important points. Omit details when possible.
Opinionated—Ego Type—Is overconfident, with strong opinions		Give these prospects "rope" by appealing to their egos. Listen attentively and guide them, using their opinions.

Selling Is You

You should present a calm rational persona. You must show a desire to understand needs and to help in their fulfillment. If you appear to be trying too hard, buyers are likely to become nervous or defensive, or both. You want to be a person whom the buyers like and trust. You can be that person and it will lead to success.

There will be times when you are not the person who can best serve a particular client. Perhaps the client is looking for a home that lies outside your market area. Or, someone may want a piece of investment property that will involve intricate tax and financing complications. The worst mistake you can make is thinking that you can serve everyone. It is far better to refer people to brokers or other individuals who have the required expertise. Even if you do refer a prospect to another agent, it would be ethical and legal to earn a referral fee from the other agent after the transaction has reached a successful close.

OBTAINING THE OFFER

Closing is simply asking for a decision.

To narrow the number of homes shown for a purchase decision, some brokers create a list. When you show a number of properties to clients, the list approach should be considered. It is a logical approach to selling. After each showing, ask the clients what they liked about the property and what they considered negatives. Then ask if the property should be added to their list for consideration. After you have three or more properties on the list, go over the pluses and minuses of the properties and let the clients tell you which properties they feel they like best. Do not be assertive and try to influence this final decision. Your personal likes and dislikes could turn a decision into no decision at all. Once they have made their choice, ask whether they would like to put an offer on the property. Selling becomes a matter of showing the prospects how and why it should be their home.

In striving to obtain an offer to purchase, you will find that each transaction is unique and has its own approach and required motivation. However, there are some general principles to apply. Understanding why customers buy and the basic steps of transactions help you prepare for a presentation that will lead to an offer. Four basic steps are illustrated in Figure 10.2. They are discussed in the following paragraphs.

Appeal to Buying Motives

Merriam-Webster's Collegiate Dictionary defines *motive* as "something (as a need or desire) that causes a person to act." Understanding a buyer's needs and wants is absolutely essential for optimum results. Remember, you are going to be selling the benefits that match those needs and wants. After all, why should an individual buy a home and be responsible for its maintenance, taxes, and so on, rather than rent for life? Why should a family skimp and save for a down payment and make monthly payments when that family could live in a public housing unit or with relatives?

Ownership of real property satisfies several basic needs or **buying motives**.

Survival.   The most basic human need is survival. If a home has no amenities other than providing shelter, it satisfies the basic human need to survive.

Security.   The desire for security is a fundamental need that has many applications in the selling process. Every licensee should appeal to it. The home often becomes the principal financial asset of many Americans. In times of financial stress, the home might be something to fall back on. People feel secure in their own homes. They do not have to worry about landlords asking them to leave because the landlords want their own children to live there.

FIGURE 10.2:   Steps in Obtaining the Offer

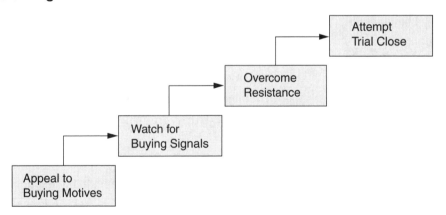

Pride of ownership/social need.   Once buyers obtain basic shelter, pride impels many to pay considerably more for additional benefits. What they feel their friends and/or family will think of the home influences many buyers. By a statement such as "Wouldn't you like to entertain your friends on this delightful patio?" you can create an image of pride in showing the home to others. Many salespeople use pride of ownership immediately by referring to the property being shown as if the prospective buyers were already the owners. Pride of ownership appeal is not limited to luxury estates. It can be used for all types of properties because most buyers are looking at properties with better amenities than they currently enjoy.

Love of family. Desirable school areas, recreational facilities, shopping conveniences, or other factors that may appeal to one or all members of the family often induce the purchase of a certain property. Many times one of the foremost factors in the buyer's mind will be how the home can help the family. Don't forget that in many families, pets are regarded as important family members.

Health. Motivation arising from health interests is closely allied to the survival instinct and can be a determining factor in a decision to buy. The quality of the environment—of the air and water, lower noise levels, the avoidance of urban congestion—often motivates a decision to buy.

Desire for profit or gain (investment). More people have started on the road to financial independence through home ownership than in any other way. Buying a home can be an investment for the future because well-located properties in the long run increase in value, a process called *appreciation*. The amount of appreciation depends on numerous factors, such as the demand for housing in the area, the supply of homes, the availability of good financing, and the area's economy. While we have seen periods of sharp declines in value in the past, property values in California historically have tended to increase an average of more than 3% a year beyond the rate of inflation. Home ownership is still likely to be the best investment or savings program the average family will ever have.

Tax benefits. Home ownership, as well as second-home ownership, offers significant tax advantages that influence many buyers. The deductibility of property taxes and interest means that true costs are significantly less than they appear. The special tax exemptions available for gains on the sale of primary residences is the frosting on the cake, because it makes home ownership extremely attractive for anyone concerned about income taxes. (See Unit 14.)

Comfort and convenience.   The human drive for comfort and convenience has less influence than some of the other, previously mentioned factors. When basic needs have been fulfilled, however, these may be considered an added dimension.

Reason versus emotion.   *Logic* makes people think, or reason. *Emotion* makes them act. Potential buyers may decide logically that a property is suited for them, but they may not act because the property does not trigger an emotional response. *In most situations, buyers do not buy simply from need, they buy what they want.* While sellers tend to sell based on logic, buyers generally buy based on emotion. The successful salesperson probes to find the buyers' desires that, when satisfied, will trigger their motivation to buy. This is why communication is so important. What a buyer says he or she wants is likely to be based on reason; what the buyer really wants may be based more on emotion than on reason. If you pay attention while showing a house, you can determine the emotional needs of the buyer and select properties to show that meet those needs. You can gain an understanding of which of several properties a buyer actually wants by questions such as "If these properties were priced identically, which property would you prefer?" Follow this up with, "Why?" By listening, you can offer knowledgeable assistance based on experience of other buyers your buyers can relate to. It is much easier to sell buyers a property that appeals to their emotions than one that appears sensible for them.

The author once showed a prospective buyer a luxury home. He could easily afford it but hesitated spending the money because he didn't need that fine a home. Giving the buyer a rational reason to buy resulted in a sale: "It's more than a home, it's an investment, and you don't have to wait to sell it to realize the appreciation. A great many homeowners have sent their children through college by refinancing their homes or using a home equity line of credit." Buyers are usually often receptive to even weak rational reasons to buy property that appeals to their emotions.

Sensory appeal.   People learn about the surrounding world through their senses, which include sound, sight, smell, taste, and touch. You can enhance your presentation by employing all the senses and by emphasizing the benefits that can be appreciated by various senses.

In appealing to the sense of *sight*, point out the restful and interesting views from the windows, the lush lawns, the lines of the house, the ample wall space. Be careful not to go overboard about certain colors; they may be your choice but not the buyer's.

The appeal of *sound* may be either its absence or its presence—perhaps it will be music, man-made or natural, to a buyer's ears. Where possible, call attention to the sound made by the ocean, a lake, a babbling brook, or birds. Also, make buyers aware that machinery in the house, such as air conditioners, water closets, and power switches, operate quietly.

To appeal to buyers' sense of *smell*, call attention to the fresh air, flower scents, or, if possible, the smell of cedar from closets or chests.

The sense of *taste* might be appealed to by testing the flavor of well water, vegetables from the garden, or fruit from the trees. If you know there is ripe fruit in the yard, an excellent technique is to bring a pen knife with you and offer a slice of fruit to the prospective buyers.

Appeal to the sense of *touch* by touching the carpeting, knocking on the solid wood paneling, or breaking up a lump of garden soil in your hand. Your prospects will likely do the same. By touching, they come a little closer to ownership.

Negative motivation. **Negative motivation** applies to knowing what someone does *not* want. There are many things we do not want: pain, hunger, fatigue, worry, strife, just to mention a few. Negative motivation can be more immediate and real to a person than positive motivation. People seem to know what they do not want better than what they do want.

To avoid a fruitless, time-wasting search, the salesperson should endeavor to learn buyers' negative motivations as well as the positive ones. Some disadvantages of home ownership are described in Figure 10.3: large initial investment, risk, increased expenses, restricted mobility, a low level of liquidity, and greater responsibility. If a buyer does not want something, the absence or mitigation of this perceived negative becomes a strong positive factor for a sale.

Watch for Buying Signals

In many situations and at various psychological moments during your presentation, prospects may signal that they are ready to buy. These **buying signals**—some action, word or phrase, or facial expression of buyers—are tip-offs to the salesperson. A buying signal says, "I'm ready to talk terms if you are." These signals are green lights. After prospects have exhibited a buying signal, follow up the opportunity with a closing statement.

Actions.   You are making a presentation, and the prospects stay mum. They do not even grunt. You start to wonder if you are talking their language. Suddenly, one of them picks up the deposit receipt and reads a clause or two. Stop your presentation and swing into your close—they are interested. Prospects also are signaling when they return to an upstairs room for a second look or to measure a room. They are envisioning their placement of furniture. If prospects seem reluctant to leave the room or the property or inspect minute details, it shows positive interest. These actions will often mean "I'm ready to buy."

Words.   Obvious buying signals would be statements such as "This is great!" "Kevin would love this back bedroom," or "I especially like the low maintenance." Even an objection or an expression of resistance can spell a buying signal: "Don't you think the price is a little too high?" The alert salesperson hears it as a signal, because it shows that the buyer actually is thinking about the purchase. Other possible signals occur if a buyer

- asks the salesperson to go over the financing details again,

- inquires about possession time,

- requests information about closing costs,

- starts to whisper with a spouse, or

- makes a statement as to a positive aspect of the property.

FIGURE 10.3: **Disadvantages of Home Ownership**

■ Large initial investment: Normally, buying a home requires a down payment of 5% to 20% of the purchase price, with the exception of VA loans, some FHA loans, and loans involving secondary financing or high rates of interest. This means the purchase price of a $400,000 home may require a down payment of $20,000 to $80,000. In addition, the closing costs could well be from $4,000 to $10,000.

■ Risk: Whenever customers invest money, they risk losing some or all of it. Changes in market conditions can affect value. However, well-located properties kept in good condition offer less risk over the long term than most other investment choices.

■ Increase in expenses: Although mortgage payments remain constant in the case of fixed-rate loans, other costs may increase. Property taxes and utility costs creep upward. Maintenance costs increase as the home ages. Adjustable-rate loans could have an increase in interest and payments. Buyers have to weigh some of these increased costs against the advantages of ownership, but they should remember that rents also increase.

■ Restricted mobility: To a degree, people are less mobile once they have bought a home. However, houses can be sold or rented out by the owner.

■ Lack of liquidity: Some say they dislike home ownership because their investment is not liquid. While an investment in a home is not as liquid as having money in the bank, homeowners can use their property as a source of cash. For example, homeowners might consider borrowing on the property by taking out a home equity loan. Or they could refinance the first mortgage once sufficient equity has been developed.

■ Greater responsibility: An investment in real property has responsibilities. Buyers must maintain the property properly. For example, they may have to climb a ladder to paint or call a painter and pay the bill. The lawn needs to be watered and cut to protect the investment.

Negative statements can be a signal to buy. A complaint about price could instead mean an offer at a lesser price is imminent. Complaining about problems that can be readily solved, coupled with a reluctance to leave the property, could be a buying tactic to justify a lower offer.

Body language. A salesperson who is not watching customers carefully may easily miss facial-expression signals. Prospects smiling as you make your presentation or nodding at each other are positive signals. A prospect sitting back in the chair and then leaning forward as you make your sales presentation is a sign of interest. Meeting your eye contact, as well as showing signs of relaxing, are also positive indicators.

Overcome Resistance

To obtain the offer, be prepared to answer any objections raised by the buyer. Buyer resistance will vary with each transaction. Typical objections might include some of the following statements:

■ "The price is too high."

■ "The water pressure is too low."

■ "The rooms are too small."

■ "The taxes are too high."

- "I can't buy until I sell."

- "I can't get occupancy soon enough."

- "I'll never get my kids into that school."

Human nature being what it is, some salespeople feel they must conquer objections by crushing them decisively. It is an unfortunate truth that many salespeople feel they must treat objections as barriers raised to block them from their goal— the sale or the offer. They see an objection as being in direct conflict with their best interests, and therefore they fear it and wish to combat it quickly.

In contrast to this, you should treat an objection as a prelude to a sale, a natural part of any sales routine. Objections may occur while showing the house or in your office before signing the offer. Before proceeding to your counterattack, determine two things in your own mind:

1. Is it really an objection or just a comment?

2. Is it an objection you can and should do something about?

There are ways to handle real objections. Five basic steps to be used in meeting objections are shown in Figure 10.4. Carefully following these steps leads to obtaining the offer and closing the sale.

When buyers are hesitant, ask a simple question or two:

What if anything would keep you from buying this house?

How could you overcome this?

If a buyer responds with a solution, you should have an offer.

Welcome objections.   An objection means that you have an interested buyer who has a concern. When you fail to get objections, it could mean that your prospect is not a serious buyer. Do not fear objections; welcome them. Encourage prospects to tell you what is on their minds. Objections help focus your talk on what matters to the prospect. They may be the prospect's way of asking for more information. They may throw some light on the prospect's thinking.

FIGURE 10.4: Meeting a Buyer's Objections

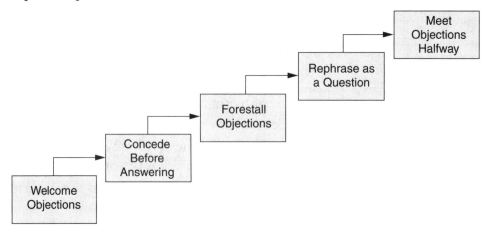

You can't overcome objections if you don't know what they are.

Concede before answering. To avoid putting the buyers on the defensive, recognize legitimate concerns. Never tell buyers who have a legitimate objection that their position is somehow not valid or less than true. This immediately creates confrontation. You might make a comment such as one of these: "Other clients have felt the same way in the past, but what they have found is that . . .," "I can appreciate your concerns," or "I understand how you feel."

Rephrase an objection as a question. The buyer might say, "I don't like tract houses," to which you could reply, "As I understand it then, Mr. and Mrs. Buyer, your question is this: 'Am I better off buying a smaller custom home in a less desirable neighborhood for the same money or would I gain greater enjoyment by owning this larger home with more amenities in a great neighborhood?'" Try to restate objections as questions. Doing so shows the buyers that you are working together and that you are most concerned with helping them.

Similarly:

> I don't like the color of this room

> If this were your house, what color would you paint it?

> Do you think [one] gallon of paint would cover it?

If the buyers can solve their own objections, you are on the path to a sale.

What you have done is minimize the objection and the prospective buyers have solved their own objection.

If a prospective buyer objects to a price, your first question should be, "What do you feel would be a fair price for this property?" If the buyer replies with a price, your response could be, "How did you arrive at that price?" Listen attentively. You could correct misconceptions and justify what you feel is a fair price, or you could state, "While I think your price is a little low, let's try it. If the owners accept, I think you'll have made a really advantageous purchase."

Meet objections halfway.   A well-known technique for answering objections is the "Yes, but . . ." technique. This technique meets objections halfway. The objection may be, "This is the smallest bedroom I've ever seen." The licensee could answer, "Yes, Ms. Buyer, you're right, that is a small bedroom, and I imagine it was intended for a young person. If this were your house, whose bedroom would this be?" You could then continue, "How would you furnish this room for your [son/daughter]?" If buyers can solve their own objections, you have gone a long way toward making a sale.

Forestall objections.   Your experience tells you to expect certain objections from your prospect. Bring up these potential objections before the prospect does. This is known as *forestalling* or *anticipating the objection*. Its effect is to reduce the objection's importance and to show the prospect that you do not fear it. "It could use a new coat of paint. Do you think 10 gallons would do the job?"

When you don't know.   If you don't know the answer to a question, never guess. It is better to say you don't know than to fabricate an answer you are unsure of. Consider this example:

"That's a good question, I'll get the answer for you by___."

Answering a question with a question.   You must handle questions as well as objections. One way to answer a question from a buyer is to use a "hook." This is the technique of answering a question with a question. It prolongs the sales interview and keeps the buyer in the act. Three examples are these:

1. **Question:** Will the sellers agree to an April 1 closing?

   Wrong answer: I'm pretty sure they will.

   Using a hook: Do you want an April 1 closing?

2. **Question:** Will the sellers consider a lower offer?

   Wrong answer: Yes, they've indicated they might listen to an offer.

   Using a hook: How much are you prepared to offer? (If you feel the figure is unreasonable, you should use it as a starting point and attempt to write a more reasonable offer. If you are a buyer's agent, then you should be recommending an offer price and be prepared to justify it.)

3. **Question:** Is the stove (refrigerator, drapery, carpeting) included?

   Wrong answer: I'll ask the seller.

   Using a hook: Do you want the stove (refrigerator, drapery, carpeting) included?

While these using-a-hook answers imply that the prospect will buy, many agents prefer a nail-down approach: "If _____, would you buy this property?" They have asked for something and the agent is asking, "If you got it, would you buy?"

Listen and minimize.   When the property meets most of the buyer's expressed needs, you can summarize benefits and attempt to minimize or overcome the objections. As an example:

This property is nearly perfect for your family.

- It is located in the Newport school district that you indicated you desired.

- It has the formal dining room you said was essential.

- It has the sunlit patio off the kitchen that you liked in the first house I showed you.

- Its size meets all your requirements: 3 bedrooms, 2½ baths, and a 3-car garage.

- The price falls within the guidelines you indicated.

- The condition, I am sure you will agree, is pristine.

- Is my analysis correct except that you don't like the tile in the kitchen and bath and that the light fixture in the dining room is way too small?

If the owner agrees with your analysis, you have emphasized the positive features and exposed the negative features in a way that tends to make them manageable. You might want to continue with, "What do you think it would cost to . . .?" You could then say, "I think an offer for this property would make sense, don't you agree?"

Attempt a Trial Close

If a salesperson successfully builds each part of the sale throughout the presentation, the close will come easily. In many cases, the buyer's reaction says, "I'm ready to make an offer." There is a psychological moment for a **trial close**, but it varies with each transaction.

Attempting a trial close often is called "test and heat." To close any sale and get the buyers' signatures on the deposit receipt, do what your great-grandmother did with the old-fashioned flatiron—test and heat. If the customer is not ready to buy, add a little "heat." This means that you present new evidence or reiterate key sales points and try again.

> With a trial close, you get the buyers to agree to something that indicates they are willing to buy.

Beginning with the first interview, the salesperson must build for this moment during every phase of the sale, because the buyer may make a decision at any time. Although all situations and all buyers are different, the following six basic closing principles can be set forth:

- Throughout the sale, use "you" and "yours" or the customers' name

- Obtain agreement on a variety of things throughout the interview

- Tell a complete story in terms of a customer's buying motives; turn the features into personal benefits and hold some talking points in reserve

- Watch for buying signals

- Say, "Let's go back to the office and see what it looks like on paper"

- Ask for their signatures if they do not volunteer to sign

Closing Techniques

Six basic closing techniques often are employed: the assumptive close, the positive choice, inducement, fear of loss, narrative, and asking for the deposit. Of course, there are hundreds of variations on these closing techniques.

Assumptive close (physical action close).   In an **assumptive close**, you assume the buyer is going to buy and you complete the deposit receipt form. This close is a natural follow-through when a buyer flashes a buying-signal question such as "Can I get possession by July 1?" You should respond, "Would you like possession by July 1? We can certainly ask for it . . ."

Other assumptive closings to consider when you are getting a positive feedback include the following:

Does 30 days for closing meet your needs? (If the answer is affirmative or another date is given, you should be writing this offer.)

The property is listed at [$], but you as the buyer decide what you wish to offer. Would you want to offer [$] and be sure you have this home, or would you want to offer a different amount? (If you are a buyer's agent, you should suggest an offer price and be prepared to justify the price with comparables.)

I think we have found your new home; let's put it on paper.

Another approach to the assumptive close would be to talk about the next steps as if the offer were signed.

When we receive confirmation of your offer, we will immediately begin finalizing the loan as well as arrange for a property inspection.

A positive choice is a choice of two factors, either of which indicate a purchase.

Positive choice.   Give the buyer a **positive choice**—that is, a choice between two things rather than between something and nothing. The skillful salesperson never asks the buyer a question that can be answered with a flat "no." Here are two examples of positive-choice questions:

Would you prefer government-backed financing with a lower down payment and higher monthly payments or conventional financing with a higher down payment and lower monthly payments?

If the seller will retile the kitchen floor, what size tile do you prefer, 18- or 20-inch?

You have seen [three] houses you really like. Which one do you feel you would be happiest in? Why? Let's see if we can make this your home.

Inducement.   If used properly, an **inducement** can be a powerful stimulant to a close. For example, consider these:

> If you buy now, I believe we can lock in the current (3.6%) interest rate. You would like a 3.6% rate, wouldn't you?

> I'm sure we could arrange the closing of escrow so you will not make double payments. You would like to save that money, wouldn't you?

Be careful when you use this technique. If the outcome of the sale hinges on a lower interest rate, a change of tile, or an added refrigerator and you cannot deliver, you may lose the sale. Try to hedge on your commitment by saying that you will do your best to obtain the inducement.

Fear of loss.   The *fear-of-loss method*, often called the *standing-room-only technique*, is effective only if it is based on fact. Buyers have built up an immunity to such statements as this: "This is the last house in this plot, and the builder doesn't plan any further development." This technique works only if it is based on facts concerning a personal, immediate, and real situation.

Here is an example of a believable fear-of-loss close that is true and is based on researched facts:

> This is the last home by this builder available in this tract. All the others are sold. When the new tract is open, the price will be $20,000 higher for the same home. Wouldn't you rather buy now and save that amount?

When a prospective buyer has made an offer or offers on other properties but lost out to other bidders, fear of loss is a strong motivation to act now. Again, it must be based on fact. "Another agent will be showing this property to an interested couple at 3:30 pm today. If you are interested in this property, I suggest an offer right now that can be accepted before the couple sees this home."

Narrative.   A *narrative close*, or storybook close, involves the use of a third party as an ally. If you are able to produce third-party verification of the fact you are trying to establish, the buyer is likely to accept what you say. For example, you could show a newspaper article stating that interest rates are expected to rise. In this situation, someone else is conveying the information. For example, the buyer may express a concern about some aspect of the property. Use the time-tested "feel, felt, found" technique. The agent might say, "I can appreciate how you FEEL; many of our clients have FELT the same way, but after examining it further, they have FOUND that . . ." Or you could say, "Mr. Jones just down the street had a question similar to yours. We were able to find a solution for him. If you wish, we can call him to verify my story."

If you live in the area, let the buyers know and explain the reasons you chose the location. This will add positive reinforcement for a choice.

Always use real experiences. From interfacing with other agents, you will find out about their experiences and how issues were resolved to the satisfaction of clients.

Ask for the deposit.   Many salespeople do an excellent job of making a presentation and even covering all objections, but they are hesitant to ask for the sale. The reason is fear; they get a battlefield fear sensation. They fear a rejection, a "no" answer. Consequently, they overlook asking or are reluctant to ask for the deposit.

> If you want a positive response, you have to ask first.

Buyers will buy if they are asked to buy, but some salespeople rarely ask. Practice and experiment with asking for the deposit. For example, say, "These units do offer an excellent appreciation potential if you're willing to do some fixing up. Why don't you get started on your investment program now? Will you give me your deposit check and let me get your purchase under way?" It's all right to ask again. A coffee salesman we know once asked a close friend, the owner of a large restaurant, why he had never purchased coffee from him. The reply was, "You never asked!"

If one closing doesn't work, continue to emphasize benefits. Suggest another look at the property and try another closing. If the property fits the buyers' needs, they like the property, and they can afford it, then treat a failure as a "maybe." A little more time might be all it takes.

"Let's jot down the issues you want to address in your offer."

Killing a Sale

A positive sales approach is to ask leading questions, gain agreement throughout the sale, then ask for the offer. A salesperson who does not use a positive approach may be the loser. The sale also can be killed by the following:

- Not listening
- Talking too much and too fast
- Being overeager to sell
- Having incomplete knowledge
- Using high-pressure tactics
- Exhibiting fear
- Criticizing competitors
- Straying from the subject
- Displaying a negative selling attitude
- Being argumentative

A Clean Offer

When a buyer is interested but "wants to sleep on it," you should set up a definite appointment, hopefully the next day, for the buyer to make an offer, or continue the home search.

Whenever possible, contingencies should be removed, as should nickel-and-dime items such as "seller to leave the workbench in the garage." Don't deviate from what the seller wants unless absolutely essential. Asking for quicker occupancy could ruin the buyer's chances. To make the offer more desirable, loan qualification information can be attached to the offer. While price is important, a clean sale is also important and a seller is likely to accept a lower offer if the sale appears more certain. Requests for changes can be made after an offer is accepted. While not required to agree to any changes after acceptance, the seller oftentimes will go along with reasonable buyer requests. If the seller counteroffers rather than accepts the offer, then other desired items can be negotiated.

When There Are Other Offers

In the event you have a prospective buyer for a property where another offer has already been made, you could suggest the following tactic to your prospective buyer: An offer for a sum over highest bona fide offer received, such as $5,000, but in no event more than a stated price, which would be the highest price your buyer is willing to pay. If your prospect's offer is accepted, your buyer's offer should allow for verification of the competing offer. This approach assures purchase unless the buyer's maximum has been exceeded.

Buyer Agent Closing

When you are representing the buyer under a buyer-agency agreement, you have a duty to best serve the interests of your principal. Those interests would include finding a house that best meets the needs of your principal at the best price and to protect the buyer against any foreseeable problems. As a buyer's agent, you should have built a trust relationship so you can ask a simple question, "Do you like this house?" and/or "Does this house meet your needs better than anything I have found for you?" Don't ask these questions unless you know the reply will be positive. You could then continue with, "I think we should offer [$] because . . ., and any offer should be contingent upon a professional inspection. Does that make sense to you?" If the response is positive, and it should be, you can begin writing up the offer. Of course, you should justify the offering price based on comparables, changes in market conditions, as well as known facts about the property, and the seller.

ESTIMATED BUYER'S COSTS

When formulating the purchase offer, provide the buyer with the good faith estimate of buyer's acquisition costs—an estimate of the total cash requirements, as well as estimated monthly payments based on the offer (Professional Publishing LLC Form 125 EBECC can be used). Although costs will vary between lenders and escrow companies, you must nevertheless strive to be realistic. Be honest and full in your disclosures. It is best for any error to be on the high side. (Keep in mind that because the dollar amount of real estate transactions is so high, surprises can make people very unhappy.)

Fine-Tuning the Offer

If buyers suggest an offer at an unrealistic price or terms, or both, consider writing up the offer. Before you give it to your prospective buyers to sign, ask the following:

Do you like this house?

You say you like the house, but you want to give an offer that doesn't indicate this. If you were the sellers, what would you think about this offer?

In this market, if you really want this property, I would advise giving your best offer. Raise this offer by just [ ]% and you'll have a chance to be an owner. Let's write it up at [$]. At that price, it is still an exceptional opportunity, and your offer at least will have a fighting chance of being accepted.

Complete this offer and hand it to the prospective buyers, along with a pen.

FIGURE 10.5: Good Faith Estimate of Buyer's Acquisition Costs

---

GOOD FAITH ESTIMATE OF BUYER'S ACQUISITION COSTS
On Acquisition of Property

Prepared by: Agent _____	**Phone** _____
Broker _____	**Email** _____

> **NOTE:** This cost sheet is prepared to assist the buyer to estimate the total cost of acquisition for a property to anticipate the amount of funds likely needed to close, and the source of these funds.
>
> The figures estimated in this cost sheet may vary at the time of closing due to periodic changes in lender demands, escrow fees, other charges and prorates, and thus constitute an opinion, not a guarantee of the preparer.
>
> If acquiring IRC §1031 replacement property, also use a §1031 Profit and Basis Recap Sheet to compute the income tax consequences of the transaction. [See **ft** Form 354]

DATE: _____, 20_____, at _____, California.

1. This is an estimate of acquisition costs and the funds required to close the following transaction:
   ☐ Purchase Agreement   ☐ Exchange agreement   ☐ Counteroffer   ☐ Escrow Instructions   ☐ Option

   1.1 entered into by _____,

   1.2 dated _____, 20_____, at _____, California,

   1.3 regarding real estate referred to as _____

   _____.

2. **EXISTING FINANCING ASSUMED:**

   2.1 First Trust Deed of Record . . . . $_____

   2.2 Second Trust Deed of Record . . . . $_____

   2.3 Other Encumbrances/Liens/Bonds . . . . $_____

   2.4 TOTAL Encumbrances Assumed [lines 2.1 to 2.4] . . . . (+)$0.00 _____

       a. If loan balance adjustments are to be made in cash, the total funds
          required to close escrow at §10 and §12 will vary.

3. **INSTALLMENT SALE FINANCING:**

   3.1 Seller Carryback Financing . . . . (+)$_____

4. **NEW FINANCING ORIGINATED:**

   4.1 New Loan Amount . . . . (+)$_____

   4.2 Points/Discount . . . . $_____

   4.3 Appraisal Fee . . . . $_____

   4.4 Credit Report Fee . . . . $_____

   4.5 Miscellaneous Origination Fees . . . . $_____

   4.6 Prepaid Interest . . . . $_____

   4.7 Mortgage Insurance Premium . . . . $_____

   4.8 Lender's Title Policy Premium . . . . $_____

   4.9 Tax Service Fee . . . . $_____

   4.10 Loan Brokerage Fee . . . . $_____

   4.11 Other _____ . . . . $_____

   4.12 TOTAL New Financing Costs [lines 4.2 to 4.11] . . . . (+)$0.00 _____

5. **PURCHASE COSTS AND CHARGES:**

   5.1 Assumption Fees (First) . . . . $_____

   5.2 Assumption Fees (Second) . . . . $_____

   5.3 Escrow Fee . . . . $_____

   5.4 Notary Fee . . . . $_____

   5.5 Document Preparation Fee . . . . $_____

   5.6 Recording Fee/Transfer Taxes . . . . $_____

   5.7 Title Insurance Premium . . . . $_____

— — — — — — — — — — — — — — — — — *PAGE ONE OF TWO — FORM 311* — — — — — — — — — — — — — — — — —

FIGURE 10.5 (continued):   Good Faith Estimate of Buyer's Acquisition Costs

— — — — — — — — — — — — — — — — *PAGE TWO OF TWO — FORM 311* — — — — — — — — — — — — — — — —

5.8   Property Condition Reports . . . . $_____

5.9   Cost of Compliance Repairs . . . . $_____

5.10   Other _____ . . . . $_____

5.11   Other _____ . . . . $_____

5.12   TOTAL Closing Costs [lines 5.1 to 5.11]. . . . . (+)$0.00_____

5.13   Down Payment on Price. . . . . (+)$_____

6.   **TOTAL ESTIMATED ACQUISITION COST** [lines 2.4, 3.1, 4.1, 4.12, 5.12 and 5.13] . . . . . (=)$0.00_____

   6.1 No post-closing repairs or renovation cost are included here.

7.   **FUNDS REQUIRED TO CLOSE ESCROW:**

7.1   Down Payment On Price (From line 5.13). . . . . (+)$_____

7.2   Closing Costs (From line 5.12) . . . . (+)$0.00_____

7.3   New Loan Proceeds (From line 4.1) . . . . (+)$_____

7.4   New Financing Costs (From line 4.12) . . . . (+)$0.00_____

7.5   Impounds for New Financing . . . . (+)$_____

7.6   Hazard Insurance Premium . . . . (+)$_____

8.   **PRORATES DUE BUYER AT CLOSE:**

8.1   Unpaid Taxes/Assessments. . . . . $_____

8.2   Interest Accrued and Unpaid . . . . $_____

8.3   Unearned Rental Income. . . . . $_____

8.4   Tenant Security Deposits. . . . . $_____

8.5   TOTAL Prorates Due Buyer [lines 8.1 to 8.4] . . . . (-)$0.00_____

9.   **PRORATES DUE SELLER AT CLOSE:**

9.1   Prepaid Taxes/Assessments . . . . $_____

9.2   Impound Account Balance. . . . . $_____

9.3   Prepaid Homeowners' Assessment . . . . $_____

9.4   Prepaid Ground Lease Rent . . . . $_____

9.5   Unpaid Rents assigned to Buyer . . . . $_____

9.6   Other _____ . . . . $_____

9.7   TOTAL Prorates Due Seller [lines 9.1 to 9.6] . . . . (+)$0.00_____

10.   **TOTAL FUNDS REQUIRED TO CLOSE ESCROW:** [lines 6, 7.1 to 7.6, less 8.5 plus 9.7]. (=)$0.00_____

   10.1   See §2.4.a. adjustments.

11.   **SOURCE OF FUNDS REQUIRED TO CLOSE ESCROW:**

11.1   New First Loan Amount (From line 4.1) . . . . $_____

11.2   New Second Loan Amount (Net loan proceeds). . . . . $_____

11.3   Third-Party Deposits . . . . $_____

11.4   Buyer's Cash . . . . $_____

12.   **TOTAL FUNDS REQUIRED TO CLOSE ESCROW:** (Same as line 10). . . . . (=)$0.00_____

I have prepared this estimate based on my knowledge and readily available data.	I have read and received a copy of this estimate.
Date: _____, 20_____	Date: _____, 20_____
Broker: _____	Buyer's Name: _____
Agent: _____	
DRE #: _____	
	Signature: _____
Signature: _____	Signature: _____

FORM 311   03-11   ©2011 **first tuesday**, P.O. BOX 20069, RIVERSIDE, CA 92516 (800) 794-0494

THE CALIFORNIA RESIDENTIAL PURCHASE AGREEMENT AND JOINT ESCROW INSTRUCTIONS

"An oral contract is not worth the paper it is written on," said Samuel Goldwyn. The California Statute of Frauds stipulates that all real estate sales contracts must be in writing to be enforceable.

When a sale has been consummated and the offer obtained, put everything in writing to avoid costly misunderstanding, bad will, and even litigation in the future. It is essential that the purchase contract include the entire agreement of the parties. There should be no "understood" provisions that are not reduced to writing. Poor draftsmanship of the purchase contract is a significant factor in lawsuits between buyer, seller, and broker, or any combination of the three. Not only must the agreement be complete, but also the parties should fully understand the agreement before signing. Many deposit receipt forms were used in California, and the buyer's offer could be submitted on any of these. However, the number of forms caused a great deal of concern in legal circles and with the California Association of REALTORS® because brokers are seldom attorneys and may be confused by the language employed. As a result, in 1985, the California Association of REALTORS®, in cooperation with the state bar and with the approval of the Bureau of Real Estate, developed a model form, the Residential Purchase Agreement [and Receipt for Deposit], which is now the **California Residential Purchase Agreement and Joint Escrow Instructions**. This form is now widely used in California. (See Figure 10.6.) It is possible to complete your purchase contract online and then print out the contract for signatures. (Other form providers also offer excellent purchasing agreements.)

Content of the Form

Essentially, the form acts as a checklist to ensure that a contract is complete in all respects. The responsible parties must comply with the requirements stipulated to help both parties avoid entangling legal complications. Any changes should be dated and initialed by the principals to the transaction.

FIGURE 10.6:   California Residential Purchase Agreement and Joint Escrow Instructions

(The following form is copyrighted by the California Association of REALTORS®, © 2014, and is reprinted under a limited license with permission. Photocopying or any other reproduction, whether electronic or otherwise, is strictly prohibited.)

CALIFORNIA
ASSOCIATION
OF REALTORS®

**CALIFORNIA
RESIDENTIAL PURCHASE AGREEMENT
AND JOINT ESCROW INSTRUCTIONS**
(C.A.R. Form RPA-CA, Revised 11/14)

Date Prepared: _____
1. **OFFER:**
    A. **THIS IS AN OFFER FROM** _____ ("Buyer").
    B. **THE REAL PROPERTY** to be acquired is _____, situated in
        _____ (City), _____ (County), California, _____ (Zip Code), Assessor's Parcel No. _____ ("Property").
    C. **THE PURCHASE PRICE** offered is _____
        _____ Dollars $ _____.
    D. **CLOSE OF ESCROW** shall occur on _____ (date)(or _____ **Days** After Acceptance).
    E. Buyer and Seller are referred to herein as the "Parties." Brokers are not Parties to this Agreement.
2. **AGENCY:**
    A. **DISCLOSURE:** The Parties each acknowledge receipt of a ☑ "Disclosure Regarding Real Estate Agency Relationships" (C.A.R. Form AD).
    B. **CONFIRMATION:** The following agency relationships are hereby confirmed for this transaction:
        Listing Agent _____ (Print Firm Name) is the agent of (check one):
        ☐ the Seller exclusively; or ☐ both the Buyer and Seller.
        Selling Agent _____ (Print Firm Name) (if not the same as the
        Listing Agent) is the agent of (check one): ☐ the Buyer exclusively; or ☐ the Seller exclusively; or ☐ both the Buyer and Seller.
    C. **POTENTIALLY COMPETING BUYERS AND SELLERS:** The Parties each acknowledge receipt of a ☑ "Possible Representation
        of More than One Buyer or Seller - Disclosure and Consent" (C.A.R. Form PRBS).
3. **FINANCE TERMS:** Buyer represents that funds will be good when deposited with Escrow Holder.
    A. **INITIAL DEPOSIT**: Deposit shall be in the amount of .... $ _____
        (1) Buyer Direct Deposit: Buyer shall deliver deposit directly to Escrow Holder by electronic funds
        transfer, ☐ cashier's check, ☐ personal check, ☐ other _____ within 3 business days
        after Acceptance (or _____);
        OR (2) ☐ **Buyer Deposit with Agent:** Buyer has given the deposit by personal check (or _____)
        to the agent submitting the offer (or to _____), made payable to
        _____. The deposit shall be held uncashed until Acceptance and then deposited
        with Escrow Holder within **3** business days after Acceptance (or _____).
        Deposit checks given to agent shall be an original signed check and not a copy.
        (Note: Initial and increased deposits checks received by agent shall be recorded in Broker's trust fund log.)
    B. **INCREASED DEPOSIT:** Buyer shall deposit with Escrow Holder an increased deposit in the amount of ....$ _____
        within _____ **Days** After Acceptance (or _____).
        If the Parties agree to liquidated damages in this Agreement, they also agree to incorporate the increased
        deposit into the liquidated damages amount in a separate liquidated damages clause (C.A.R. Form RID)
        at the time the increased deposit is delivered to Escrow Holder.
    C. ☐ **ALL CASH OFFER:** No loan is needed to purchase the Property. This offer is NOT contingent on Buyer
        obtaining a loan. Written verification of sufficient funds to close this transaction IS ATTACHED to this offer
        or ☐ Buyer shall, within **3 (or _____) Days** After Acceptance, Deliver to Seller such verification.
    D. **LOAN(S):**
        (1) FIRST LOAN: in the amount of .... $ _____
        This loan will be conventional financing or ☐ FHA, ☐ VA, ☐ Seller financing (C.A.R. Form SFA),
        ☐ assumed financing (C.A.R. Form AFA), ☐ Other _____ This loan shall be at a fixed
        rate not to exceed _____% or, ☐ an adjustable rate loan with initial rate not to exceed _____%.
        Regardless of the type of loan, Buyer shall pay points not to exceed _____% of the loan amount.
        (2) ☐ **SECOND LOAN** in the amount of .... $ _____
        This loan will be conventional financing or ☐ Seller financing (C.A.R. Form SFA), ☐ assumed
        financing (C.A.R. Form AFA), ☐ Other _____. This loan shall be at a fixed rate not to
        exceed _____% or, ☐ an adjustable rate loan with initial rate not to exceed _____%. Regardless of
        the type of loan, Buyer shall pay points not to exceed _____% of the loan amount.
        (3) FHA/VA: For any FHA or VA loan specified in 3D(1), Buyer has **17 (or ___) Days** After Acceptance
        to Deliver to Seller written notice (C.A.R. Form FVA) of any lender-required repairs or costs that
        Buyer requests Seller to pay for or otherwise correct. Seller has no obligation to pay or satisfy lender
        requirements unless agreed in writing. A FHA/VA amendatory clause (C.A.R. Form FVAC) shall be a
        part of this transaction.
    E. **ADDITIONAL FINANCING TERMS:** _____
        _____
    F. **BALANCE OF DOWN PAYMENT OR PURCHASE PRICE** in the amount of.......................................$ _____
        to be deposited with Escrow Holder pursuant to Escrow Holder instructions.
    G. **PURCHASE PRICE (TOTAL):** ....$ _____

Buyer's Initials (_____)(_____)   Seller's Initials (_____)(_____)

RPA-CA REVISED 11/14 (PAGE 1 OF 10) Print Date

EQUAL HOUSING OPPORTUNITY

CALIFORNIA RESIDENTIAL PURCHASE AGREEMENT (RPA-CA PAGE 1 OF 10)

FIGURE 10.6 (continued):   California Residential Purchase Agreement and Joint Escrow Instructions

Property Address: _____   Date: _____

- **H. VERIFICATION OF DOWN PAYMENT AND CLOSING COSTS:** Buyer (or Buyer's lender or loan broker pursuant to paragraph 3J(1)) shall, within **3 (or ___) Days** After Acceptance, Deliver to Seller written verification of Buyer's down payment and closing costs. (☐ Verification attached.)
- **I. APPRAISAL CONTINGENCY AND REMOVAL:** This Agreement is (or ☐ is NOT) contingent upon a written appraisal of the Property by a licensed or certified appraiser at no less than the purchase price. Buyer shall, as specified in paragraph 14B(3), in writing, remove the appraisal contingency or cancel this Agreement within **17 (or ___) Days** After Acceptance.
- **J. LOAN TERMS:**
  - **(1) LOAN APPLICATIONS:** Within **3 (or ___) Days** After Acceptance, Buyer shall Deliver to Seller a letter from Buyer's lender or loan broker stating that, based on a review of Buyer's written application and credit report, Buyer is prequalified or preapproved for any NEW loan specified in paragraph 3D. If any loan specified in paragraph 3D is an adjustable rate loan, the prequalification or preapproval letter shall be based on the qualifying rate, not the initial loan rate. (☐ Letter attached.)
  - **(2) LOAN CONTINGENCY:** Buyer shall act diligently and in good faith to obtain the designated loan(s). Buyer's qualification for the loan(s) specified above **is a contingency** of this Agreement unless otherwise agreed in writing. If there is no appraisal contingency or the appraisal contingency has been waived or removed, then failure of the Property to appraise at the purchase price does not entitle Buyer to exercise the cancellation right pursuant to the loan contingency if Buyer is otherwise qualified for the specified loan. Buyer's contractual obligations regarding deposit, balance of down payment and closing costs **are not contingencies** of this Agreement.
  - **(3) LOAN CONTINGENCY REMOVAL:**
    Within **21 (or ___) Days** After Acceptance, Buyer shall, as specified in paragraph 14, in writing, remove the loan contingency or cancel this Agreement. If there is an appraisal contingency, removal of the loan contingency shall not be deemed removal of the appraisal contingency.
  - **(4)** ☐ **NO LOAN CONTINGENCY:** Obtaining any loan specified above is NOT a contingency of this Agreement. If Buyer does not obtain the loan and as a result does not purchase the Property, Seller may be entitled to Buyer's deposit or other legal remedies.
  - **(5) LENDER LIMITS ON BUYER CREDITS:** Any credit to Buyer, from any source, for closing or other costs that is agreed to by the Parties ("Contractual Credit") shall be disclosed to Buyer's lender. If the total credit allowed by Buyer's lender ("Lender Allowable Credit") is less than the Contractual Credit, then (i) the Contractual Credit shall be reduced to the Lender Allowable Credit, and (ii) in the absence of a separate written agreement between the Parties, there shall be no automatic adjustment to the purchase price to make up for the difference between the Contractual Credit and the Lender Allowable Credit.
- **K. BUYER STATED FINANCING:** Seller is relying on Buyer's representation of the type of financing specified (including but not limited to, as applicable, all cash, amount of down payment, or contingent or non-contingent loan). Seller has agreed to a specific closing date, purchase price and to sell to Buyer in reliance on Buyer's covenant concerning financing. Buyer shall pursue the financing specified in this Agreement. Seller has no obligation to cooperate with Buyer's efforts to obtain any financing other than that specified in the Agreement and the availability of any such alternate financing does not excuse Buyer from the obligation to purchase the Property and close escrow as specified in this Agreement.
- **4. SALE OF BUYER'S PROPERTY:**
  - **A.** This Agreement and Buyer's ability to obtain financing are NOT contingent upon the sale of any property owned by Buyer.
- **OR   B.** ☐ This Agreement and Buyer's ability to obtain financing are contingent upon the sale of property owned by Buyer as specified in the attached addendum (C.A.R. Form COP).
- **5. ADDENDA AND ADVISORIES:**
  - A. ADDENDA: ☐ Addendum #_____(C.A.R. Form ADM)
    - ☐ Back Up Offer Addendum (C.A.R. Form BUO)   ☐ Court Confirmation Addendum (C.A.R. Form CCA)
    - ☐ Septic, Well and Property Monument Addendum (C.A.R. Form SWPI)
    - ☐ Short Sale Addendum (C.A.R. Form SSA)   ☐ Other _____

  - B. BUYER AND SELLER ADVISORIES: ☑ Buyer's Inspection Advisory (C.A.R. Form BIA)
    - ☐ Probate Advisory (C.A.R. Form PAK)   ☐ Statewide Buyer and Seller Advisory (C.A.R. Form SBSA)
    - ☐ Trust Advisory (C.A.R. Form TA)   ☐ REO Advisory (C.A.R. Form REO)
    - ☐ Short Sale Information and Advisory (C.A.R. Form SSIA) ☐ Other _____
- **6. OTHER TERMS:**_____
  _____
  _____
  _____

- **7. ALLOCATION OF COSTS**
  - **A. INSPECTIONS, REPORTS AND CERTIFICATES:** Unless otherwise agreed in writing, this paragraph only determines who is to pay for the inspection, test, certificate or service ("Report") mentioned; it **does not determine who is to pay for any work recommended or identified in the Report.**
    - **(1)** ☐ Buyer ☐ Seller shall pay for a natural hazard zone disclosure report, including tax ☐ environmental ☐ Other: _____
      _____ prepared by _____.
    - **(2)** ☐ Buyer ☐ Seller shall pay for the following Report _____
      prepared by_____.
    - **(3)** ☐ Buyer ☐ Seller shall pay for the following Report _____
      prepared by _____.

Buyer's Initials (_____)(_____)   Seller's Initials (_____)(_____)

RPA-CA REVISED 11/14 (PAGE 2 OF 10) Print Date

CALIFORNIA RESIDENTIAL PURCHASE AGREEMENT (RPA-CA PAGE 2 OF 10)

FIGURE 10.6 (continued):   California Residential Purchase Agreement and Joint Escrow Instructions

Property Address: _____   Date: _____

B.   GOVERNMENT REQUIREMENTS AND RETROFIT:

(1) ☐ Buyer ☐ Seller shall pay for smoke alarm and carbon monoxide device installation and water heater bracing, if required by Law. Prior to Close Of Escrow ("COE"), Seller shall provide Buyer written statement(s) of compliance in accordance with state and local Law, unless Seller is exempt.

(2) (i) ☐ Buyer ☐ Seller shall pay the cost of compliance with any other minimum mandatory government inspections and reports if required as a condition of closing escrow under any Law.

(ii) ☐ Buyer ☐ Seller shall pay the cost of compliance with any other minimum mandatory government retrofit standards required as a condition of closing escrow under any Law, whether the work is required to be completed before or after COE.

(iii) Buyer shall be provided, within the time specified in paragraph 14A, a copy of any required government conducted or point-of-sale inspection report prepared pursuant to this Agreement or in anticipation of this sale of the Property.

C.   ESCROW AND TITLE:

(1) (a) ☐ Buyer ☐ Seller shall pay escrow fee _____

(b) Escrow Holder shall be _____.

(c) The Parties shall, within **5 (or ___) Days** After receipt, sign and return Escrow Holder's general provisions.

(2) (a) ☐ Buyer ☐ Seller shall pay for **owner's** title insurance policy specified in paragraph 13E _____

(b) Owner's title policy to be issued by _____.

(Buyer shall pay for any title insurance policy insuring Buyer's **lender**, unless otherwise agreed in writing.)

D.   OTHER COSTS:

(1) ☐ Buyer ☐ Seller shall pay County transfer tax or fee _____.

(2) ☐ Buyer ☐ Seller shall pay City transfer tax or fee _____.

(3) ☐ Buyer ☐ Seller shall pay Homeowners' Association ("HOA") transfer fee _____.

(4) Seller shall pay HOA fees for preparing documents required to be delivered by Civil Code §4525.

(5) ☐ Buyer ☐ Seller shall pay HOA fees for preparing all documents other than those required by Civil Code §4525.

(6) Buyer to pay for any HOA certification fee.

(7) ☐ Buyer ☐ Seller shall pay for any private transfer fee _____.

(8) ☐ Buyer ☐ Seller shall pay for _____.

(9) ☐ Buyer ☐ Seller shall pay for _____.

(10) ☐ Buyer ☐ Seller shall pay for the cost, not to exceed $ _____, of a standard (or ☐ upgraded) one-year home warranty plan, issued by _____, with the following optional coverages: ☐ Air Conditioner ☐ Pool/Spa ☐ Other: _____.

Buyer is informed that home warranty plans have many optional coverages in addition to those listed above. Buyer is advised to investigate these coverages to determine those that may be suitable for Buyer.

OR ☐ **Buyer waives the purchase of a home warranty plan. Nothing in this paragraph precludes Buyer's purchasing a home warranty plan during the term of this Agreement.**

8.   ITEMS INCLUDED IN AND EXCLUDED FROM SALE:

A.   NOTE TO BUYER AND SELLER: Items listed as included or excluded in the MLS, flyers or marketing materials are **not** included in the purchase price or excluded from the sale unless specified in paragraph 8 B or C.

B.   ITEMS INCLUDED IN SALE: Except as otherwise specified or disclosed,

(1) All EXISTING fixtures and fittings that are attached to the Property;

(2) EXISTING electrical, mechanical, lighting, plumbing and heating fixtures, ceiling fans, fireplace inserts, gas logs and grates, solar power systems, built-in appliances, window and door screens, awnings, shutters, window coverings, attached floor coverings, television antennas, satellite dishes, air coolers/conditioners, pool/spa equipment, garage door openers/remote controls, mailbox, in-ground landscaping, trees/shrubs, water features and fountains, water softeners, water purifiers, security systems/alarms and the following if checked: ☐ all stove(s), except _____; ☐ all refrigerator(s) except _____; ☐ all washer(s) and dryer(s), except _____;

(3) The following additional items: _____

(4) Existing integrated phone and home automation systems, including necessary components such as intranet and Internet-connected hardware or devices, control units (other than non-dedicated mobile devices, electronics and computers) and applicable software, permissions, passwords, codes and access information, are (☐ are NOT) included in the sale.

(5)   LEASED OR LIENED ITEMS AND SYSTEMS: Seller shall, within the time specified in paragraph 14A, (i) disclose to Buyer if any item or system specified in paragraph 8B or otherwise included in the sale is leased, or not owned by Seller, or specifically subject to a lien or other encumbrance, and (ii) Deliver to Buyer all written materials (such as lease, warranty, etc.) concerning any such item. Buyer's ability to assume any such lease, or willingness to accept the Property subject to any such lien or encumbrance, is a contingency in favor of Buyer and Seller as specified in paragraph 14B and C.

(6) Seller represents that all items included in the purchase price, unless otherwise specified, (i) are owned by Seller and shall be transferred free and clear of liens and encumbrances, except the items and systems identified pursuant to 8B(4) and _____ , and (ii) are transferred without Seller warranty regardless of value.

C.   ITEMS EXCLUDED FROM SALE: Unless otherwise specified, the following items are excluded from sale: (i) audio and video components (such as flat screen TVs, speakers and other items) if any such item is not itself attached to the Property, even if a bracket or other mechanism attached to the component or item is attached to the Property; (ii) furniture and other items secured to the Property for earthquake purposes; and (iii) _____

_____. **Brackets attached to walls, floors or ceilings for any such component, furniture or item shall remain with the Property (or** ☐ **will be removed and holes or other damage shall be repaired, but not painted).**

Buyer's Initials (_____)(_____)   Seller's Initials (_____)(_____)

RPA-CA REVISED 11/14 (PAGE 3 OF 10) Print Date

CALIFORNIA RESIDENTIAL PURCHASE AGREEMENT (RPA-CA PAGE 3 OF 10)

FIGURE 10.6 (continued): **California Residential Purchase Agreement and Joint Escrow Instructions**

Property Address: _____   Date: _____

9. **CLOSING AND POSSESSION:**
    A. Buyer intends (or ☐ does not intend) to occupy the Property as Buyer's primary residence.
    B. **Seller-occupied or vacant property:** Possession shall be delivered to Buyer: (i) at 6 PM or (_____ ☐ AM/☐ PM) on the date of Close Of Escrow; (ii) ☐ no later than ___ calendar days after Close Of Escrow; or (iii) ☐ at ____ ☐ AM/☐ PM on _____.
    C. **Seller remaining in possession After Close Of Escrow:** If Seller has the right to remain in possession after Close Of Escrow, (i) the Parties are advised to sign a separate occupancy agreement such as ☐ C.A.R. Form SIP, for Seller continued occupancy of less than 30 days, ☐ C.A.R. Form RLAS for Seller continued occupancy of 30 days or more; and (ii) the Parties are advised to consult with their insurance and legal advisors for information about liability and damage or injury to persons and personal and real property; and (iii) Buyer is advised to consult with Buyer's lender about the impact of Seller's occupancy on Buyer's loan.
    D. **Tenant-occupied property: Property shall be vacant** at least **5 (or ___) Days** Prior to Close Of Escrow, unless otherwise agreed in writing. **Note to Seller: If you are unable to deliver Property vacant in accordance with rent control and other applicable Law, you may be in breach of this Agreement.**
        OR ☐ **Tenant to remain in possession** (C.A.R. Form TIP).
    E. At Close Of Escrow, Seller assigns to Buyer any assignable warranty rights for items included in the sale; and Seller shall Deliver to Buyer available Copies of any such warranties. Brokers cannot and will not determine the assignability of any warranties.
    F. At Close Of Escrow, unless otherwise agreed in writing, Seller shall provide keys, passwords, codes and/or means to operate all locks, mailboxes, security systems, alarms, home automation systems and intranet and Internet-connected devices included in the purchase price, and garage door openers. If the Property is a condominium or located in a common interest subdivision, Buyer may be required to pay a deposit to the Homeowners' Association ("HOA") to obtain keys to accessible HOA facilities.

10. **STATUTORY AND OTHER DISCLOSURES (INCLUDING LEAD-BASED PAINT HAZARD DISCLOSURES) AND CANCELLATION RIGHTS:**
    A. **(1)** Seller shall, within the time specified in paragraph 14A, Deliver to Buyer: (i) if required by Law, a fully completed: Federal Lead-Based Paint Disclosures (C.A.R. Form FLD) and pamphlet ("Lead Disclosures"); and **(ii)** unless exempt, fully completed disclosures or notices required by sections 1102 et. seq. and 1103 et. seq. of the Civil Code ("Statutory Disclosures"). Statutory Disclosures include, but are not limited to, a Real Estate Transfer Disclosure Statement ("TDS"), Natural Hazard Disclosure Statement ("NHD"), notice or actual knowledge of release of illegal controlled substance, notice of special tax and/or assessments (or, if allowed, substantially equivalent notice regarding the Mello-Roos Community Facilities Act of 1982 and Improvement Bond Act of 1915) and, if Seller has actual knowledge, of industrial use and military ordnance location (C.A.R. Form SPQ or SSD).
        (2) Any Statutory Disclosure required by this paragraph is considered fully completed if Seller has answered all questions and completed and signed the Seller section(s) and the Listing Agent, if any, has completed and signed the Listing Broker section(s), or, if applicable, an Agent Visual Inspection Disclosure (C.A.R. Form AVID). Nothing stated herein relieves a Buyer's Broker, if any, from the obligation to (i) conduct a reasonably competent and diligent visual inspection of the accessible areas of the Property and disclose, on Section IV of the TDS, or an AVID, material facts affecting the value or desirability of the Property that were or should have been revealed by such an inspection or (ii) complete any sections on all disclosures required to be completed by Buyer's Broker.
        (3) Note to Buyer and Seller: Waiver of Statutory and Lead Disclosures is prohibited by Law.
        (4) Within the time specified in paragraph 14A, (i) Seller, unless exempt from the obligation to provide a TDS, shall, complete and provide Buyer with a Seller Property Questionnaire (C.A.R. Form SPQ); (ii) if Seller is not required to provide a TDS, Seller shall complete and provide Buyer with a Supplemental Contractual and Statutory Disclosure (C.A.R. Form SSD).
        (5) Buyer shall, within the time specified in paragraph 14B(1), return Signed Copies of the Statutory, Lead and other disclosures to Seller.
        (6) In the event Seller or Listing Broker, prior to Close Of Escrow, becomes aware of adverse conditions materially affecting the Property, or any material inaccuracy in disclosures, information or representations previously provided to Buyer, Seller shall promptly provide a subsequent or amended disclosure or notice, in writing, covering those items. **However, a subsequent or amended disclosure shall not be required for conditions and material inaccuracies** of which Buyer is otherwise aware, or which are **disclosed in reports provided to or obtained by Buyer or ordered and paid for by Buyer.**
        (7) If any disclosure or notice specified in paragraph 10A(1), or subsequent or amended disclosure or notice is Delivered to Buyer after the offer is Signed, Buyer shall have the right to cancel this Agreement within **3 Days** After Delivery in person, or **5 Days** After Delivery by deposit in the mail, by giving written notice of cancellation to Seller or Seller's agent.
    B. **NATURAL AND ENVIRONMENTAL HAZARD DISCLOSURES AND OTHER BOOKLETS:** Within the time specified in paragraph 14A, Seller shall, if required by Law: **(i)** Deliver to Buyer earthquake guide(s) (and questionnaire), environmental hazards booklet, and home energy rating pamphlet; **(ii)** disclose if the Property is located in a Special Flood Hazard Area; Potential Flooding (Inundation) Area; Very High Fire Hazard Zone; State Fire Responsibility Area; Earthquake Fault Zone; and Seismic Hazard Zone; and **(iii)** disclose any other zone as required by Law and provide any other information required for those zones.
    C. **WITHHOLDING TAXES:** Within the time specified in paragraph 14A, to avoid required withholding, Seller shall Deliver to Buyer or qualified substitute, an affidavit sufficient to comply with federal (FIRPTA) and California withholding Law (C.A.R. Form AS or QS).
    D. **MEGAN'S LAW DATABASE DISCLOSURE:** Notice: Pursuant to Section 290.46 of the Penal Code, information about specified registered sex offenders is made available to the public via an Internet Web site maintained by the Department of Justice at **www.meganslaw.ca.gov**. Depending on an offender's criminal history, this information will include either the address at which the offender resides or the community of residence and ZIP Code in which he or she resides. (Neither Seller nor Brokers are required to check this website. If Buyer wants further information, Broker recommends that Buyer obtain information from this website during Buyer's inspection contingency period. Brokers do not have expertise in this area.)
    E. **NOTICE REGARDING GAS AND HAZARDOUS LIQUID TRANSMISSION PIPELINES:** This notice is being provided simply to inform you that information about the general location of gas and hazardous liquid transmission pipelines is available to the public via the National Pipeline Mapping System (NPMS) Internet Web site maintained by the United States Department of Transportation at **http://www.npms.phmsa.dot.gov/**. To seek further information about possible transmission pipelines near the Property, you may contact your local gas utility or other pipeline operators in the area. Contact information for pipeline operators is searchable by ZIP Code and county on the NPMS Internet Web site.

Buyer's Initials (_____)(_____)   Seller's Initials (_____)(_____)

RPA-CA REVISED 11/14 (PAGE 4 OF 10) Print Date
CALIFORNIA RESIDENTIAL PURCHASE AGREEMENT (RPA-CA PAGE 4 OF 10)

FIGURE 10.6 (continued):   California Residential Purchase Agreement and Joint Escrow Instructions

Property Address: _____   Date: _____

F. CONDOMINIUM/PLANNED DEVELOPMENT DISCLOSURES:
(1) SELLER HAS: 7 (or ___) Days After Acceptance to disclose to Buyer if the Property is a condominium, or is located in a planned development or other common interest subdivision (C.A.R. Form SPQ or SSD).
(2) If the Property is a condominium or is located in a planned development or other common interest subdivision, Seller has **3 (or ___) Days** After Acceptance to request from the HOA (C.A.R. Form HOA1): **(i)** Copies of any documents required by Law; **(ii)** disclosure of any pending or anticipated claim or litigation by or against the HOA; **(iii)** a statement containing the location and number of designated parking and storage spaces; **(iv)** Copies of the most recent 12 months of HOA minutes for regular and special meetings; and **(v)** the names and contact information of all HOAs governing the Property (collectively, "CI Disclosures"). Seller shall itemize and Deliver to Buyer all CI Disclosures received from the HOA and any CI Disclosures in Seller's possession. Buyer's approval of CI Disclosures is a contingency of this Agreement as specified in paragraph 14B(3). The Party specified in paragraph 7, as directed by escrow, shall deposit funds into escrow or direct to HOA or management company to pay for any of the above.
11. CONDITION OF PROPERTY: Unless otherwise agreed in writing: **(i)** the Property is sold (a) "AS-IS" in its PRESENT physical condition as of the date of Acceptance and (b) subject to Buyer's Investigation rights; **(ii)** the Property, including pool, spa, landscaping and grounds, is to be maintained in substantially the same condition as on the date of Acceptance; and **(iii)** all debris and personal property not included in the sale shall be removed by Close Of Escrow.
  A. Seller shall, within the time specified in paragraph 14A, DISCLOSE KNOWN MATERIAL FACTS AND DEFECTS affecting the Property, including known insurance claims within the past five years, and make any and all other disclosures required by law.
  B. Buyer has the right to conduct Buyer Investigations of the Property and, as specified in paragraph 14B, based upon information discovered in those investigations: (i) cancel this Agreement; or (ii) request that Seller make Repairs or take other action.
  C. Buyer is strongly advised to conduct investigations of the entire Property in order to determine its present condition. Seller may not be aware of all defects affecting the Property or other factors that Buyer considers important. Property improvements may not be built according to code, in compliance with current Law, or have had permits issued.
12. BUYER'S INVESTIGATION OF PROPERTY AND MATTERS AFFECTING PROPERTY:
  A. Buyer's acceptance of the condition of, and any other matter affecting the Property, is a contingency of this Agreement as specified in this paragraph and paragraph 14B. Within the time specified in paragraph 14B(1), Buyer shall have the right, at Buyer's expense unless otherwise agreed, to conduct inspections, investigations, tests, surveys and other studies ("Buyer Investigations"), including, but not limited to, the right to: **(i)** inspect for lead-based paint and other lead-based paint hazards; **(ii)** inspect for wood destroying pests and organisms. Any inspection for wood destroying pests and organisms shall be prepared by a registered Structural Pest Control company; shall cover the main building and attached structures; may cover detached structures; shall NOT include water tests of shower pans on upper level units unless the owners of property below the shower consent; shall NOT include roof coverings; and, if the Property is a unit in a condominium or other common interest subdivision, the inspection shall include only the separate interest and any exclusive-use areas being transferred, and shall NOT include common areas; and shall include a report ("Pest Control Report") showing the findings of the company which shall be separated into sections for evident infestation or infections (Section 1) and for conditions likely to lead to infestation or infection (Section 2); **(iii)** review the registered sex offender database; **(iv)** confirm the insurability of Buyer and the Property including the availability and cost of flood and fire insurance; **(v)** review and seek approval of leases that may need to be assumed by Buyer; and **(vi)** satisfy Buyer as to any matter specified in the attached Buyer's Inspection Advisory (C.A.R. Form BIA). Without Seller's prior written consent, Buyer shall neither make nor cause to be made: (i) invasive or destructive Buyer Investigations except for minimally invasive testing required to prepare a Pest Control Report; or (ii) inspections by any governmental building or zoning inspector or government employee, unless required by Law.
  B. Seller shall make the Property available for all Buyer Investigations. Buyer shall **(i)** as specified in paragraph 14B, complete Buyer Investigations and either remove the contingency or cancel this Agreement, and **(ii)** give Seller, at no cost, complete Copies of all such Investigation reports obtained by Buyer, which obligation shall survive the termination of this Agreement.
  C. Seller shall have water, gas, electricity and all operable pilot lights on for Buyer's Investigations and through the date possession is made available to Buyer.
  D. Buyer indemnity and seller protection for entry upon property: Buyer shall: **(i)** keep the Property free and clear of liens; **(ii)** repair all damage arising from Buyer Investigations; and **(iii)** indemnify and hold Seller harmless from all resulting liability, claims, demands, damages and costs. Buyer shall carry, or Buyer shall require anyone acting on Buyer's behalf to carry, policies of liability, workers' compensation and other applicable insurance, defending and protecting Seller from liability for any injuries to persons or property occurring during any Buyer Investigations or work done on the Property at Buyer's direction prior to Close Of Escrow. Seller is advised that certain protections may be afforded Seller by recording a "Notice of Non-Responsibility" (C.A.R. Form NNR) for Buyer Investigations and work done on the Property at Buyer's direction. Buyer's obligations under this paragraph shall survive the termination of this Agreement.
13. TITLE AND VESTING:
  A. Within the time specified in paragraph 14, Buyer shall be provided a current preliminary title report ("Preliminary Report"). The Preliminary Report is only an offer by the title insurer to issue a policy of title insurance and may not contain every item affecting title. Buyer's review of the Preliminary Report and any other matters which may affect title are a contingency of this Agreement as specified in paragraph 14B. The company providing the Preliminary Report shall, prior to issuing a Preliminary Report, conduct a search of the General Index for all Sellers except banks or other institutional lenders selling properties they acquired through foreclosure (REOs), corporations, and government entities. Seller shall within 7 Days After Acceptance, give Escrow Holder a completed Statement of Information.
  B. Title is taken in its present condition subject to all encumbrances, easements, covenants, conditions, restrictions, rights and other matters, whether of record or not, as of the date of Acceptance except for: **(i)** monetary liens of record (which Seller is obligated to pay off) unless Buyer is assuming those obligations or taking the Property subject to those obligations; and **(ii)** those matters which Seller has agreed to remove in writing.
  C. Within the time specified in paragraph 14A, Seller has a duty to disclose to Buyer all matters known to Seller affecting title, whether of record or not.
  D. At Close Of Escrow, Buyer shall receive a grant deed conveying title (or, for stock cooperative or long-term lease, an assignment of stock certificate or of Seller's leasehold interest), including oil, mineral and water rights if currently owned by Seller. Title shall vest as designated in Buyer's supplemental escrow instructions. THE MANNER OF TAKING TITLE MAY HAVE SIGNIFICANT LEGAL AND TAX CONSEQUENCES. CONSULT AN APPROPRIATE PROFESSIONAL.

Buyer's Initials (_____)(_____)   Seller's Initials (_____)(_____)

RPA-CA REVISED 11/14 (PAGE 5 OF 10) Print Date
CALIFORNIA RESIDENTIAL PURCHASE AGREEMENT (RPA-CA PAGE 5 OF 10)

FIGURE 10.6 (continued):   California Residential Purchase Agreement and Joint Escrow Instructions

Property Address: _____   Date: _____

E.   Buyer shall receive a CLTA/ALTA "Homeowner's Policy of Title Insurance", if applicable to the type of property and buyer. If not, Escrow Holder shall notify Buyer. A title company can provide information about the availability, coverage, and cost of other title policies and endorsements. If the Homeowner's Policy is not available, Buyer shall choose another policy, instruct Escrow Holder in writing and shall pay any increase in cost.

14. **TIME PERIODS; REMOVAL OF CONTINGENCIES; CANCELLATION RIGHTS: The following time periods may only be extended, altered, modified or changed by mutual written agreement. Any removal of contingencies or cancellation under this paragraph by either Buyer or Seller must be exercised in good faith and in writing (C.A.R. Form CR or CC).**

A.   **SELLER HAS: 7 (or ___) Days** After Acceptance to Deliver to Buyer all Reports, disclosures and information for which Seller is responsible under paragraphs 5, 6, 7, 8B(4), 10A, B, C, and F, 11A and 13A. If, by the time specified, Seller has not Delivered any such item, Buyer after first Delivering to Seller a Notice to Seller to Perform (C.A.R. Form NSP) may cancel this Agreement.

B.   **(1) BUYER HAS: 17 (or ___) Days** After Acceptance, unless otherwise agreed in writing, to:

(i) complete all Buyer Investigations; review all disclosures, reports, lease documents to be assumed by Buyer pursuant to paragraph 8B(4), and other applicable information, which Buyer receives from Seller; and approve all matters affecting the Property; and **(ii)** Deliver to Seller Signed Copies of Statutory and Lead Disclosures and other disclosures Delivered by Seller in accordance with paragraph 10A.

(2) Within the time specified in paragraph 14B(1), Buyer may request that Seller make repairs or take any other action regarding the Property (C.A.R. Form RR). Seller has no obligation to agree to or respond to (C.A.R. Form RRRR) Buyer's requests.

(3) By the end of the time specified in paragraph 14B(1) (or as otherwise specified in this Agreement), Buyer shall Deliver to Seller a removal of the applicable contingency or cancellation (C.A.R. Form CR or CC) of this Agreement. However, if any report, disclosure or information for which Seller is responsible is not Delivered within the time specified in paragraph 14A, then Buyer has **5 (or ___) Days** After Delivery of any such items, or the time specified in paragraph 14B(1), whichever is later, to Deliver to Seller a removal of the applicable contingency or cancellation of this Agreement.

(4) Continuation of Contingency: Even after the end of the time specified in paragraph 14B(1) and before Seller cancels, if at all, pursuant to paragraph 14C, Buyer retains the right, in writing, to either (i) remove remaining contingencies, or (ii) cancel this Agreement based on a remaining contingency. Once Buyer's written removal of all contingencies is Delivered to Seller, Seller may not cancel this Agreement pursuant to paragraph 14C(1).

C.   **SELLER RIGHT TO CANCEL:**

(1) Seller right to Cancel; Buyer Contingencies: If, by the time specified in this Agreement, Buyer does not Deliver to Seller a removal of the applicable contingency or cancellation of this Agreement, then Seller, after first Delivering to Buyer a Notice to Buyer to Perform (C.A.R. Form NBP), may cancel this Agreement. In such event, Seller shall authorize the return of Buyer's deposit, except for fees incurred by Buyer.

(2) Seller right to Cancel; Buyer Contract Obligations: Seller, after first delivering to Buyer a NBP, may cancel this Agreement if, by the time specified in this Agreement, Buyer does not take the following action(s): **(i)** Deposit funds as required by paragraph 3A, or 3B or if the funds deposited pursuant to paragraph 3A or 3B are not good when deposited; **(ii)** Deliver a notice of FHA or VA costs or terms as required by paragraph 3D(3) (C.A.R. Form FVA); **(iii)** Deliver a letter as required by paragraph 3J(1); **(iv)** Deliver verification, or a satisfactory verification if Seller reasonably disapproves of the verification already provided, as required by paragraph 3C or 3H; **(v)** In writing assume or accept leases or liens specified in 8B5; **(vi)** Return Statutory and Lead Disclosures as required by paragraph 10A(5); or **(vii)** Sign or initial a separate liquidated damages form for an increased deposit as required by paragraphs 3B and 21B; or **(viii)** Provide evidence of authority to sign in a representative capacity as specified in paragraph 19. In such event, Seller shall authorize the return of Buyer's deposit, except for fees incurred by Buyer.

D.   **NOTICE TO BUYER OR SELLER TO PERFORM:** The NBP or NSP shall: **(i)** be in writing; **(ii)** be signed by the applicable Buyer or Seller; and **(iii)** give the other Party at least **2 (or ___) Days** After Delivery (or until the time specified in the applicable paragraph, whichever occurs last) to take the applicable action. A NBP or NSP may not be Delivered any earlier than **2 Days** Prior to the expiration of the applicable time for the other Party to remove a contingency or cancel this Agreement or meet an obligation specified in paragraph 14.

E.   **EFFECT OF BUYER'S REMOVAL OF CONTINGENCIES:** If Buyer removes, in writing, any contingency or cancellation rights, unless otherwise specified in writing, Buyer shall conclusively be deemed to have: **(i)** completed all Buyer Investigations, and review of reports and other applicable information and disclosures pertaining to that contingency or cancellation right; **(ii)** elected to proceed with the transaction; and **(iii)** assumed all liability, responsibility and expense for Repairs or corrections pertaining to that contingency or cancellation right, or for the inability to obtain financing.

F.   **CLOSE OF ESCROW:** Before Buyer or Seller may cancel this Agreement for failure of the other Party to close escrow pursuant to this Agreement, Buyer or Seller must first Deliver to the other Party a demand to close escrow (C.A.R. Form DCE). The DCE shall: **(i)** be signed by the applicable Buyer or Seller; and **(ii)** give the other Party at least **3 (or ___) Days** After Delivery to close escrow. A DCE may not be Delivered any earlier than **3 Days** Prior to the scheduled close of escrow.

G.   **EFFECT OF CANCELLATION ON DEPOSITS:** If Buyer or Seller gives written notice of cancellation pursuant to rights duly exercised under the terms of this Agreement, the Parties agree to Sign mutual instructions to cancel the sale and escrow and release deposits, if any, to the party entitled to the funds, less fees and costs incurred by that party. Fees and costs may be payable to service providers and vendors for services and products provided during escrow. Except as specified below, **release of funds will require mutual Signed release instructions from the Parties, judicial decision or arbitration award.** If either Party fails to execute mutual instructions to cancel escrow, one Party may make a written demand to Escrow Holder for the deposit (C.A.R. Form BDRD or SDRD). Escrow Holder, upon receipt, shall promptly deliver notice of the demand to the other Party. If, within 10 Days After Escrow Holder's notice, the other Party does not object to the demand, Escrow Holder shall disburse the deposit to the Party making the demand. If Escrow Holder complies with the preceding process, each Party shall be deemed to have released Escrow Holder from any and all claims or liability related to the disbursal of the deposit. Escrow Holder, at its discretion, may nonetheless require mutual cancellation instructions. **A Party may be subject to a civil penalty of up to $1,000 for refusal to sign cancellation instructions if no good faith dispute exists as to who is entitled to the deposited funds (Civil Code §1057.3).**

15. **FINAL VERIFICATION OF CONDITION:** Buyer shall have the right to make a final verification of the Property within **5 (or ☐ ___) Days** Prior to Close Of Escrow, NOT AS A CONTINGENCY OF THE SALE, but solely to confirm: **(i)** the Property is maintained

Buyer's Initials (_____)(_____)   Seller's Initials (_____)(_____)

RPA-CA REVISED 11/14 (PAGE 6 OF 10) Print Date

CALIFORNIA RESIDENTIAL PURCHASE AGREEMENT (RPA-CA PAGE 6 OF 10)

FIGURE 10.6 (continued):   **California Residential Purchase Agreement and Joint Escrow Instructions**

Property Address: _____   Date: _____

pursuant to paragraph 11; **(ii)** Repairs have been completed as agreed; and **(iii)** Seller has complied with Seller's other obligations under this Agreement (C.A.R. Form VP).

16. **REPAIRS:** Repairs shall be completed prior to final verification of condition unless otherwise agreed in writing. Repairs to be performed at Seller's expense may be performed by Seller or through others, provided that the work complies with applicable Law, including governmental permit, inspection and approval requirements. Repairs shall be performed in a good, skillful manner with materials of quality and appearance comparable to existing materials. It is understood that exact restoration of appearance or cosmetic items following all Repairs may not be possible. Seller shall: **(i)** obtain invoices and paid receipts for Repairs performed by others; **(ii)** prepare a written statement indicating the Repairs performed by Seller and the date of such Repairs; and **(iii)** provide Copies of invoices and paid receipts and statements to Buyer prior to final verification of condition.

17. **PRORATIONS OF PROPERTY TAXES AND OTHER ITEMS:** Unless otherwise agreed in writing, the following items shall be PAID CURRENT and prorated between Buyer and Seller as of Close Of Escrow: real property taxes and assessments, interest, rents, HOA regular, special, and emergency dues and assessments imposed prior to Close Of Escrow, premiums on insurance assumed by Buyer, payments on bonds and assessments assumed by Buyer, and payments on Mello-Roos and other Special Assessment District bonds and assessments that are now a lien. The following items shall be assumed by Buyer WITHOUT CREDIT toward the purchase price: prorated payments on Mello-Roos and other Special Assessment District bonds and assessments and HOA special assessments that are now a lien but not yet due. Property will be reassessed upon change of ownership. Any supplemental tax bills shall be paid as follows: **(i)** for periods after Close Of Escrow, by Buyer; and **(ii)** for periods prior to Close Of Escrow, by Seller (see C.A.R. Form SPT or SBSA for further information). TAX BILLS ISSUED AFTER CLOSE OF ESCROW SHALL BE HANDLED DIRECTLY BETWEEN BUYER AND SELLER. Prorations shall be made based on a 30-day month.

18. **BROKERS:**
    A. **COMPENSATION:** Seller or Buyer, or both, as applicable, agree to pay compensation to Broker as specified in a separate written agreement between Broker and that Seller or Buyer. Compensation is payable upon Close Of Escrow, or if escrow does not close, as otherwise specified in the agreement between Broker and that Seller or Buyer.
    B. **SCOPE OF DUTY:** Buyer and Seller acknowledge and agree that Broker: **(i)** Does not decide what price Buyer should pay or Seller should accept; **(ii)** Does not guarantee the condition of the Property; **(iii)** Does not guarantee the performance, adequacy or completeness of inspections, services, products or repairs provided or made by Seller or others; **(iv)** Does not have an obligation to conduct an inspection of common areas or areas off the site of the Property; **(v)** Shall not be responsible for identifying defects on the Property, in common areas, or offsite unless such defects are visually observable by an inspection of reasonably accessible areas of the Property or are known to Broker; **(vi)** Shall not be responsible for inspecting public records or permits concerning the title or use of Property; **(vii)** Shall not be responsible for identifying the location of boundary lines or other items affecting title; **(viii)** Shall not be responsible for verifying square footage, representations of others or information contained in Investigation reports, Multiple Listing Service, advertisements, flyers or other promotional material; **(ix)** Shall not be responsible for determining the fair market value of the Property or any personal property included in the sale; **(x)** Shall not be responsible for providing legal or tax advice regarding any aspect of a transaction entered into by Buyer or Seller; and **(xi)** Shall not be responsible for providing other advice or information that exceeds the knowledge, education and experience required to perform real estate licensed activity. Buyer and Seller agree to seek legal, tax, insurance, title and other desired assistance from appropriate professionals.

19. **REPRESENTATIVE CAPACITY:** If one or more Parties is signing this Agreement in a representative capacity and not for him/ herself as an individual then that Party shall so indicate in paragraph 31 or 32 and attach a Representative Capacity Signature Disclosure (C.A.R. Form RCSD).   Wherever the signature or initials of the representative identified in the RCSD appear on this Agreement or any related documents, it shall be deemed to be in a representative capacity for the entity described and not in an individual capacity, unless otherwise indicated. The Party acting in a representative capacity (i) represents that the entity for which that party is acting already exists and (ii) shall Deliver to the other Party and Escrow Holder, within 3 Days After Acceptance, evidence of authority to act in that capacity (such as but not limited to: applicable portion of the trust or Certification Of Trust (Probate Code §18100.5), letters testamentary, court order, power of attorney, corporate resolution, or formation documents of the business entity).

20. **JOINT ESCROW INSTRUCTIONS TO ESCROW HOLDER:**
    A. **The following paragraphs, or applicable portions thereof, of this Agreement constitute the joint escrow instructions of Buyer and Seller to Escrow Holder,** which Escrow Holder is to use along with any related counter offers and addenda, and any additional mutual instructions to close the escrow: paragraphs 1, 3, 4B, 5A, 6, 7, 10C, 13, 14G, 17, 18A, 19, 20, 26, 29, 30, 31, 32 and paragraph D of the section titled Real Estate Brokers on page 10. If a Copy of the separate compensation agreement(s) provided for in paragraph 18A, or paragraph D of the section titled Real Estate Brokers on page 10 is deposited with Escrow Holder by Broker, Escrow Holder shall accept such agreement(s) and pay out from Buyer's or Seller's funds, or both, as applicable, the Broker's compensation provided for in such agreement(s). The terms and conditions of this Agreement not set forth in the specified paragraphs are additional matters for the information of Escrow Holder, but about which Escrow Holder need not be concerned. Buyer and Seller will receive Escrow Holder's general provisions, if any, directly from Escrow Holder and will execute such provisions within the time specified in paragraph 7C(1)(c). To the extent the general provisions are inconsistent or conflict with this Agreement, the general provisions will control as to the duties and obligations of Escrow Holder only. Buyer and Seller will execute additional instructions, documents and forms provided by Escrow Holder that are reasonably necessary to close the escrow and, as directed by Escrow Holder, within 3 (or ___) Days, shall pay to Escrow Holder or HOA or HOA management company or others any fee required by paragraphs 7, 10 or elsewhere in this Agreement.
    B. A Copy of this Agreement including any counter offer(s) and addenda shall be delivered to Escrow Holder within **3** Days After Acceptance (or _____). Buyer and Seller authorize Escrow Holder to accept and rely on Copies and Signatures as defined in this Agreement as originals, to open escrow and for other purposes of escrow. The validity of this Agreement as between Buyer and Seller is not affected by whether or when Escrow Holder Signs this Agreement. Escrow Holder shall provide Seller's Statement of Information to Title company when received from Seller. If Seller delivers an affidavit to Escrow Holder to satisfy Seller's FIRPTA obligation under paragraph 10C, Escrow Holder shall deliver to Buyer a Qualified Substitute statement that complies with federal Law.
    C. Brokers are a party to the escrow for the sole purpose of compensation pursuant to paragraph 18A and paragraph D of the section titled Real Estate Brokers on page 10. Buyer and Seller irrevocably assign to Brokers compensation specified in paragraph 18A, and irrevocably instruct Escrow Holder to disburse those funds to Brokers at Close Of Escrow or pursuant to any

Buyer's Initials (_____)(_____)   Seller's Initials (_____)(_____)

RPA-CA REVISED 11/14 (PAGE 7 OF 10) Print Date
CALIFORNIA RESIDENTIAL PURCHASE AGREEMENT (RPA-CA PAGE 7 OF 10)

FIGURE 10.6 (continued): **California Residential Purchase Agreement and Joint Escrow Instructions**

Property Address: _____ Date: _____

other mutually executed cancellation agreement. Compensation instructions can be amended or revoked only with the written consent of Brokers. Buyer and Seller shall release and hold harmless Escrow Holder from any liability resulting from Escrow Holder's payment to Broker(s) of compensation pursuant to this Agreement.

D. Upon receipt, Escrow Holder shall provide Seller and Seller's Broker verification of Buyer's deposit of funds pursuant to paragraph 3A and 3B. Once Escrow Holder becomes aware of any of the following, Escrow Holder shall immediately notify all Brokers: **(i)** if Buyer's initial or any additional deposit or down payment is not made pursuant to this Agreement, or is not good at time of deposit with Escrow Holder; or **(ii)** if Buyer and Seller instruct Escrow Holder to cancel escrow.

E. A Copy of any amendment that affects any paragraph of this Agreement for which Escrow Holder is responsible shall be delivered to Escrow Holder within **3** Days after mutual execution of the amendment.

21. REMEDIES FOR BUYER'S BREACH OF CONTRACT:

A. Any clause added by the Parties specifying a remedy (such as release or forfeiture of deposit or making a deposit non-refundable) for failure of Buyer to complete the purchase in violation of this Agreement shall be deemed invalid unless the clause independently satisfies the statutory liquidated damages requirements set forth in the Civil Code.

B. LIQUIDATED DAMAGES: If Buyer fails to complete this purchase because of Buyer's default, Seller shall retain, as liquidated damages, the deposit actually paid. If the Property is a dwelling with no more than four units, one of which Buyer intends to occupy, then the amount retained shall be no more than 3% of the purchase price. Any excess shall be returned to Buyer. Except as provided in paragraph 14G, release of funds will require mutual, Signed release instructions from both Buyer and Seller, judicial decision or arbitration award. AT THE TIME OF ANY INCREASED DEPOSIT BUYER AND SELLER SHALL SIGN A SEPARATE LIQUIDATED DAMAGES PROVISION INCORPORATING THE INCREASED DEPOSIT AS LIQUIDATED DAMAGES (C.A.R. FORM RID).

Buyer's Initials _____/_____   Seller's Initials _____/_____

22. DISPUTE RESOLUTION:

A. MEDIATION: The Parties agree to mediate any dispute or claim arising between them out of this Agreement, or any resulting transaction, before resorting to arbitration or court action through the C.A.R. Real Estate Mediation Center for Consumers (**www.consumermediation.org**) or through any other mediation provider or service mutually agreed to by the Parties. The Parties **also agree to mediate any disputes or claims with Broker(s), who, in writing, agree to such mediation prior to, or within a reasonable time after, the dispute or claim is presented to the Broker.** Mediation fees, if any, shall be divided equally among the Parties involved. If, for any dispute or claim to which this paragraph applies, any Party (i) commences an action without first attempting to resolve the matter through mediation, or (ii) before commencement of an action, refuses to mediate after a request has been made, then that Party shall not be entitled to recover attorney fees, even if they would otherwise be available to that Party in any such action. THIS MEDIATION PROVISION APPLIES WHETHER OR NOT THE ARBITRATION PROVISION IS INITIALED. **Exclusions from this mediation agreement are specified in paragraph 22C.**

B. ARBITRATION OF DISPUTES:

The Parties agree that any dispute or claim in Law or equity arising between them out of this Agreement or any resulting transaction, which is not settled through mediation, shall be decided by neutral, binding arbitration. The Parties also agree to arbitrate any disputes or claims with Broker(s), who, in writing, agree to such arbitration prior to, or within a reasonable time after, the dispute or claim is presented to the Broker. The arbitrator shall be a retired judge or justice, or an attorney with at least 5 years of residential real estate Law experience, unless the parties mutually agree to a different arbitrator. The Parties shall have the right to discovery in accordance with Code of Civil Procedure §1283.05. In all other respects, the arbitration shall be conducted in accordance with Title 9 of Part 3 of the Code of Civil Procedure. Judgment upon the award of the arbitrator(s) may be entered into any court having jurisdiction. Enforcement of this agreement to arbitrate shall be governed by the Federal Arbitration Act. Exclusions from this arbitration agreement are specified in paragraph 22C.

"NOTICE: BY INITIALING IN THE SPACE BELOW YOU ARE AGREEING TO HAVE ANY DISPUTE ARISING OUT OF THE MATTERS INCLUDED IN THE 'ARBITRATION OF DISPUTES' PROVISION DECIDED BY NEUTRAL ARBITRATION AS PROVIDED BY CALIFORNIA LAW AND YOU ARE GIVING UP ANY RIGHTS YOU MIGHT POSSESS TO HAVE THE DISPUTE LITIGATED IN A COURT OR JURY TRIAL. BY INITIALING IN THE SPACE BELOW YOU ARE GIVING UP YOUR JUDICIAL RIGHTS TO DISCOVERY AND APPEAL, UNLESS THOSE RIGHTS ARE SPECIFICALLY INCLUDED IN THE 'ARBITRATION OF DISPUTES' PROVISION. IF YOU REFUSE TO SUBMIT TO ARBITRATION AFTER AGREEING TO THIS PROVISION, YOU MAY BE COMPELLED TO ARBITRATE UNDER THE AUTHORITY OF THE CALIFORNIA CODE OF CIVIL PROCEDURE. YOUR AGREEMENT TO THIS ARBITRATION PROVISION IS VOLUNTARY."

"WE HAVE READ AND UNDERSTAND THE FOREGOING AND AGREE TO SUBMIT DISPUTES ARISING OUT OF THE MATTERS INCLUDED IN THE 'ARBITRATION OF DISPUTES' PROVISION TO NEUTRAL ARBITRATION."

Buyer's Initials _____/_____   Seller's Initials _____/_____

C. ADDITIONAL MEDIATION AND ARBITRATION TERMS:

(1) EXCLUSIONS: The following matters are excluded from mediation and arbitration: (i) a judicial or non-judicial foreclosure or other action or proceeding to enforce a deed of trust, mortgage or installment land sale contract as defined in Civil Code §2985; (ii) an unlawful detainer action; and (iii) any matter that is within the jurisdiction of a probate, small claims or bankruptcy court.

(2) PRESERVATION OF ACTIONS: The following shall not constitute a waiver nor violation of the mediation and arbitration provisions: (i) the filing of a court action to preserve a statute of limitations; (ii) the filing of a court action to enable the recording of a notice of pending action, for order of attachment, receivership, injunction, or other provisional remedies; or (iii) the filing of a mechanic's lien.

(3) BROKERS: Brokers shall not be obligated nor compelled to mediate or arbitrate unless they agree to do so in writing. Any Broker(s) participating in mediation or arbitration shall not be deemed a party to this Agreement.

Buyer's Initials (_____)(_____)   Seller's Initials (_____)(_____)

RPA-CA REVISED 11/14 (PAGE 8 of 10)   Print Date

CALIFORNIA RESIDENTIAL PURCHASE AGREEMENT (RPA-CA PAGE 8 OF 10)

FIGURE 10.6 (continued): California Residential Purchase Agreement and Joint Escrow Instructions

Property Address: _____ Date: _____

23. SELECTION OF SERVICE PROVIDERS: Brokers do not guarantee the performance of any vendors, service or product providers ("Providers"), whether referred by Broker or selected by Buyer, Seller or other person. Buyer and Seller may select ANY Providers of their own choosing.

24. MULTIPLE LISTING SERVICE ("MLS"): Brokers are authorized to report to the MLS a pending sale and, upon Close Of Escrow, the sales price and other terms of this transaction shall be provided to the MLS to be published and disseminated to persons and entities authorized to use the information on terms approved by the MLS.

25. ATTORNEY FEES: In any action, proceeding, or arbitration between Buyer and Seller arising out of this Agreement, the prevailing Buyer or Seller shall be entitled to reasonable attorney fees and costs from the non-prevailing Buyer or Seller, except as provided in paragraph 22A.

26. ASSIGNMENT: Buyer shall not assign all or any part of Buyer's interest in this Agreement without first having obtained the separate written consent of Seller to a specified assignee. Such consent shall not be unreasonably withheld. Any total or partial assignment shall not relieve Buyer of Buyer's obligations pursuant to this Agreement unless otherwise agreed in writing by Seller (C.A.R. Form AOAA).

27. EQUAL HOUSING OPPORTUNITY: The Property is sold in compliance with federal, state and local anti-discrimination Laws.

28. TERMS AND CONDITIONS OF OFFER:
This is an offer to purchase the Property on the above terms and conditions. The liquidated damages paragraph or the arbitration of disputes paragraph is incorporated in this Agreement if initialed by all Parties or if incorporated by mutual agreement in a counter offer or addendum. If at least one but not all Parties initial, a counter offer is required until agreement is reached. Seller has the right to continue to offer the Property for sale and to accept any other offer at any time prior to notification of Acceptance. The Parties have read and acknowledge receipt of a Copy of the offer and agree to the confirmation of agency relationships. If this offer is accepted and Buyer subsequently defaults, Buyer may be responsible for payment of Brokers' compensation. This Agreement and any supplement, addendum or modification, including any Copy, may be Signed in two or more counterparts, all of which shall constitute one and the same writing.

29. TIME OF ESSENCE; ENTIRE CONTRACT; CHANGES: Time is of the essence. All understandings between the Parties are incorporated in this Agreement. Its terms are intended by the Parties as a final, complete and exclusive expression of their Agreement with respect to its subject matter, and may not be contradicted by evidence of any prior agreement or contemporaneous oral agreement. If any provision of this Agreement is held to be ineffective or invalid, the remaining provisions will nevertheless be given full force and effect. Except as otherwise specified, this Agreement shall be interpreted and disputes shall be resolved in accordance with the Laws of the State of California. **Neither this Agreement nor any provision in it may be extended, amended, modified, altered or changed, except in writing Signed by Buyer and Seller.**

30. DEFINITIONS: As used in this Agreement:
A. **"Acceptance"** means the time the offer or final counter offer is accepted in writing by a Party and is delivered to and personally received by the other Party or that Party's authorized agent in accordance with the terms of this offer or a final counter offer.
B. **"Agreement"** means this document and any counter offers and any incorporated addenda, collectively forming the binding agreement between the Parties. Addenda are incorporated only when Signed by all Parties.
C. **"C.A.R. Form"** means the most current version of the specific form referenced or another comparable form agreed to by the parties.
D. **"Close Of Escrow"**, including "COE", means the date the grant deed, or other evidence of transfer of title, is recorded.
E. **"Copy"** means copy by any means including photocopy, NCR, facsimile and electronic.
F. **"Days"** means calendar days. However, after Acceptance, the last **Day** for performance of any act required by this Agreement (including Close Of Escrow) shall not include any Saturday, Sunday, or legal holiday and shall instead be the next Day.
G. **"Days After"** means the specified number of calendar days after the occurrence of the event specified, not counting the calendar date on which the specified event occurs, and ending at 11:59 PM on the final day.
H. **"Days Prior"** means the specified number of calendar days before the occurrence of the event specified, not counting the calendar date on which the specified event is scheduled to occur.
I. **"Deliver"**, **"Delivered"** or **"Delivery"**, unless otherwise specified in writing, means and shall be effective upon: personal receipt by Buyer or Seller or the individual Real Estate Licensee for that principal as specified in the section titled Real Estate Brokers on page 10, regardless of the method used (i.e., messenger, mail, email, fax, other).
J. **"Electronic Copy" or "Electronic Signature"** means, as applicable, an electronic copy or signature complying with California Law. Buyer and Seller agree that electronic means will not be used by either Party to modify or alter the content or integrity of this Agreement without the knowledge and consent of the other Party.
K. **"Law"** means any law, code, statute, ordinance, regulation, rule or order, which is adopted by a controlling city, county, state or federal legislative, judicial or executive body or agency.
L. **"Repairs"** means any repairs (including pest control), alterations, replacements, modifications or retrofitting of the Property provided for under this Agreement.
M. **"Signed"** means either a handwritten or electronic signature on an original document, Copy or any counterpart.

31. EXPIRATION OF OFFER: This offer shall be deemed revoked and the deposit, if any, shall be returned to Buyer unless the offer is Signed by Seller and a Copy of the Signed offer is personally received by Buyer, or by _____, who is authorized to receive it, by 5:00 PM on the third Day after this offer is signed by Buyer (or by ☐ _____ ☐AM/☐PM, on _____ (date)).
☐ One or more Buyers is signing this Agreement in a representative capacity and not for him/herself as an individual. See attached Representative Capacity Signature Disclosure (C.A.R. Form RCSD) for additional terms.

Date _____ BUYER _____

(Print name) _____

Date _____ BUYER _____

(Print name) _____

☐ Additional Signature Addendum attached (C.A.R. Form ASA).

RPA-CA REVISED 11/14 (PAGE 9 of 10) Print Date   Seller's Initials (_____)(_____)

CALIFORNIA RESIDENTIAL PURCHASE AGREEMENT (RPA-CA PAGE 9 OF 10)

FIGURE 10.6 (continued): **California Residential Purchase Agreement and Joint Escrow Instructions**

Property Address: _____ Date: _____

32. **ACCEPTANCE OF OFFER:** Seller warrants that Seller is the owner of the Property, or has the authority to execute this Agreement. Seller accepts the above offer and agrees to sell the Property on the above terms and conditions. Seller has read and acknowledges receipt of a Copy of this Agreement, and authorizes Broker to Deliver a Signed Copy to Buyer.

☐ (If checked) SELLER'S ACCEPTANCE IS **SUBJECT TO ATTACHED COUNTER OFFER (C.A.R. Form SCO or SMCO) DATED:**
_____.

☐ One or more Sellers is signing this Agreement in a representative capacity and not for him/herself as an individual. See attached Representative Capacity Signature Disclosure (C.A.R. Form RCSD) for additional terms.

Date _____ SELLER _____

(Print name) _____

Date _____ SELLER _____

(Print name) _____

☐ Additional Signature Addendum attached (C.A.R. Form ASA).

(___/___) **(Do not initial if making a counter offer.) CONFIRMATION OF ACCEPTANCE:** A Copy of Signed Acceptance was
(Initials) personally received by Buyer or Buyer's authorized agent on (date) _____ at _____ ☐ AM/ ☐ PM. **A binding Agreement is created when a Copy of Signed Acceptance is personally received by Buyer or Buyer's authorized agent whether or not confirmed in this document. Completion of this confirmation is not legally required in order to create a binding Agreement; it is solely intended to evidence the date that Confirmation of Acceptance has occurred.**

REAL ESTATE BROKERS:
A. Real Estate Brokers are not parties to the Agreement between Buyer and Seller.
B. Agency relationships are confirmed as stated in paragraph 2.
C. If specified in paragraph 3A(2), Agent who submitted the offer for Buyer acknowledges receipt of deposit.
D. **COOPERATING BROKER COMPENSATION:** Listing Broker agrees to pay Cooperating Broker **(Selling Firm)** and Cooperating Broker agrees to accept, out of Listing Broker's proceeds in escrow, the amount specified in the MLS, provided Cooperating Broker is a Participant of the MLS in which the Property is offered for sale or a reciprocal MLS. If Listing Broker and Cooperating Broker are not both Participants of the MLS, or a reciprocal MLS, in which the Property is offered for sale, then compensation must be specified in a separate written agreement (C.A.R. Form CBC). Declaration of License and Tax (C.A.R. Form DLT) may be used to document that tax reporting will be required or that an exemption exists.

Real Estate Broker (Selling Firm) _____ CalBRE Lic. # _____
By _____ CalBRE Lic. # _____ Date _____
By _____ CalBRE Lic. # _____ Date _____
Address _____ City _____ State _____ Zip _____
Telephone _____ Fax _____ E-mail _____
Real Estate Broker (Listing Firm) _____ CalBRE Lic. # _____
By _____ CalBRE Lic. # _____ Date _____
By _____ CalBRE Lic. # _____ Date _____
Address _____ City _____ State _____ Zip _____
Telephone _____ Fax _____ E-mail _____

ESCROW HOLDER ACKNOWLEDGMENT:
Escrow Holder acknowledges receipt of a Copy of this Agreement, (if checked, ☐ a deposit in the amount of $ _____),
counter offer numbers _____ ☐ Seller's Statement of Information and
_____, and agrees to act as Escrow Holder subject to paragraph 20 of this Agreement, any supplemental escrow instructions and the terms of Escrow Holder's general provisions.

Escrow Holder is advised that the date of Confirmation of Acceptance of the Agreement as between Buyer and Seller is _____

Escrow Holder _____ Escrow # _____
By _____ Date _____
Address _____
Phone/Fax/E-mail _____
Escrow Holder has the following license number # _____
☐ Department of Business Oversight, ☐ Department of Insurance, ☐ Bureau of Real Estate.

PRESENTATION OF OFFER: (_____) Listing Broker presented this offer to Seller on _____ (date).
Broker or Designee Initials

REJECTION OF OFFER: (_____)(_____) No counter offer is being made. This offer was rejected by Seller on _____ (date).
Seller's Initials

Buyer's Acknowledge that page 10 is part of
this Agreement (_____)(_____)

Reviewed by _____
Broker or Designee _____

RPA-CA REVISED 11/14 (PAGE 10 of 10) **Print Date**

CALIFORNIA RESIDENTIAL PURCHASE AGREEMENT (RPA-CA PAGE 10 OF 10)

Understanding the Purchase Agreement Form

Paragraph 1: Basic offer.   1A shows the buyer or buyers; 1B describes the property by address, legal description, and/or assessor's parcel number and further indicates the city or county where the property is located; 1C sets forth the purchase price; and 1D sets the time for close of escrow to complete the transaction.

Paragraph 2: Agency.

   A.   This is acknowledgment by buyer and seller as to receipt of agency disclosure.

   B.   The agency relations selected are confirmed.

   C.   The possibility of multiple representations is explained.

Paragraph 3: Finance terms.   Buyer represents that funds will be good when deposited in escrow (cash, cashier's check, etc.).

Subparagraphs A through K under Financing are explained below.

   A.   This provides for the initial earnest money deposit, its form, and if it is to be deposited (escrow or trust account) or held uncashed.

   B.   Provision is made for increasing the earnest money (used in cases of low initial deposits).

   C.   Can be checked if it is an all-cash offer without financial contingencies.

   D.   Paragraph (1) states the requirements of the new first loan on which this offer is contingent. If the buyer cannot obtain the loan, the buyer is relieved of any purchase obligation. For this paragraph, consider setting the interest rate and points above current market interest, so that a minor fluctuation will not relieve the buyer from the purchase obligation. Paragraph (2) applies to conditions of any second loan. Paragraph (3) applies to terms if FHA or VA financing is sought.

E. This provides for additional financing terms, such as seller financing, loan assumptions, balloon payments, et cetera.

F. Provision is made for the balance of the purchase price to be deposited in escrow before closing.

G. This paragraph shows the total purchase price. (**Note:** The down payment and loans assumed and/or new loans by lenders or seller should equal the purchase price.)

H. This paragraph requires the buyers to verify that they have the down payment and closing costs.

I. This paragraph provides, by checking, whether or not the agreement is to be contingent upon an appraisal equal to or greater than the purchase price.

J. Loan terms (1) require providing evidence of prequalification or preapproval for the loan, (2) require the buyer to act diligently to obtain the loan, (3) provides for removal of loan contingency, or if checked, no loan contingency.

K. Provides that the seller has relied upon buyer representation as to financing sought and failure to obtain alternative type of financing will not excuse the buyer.

Paragraph 4: Sale of buyer's property. If checked, the sale is contingent upon the sale of the buyer's property.

Paragraph 5: Addendum and advisories. Addendums and advisory notices to buyer are checked if they are to be included in the offer.

Paragraph 6: Other terms. Space is provided for other terms of the offer.

Paragraph 7: Allocation of costs.

A. Subparagraph A. Checking the appropriate box determines who is to pay which costs as to inspection reports and certificates.

B.   Subparagraph B sets forth who is responsible. Compliance with government inclusion requirements and retrofit.

C.   Subparagraph C determines responsibility for escrow fees, the escrow holder and time period to sign and return escrow provisions, as well as responsibility for title insurance.

D.   Subparagraph D determines, by checking appropriate boxes, who shall be responsible for other costs and fees.

Paragraph 8: Items included and excluded.   This paragraph makes it clear that designated fixtures remain with the property, but it also provides for inclusion of other items in the sale, as well as exclusion of designated items from the sale. The agent should make certain that questionable items such as installed TVs, et cetera, are covered.

Paragraph 9: Closing and possession.

A.   This paragraph states whether the buyer intends to occupy the premises as a principal residence. If the buyer intends the property to be a principal residence, then liquidated damages resulting from buyer default cannot exceed 3% of the purchase price. (See paragraph 21B.)

(If a buyer falsely indicates a property will be the principal residence for the purpose of obtaining a loan at a lower rate of interest, it would be fraud against the lender.)

B.   This paragraph provides the date on which seller-occupied or vacant property will be turned over to the buyer.

C.   Subparagraph C provides for conditions of the seller remaining in possession after close of escrow.

D.   This paragraph provides that tenant-occupied property will be vacant before close of escrow unless agreed otherwise. If the property is not vacated, the seller could be in breach of contract. If the box allowing the tenant to remain in possession is checked, the buyer and the seller are to enter into a written occupancy agreement. If they do not reach an occupancy agreement, either the buyer or the seller may cancel the purchase agreement in writing.

E.   This paragraph provides that the seller will assign to the buyer any assignable warranty rights.

F.   This paragraph provides that keys, openers, et cetera, will be given to the buyer.

Paragraph 10: Statutory and other disclosures. This paragraph requires the seller to provide all required statutory and other disclosures, including lead paint, transfer disclosure statement, natural and environmental hazard disclosures and booklets, withholding as to FIRPTA, Megan's Law database, notice regarding gas and hazardous liquids, transmission lines, as well as condominium and planned development disclosures

Paragraph11: Conditions of property. Unless otherwise indicated, property is sold in present condition, subject to buyer's inspection rights, and will be maintained in substantially the same condition.

A.   The seller will disclose known material facts and defects.

B.   The buyer has the right of inspection and may cancel the agreement or request corrective action based on defects discovered.

C.   The buyer is strongly advised to conduct an investigation of the property.

Paragraph 12: Buyer's investigation of property and matters affecting property. This paragraph provides for the buyer's rights to inspection and provides for either the removal of the inspection contingency or cancellation of the agreement. Utilities must be on for the buyer's inspection. The buyer agrees to keep the property free from liens (pay for investigative work), repair any damage and costs associated with inspection, and protect the owner from any liability because of such investigations and inspections.

Paragraph 13: Title and vesting.

A. This paragraph provides that the buyer will receive a preliminary title report.

B. This paragraph indicates that title will be taken in present condition and subject to stated nonmonetary encumbrances.

C. This paragraph sets forth the seller's duty to disclose all matters known to the seller affecting title.

D. This paragraph provides that title will be transferred by a grant deed, and the buyer is notified to obtain professional advice as to the manner of taking title.

E. This paragraph provides that the buyer will receive a homeowners policy of title insurance.

Paragraph 14: Time periods; removal of contingencies; cancellation rights.   This paragraph sets forth all time periods for compliance and disclosures. Modification of time periods must be in writing. If the seller removes contingencies, this will be conclusive evidence of the buyer's election to proceed with the transaction. If the buyer and seller agree to cancellation of the agreement, release of the funds will require mutual signed agreement (with a civil penalty of up to $1,000 for refusal to sign the agreement if no good faith dispute exists).

In November 2014, the California Association of REALTORS® made a pretty significant change to the purchase contract. Previously in the event of a failed escrow, the release of the buyer's deposit could only be released after receiving mutually signed cancellation instructions. However, the current iteration of the purchase contract allows the escrow company to make a demand on a party for cancellation of the escrow. If the party fails to respond within 10 days, the escrow company is permitted to release the buyer's deposit. This is a massive shift from all previous versions of the purchase contract because it allows either the buyers or the sellers to tell escrow that they want to cancel a given transaction, and theoretically if the other party didn't respond for whatever reason for 10 days, the escrow company can unilaterally release funds without a subsequent signature.

Paragraph 15: Final verification of condition. This paragraph provides the buyer the right to conduct a final inspection before close of escrow to confirm that the property has been properly maintained and repairs have been made, and that the seller has complied with other contractual obligations.

Paragraph 16: Repairs. Seller repairs will be performed in accordance with governmental requirements in a skillful manner.

Paragraph 17: Prorations of property taxes and other items. This paragraph provides for proration of taxes and other items based on a 30-day month. Bonds will be assumed without buyer credit if not yet due.

Paragraph 18: Brokers. Parties agree to pay brokers as determined in a separate written agreement. Subparagraph B points out what the broker doesn't do and is not responsible for.

Paragraph 19: Representative capacity. If a party is acting as a representative, the party will so indicate and deliver supporting documentation to escrow.

Paragraph 20: Joint escrow instructions to escrow holder. This paragraph provides that designated paragraphs of the agreement are joint escrow instructions and that the agreement will be delivered to the escrow within a designated period. It makes clear that the broker is a party to the escrow only so far as those commission rights are concerned that have been irrevocably assigned to the broker.

Paragraph 21: Remedies for buyer's breach of contract. Any added remedy for buyer breach will be invalid unless the clause added satisfies the statutory liquidated damages requirement. For 1-4 residential units that buyer intends to occupy, the liquidated damages cannot exceed 3% of the sale price.

Paragraph 22: Dispute resolution. The parties agree to try to settle any dispute by mediation. By initialing, the parties agree to binding arbitration of any dispute not settled by mediation. (If it is not initialed, the parties could settle disputes through the courts.)

Disputes with brokers are subject to mediation and arbitration only if the brokers agree to such resolution.

Paragraph 23: Selection of service providers.   The broker does not guarantee performance of any service provider she may have referred to the buyer and/or seller.

Paragraph 24: Multiple listing service.   This paragraph gives the broker the right to report the sale terms to an MLS to be published. Without this authorization, release of information by an agent could breach the duty of confidentiality.

Paragraph 25: Attorney's fees.   In the event of a legal proceeding or arbitration, the prevailing party will be entitled to reasonable attorney's fees.

Paragraph 26: Assignment.   The buyer agrees not to assign any portion of this agreement to a named party without the written permission of seller. Permission will not be unreasonably withheld toward the buyer's obligation unless otherwise agreed.

Paragraph 27: Equal housing opportunity.   This paragraph states that the sale is being made in compliance with antidiscrimination laws.

Paragraph 28: Terms and conditions of offer.   This paragraph makes it clear it is an offer that includes initialed paragraphs and provides that should the buyer default after acceptance, the buyer may be responsible for the broker's commission.

Paragraph 29: Time of essence; entire contract; changes.   This is the complete agreement and may not be contradicted by prior agreements or contemporaneous oral agreements. It cannot be extended, modified, or changed except in writing signed by both buyer and seller.

Paragraph 30: Definitions.   This paragraph provides definitions of terms used.

Paragraph 31: Expiration of offer.   This paragraph provides a definite termination time and date if the offer is not accepted by that time and date. The buyer's signature as to the offer is included in this paragraph.

Paragraph 32: Acceptance of offer.   The seller warrants ownership and accepts the offer on terms indicated, or by checking the appropriate block indicates acceptance subject to attached counteroffer.

The buyer initials confirmation of receipt of acceptance.

There is a block for the broker to sign in which the broker agrees to cooperating broker compensation.

Another block is signed by the escrow holder acknowledging receipt of copy of the agreement.

SUMMARY

Selling is helping others meet their needs. Selling can give buyers the security of home ownership.

Selling involves elements such as persuasion, communication, discovery, and knowledge of the customer and knowledge of the product. Your strategy should be based on the type of prospect and the prospect's attitude toward purchasing in general and purchasing a special property in particular.

To close a sale you must appeal to buying motives, watch for buying signals, overcome any resistance that is raised, and attempt a trial close. Buying motives include survival, security, pride of ownership, love of family, health, desire for profit or gain, and desire for comfort and convenience.

If you understand buying signals, you know when to close. Timing can be essential. Treat objections as a natural part of a sale. Welcome the objection, concede before answering, rephrase the objection as a question, and meet the objection. You can forestall an obvious objection by bringing it up yourself and covering it.

You have a choice of six basic techniques with untold variations for closing:

1. An assumptive close asks a question that assumes the prospect will buy.

2. The positive choice gives the prospect a choice between positive actions.

3. The inducement technique contains a benefit for buying now.

4. The fear of loss or approval is based on a "last chance."

5. The narrative close uses third-party verification.

6. The ask-for-a-deposit close gets right to the heart of the matter.

Sales can be lost for many reasons. Generally, salespeople lose sales by talking when they should be listening and not knowing when they should be silent. Overeagerness, incomplete knowledge, too much pressure, appearing frightened, criticizing competitors, wandering from your purpose, displaying a negative attitude, and being argumentative or negative are all reasons why salespeople fail.

The estimated buyer's closing cost should be given to the buyer before the offer is complete. Buyers don't like to be surprised. Be realistic in estimating buyer costs.

The eight-page California Residential Purchase Agreement and Joint Escrow Instructions form is a complete agreement that you must fully understand before attempting to sell a property. The form is designed to aid you in explaining the agreement and in meeting your obligations.

CLASS DISCUSSION TOPICS

1. How would you overcome the following buyer objections?

   a. I wanted a house with a [pool] and this house doesn't have a [pool].

   b. I didn't want an older house.

   c. I don't like the location.

   d. The price is too high.

   e. The monthly assessments are way too high.

   f. The interest rate is too high; I better wait.

   g. The mortgage payments are more than my rent.

   h. The financing is too complicated.

   i. I'm worried about [my job/the economy].

   j. I want to sell my present home first.

   k. We want to think it over.

   l. I'd like to discuss it with [my accountant/lawyer/son-in-law].

2. Using another student to represent a buyer, demonstrate a closing (no more than three minutes).

3. Complete a Residential Purchase Agreement for the residential property in Unit 6, Class Discussion Topic 5, according to the following:

   Buyers: Orem and Melody Rosatta

   Deposit: Personal check for $15,000

   Purchase price: $500,000

   Financing contingency: Contingent on obtaining a new 80% fixed-rate loan at no more than 5¼% interest and no more than $8,000 in loan fees and discount points. Buyers will provide evidence that they are prequalified for a loan, meeting above terms within five days of acceptance.

   Appraisal contingency: Offer contingent on property appraisal for no less than purchase price (there are no other contingencies).

Closing: Within 60 days of acceptance. Possession at closing.

Occupancy: Buyers intend property as their permanent residence.

Fees and costs: Seller will pay transfer fees and title insurance. Escrow fees shall be split equally. Apex Escrow shall be the escrow for the transaction. Sewer and well costs are not applicable. Seller will pay for smoke detector and water heater bracing as required. All other costs are to be borne by seller. Seller will pay for a one-year home warranty, as well as a pest control inspection, and seller will pay for any corrective work indicated.

Condition: Seller will pay for inspections and reports set forth in paragraph 7 of the purchase contract.

Personal property included: Refrigerator, pool equipment, fireplace accessories, window coverings, portable steel garden building, and riding lawn mower.

Time periods specified in paragraph 14 are adequate.

4. Bring to class one current-events article dealing with some aspect of real estate practice for class discussion.

UNIT 10 QUIZ

1. A good salesperson
    a. uses technical terms whenever possible to impress buyers.
    b. speaks fast so she can reach the closing.
    c. approaches every customer in the same way.
    d. does none of these.

2. A salesperson appeals to buying motives. Which of the following is a buying motive?
    a. Love of family
    b. Comfort and convenience
    c. Security
    d. All of these

3. Disadvantages of home ownership include
    a. increase in expenses.
    b. risk.
    c. lack of liquidity.
    d. all of these.

4. Buying signals might include a buyer's
    a. whispering with a spouse.
    b. pacing off a room.
    c. seeming reluctant to leave a property.
    d. doing all of these.

5. A prospective buyer says, "The price is too high." The *BEST* response is
    a. "I think the price is fair."
    b. "Why don't you offer less?"
    c. "The comparable sales don't bear that out."
    d. "Why do you feel that the price is too high?"

6. A professional salesperson knows that
   a. telling is more effective than asking.
   b. appealing to emotions should be avoided.
   c. in dealing with a cautious buyer, you should be assertive and push for a decision.
   d. none of these apply.

7. When you ask prospective buyers if they prefer June 1, July 1, or August 1 for possession, what type of closing technique are you using?
   a. Inducement
   b. Positive choice
   c. Fear of loss
   d. Narrative close

8. The paragraph in the purchase contract in which the buyer indicates an intention to occupy the property (applies to 1–4-unit residential properties) is important because it relates to
   a. liquidated damages.
   b. vesting of title.
   c. smoke detectors.
   d. home protection plans.

9. Who can modify an accepted offer to purchase?
   a. The selling broker
   b. The listing broker
   c. The listing broker and the seller
   d. The buyer and the seller by mutual agreement

10. In making a property inspection, the inspector hired by the buyer negligently damaged the air-conditioning unit. Who is responsible for the damage based on the California Residential Purchase Agreement and Joint Escrow Instructions?
    a. The seller
    b. The buyer
    c. The buyer's agent
    d. The seller's agent

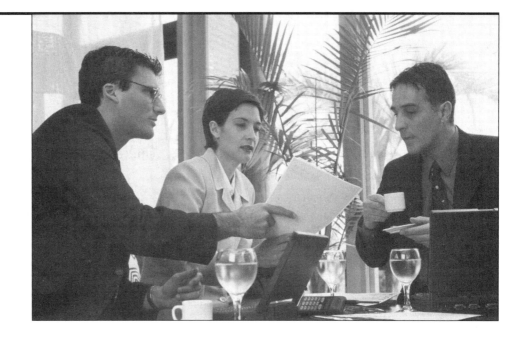

FROM OFFER TO CLOSING

LEARNING OBJECTIVES

When you have completed this unit, you will be able to

- describe the preparation required before presentation of the offer,

- explain how to deal with multiple offers and how to present offers to owners,

- understand your agency duties to your principal as to recommendations,

- demonstrate how ow to deal with objections,

- explain when and how to prepare a counteroffer and what to do when an offer is accepted, and

- explain the importance of checklists for closing.

KEY TERMS

acceptance	history of the sale	rent skimming
buyer's remorse	multiple offers	seller objections
cash-out scheme	price	subordination clause
closing	rejection	terms
counteroffer	release of contract	

THE OFFER TO PURCHASE

The offer to purchase is really the California Residential Purchase Agreement and Joint Escrow Instructions that was covered in Unit 10. When it is signed by the buyers, we customarily call it an *offer to purchase*. Keep in mind that selling real estate really involves the following three separate sales:

1. Selling the owner on a listing or the buyer on agency representation

2. Selling the buyer on an offer

3. Selling the seller on an acceptance

While two out of three might be a tremendous average in baseball, you have totally failed if the third sale is not completed.

A seller's agent must continue sales efforts until an offer has been accepted. To cease working to sell a property merely because an offer was received is not in the owners' best interest. It could be regarded as unethical conduct.

Preparing to Submit the Offer

After you receive an offer to purchase, preparation is normally necessary for your presentation of the offer to the owners.

> The third sale—acceptance of the offer—is the one that means success.

The appointment. When you have a signed offer to purchase, notify the listing office immediately and deliver the offer to the listing office as soon as possible. Provide information you have about the buyers and whether they have qualified or been approved for a loan. If the offer is for less than the list price, you might want to include any data you have that justifies the price.

The listing agent has a fiduciary relationship with the owner. The listing agent should present the offer to the owner. There might be circumstances where the listing agent would want the selling agent present when making the offer. Keep in mind that a listing agent, who has sole agency duties to the seller, has different objectives than an agent whose sole agency is to the buyer. It is the listing agent's responsibility to make an appointment with the owners to present the offer to them.

Avoid giving any details about an offer to an owner until you can present the offer in its entirety.

It is a good idea to set up an appointment with the owner so as not to be questioned by the owner over the phone about price. You need to present the entire offer, not just the price. Revealing only one aspect of an offer, when not presented as part of the total package, could result in antagonistic owners rejecting an offer, an action that could be to their detriment.

When viewed as a whole, the offer at what an owner regards as too low a price might appear much more acceptable, or it could be the starting point for an acceptable counteroffer.

You want to be able to present the offer to all the owners at once. Whenever possible, schedule the presentation after small children have gone to bed, because any interruptions can make your job extremely difficult.

Should the owners contact you before you present the offer and ask you what the offer is, we suggest this answer:

> It wouldn't be fair to you or the buyers to condense the offer into a minute or two. This offer deserves careful consideration as well as explanation. You will want to see this offer.

If the owner persists, ask "Can you and [spouse or co-owner, if applicable] meet with me right now?"

Owners can't accept offers over the phone, so try to avoid presenting them over the phone.

Generally, you should not present an offer over the telephone. The sellers can't accept over the phone, but they can say no. A phone presentation also gives owners time to talk to others about the offer before your presentation to them. Unfortunately, friends tend to give uninformed advice they think the owners want to hear, such as "Oh! Your home is worth more than that!"

If you must present the offer by phone, you should also fax or email the offer. The offer cannot be accepted until a signed copy is transmitted electronically or placed in the mail.

If the listing agent does not have much experience, the agent's broker may want to be present.

> Make certain the sellers know what they will receive.

Estimated seller's proceeds.   For an offer less than list price, prepare an Estimated Seller Proceeds form, based on the offer received. Show the owners what they will net from the offer. Use of this form shows the owners that you are being straightforward in your dealings with them. Your recommendations will bear more weight when it is clear to the owners that you are being totally aboveboard in your dealings.

Comparative market analysis.   If market values have been falling and the property has been on the market for several months, update the comparative market analysis (CMA) that you prepared when you took the listing. If a comparable used for the CMA has been sold, you want to be able to present the sale information.

Anticipate problems.   Role-playing exercises such as those discussed in Unit 1 can be an important part of your preparation. From analysis of the offer, you can anticipate the objections you will receive. Decide how you are going to help the owners overcome problem areas (if you believe it is in their best interests to accept the offer).

Some agents lose sight of their agency duties and give priority to their own interests over those of their principals. This is unethical conduct and cannot be tolerated. It might mean a commission now, but in the long run, it will have far greater negative impact on your reputation and future business.

Multiple offers.   When more than one offer has been received on a property, you must present the **multiple offers** together. If you know of another offer that has not yet been received, you have a duty to inform the owners of it. You even have a duty to inform owners of verbal offers, although they're not binding, nor can they be accepted.

Keep in mind that as a listing agent your first duty is to your seller, not to your firm or for your personal gain. Offers should be presented in a non-prejudicial manner so that owners can compare the offers and make their decision. With multiple offers, you might want to suggest obtaining loan preapproval on the prospective purchasers. The owners might otherwise accept an offer from a buyer who is unable to obtain financing and reject the offer from a prospective buyer who would have no difficulty obtaining the necessary loan.

A listing agent might want to encourage multiple offers so that the seller is able to take advantage of competition. The listing agent may want to obtain the seller's permission to inform all offerors of the fact that there are multiple offers. The agent could suggest to the owner that a deadline be set for improved offers. In a seller's market, this could be beneficial to the seller.

Present multiple offers in an impartial manner.

A selling agent wants the buyer to be successful in a competitive situation, as long as the successful purchase is in the best interests of the buyer. Price is important to the seller, as is the cleanest deal, which is the sale that will most likely avoid problems. Besides increasing price, even if above list price, sellers are likely to react favorably to an offer where the buyer pays all escrow fees and other closing costs. Therefore, it is important for the listing agent to prepare a seller's net sheet to show the seller the net from a successful sale, including any concessions to the buyer.

Setting the mood.   You should present the offer to the owners at your office or the owners' home. If at the home, a good place to present the offer is at the kitchen table (likely in the same location where you took the listing). This is a nonthreatening environment, and the listing and selling agent can physically be quite close to the owners. If presented in any other room, use a table such as a cocktail table and sit close together with direct eye contact with the owners.

To set a positive mood, mention some feature that played a part in the sale and that the owners can be proud of. For example:

> Frankly, I think the reason I have an offer on the house is because of your delightful garden. The buyers fell in love with your rose bushes.

> While [Mrs. Wilson] loves your light and bright decorating, [Mr. Wilson] was sold on your house because of the workroom in the garage. It's something he has always wanted.

This is also the time to confirm agency election and obtain the seller's signature on the confirmation, unless it is part of the purchase contract.

Stages of the presentation.   Professional presentations are well organized. One organization plan is a three-stage presentation, as follows:

1. A history of the property sales effort and any problems with the property

2. Information about the buyers—humanize the buyers so that they can be seen as people the sellers would like

3. The offer itself

As in a sale, agents should use a closing if they feel acceptance of the offer is in the best interest of the sellers.

History of the sale.   If the property has been on the market for several months or longer, go over the **history of the sale**.

Cover the following:

- The length of time on the market (in days)

- Previous listings or sale efforts (for sale by owner)

- Advertising (all types)

- The role of the multiple listing service

- Internet postings

- Agent caravans

- Open houses

- Showings

- Responses to showings—reasons why other buyers rejected the home (negative features or lack of features)

- Any other offers received

If the property was recently listed and you already have received an offer, it is possible the owners may feel that they must have set their sale price too low. These owners can become adamant about not giving one inch.

Consider the following approach:

[Mr. and Mrs. Finch], when you listed the property with me, I explained that offers are very often received within a few days of the property being placed on the market. When this happens, you are fortunate, and you're fortunate today. Real estate agents, as well as buyers, get excited over new listings, because they feel they're getting first chance at a home rather than it being shopworn merchandise that hundreds of buyers have rejected. In fact, the most active sale period for a listing is the first 30 days it is on the market. When it's on the market longer than that, it can become much harder work to locate a buyer. For this reason, it is important to avoid listing a property at a price that is too high because you will lose much of the momentum resulting from taking a new listing. Steer clear of the trap to "list high and then come down later."

Often, owners reject offers that they receive within days of the listing and then go for a long time without another offer. Do you know what happens then? In most cases, when they do get an offer, it is for less than they received earlier. I'm telling you this so you don't respond emotionally to this offer but rather receive it with reason.

About the buyers. Whenever possible, paint a verbal picture of the buyers that will make the sellers feel they are likable people who will appreciate the home. For example:

> The buyers are the [Henleys], the young family who came here last Thursday and then again yesterday. [Tom Henley] is [chief of security] at the [Nesco Corporation] and [Mary Henley] is an [associate editor] for the [Daily News].

> Their daughter [, Tricia,] [age nine,] goes to [Sunnyvale School]. One of the reasons they like your home is that the children would not have to change schools. Their son [, Jeffrey,] is just four years old and is in preschool.

Note: Obtain the buyers' permission before you reveal any personal information about the buyers.

Keep in mind that a home sale is emotional, and although owners have logical reasons to sell, there is often emotional reluctance at the same time.

In addition to reassuring sellers that the prospective buyers are nice people, you also want their offer to appear reasonable. If the buyers also are interested in another property, and most buyers are, point this out. When they receive an offer, owners tend to forget that they're competing with many other sellers:

> The [Henleys] were undecided between your house and a three-bedroom, two-and-one-half-bath Spanish-style home off [Wedgewood Way]. That house has two and a half baths, while your home has two baths, and had concrete block walls, but I was able to convince the [Henleys] that your house met their total needs better because it doesn't require [Tricia] to change schools, and the workroom in the garage was just what [Tom] wanted for his woodworking. He carves duck decoys.

Cover all three steps:
1. History
2. Buyers
3. Offer

With this kind of comparison, you have shown the owners to be winners over the competition (the house off Wedgewood Way). The owners will feel their house is appreciated and that you have been working for them. Never use an imaginary competitive house. Remember, be honest. All you need to do is to tell the owners why they are winners.

The Offer

We recommend that you gain agreement on the little things before you hand the offer to the sellers. As an example, get agreement about the following:

- The occupancy date

- What stays with the house or goes

- Seller preparing a transfer disclosure statement

- Name of escrow and if costs are to be split

- Prorating of taxes

- Keys and openers to be turned over

- Other pertinent terms

Then hand copies of the offer to each owner. If everything else has been agreed upon, then the only obstacle to a sale is the price.

Some agents like to use a silent approach and wait for owners to react. If the offer is substantially in accordance with the listing, you could go through the offer paragraph by paragraph with the owners. Answer any questions they may have. When you are finished, ask them to initial clauses where appropriate and to approve the agreement by signing where you have indicated.

Justify the Offer

When an offer is less than the list price, you must be able to justify the offer, or you risk that the sellers will regard the buyers as arbitrary. Explain how or why the buyer decided on the offering price. When sellers and buyers have a high regard for each other, there is less likelihood of a sale's failing during escrow. An example of such an explanation is:

> You don't want the buyer to appear arbitrary as to price.

> While the offer I have is less than the list price, I believe it is a fair offer. Even though I convinced the [Henleys] that your home met their needs better than [the house off Wedgewood Way], they didn't feel they should pay more than what they would have paid for the [Wedgewood Way] house.

Not only does this statement justify the price, it again emphasizes that the sellers are in competition with other sellers. In cases in which an offer is reasonable, acceptance rather than a counteroffer should be sought. By accepting, your sellers will be the winners over the owners of the competing house. Always be completely honest in justifying acceptance of an offer.

Agent Recommendations—Accept, Reject, or Counteroffer

It is unethical for a seller's agent to recommend to owners that an offer be accepted if the agent does not feel that the offer is in the best interests of the owners, considering the market, the property, and their needs. If an offer is clearly not in the owners' best interests, tell them. This is part of your fiduciary duty. The less sophisticated the owners, the greater is your duty to advise them. The name of the game is not "a commission by any means."

Owners' Responses to Offers

Keep in mind that owners have three choices when an offer is received:

1. Acceptance
2. Rejection
3. Counteroffer

It would be unusual if you were to recommend outright rejection. This recommendation likely would be made only in cases of clearly frivolous offers or offers in which the buyers are attempting to take unconscionable advantage of the sellers.

If an offer is fair, work for its acceptance rather than for a counteroffer. Many agents are too quick to suggest a counteroffer when it isn't necessarily in the owners' best interests. Some agents like to push for a counteroffer because it is relatively easy and avoids further confrontation with the owners. If you truly represent the owners, you have a duty to try to make them understand that a counteroffer rejects the offer and gives the buyers an out. Once an offer is rejected, the owners have lost their right to accept and form a contract. The offer is dead.

Until accepted, an offer can be withdrawn.

Explain **buyer's remorse**. Buyer's remorse is like a virus. Most buyers get it—some worse than others. They question their wisdom in having made the offer at the price they did and wonder whether it should have been made at all. They wonder if they should have spent more time looking. To some, a counteroffer is like a heaven-sent escape.

Even buyers who intend to accept a counteroffer frequently decide to spend one more day looking before they sign. All too often, they find something they like. A great many owners have lost advantageous deals because they tried to squeeze just a little more out of buyers. A counteroffer gives up the "bird in the hand."

It is not unethical conduct to use your persuasive skills to persuade an owner to accept an offer you believe is reasonable. In fact, it is the only truly ethical way to deal with the situation.

If owners want "to sleep on it" and you feel acceptance is in their best interests, you should consider a response such as this: "Let's take a moment to go over the sale again. You placed your home on the market because . . . Are your reasons for selling still valid?" Then continue with a logical summary of the benefits of the offer and go to a closing such as this one: "Don't you agree that accepting this offer now makes sense rather than allowing the buyers an opportunity to change their minds?" You could then hand them a pen.

Duties as a Buyer's Agent

If an agent does not represent the seller, then the agent has a duty to try to get his client's offer accepted. However, the agent must be absolutely honest about any facts presented to influence the seller. An agent must never aid the buyer in fraud. The buyer's agent should fully explain the offer to the seller's agent, especially any provision that is unusual or provides the buyer with a right to cancel the agreement. It is important that the seller understand that the agent represents the buyer as a buyer's agent.

Protecting the Seller

As the sellers' agent, you have a duty to protect them from fraudulent or "shady" practices. There are offers that on careful reading do not actually state what you expect them to.

If you are unsure of the meaning of an offer that has come through another agent, suggest the owners obtain legal help or reword the offer in a counter-offer. Be especially wary of any offer received on an offer form you are not familiar with. Some sharp operators use their own forms printed with a computer printer. They may even label the form with a designation number so it looks like a standard form. By submitting forms that contain what appear to be standard or "boilerplate" clauses, they could, for example, require that the sellers pay all the buyers' loan costs, as well as all closing costs.

Be wary of offers with low earnest money deposits coupled with lengthy escrow periods. The buyer may be using the purchase offer more as an option than as a purchase with the hope of reselling it before closing. You should ask for an increased down payment and either verification of funds or the buyers' loan preapproval.

Be particularly alert for any purchase in which it appears the buyer could be promoting a **cash-out scheme**. While there are a number of ways this can be done, the most popular is by use of a **subordination clause**. Where the property is owned free and clear or the sellers have substantial equity, the buyer offers a large cash amount and asks the sellers to carry the balance with a short-term trust deed. The catch is that the trust deed is a "subordinate" trust deed.

EXAMPLE Ina Cent owns her home free and clear. She wants to sell it for $400,000. After the home has been on the market for several months, Cent receives an offer from Joe Sharp. Sharp offers her full price for the home, with $100,000 down. He asks that she carry a subordinate trust deed for the $300,000 balance at 10% interest, all due and payable in one year. This offer looks terrific to Ina Cent, so she accepts the offer. Sharp arranges for a first trust deed at $250,000. Because the trust deed for $300,000 is subordinate, the lender is protected by the full value of the property (a $250,000 loan on a property having value of $400,000).

Even though Sharp's scheme would be apparent to a lender, there are lenders who will make the new loan but would likely charge high loan origination costs, as well as a high rate of interest. As far as the lender is concerned, Sharp has a $250,000 equity in the home. Sharp uses $100,000 for his down payment and has $150,000 left. He is a cash-out buyer.

The normal scenario is that Sharp would make no payments on the $250,000 first trust deed or the $300,000 subordinate (second) trust deed. The first trust deed would either foreclose and wipe out Ina Cent's equity or she would have to cure the first trust deed and foreclose on her second trust deed, leaving her in possession of her house but with a $250,000 trust deed against it. Joe Sharp, in the meantime, is spending his money.

Other buyers to be on the alert for are those who enter into a purchase with no investment. While many no-down-payment sales are legitimate, there have been horror cases. No-down buyers have rented the property, collecting rent without making payments on the trust deed obligation. This is called **rent skimming**. Rent skimming is illegal in California and subject to criminal penalties, but violations still occur. The definition of rent skimming has been expanded to cover collecting rents and deposits on property not owned or controlled by the renter. The penalty for renting a unit without the owner's permission is up to one year of imprisonment plus a $2,500 fine. While this form of rent skimming usually involves a party who rents out a vacant property, usually in foreclosure, a variation occurs when a buyer with low or no earnest money is given possession prior to closing. The buyer rents out the property, delays closing, and eventually the purchase fails. Other no-down buyers have harvested trees and sold personal property that was included in the sale but was not separately secured by a lien.

At the very least, you have a duty to warn the owners of negative possibilities. You also might suggest that a check be made of court dockets to determine whether such potential buyers have been defendants in lawsuits.

Be wary of offers in which buyers want to exchange personal property or real property. Again, many exchanges are valid transactions, but there also have been many sharp deals. Make certain the value of the property being received has been properly verified. Don't accept at face value appraisals provided by the buyers. Be particularly careful if a property profile indicates that buyers have only recently acquired the property. If a trust deed is being traded for property, be on guard if it is a new trust deed. It is important to determine the creditworthiness of the trustor and if the trustor has personal liability. Also, determine the value of the property. Some buyers have created trust deeds on nearly worthless property to use as trading material for valuable property.

A few years ago, sharp buyers were using uncut diamonds and colored gemstones as trading material. They also were including appraisals. Sellers who accepted the stones often found they had sold their properties for less than 10 cents on the dollar.

Because real estate involves large amounts of money, it can attract some very unscrupulous people. Many of these people are very intelligent and will devise elaborate schemes to get something for as close to nothing as possible. Some seminars have explained these unethical and often illegal schemes to attendees as a get-rich-quick answer to all their dreams. It is your duty as a real estate professional to look carefully at any deal that looks too good to be true. You have a fiduciary duty to protect your principal against the devious schemes of others. Of course, this points out why sellers should be represented by agents. (Even if you are a buyer's agent, you don't want to be an accomplice in an unethical and/or fraudulent scheme.)

Gaining an Acceptance

Many sellers will accept your recommendations for acceptance when those recommendations are logical and you have built up a relationship of trust with the owners. However, a home sale is not all logic. Emotions play a significant role in acceptance or rejection of a purchase offer. The primary **seller objections** concern price.

Price.   The most common objection to an offer is about **price**. The sellers might have counted on obtaining a specified price, and they feel that accepting less is a price cut. You can answer this objection by minimizing the difference. The goal of minimizing the difference is to make the difference—the unattained portion—appear small in relation to the whole:

> Buyers, not sellers, determine price. A price set by sellers is merely a wish unless they have a buyer. Right now, we have a buyer. While the offer is less than we had hoped, it is within [7%] of the comparative market

analysis, which places the offer in the realm of reasonableness. You are being offered [93%] of what you hoped for. You are only a signature away from a sale.

An excellent approach when sellers are adamant on a price is:

[Mr. and Mrs. Jones], if you did not own this house and you were given the opportunity to buy it right now, would you buy the house if it could be yours for [the price of the offer]?

The answer to such a question probably will be, "No, we don't need the house; that's why we are selling it!" You should now continue with the very logical:

Then why are you bidding on it? When you turn down an offer for [$489,000], you're really saying that the house is worth more to you than has been offered. You're an active bidder competing against this buyer. If you wouldn't pay [$489,000] for this house today, then you should be accepting an offer to sell it at [$489,000].

If the owners indicate that a reasonable offer is ridiculous, point out the following:

Right now I have a check for [$10,000]; now that's not ridiculous. I also have an offer for [$489,000]. It may be less than you had hoped for, but it is only [7%] less than the value established by our comparative market analysis. That to me is not ridiculous. It is a serious offer deserving serious consideration.

You will likely hear the "our friend said . . ." response. Basically, it is that someone they know who is "very knowledgeable" about real estate told them, "Don't take a dollar less than [$500,000] for your home." The way to deal with this invisible friend is:

[Mr. and Mrs. Jones], let us assume that you reject this offer, and that, despite my best efforts, months pass without another offer on your house. Let us also assume we finally obtain another offer at less than the present offer. Now assume you accept this offer. Will your friend make up your loss?

This shows that the owners alone bear the results of the decision and that it should not be made by anyone else. You can point out actual case histories that sellers can relate to. Chances are your broker can tell you many stories that follow this identical scenario.

When sellers are adamant about a set price and refuse an offer that almost gives them what they want, an approach you could raise is the following:

> Right now, you are willing to wait until you get what you are asking. Suppose we are able to find a buyer willing to meet your price but it takes us three months to do so, acceptance of the offer before us will likely mean more dollars in your pockets than the full price in three months. Consider the costs of taxes, insurance, (utilities), maintenance, and the lost opportunity in not having ($_____) right now. Coupled with these costs are additional risks of future offers at even lower prices.

| Put the difference in perspective; show it as a percentage. |

The sellers may be thinking in terms of thousands of dollars less than they had hoped for; however, you must present the positive side of a reasonable offer. You can do this by showing the difference not in dollars but in a percentage:

> Right now we have an offer giving you 93% of what you wanted to receive for your home. I think that's a pretty good offer.

The following "gambler" argument is also an excellent approach that uses percentages:

> [Mr. and Mrs. Jones], you certainly are gamblers. By accepting the offer before us, you can tie the buyers to this agreement. You are proposing a counteroffer that will give you [7%] more than this offer. You are wagering [93%] against [7%]. To me those seem like pretty long odds. I know I wouldn't gamble [93 cents] to make [7 cents], and I don't think you should either.

THE COUNTEROFFER

> A little more work on the offer might eliminate the need for a counteroffer.

If agents worked harder with buyers in formulating offers, the need for **counteroffers** would be diminished. Unfortunately, some agents accept unreasonable offers from potential purchasers without expending much effort to improve the offer. This allows prospective buyers to believe that a terrific bargain is possible. What the agent is hoping for isn't acceptance but a counteroffer that might be accepted. Unfortunately, it can be difficult to get a reasonable counteroffer accepted, once prospective buyers have been given these false hopes. Nevertheless, an unreasonable offer should be countered rather than rejected, because there is still the chance of a sale. Try to structure the counteroffer in such a manner that it will be met with acceptance.

What Is a Reasonable Offer?

What is a reasonable offer will vary, depending on the market. In a seller's market with many buyers and relatively few sellers, an offer of 10% below the CMA might be viewed as unreasonable. However, in a buyer's market with many sellers, such an offer might be regarded as reasonable. As a rule of thumb, a reasonable and acceptable offer falls within 10% of the value established by the CMA, again depending on the market.

If the listing agent does not feel acceptance of an offer is in the principal's best interest, the agent should advise against acceptance and make suggestions for a counteroffer that will serve the principal's interests. However, when an agent feels that the principal's best interests would be served by acceptance of an offer, the agent should strongly recommend acceptance and explain the reasons for the recommendation.

When all other efforts have failed to obtain acceptance of the offer in its present form, persuade the seller to make a counteroffer or a new offer in response to a potential buyer's offer. Any alteration to an offer, even a change in date or time of close, is considered a counteroffer. A counteroffer is a new offer where the seller becomes the offeror.

The following are the most common conditions desired by the seller when making a counteroffer:

- Increase in purchase price and/or cash deposit

- Safeguard provisions for the seller when the buyer's offer is conditional on sale of other property

- Limitations on the seller's warranties or demands that the buyer accept property as is

- Change of amount, terms, and conditions relating to loans to be carried

- Limitations on time allowed to obtain financing and the right of the seller to assist in locating a lender

Limitation on the liability for termite work, repairs, and the like

- Change in date of possession and demand for free occupancy

- The seller's right to accept other offers until the counteroffer is accepted

The following *dos* and *don'ts* will help you prepare and present a legitimate counteroffer:

- *Do* start by amending the acceptance clause to incorporate reference to the counteroffer

- *Do* have the seller sign the printed acceptance clause as amended if a separate acceptance clause is not inserted in the provisions of the counteroffer

- *Don't* make changes in the contract simply for the sake of change

- *Don't* pressure your principal to agree when the other party wishes to have some particular right or remedy inserted

- *Do* make sure that the addendum is dated and proper reference is made to the contract of which it is a part

- *Don't* make piecemeal changes in important terms; instead, rewrite the whole paragraph in which the terms occur for better clarity

- *Do* number the items of the counteroffer and refer to the contract paragraph where possible

- *Don't* let disagreement concerning language terminate the sale

- *Do* use a simple checklist for all points to be included in the counteroffer when drafting it

- *Do* be sure that all changes are initialed or signed properly and that all parties receive copies of the final contract executed by both sides

If you recommend a counteroffer, we suggest using a separate counteroffer, such as form 101-A prepared by Professional Publishing (Figure 11.1). Do not make changes on the purchase contract. If you change the purchase contract and the buyers counter the counteroffer and the sellers then counter the counter-counteroffer, you have a form that becomes difficult to understand. Tracing the chronological order of the sale also becomes difficult. If you use separate dated forms, what was agreed to and when will be clear. You may wish to number each counteroffer for clarity as to what the final agreement is.

FIGURE 11.1:   Counter Offer

COUNTER OFFER

In response to the Offer concerning the property located at _____
_____ made by, _____, Buyer,
dated _____ **the following Counter Offer is submitted:**

_____
_____
_____
_____
_____
_____
_____
_____
_____
_____
_____
_____
_____
_____
_____
_____
_____
_____
_____

OTHER TERMS: All other terms to remain the same.
RIGHT TO ACCEPT OTHER OFFERS: Seller reserves the right to accept any other offer prior to Buyer's written
acceptance of this Counter Offer. Acceptance shall not be effective until a copy of this Counter Offer, dated and signed by
Buyer, is received by Seller or _____, the Agent of the Seller.
EXPIRATION: This Counter Offer shall expire unless written acceptance is delivered to Seller or his or her Agent on or
before _____ ☐ a.m., ☐ p.m., on (date) _____.

Seller _____   Date _____ Time _____

Seller _____   Date _____ Time _____

ACCEPTANCE

The undersigned Buyer accepts the above Counter Offer (if checked ☐, subject to the attached Counter to Counter Offer).

Buyer _____   Date _____ Time _____

Buyer _____   Date _____ Time _____

Receipt of acceptance is acknowledged.

Seller _____   Seller _____

Use a separate form for a counteroffer. Do not make changes on the purchase contract.

A counteroffer at full asking price isn't much of a counteroffer, even if the original price was fair or below market value. You must allow the buyers to receive some advantage from the negotiations. Many sales are lost because of stubborn buyers and sellers. Sellers refuse to give an inch, and buyers want to "save face" by gaining some concession. Many buyers will walk away from an advantageous purchase rather than pay the full price.

Unless care is exercised in negotiations, a psychological wall may be built between the buyer and the seller. Figure 11.2 shows the bricks of a psychological wall between two principals.

A good approach to use when sellers do not want to give buyers a concession on a counteroffer is the following:

> Why not split the difference? The offer is for [$430,000] and you want [$490,000]. Why not counter at [$460,000]?

In presenting the counteroffer to the buyers, you can make the sellers appear reasonable, because "splitting the difference" is often considered fair. Although there is no rational justification for splitting the difference, very often it is accepted.

There are often counters to counteroffers and counters to the counters to the counteroffers. You can feel like a messenger. Much of the running from seller to buyer could ordinarily have been avoided by pressing to improve the offer when originally prepared.

THE ACCEPTANCE

Acceptance of an offer must be unqualified; a *qualified acceptance* must be considered as a new offer or a counteroffer. The legal effect of any changes is to reject the original offer and bar its later acceptance.

Acceptance must be unqualified or it becomes a counteroffer.

Keep in mind that acceptance does not take place until the person making the offer is notified of the acceptance. Until that time, the offeror is free to revoke the offer. Notification of acceptance is the delivery of a signed copy of the acceptance to the offeror. The CAR Residential Purchase Agreement allows notification of acceptance to be to the buyer's agent (broker).

Placing the acceptance in the mail constitutes notification. We recommend that you notify buyers of the acceptance immediately on receiving it.

Leave a completed offer form with the buyers, and let them know the procedure to be followed, as well as when you will contact them again. Be certain to give the buyers assurances of value and that they have purchased a fine house. People need to feel that they have done the right thing.

FIGURE 11.2: Building a Psychological Wall Between Principals

If buyers enjoy a home, they will not feel that they have overpaid, no matter what the price. On the other hand, if buyers are not happy in their home, even though they thought the home was a bargain—they overpaid. What really counts in the long run are the benefits, not the price tag.

Fax and Email Acceptance

There will be circumstances where you will be unable to present offers in person. In California, an electronic acceptance can be used. When you present an offer by fax, you should put your recommendations and your reasoning in a cover letter. If the offer is accepted by fax or a counteroffer is made, the seller should generate a transmission report reflecting the accurate transmission of the document.

Because email is considered an increasingly common means of modern communication, email acceptances of offers are now considered possible. The accepted offer can be an attachment to the email. Nevertheless, a signed copy of the acceptance should be placed in the mail to avoid any problems of delayed or claimed nonreceipt of electronic acceptance.

Advise the buyer

Advise the buyer to put off any large credit purchases until after closing. Buying a new car on credit for that new garage could mean the buyer is no longer qualified for the loan and will have a new car without a garage.

CHECKLIST FOR CLOSING

Your job isn't finished with the accepted offer. Because you don't receive compensation until the escrow closes, you must make certain the **closing** actually takes place. There are many things you must do to be sure no delays occur during closing. When there are delays, the likelihood of something happening to "kill" the sale tends to increase.

Because the individuals involved in the closing of a transaction may miss certain details and errors may creep in, it is your job to check frequently to uncover small problems before they become big ones. Check frequently to see if everything is moving according to schedule. Keep all parties fully informed of all events and conclusions. Remember, referrals depend on good follow-through. Some agents and teams have personal assistants that specialize in handling the required disclosures and paperwork of closing. They keep the lines of communication open with buyers, sellers, lenders, and escrow and prevent the occurrence of many problems.

Some agents tend to lose a great many deals during escrow. They like to blame it on bad luck, but they would be surprised how much luckier they could have been if they had worked just a little harder during escrow. There are a number of low-cost computer programs available to aid you in tracking the progress of escrows.

Closing Checklist

The following checklist contains some of the things you should be doing:

- ■ Provide information or purchase contract to escrow so the escrow holder can prepare escrow instructions.

- ■ Make certain all applicable disclosures discussed in Unit 3 or stated in the purchase contract are made.

- ■ If the offer calls for a structural pest control inspection, make certain that it is ordered as soon as possible.

- ■ If the offer provides for a professional home inspection, make certain that arrangements are made and that any problems be promptly resolved.

- ■ Make certain that parties sign the escrow instructions as soon as they are available (if they are not part of the purchase contract), as well as the necessary transfer documentation.

- ■ Keep in touch with the lender and make certain that this entity has everything needed to complete the loan.

- ■ Communicate with both buyer and seller at least once each week. Let both know what is happening and what you are doing for them. If there are any problems, disclose them and work with both parties toward a solution.

- ■ If there is a walk-through final inspection, you should be there. You don't want a nervous buyer and seller getting together without you.

- ■ Make certain the seller has labeled all keys and left behind any applicable appliance manuals, warranties, matching paint, garage-door openers, et cetera. Also, be sure the property is in clean condition. If necessary, suggest that the seller have the carpet cleaned as soon as the house is vacated.

- ■ Communicate with the escrow on a weekly basis. You want to know if a party has not done something or if there is a problem.

- ■ Contact the lending officer on a regular basis to make certain things are running smoothly.

- ■ After closing, thank both buyer and seller for their faith in you.

Some buyers will use their property inspection as the basis for another "bite at the apple" or a renegotiation of the price. They may seek disproportionate adjustment in price for real or perceived problems revealed by the inspection. You can point out to such buyers that they could be giving the seller the opportunity to get out of the contract and, if they really want the property, they should not take this risk.

Should the buyer or the seller, or both, be unable or unwilling to complete the purchase, you will want the buyer and the seller to agree, as soon as possible, as to the disposition of the deposit. By immediately addressing the problem, you will reduce the likelihood of legal action. A Cancellation of Agreement form is shown in Figure 11.3. This form calls for return of funds to parties depositing the funds, as well as a waiver of all rights pertaining to the agreement and who will pay required costs and fees incurred. A lawsuit means time spent testifying as a witness or, possibly, a defendant.

FIGURE 11.3:   **Cancellation of Agreement**

CANCELLATION OF AGREEMENT
Release and Waiver of Rights with Distribution of Funds in Escrow

| Prepared by: Agent _____ | Phone _____ |
| Broker _____ | Email _____ |

DATE: _____, 20_____, at _____, California.
Items left blank or unchecked are not applicable.
FACTS:

1. This mutual cancellation and release agreement with waiver of rights pertains to the following agreement:
    - ☐ Purchase agreement
    - ☐ Exchange agreement
    - ☐ _____

    1.1   dated _____, 20_____, at _____, California,
    1.2   entered into by _____, as the Buyer, and
          _____, as the Seller,
    1.3   whose real estate brokers (agents) are
          Buyer's Broker_____
          Seller's Broker _____,
          a. If an exchange is involved, the first and second parties to the exchange are here identified as Buyer
             and Seller, respectively.
    1.4   regarding real estate referred to as _____
          _____.
    1.5   Escrow Agent _____ Escrow Number _____

AGREEMENT:

2. Buyer and Seller hereby cancel and release each other and their agents from all claims and obligations, known or unknown, arising out of the above referenced agreement.
3. The real estate broker(s) and escrow agent(s) are hereby instructed to return all instruments and funds to the parties depositing them.
4. Costs and fees to be disbursed and charged to ☐ Seller, or ☐ Buyer.
    4.1 $_____ to _____
    4.2 $_____ to _____
    4.3   _____
          _____
          _____
          _____
          _____
          _____
5. The parties hereby waive any rights provided by Section 1542 of the California Civil Code, which provides:
    "A general release does not extend to claims which the creditor does not know or suspect to exist in his or her favor at the time of executing the release, which if known by him or her must have materially affected his or her settlement with the debtor."

I agree to the terms stated above.	**I agree to the terms stated above.**
☐ See attached Signature Page Addendum. [ft Form 251]	☐ See attached Signature Page Addendum. [ft Form 251]
Date: _____, 20_____	Date: _____, 20_____
Buyer's Name: _____	Seller's Name: _____
Signature: _____	Signature: _____
Buyer's Name: _____	Seller's Name: _____
Signature: _____	Signature: _____

FORM 181   03-11   ©2011 **first tuesday**, P.O. BOX 20069, Riverside, CA 92516 (800) 794-0494

©2015 RPI — Realty Publications, Inc., P.O. BOX 5707, RIVERSIDE, CA 92517

SUMMARY

It is important that the owners not know the details of any offer you have until you present it, so they can see the entire offer. Otherwise, they may build psychological walls that will make communication difficult. Before meeting with the owners, you should prepare a new Estimated Seller Proceeds form, and you might want to update the comparative market analysis.

Multiple offers should be presented in a fair and honest manner. A listing agent might encourage bidding by the offerees to raise the price.

Before you present the offer, set the mood by discussing what sold the buyers on the house. You also want the owners to sign the agency confirmation, if not covered in the offer form. The presentation process involves three stages:

1. The history of the sale

2. About the buyers

3. The offer itself

By covering the history of the sale, you will bring out the problems, if any, with the property that led other prospective buyers to reject the property. This helps deflate unrealistic expectations.

When you tell the owners about the buyers, make the buyers appear to be nice people that the sellers would like in their home. The buyers cannot appear to be arbitrary.

After covering the minor points, explain how the offer was arrived at. Recommend acceptance of a reasonable offer rather than advising a counteroffer. If the offer is not in the owners' best interests, however, recommend rejection or a counteroffer. If multiple offers are obtained, they should be presented in a nonprejudicial manner. Consider prequalifying buyers when multiple offers are received.

You must protect owners against fraud and sharp operators. Be on the alert for buyers who use their own forms, who want the sellers to carry a subordinate note, or who might otherwise be cash-out buyers. Also, be concerned if buyers are to obtain possession without any cash investment or if buyers want to exchange real or personal property for the owners' property. Don't place any value on appraisals provided by the buyers—verify everything. Be on the alert for buyers who recently acquired trust deeds or property and want to use them as trade property.

The most common objection raised by sellers to buyers' offers is price. It is in the owners' best interests to accept a reasonable offer rather than make a counteroffer that frees the buyers from the agreement. Counteroffers should consider benefits to both buyers and sellers and should be written on a separate form rather than added to the purchase contract. In this way, it will be easier to determine what exactly was agreed on and when.

Buyers can withdraw an offer anytime before acceptance. Acceptance does not take place until the accepted offer is mailed or delivered to the buyers.

Prepare a checklist of what must be done before closing.

Monitor the sale closely from acceptance to close of escrow while communicating with the buyers, the sellers, the escrow officer, and the loan officer on a regular basis. You must help the parties and make certain everything gets done; remember, a commission is not received until the closing.

CLASS DISCUSSION TOPICS

1. (If assigned by instructor) present a completed offer to an owner (another student). Your presentation will be either

   a. the history of the sale,

   b. information about the buyer, or

   c. the offer itself.

2. How would you handle the following objections of the seller to an offer?

   a. "That's $20,000 less than I paid."

   b. "Last year the house across the street from me sold for $10,000 more than this offer, and my house is nicer than their house."

   c. "If I have to cut my price, then you have to cut your commission or I won't accept the offer."

   d. "We would like to think it over."

   e. "The house is paid for. We can wait until we receive our price."

3. Bring to class one current-events article dealing with some aspect of real estate practice for class discussion.

UNIT 11 QUIZ

1. For listing agents, selling real estate involves three separate sales. Which is *NOT* one of them?
   a. Obtaining the listing
   b. Advertising for buyers
   c. Selling the buyer as to an offer
   d. Selling the seller on acceptance

2. You receive two offers on a property you have listed. One is from your own firm and the other, which was received an hour earlier, is from another firm. You should
   a. present the offers in the order received.
   b. present the highest-price offer first and, if not accepted, present the next offer.
   c. present the offers at the same time.
   d. always present your firm's offer before offers from other firms.

3. It would be *MOST* difficult to persuade an owner to accept a reasonable offer received
   a. 3 days after listing the property.
   b. 30 days after listing the property.
   c. 90 days after listing the property.
   d. 180 days after listing the property.

4. When presenting an offer on your listing for less than list price, it is good policy to
   a. immediately tell the seller what the offer is.
   b. not recommend acceptance or rejection.
   c. recommend that sellers counter or reject offers when acceptance is not in their best interest.
   d. have a number of your office staff present to intimidate the sellers.

5. Many buyers have second thoughts after placing an offer. This buyer apprehension is commonly known as
   a. feedback.
   b. the gambler syndrome.
   c. buyer's remorse.
   d. negative motivation.

6.   Which statement regarding counteroffers is *NOT* true?
     a.   A counteroffer serves as a rejection of an offer.
     b.   If the counteroffer is not accepted, the owner has the option of accepting the original offer.
     c.   A counteroffer turns the original offeree (the owner) into an offeror.
     d.   Both a and c.

7.   You should be particularly wary if an offer is received on your listing that contains the word(s)
     a.   "subordination."
     b.   "transfer disclosure."
     c.   "time is of the essence."
     d.   "liquidated damages."

8.   Rent skimming is
     a.   charging minorities an exorbitant rent.
     b.   a property manager's failure to disclose all rents received.
     c.   a buyer's failure to apply rents to loans that were assumed.
     d.   a tenant making monthly rent payments every 40 days.

9.   After two months, you receive an offer on one of your listings. Although for less than the listing amount, the offer is certainly reasonable based on the CMA. You should recommend to the owners that
     a.   they counteroffer at a price halfway between list price and the offer to split the difference.
     b.   the offer be rejected so that the offeror will raise the offer to the list price.
     c.   they let the offer period expire without taking any action to make the offeror anxious.
     d.   they accept the offer.

10. After an offer is accepted, the listing agent should
     a.   keep track of escrow progress.
     b.   make certain all papers are signed by the parties.
     c.   make certain that conditions are being met.
     d.   do all of these.

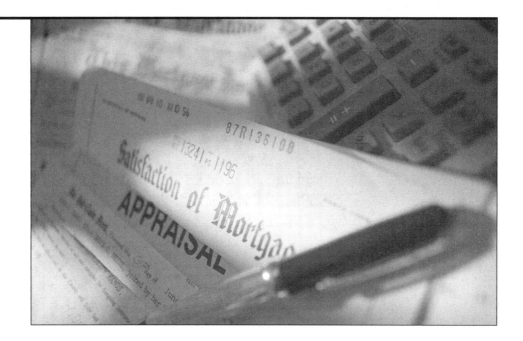

REAL ESTATE FINANCING

LEARNING OBJECTIVES

When you have completed this unit, you will be able to

- explain how the monetary policy of the Federal Reserve and the government's fiscal policy can affect the availability of funds for mortgage lending;

- describe the effect interest rates have on the real estate marketplace;

- explain the difference between primary and secondary financing and primary and secondary mortgage markets;

- explain the difference between conventional and government-involved financing;

- compare and contrast FHA, VA, and CalVet loans;

- describe different types of loans, including advantages and disadvantages of each; and

- explain the loan-qualifying process, the use of ratios and FICO scores, and the regulations that pertain to real estate finance.

KEY TERMS

adjustable-rate mortgage

adjustment period

affordability index

annual percentage rate (APR)

back-end ratio

blanket trust deed

California Housing Finance Agency loans

CalVet loans

closing the loan

commercial banks

computerized loan origination

conforming loans

construction loan

controlled business arrangement

conventional loans

convertible ARM

cosigner

credit union

direct endorsement

discount points

discount rate

Dodd-Frank

due-on-sale clause

Equal Credit Opportunity Act

Fair Credit Reporting Act

Fannie Mae

Farmer Mac

Federal Reserve

FHA-insured loan

FICO score

fixed-rate loan

Freddie Mac

front-end ratio

Ginnie Mae

hard money loans

hybrid loans

index rate

institutional lenders

insurance

interest-only loans

jumbo loans

life insurance company

Loan Estimate

margin

monetary policy

mortgage banker

mortgage broker

mortgage companies

mortgage loan broker

mortgage loan disclosure

mortgage warehousing

negative amortization

nonconforming loans

noninstitutional lenders

open market transactions

open-end trust deed

option ARM

origination points

packaged loan

participation loan

payment shock

pension fund

points

portfolio loans

predatory lending

primary financing

primary mortgage market

private mortgage

qualified mortgage

qualifying borrowers

real estate investment trust

release clause

renegotiable-rate mortgage

reserve requirements

reverse mortgage

SAFE

savings associations

secondary financing

secondary mortgage market

seller carryback financing

Service Members Civil Relief Act

statement

subprime lender

take-out loan

third-party originator

TILA-RESPA Integrated Disclosure (TRID) rule

Truth in Lending Act

Truth in Savings Act

VA-guaranteed loan

verification of employment

wraparound trust deed

FEDERAL RESERVE

The **Federal Reserve** is responsible for our **monetary policy**. It seeks to adjust the availability and cost of money so there is steady economic growth with minimum unemployment and inflation in check. The Federal Reserve has three basic controls:

1. **Discount rate.** By raising and lowering the discount rate charged to member banks to borrow funds, the Federal Reserve affects long-term rates charged by lenders. Lower rates fuel the economy, but higher rates are a contractionary economic policy.

2. **Reserve requirements.** By raising and lowering reserve requirements of banks, the amount of available funds to loan is regulated. Less funds for lending means higher interest based on supply and demand factors.

3. **Open market transactions.** The Federal Reserve can buy government securities on the open market to put money into the economy or to sell government securities to take money from the economy to slow growth.

INTEREST RATES AND THE REAL ESTATE MARKET

The health of the real estate industry is directly related to the cost of money or interest rates. Lower interest rates mean lower payments, which in turn means that more people become qualified for loans. With more buyers, we tend to have a seller's market and see real estate prices increase.

Real estate sales had been strong because of affordability brought about by low interest rates. Strong real estate sales also aided construction-related industries, as well as sales of furniture, appliances, and textiles for households.

When interest rates increase, real estate sales tend to decrease. (Sales are related inversely to interest rates.) Rising interest rates affect affordability.

LOAN POINTS

Points are percentages of the loan. They are charged to the borrower at the time the loan is made. One point would be 1% of the loan amount.

Points are either discount points or origination points.

Discount points are monies paid at the time of loan origination that allow the borrower a rate of interest less than originally offered by the lender. Therefore, discount points could be considered prepaid interest. As a rule of thumb, a lender considers eight points equivalent to 1% difference in a fixed rate loan. So a lender would want two points on a 6¼% loan if the lender wanted a 6½% yield.

Origination points are fees to cover administrative loan costs and lender compensation. As an example, a mortgage broker may want one point to make the loan even though the lender intends to sell the loan at face amount to another lender.

The **affordability index** from the National Association of REALTORS® measures the median family income necessary to support a mortgage for the median-priced home. The index is based on a 30-year fixed-rate mortgage with a 20% down payment at the current Freddie Mac mortgage rate. It is also based on the assumption that total monthly house payments, including taxes and insurance, cannot exceed 30% of gross household income. Because lenders allowed families to pay more than 30% of gross income and because of the variety of loan products offering lower payments, the affordability index best measures changes in housing affordability.

According to the California Association of REALTORS®, only 30% of California homebuyers can afford the median-priced home in California. In order to afford the median-priced house, a household would have to have income of $95,980 annually to make monthly payments of $2,400. A rapid rise in property values from 2012 to early 2016 has made housing less affordable.[1]

---

1   California Association of REALTORS®, "Growth in spring home prices leads to sizable drop in California housing affordability, C.A.R. reports," August 22, 2015, 2nd Qtr 2015 Housing Affordabiity report, news release, www.car.org/newsstand/newsreleases/2015releases/2q2015hai.

SOURCES OF FUNDS

Almost everyone is at some time a user, a buyer, or a seller of real estate. The average American spends more than 20% of his lifetime income on some form of real estate, either for rental or for purchase as an investment or as a residence. Because real estate is the largest purchase most people make in their lifetimes, few are prepared to pay cash. Thus, the completion of most real estate sales will depend on funds available in the money market at the time of the transaction.

Because most buyers are unable or unwilling to pay cash for real property, long-term financing in the form of a mortgage (or trust deed) loan is necessary. Understanding the use of real estate mortgage money requires an understanding of the sources of these funds. Money to finance real estate purchases is available through three primary money market areas: *directly* from someone or some institution that has accumulated this money, *indirectly* from a lending institution that loans money deposited in customers' accounts, or from investors who purchase loans or collateralized mortgage securities. You should be constantly aware of the status of the money market in your area, including policies of lenders, interest rates, points, and lending costs.

Different lenders offer variations in products (loans) and have different underwriting standards for different types of properties. An experienced agent will help clients select a lender and type of loan whose standards meet the property being purchased, as well as the specific client needs.

PRIMARY AND SECONDARY FINANCING

Primary financing refers to the first loan recorded against the property. Because interest rates are related to risk, primary financing generally has lower interest rates than other loans in which the security interest is secondary (i.e., second trust deeds).

> Primary financing refers to first trust deeds, secondary financing to junior loans.

Any junior trust deed is **secondary financing**. Holders of a second trust deed bear a greater risk than holders of a first trust deed; therefore, second trust deeds customarily bear a higher rate of interest. In the event of default of the first trust deed, the holders of the second have to either cure the default and foreclose on the second trust deed or wait until the foreclosure and bid cash. If holders of the second trust deed fail to do either, they may lose their security.

PRIMARY AND SECONDARY MORTGAGE MARKETS

While primary financing refers to first trust deeds, the **primary mortgage market** refers to loans being made directly to borrowers, either first or second trust deeds. The **secondary mortgage market** refers to the resale of existing mortgages and trust deeds.

Four agencies—Fannie Mae (FNMA), Ginnie Mae (GNMA), and Freddie Mac (FHLMC), and Farmer Mac—are responsible for creating and establishing a viable secondary mortgage market. They buy loans originated by others and resell mortgage-backed securities. Their operations have created a national securities market for the sale of real estate debt instruments by the originators to second buyers. Selling the loans frees capital to create more real estate mortgages. The secondary market also minimizes the effects of regional cycles and redistributes the funds from cash-rich areas to cash-poor ones, thus stabilizing the money market.

Fannie Mae

Fannie Mae, formerly the Federal National Mortgage Association (FNMA), was established in 1938 to stimulate the secondary mortgage market by buying FHA-insured and VA-guaranteed mortgages made by private lenders. In 1968, Fannie Mae evolved into a private, profit-oriented corporation that markets its own securities and handles a variety of real estate loans. These loans are purchased (sometimes at a discount) and can be resold to other lenders or investors. Stabilizing the market gives lenders a sense of security and encourages them to make more loans. Because of loan problems, Fannie Mae is again under government conservatorship.

Freddie Mac

Freddie Mac, formerly the Federal Home Loan Mortgage Corporation (FHLMC), was founded with money provided by the 12 Federal Home Loan Banks when new mortgage loans could not be made because money was flowing out of the savings and loan associations (S&Ls). Freddie Mac created needed funds by floating its own securities backed by its pool of mortgages and guaranteed by Ginnie Mae. This gave S&Ls a secondary market for selling their conventional mortgages. Freddie Mac buys loans that have been closed within one year at specified discount rates.

Both Fannie Mae and Freddie Mac ran into serious financial difficulties because of their purchases of high-risk loans.

Federal Takeover of Fannie Mae and Freddie Mac

In September 2008, the federal government placed a conservatorship over Freddie Mac and Fannie Mae. The conservatorship of these government-sponsored agencies was to be run by the Federal Housing Finance Agency (FHFA). Huge losses and concerns that the agencies could no longer raise capital to support the U.S. housing market necessitated the takeover. Both agencies are now operating at a profit, and there is political pressure to again place them under private control.

Ginnie Mae

Ginnie Mae, once the Government National Mortgage Association (GNMA), is presently a wholly government-owned agency, but privatization is being considered. Higher-risk—but important—programs, such as urban renewal, low-income housing, and other special-purpose government-backed programs, are financed through this agency. Ginnie Mae participates in the secondary mortgage market through its mortgage-backed securities programs. Qualified mortgage lenders and approved dealers can obtain additional capital for mortgages by pooling a group of homogeneous existing loans and pledging them as collateral. Ginnie Mae guarantees that holders of these securities will receive timely principal and interest payments.

Federal Agricultural Mortgage Corporation

Farmer Mac, the Federal Agricultural Mortgage Corporation, is a government-chartered, but now private, corporation that provides a secondary mortgage market for farm property and rural housing.

CONFORMING LOANS

Conforming loans meet Fannie Mae and Freddie Mac purchase criteria.

A lender that makes a loan either keeps the loan in its portfolio or sells the loan in the secondary mortgage market. Loans that the lender keeps (does not sell) are called **portfolio loans**. Loans that the lender sells are called *nonportfolio loans*. **Conforming loans** are conventional loans that meet the underwriting standards for purchase by Fannie Mae or Freddie Mac. These loans are written for 15-year or 30-year terms and are not assumable. They have strict guidelines regarding down payments and maximum amounts. In 2015, a single-family loan had a limit to $417,000 to be eligible for purchase by Fannie Mae or Freddie Mac (this amount is revised on January 1 of each year) and is higher in some high-housing-cost areas. Because of the ready market for these loans, lenders are willing to make them and to purchase them on the secondary mortgage market. Because of their strict underwriting requirements, the interest rates for conforming loans are generally less than rates charged for **nonconforming loans**.

Loans for amounts of $417,000 and more are customarily called jumbo loans. Interest rates on **jumbo loans** are higher than rates for conforming loans.

LENDERS

All lenders are interested in the value of the property, the character of the borrower reflected in the FICO score, and the buyers' ability to make the payments.

Lenders can be divided into two groups: institutional lenders and noninstitutional lenders.

Institutional Lenders

Institutional lenders are subject to government regulations. These are major commercial banks, savings associations, and life insurance companies. (See Figure 12.1.)

Commercial banks. **Commercial banks** are familiarly known as the "department stores" of financial institutions because of the variety of operations in which they engage. A principal activity of commercial banks is lending money. Commercial banks prefer to make loans to their customers because this preference helps create depositors.

Banks often charge lower loan fees than other institutional lenders. They are quite versatile in the type of loans they may consider, but they seldom allow secondary financing at the time of providing a purchase-money loan.

Commercial banks have been a major source for construction loans. They like the shorter term and higher interest rates of these loans.

Banks have been expanding their home equity loans (second trust deeds). Some offer an open-end line of credit secured by the borrowers' home equity.

Banks in California

In California, banks are either federally chartered or state chartered and are regulated by federal and state laws, respectively. They tend to favor short-term loans and follow relatively conservative appraisal and lending practices. Their real estate loans generally are 80% or less of the appraised value of the property. Borrowers who are unable to put at least 20% down will likely be required to buy **private mortgage insurance** (PMI). A homeowner can request cancellation of the mortgage insurance when the homeowner's equity reaches 20%, payments are current, and there has not been more than one late payment in the prior year. The insurance must be canceled when the homeowner's equity reaches 22% (based on purchase price).

FIGURE 12.1:   Institutional Lenders

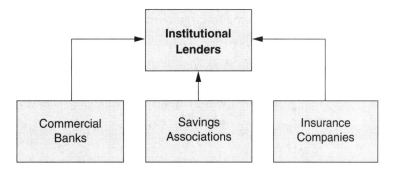

Many banks have also gone into the mortgage banking business. They make loans, which they then sell to other lenders or investors such as pension funds. They may continue to service loans that they sell.

Savings associations. Savings associations, also known as "thrifts" and originally known as savings and loan associations (S&Ls), formerly accounted for more home loans than any other source. After deregulation in the 1980s, they branched into other higher-yielding but higher-risk loans, which led to a great many S&L failures. Like banks, savings associations are state or federally chartered. They are allowed to loan up to 95% of the property's appraised value, although an 80% loan-to-value ratio (LTV) is most usual. The distinction between banks and savings associations has almost disappeared. Most California S&Ls have now become state- or federally chartered banks

Life insurance companies. The lending policies of **life insurance companies** are governed by the laws of the state in which the company is chartered, the laws of the state in which the loan originates, the policies of management, and the availability of loan funds.

Insurance companies supply many of the loans on properties for which huge loans are required (commercial properties, shopping centers, industrial properties, and hotels). In California, they make loans for up to 75% of the property's market value. Their commercial loans are commonly for 25 to 30 years. Insurance companies' interest rates often are lower than those of banks or savings associations. These loans seldom have due-on-sale clauses.

Insurance companies frequently demand an equity position as a limited partner as a condition of making a loan (**participation loan**). Many insurance companies were motivated by the benefit of an equity position coupled with the rapid depreciation allowed by the Tax Reform Act of 1981 to make large commercial loans. (Insurance company lending in the mid-1980s contributed to the overbuilding of shopping centers and office structures in many areas of the country.)

Noninstitutional lenders that make real estate loans include pension funds, credit unions, private individuals, and real estate investment trusts. (See Figure 12.2.)

FIGURE 12.2:   Noninstitutional Lenders

Mortgage Bankers or Mortgage Companies

Mortgage bankers can be licensed in California by either the Bureau of Real Estate or the Department of Corporations.

Mortgage bankers make loans using a line of credit from another lending institution and usually resell the loans on the secondary mortgage market. This resale of existing loans allows mortgage bankers to free up capital on their line of credit in order to make new loans. They usually have a close working relationship with one or more lenders and receive daily rate sheets. **Mortgage companies** are currently the largest single source of residential mortgage loan origination in California. You will see that the lender websites listed in the appendix are primarily mortgage bankers.

Mortgage companies make money on origination fees, as well as on loan servicing fees. Though they generally resell the loans that they originate, mortgage companies often continue to service these loans.

Mortgage companies might hold off selling mortgages that they originated if they believe that mortgage interest rates will drop. If they are right, mortgages made at higher rates could be sold at a premium above face value. The mortgage banker might borrow on this inventory of loans held for resale. This is known as **mortgage warehousing**.

Mortgage companies are careful in qualifying borrowers because loans that fail to conform to Fannie Mae and Freddie Mac purchase requirements are difficult to sell on the secondary mortgage market. Mortgage bankers will generally only make loans when they have a buyer for them. They seldom make loans that they do not intend to resell.

Mortgage companies are able to make many difficult loans that most banks would decline, such as loans for mixed-use properties or loans where buyers have had credit problems or low FICO scores. They might place such loans with **subprime lenders** that make difficult loans at a higher rate of interest. Many of the financial problems, beginning in 2008, were the result of high-risk loans originated by mortgage companies because there were buyers for them. In many cases the loans were used to back securities that were sold throughout the world. Nonperforming loans and foreclosure have led to severe financial difficulties by those holding those loans and/or their mortgage backed securities.

Mortgage Loan Broker

> Mortgage brokers are strictly middlemen who bring lenders and borrowers together.

According to the state's Mortgage Loan Brokerage Law, a **mortgage loan broker** is a person who acts for compensation in negotiating a new loan and is required to be licensed as a real estate broker or salesperson. No separate license is required. Real estate brokers who negotiate mortgage loans under the Mortgage Loan Brokerage Law are limited in the amount that they may charge as a commission for arranging the loan and for costs and expenses of making the loan. Loans on first trust deeds of $30,000 or more or on second trust deeds of $20,000 or more do not come within the purview of the law, but commissions and expenses are negotiable between the broker and the buyer.

Commission maximums under the law are as follows:

- First trust deeds (less than $30,000)—5% of the loan if less than three years; 10% if three years or more

- Second trust deeds (less than $20,000)—5% of the loan if less than two years; 10% if at least two years but less than three years; 15% if three years or more

If the loan comes under the purview of the law, the expenses of making the loan charged to the borrower (i.e., appraisal fees, escrow fees, title charges, notary fees, recording fees, and credit investigation fees) cannot exceed 5% of the principal amount of the loan. However, if 5% of the loan is less than $390, the broker may charge up to that amount. Regardless of the size of the loan, the buyer (borrower) cannot be charged more than $700 for costs and expenses. In no event may the maximum be charged if it exceeds the actual costs and expenses incurred.

Because mortgage loan brokers can arrange loans for noninstitutional as well as institutional lenders, they are often able to place loans that many direct lenders turn down because of perceived problems with the borrower or the loan security. These loans could require higher loan costs and/or a higher rate of interest. Mortgage loan brokers are required to provide a **mortgage loan disclosure statement** to borrowers (see Figure 12.3).

Because most loans arranged by mortgage loan brokers are first trust deeds of $30,000 or more or second trust deeds of $20,000 or more, the limitations on loan cost and commissions seldom become an issue. The lender can charge whatever the market will bear for loans above the amounts stated.

Mortgage loan brokers arrange a wide variety of loans. Because the mortgage loan broker is a middleman, the security for the loan must satisfy the *lender's criteria* for the loan. Mortgage loan brokers generally do not service the loans they arrange.

FIGURE 12.3:   Mortgage Loan Disclosure Statement (Borrower)

MORTGAGE LOAN DISCLOSURE STATEMENT
(Traditional) (DRE 882)

Prepared by: Agent _____   **Phone** _____

Broker _____   **Email** _____

BORROWER'S NAME(S)

REAL PROPERTY COLLATERAL: THE INTENDED SECURITY FOR THIS PROPOSED LOAN WILL BE A DEED OF TRUST OR MORTGAGE ON (STREET ADDRESS OR LEGAL DESCRIPTION)

THIS MORTGAGE LOAN DISCLOSURE STATEMENT IS BEING PROVIDED BY THE FOLLOWING CALIFORNIA REAL ESTATE BROKER ACTING AS A MORTGAGE BROKER

INTENDED LENDER TO WHOM YOUR LOAN APPLICATION WILL BE DELIVERED (IF KNOWN)   ☐ Unknown

❖ For any federally related mortgage loans, HUD/RESPA laws require that a Good Faith Estimate (GFE) be provided. A RE 882 Mortgage Loan Disclosure Statement (MLDS) is required by California law and must also be provided.

❖ The information provided below reflects estimates of the charges you are likely to incur at the settlement of your loan. The fees, commissions, costs and expenses listed are estimates; the actual charges may be more or less. Your transaction may not involve a charge for every item listed and any additional items charged will be listed.

Item	Paid to Others	Paid to Broker
Items Payable in Connection with Loan		
Mortgage Broker Commission/Fee	▓▓▓▓▓▓▓▓	$
Lender's Loan Origination Fee	$	▓▓▓▓▓▓▓▓
Lender's Loan Discount Fee	$	
Appraisal Fee	$	$
Credit Report	$	$
Lender's Inspection Fee	$	$
Tax Service Fee	$	$
Processing Fee	$	$
Underwriting Fee	$	$
Wire Transfer Fee	$	$
Items Required by Lender to be Paid in Advance		
Interest for _____ days at $_____ per day	$ 0.00	$
Hazard Insurance Premiums	$	$
County Property Taxes	$	$
Mortgage Insurance Premiums	$	$
VA Funding Fee/FHA MIP/PMI	$	$
Other:_____	$	$
Reserves Deposited with Lender		
Hazard Insurance: _____ months at $_____ /mo.	$ 0	$
Co. Property Taxes: _____ months at $_____ /mo.	$ 0	$
Mortgage Insurance: _____ months at $_____ /mo.	$ 0	$
Other:_____	$	$
Title Charges		
Settlement or Closing/Escrow Fee	$	$
Document Preparation Fee	$	$
Notary Fee	$	$
Title Insurance	$	$
Other:_____	$	$

— — — — — — — — — — — — — — — PAGE ONE OF FOUR — FORM 204 (DRE 882) — — — — — — — — — — — — — — — —

FIGURE 12.3 (continued):   Mortgage Loan Disclosure Statement (Borrower)

— — — — — — — — — — — — — — — — — *PAGE TWO OF FOUR — FORM 204 (DRE 882)* — — — — — — — — — — — — — — — — — —

<u>*Government Recording and Transfer Charges*</u>

Recording Fees	$_____	$_____
City/County Tax/Stamps	$_____	$_____
Other:_____	$_____	$_____

<u>*Additional Settlement Charges*</u>

Pest Inspection	$_____	$_____
Credit Life, and/or Disabilty Insurance (See Note below)✳	$_____	$_____
Subtotals of Initial Fees, Commissions, Costs and Expenses	$0.00	$0.00

Total of Initial Fees, Commissions, Costs and Expenses $ 0.00

<u>*Compensation to Broker (Not Paid Out of Loan Proceeds)*</u>

Yield Spread Premium, Service Release Premium or Other Rebate <u>Received from Lender</u> $_____

Yield Spread Premium, Service Release Premium or Other Rebate <u>Credited to Borrower</u> $_____

Total Amount of Compensation <u>Retained by Broker</u> $_____

✳ **Note: The purchase of Credit Life and/or Disability Insurance is NOT required as a condition of making this proposed loan.**

ADDITIONAL REQUIRED CALIFORNIA DISCLOSURES

Proposed Loan Amount	$_____
Initial Commissions, Fees, Costs, and Expenses Summarized on Page 1	$_____
Down Payment or Loan Payoffs/Creditors (List):	$_____
_____	$_____
_____	$_____
_____	$_____
Subtotal of All Deductions	$_____
Estimated Cash at Closing ☐ To You ☐ That You Must Pay	$_____

GENERAL INFORMATION ABOUT LOAN	
PROPOSED INTEREST RATE: _____% ☐ FIXED RATE ☐ INITIAL VARIABLE RATE	Proposed Monthly Loan Payments: $_____ Principal & Interest (P&I) If the loan is a variable interest rate loan, the payment will vary. See loan documents for details. Total Number of Installments: _____ Loan Term _____ Years _____ Months

BALLOON PAYMENT INFORMATION		
IS THIS LOAN SUBJECT TO A BALLOON PAYMENT? ☐ Yes ☐ No	DUE DATE OF FINAL BALLOON PAYMENT (ESTIMATED MONTH/DAY/YEAR)	AMOUNT OF BALLOON PAYMENT $

IF YES, THE FOLLOWING PARAGRAPH APPLIES:

NOTICE TO BORROWER: IF YOU DO NOT HAVE THE FUNDS TO PAY THE BALLOON PAYMENT WHEN IT COMES DUE, YOU MAY HAVE TO OBTAIN A NEW LOAN AGAINST YOUR PROPERTY TO MAKE THE BALLOON PAYMENT. IN THAT CASE, YOU MAY AGAIN HAVE TO PAY COMMISSIONS, FEES, AND EXPENSES FOR THE ARRANGING OF THE NEW LOAN. IN ADDITION, IF YOU ARE UNABLE TO MAKE THE MONTHLY PAYMENTS OR THE BALLOON PAYMENT, YOU MAY LOSE THE PROPERTY AND ALL OF YOUR EQUITY THROUGH FORECLOSURE. KEEP THIS IN MIND IN DECIDING UPON THE AMOUNT AND TERMS OF THIS LOAN.

PREPAYMENT INFORMATION		
PREPAYMENT PENALTY? ☐ Yes ☐ No	# OF YEARS THAT PREPAYMENT PENALTY IS IN EFFECT	MAXIMUM DOLLAR AMOUNT OF PENALTY

IS THERE A PREPAYMENT PENALTY FOR PAYING IN EXCESS OF 20% OF THE ORIGINAL OR UNPAID LOAN BALANCE?

☐ Yes ☐ No   If Yes, see loan documents for details.

TAXES AND INSURANCE	
IMPOUND ACCOUNT? ☐ Yes ☐ No **APPROXIMATE** AMOUNT THAT WILL BE COLLECTED MONTHLY $	IMPOUND ACCOUNT WILL INCLUDE County Property Taxes ☐ Yes ☐ No Mortgage Insurance ☐ Yes ☐ No Hazard Insurance ☐ Yes ☐ No Flood Insurance ☐ Yes ☐ No Other:_____ ☐ Yes ☐ No

— — — — — — — — — — — — — — — — *PAGE TWO OF FOUR — FORM 204 (DRE 882)* — — — — — — — — — — — — — — — — — —

FIGURE 12.3 (continued):   Mortgage Loan Disclosure Statement (Borrower)

— — — — — — — — — — — — — — — — — *PAGE THREE OF FOUR — FORM 204 (DRE 882)* — — — — — — — — — — — — — — — —

IF NO, PLAN FOR THESE PAYMENTS ACCORDINGLY	BORROWER MUST PLAN FOR PAYMENTS OF THE FOLLOWING ITEMS
→	County Property Taxes Mortgage Insurance Hazard Insurance Flood Insurance Other: _____ ☐ Yes ☐ No ☐ Yes ☐ No ☐ Yes ☐ No ☐ Yes ☐ No ☐ Yes ☐ No

Note: In a purchase transaction, county property taxes are calculated based on the sales price of the property and may require the payment of an additional (supplemental) tax bill issued by the county tax authority. The payment of county property taxes (including supplemental bills) may be paid by your lender if an impound/escrow account has been established.

If an impound/escrow account has not been established, the payment of all tax bills including any and all supplemental tax bills will be the responsibility of the borrower(s).

OTHER LIENS

LIENS CURRENTLY ON THIS PROPERTY FOR WHICH THE BORROWER IS OBLIGATED

Lienholder's Name	*Amount Owing*	*Priority*

LIST LIENS THAT WILL REMAIN OR ARE ANTICIPATED TO REMAIN ON THIS PROPERTY AFTER THE PROPOSED LOAN FOR WHICH YOU ARE APPLYING IS MADE OR ARRANGED (INCLUDING THE PROPOSED LOAN FOR WHICH YOU ARE APPLYING):

Lienholder's Name	*Amount Owing*	*Priority*

NOTICE TO BORROWER: BE SURE THAT YOU STATE THE AMOUNT OF ALL LIENS AS ACCURATELY AS POSSIBLE. IF YOU CONTRACT WITH THE BROKER TO ARRANGE THIS LOAN, BUT IT CANNOT BE ARRANGED BECAUSE YOU DID NOT STATE THESE LIENS CORRECTLY, YOU MAY BE LIABLE TO PAY COMMISSIONS, COSTS, FEES, AND EXPENSES EVEN THOUGH YOU DO NOT OBTAIN THE LOAN.

ARTICLE 7 COMPLIANCE

If this proposed loan is secured by a first deed of trust in a principal amount of less than $30,000 or secured by a junior lien in a principal amount of less than $20,000, the undersigned broker certifies that the loan will be made in compliance with Article 7 of Chapter 3 of the Real Estate Law.

WILL THIS LOAN BE MADE WHOLLY OR IN PART FROM BROKER CONTROLLED FUNDS AS DEFINED IN SECTION 10241(J) OF THE BUSINESS AND PROFESSIONS CODE?

☐ May   ☐ Will   ☐ Will Not

Note: If the broker indicates in the above statement that the loan "may" be made out of broker-controlled funds, the broker must inform the borrower prior to the close of escrow if the funds to be received by the borrower are in fact broker-controlled funds.

STATED INCOME

IS THIS LOAN BASED ON LIMITED OR NO DOCUMENTATION OF YOUR INCOME AND/OR ASSETS?

☐ Yes ☐ No   If Yes, be aware that this loan may have a higher interest rate or more points or fees than other products requiring documentation.

NOTICE TO BORROWER: THIS IS NOT A LOAN COMMITMENT

Do not sign this statement until you have read and understood all of the information in it. All parts of this form must be completed before you sign it. Borrower hereby acknowledges the receipt of a copy of this statement.

NAME OF BROKER	LICENSE ID NUMBER	BROKER'S REPRESENTATIVE	LICENSE ID NUMBER
	NMLS ID NUMBER		NMLS ID NUMBER

BROKER'S ADDRESS			

BROKER'S SIGNATURE	DATE	OR SIGNATURE OF REPRESENTATIVE	DATE
BORROWER'S SIGNATURE	DATE	BORROWER'S SIGNATURE	DATE

FIGURE 12.3 (continued):   Mortgage Loan Disclosure Statement (Borrower)

— — — — — — — — — — — — — — — — *PAGE FOUR OF FOUR — FORM 204 (DRE 882)* — — — — — — — — — — — — — — — —

Department of Real Estate license information telephone number: 877-373-4542, or check license status at www.dre.ca.gov

NMLS - http://mortgage.nationwidelicensingsystem.org/about/pages/nmlsconsumeraccess.aspx

The Real Estate Broker negotiating the loan shall retain on file for a period of three years a true and correct copy of this disclosure signed and dated by the borrower(s).

THE RE 855 MORTGAGE LOAN DISCLOSURE STATEMENT, NON-TRADITIONAL MORTGAGE MUST BE USED FOR NON-TRADITIONAL MORTGAGE LOANS OF RESIDENTIAL PROPERTY (1-4 UNITS).

Non-Traditional Mortgage Loans are loan products that allow the borrower to defer payments of principal or interest. If any of the payments are not full principal and interest payments, then it is considered a Non-Traditional Mortgage Loan.

FORM 204 (DRE 882)   3-11   ©2011 first tuesday, P.O. BOX 20069, RIVERSIDE, CA 92516 (800) 794-0494

©2015 RPI — Realty Publications, Inc., P.O. BOX 5707, RIVERSIDE, CA 92517

Scope of lending activity—real estate brokers.

There are three distinct areas of lending activity that a real estate broker can engage in:

> The mortgage broker brings together individual lenders and borrowers.

1. **Hard money makers and arrangers**—A **hard money loan** is a cash loan rather than an extension, such as seller financing. Articles V and VII of the real estate law primarily deal with hard money loans where the mortgage broker acts as an intermediary, bringing together lenders and borrowers. This activity is commonly known as *mortgage brokerage*, and the real estate licensee is acting as a **mortgage broker**.

   The loans are not made in the broker's name. They are made in the name of the lender. Most of the hard money loans are equity loans rather than purchase loans. Lenders are often private individuals.

2. **Third-party originators**—Third-party originators prepare loan applications for borrowers, which they submit to lenders. They may be agents of the borrower or the lender or dual agents of both borrower and lender. Out-of-state lenders that wish to invest directly in California mortgages frequently use third-party originators, as do pension plans and trusts. Thus, lenders that are not prepared to take loan applications in California can be direct lenders rather than having to purchase loans that were originated by others in the secondary mortgage market. They primarily deal in purchase-money loans.

> Mortgage bankers are regulated by either the Bureau of Real Estate or the Department of Corporations.

3. **Mortgage bankers**—Not all mortgage bankers are real estate brokers. Some mortgage bankers are licensed under the California Residential Mortgage Lending Act, which is administered by the Department of Corporations. A mortgage banker must elect which license to operate under. Thus, we have two state agencies, the Bureau of Real Estate and the Department of Corporations, regulating the same type of activity, depending on which license the mortgage banker is operating under. (The broker makes loans while operating as a mortgage banker; however, the broker only arranges loans as a third party when operating as a mortgage broker.)

Real estate investment trusts. The **real estate investment trust** (REIT) was created in 1960 to encourage small investors to pool their resources with others to raise venture capital for real estate transactions. To qualify as a REIT, the trust must have at least 100 investors, and 90% of the trust's income must be distributed annually to its investors.

While a number of equity trusts invests solely in ownership of real property, there are many mortgage trusts that invest their money in mortgages, either directly or through a mortgage company. There also are hybrid trusts that invest in both equity ownership and mortgages.

Pension funds. At one time, **pension funds** invested primarily in stocks. However, they perceived mortgages to be safe yet high-return investments and they became important players in the mortgage market. They made loans on large projects. Pension funds generally purchased loans originated by mortgage companies or worked through mortgage brokers. They often take an equity position in large developments.

Credit unions. At one time, **credit unions** offered mostly low-dollar loans for consumer purchases. Credit unions have evolved to become major lenders. While they limit loans to members, they have expanded their loan activity. Unlike profit-oriented lenders, their loans are more community based. Besides home equity loans and home purchase loans, credit unions have expanded their community lender role to include construction and development loans. Credit unions in many ways now resemble commercial banks.

Seller Carryback Financing

When conventional financing is not available to a buyer in the amount required or is too costly, a seller often can be persuaded to carry back a first or second mortgage on property to facilitate a sale. If a seller does not need the cash and the purchaser will pay a rate of interest higher than that provided by a certificate of deposit, the seller is a likely candidate for carryback financing.

Generally, **seller carryback financing** is customized to the needs of the parties. Such loans are generally fixed-rate loans with payments based on a 30-year amortization but due and payable in five to seven years. Most sellers are not interested in having their money tied up for longer periods of time.

Because most loans now have due-on-sale clauses, seller carryback financing is limited to situations where the property is owned by the seller free of loans, where the lender will agree to a loan assumption, where the existing loan does not have a due-on-sale clause, or where the seller will hold a secondary loan after the buyer obtains primary financing.

SAFE Act

The Federal Secure and Fair Enforcement Mortgage Licensing Act (SAFE).   SAFE was enacted for consumer protection and to reduce fraud. The act requires licensing for mortgage loan originators. Anyone who accepts compensation for taking a loan application, offers or negotiates terms of a 1–4-residential-unit mortgage loan, or who is compensated by a mortgage originator must have an **MLO endorsement** on their license. The endorsement requires education, testing, and reporting.

TYPES OF LOANS

While most 1–4-unit dwellings still are financed by conventional loans, the choice of a loan is no longer a foregone conclusion. Both buyers and sellers need to know what is currently available, which loan best suits their requirements, and even where to go for financing. With real estate firms allying themselves with financial institutions, even the players are changing every day.

CONVENTIONAL LOANS

By definition, a **conventional loan** is any loan that does not involve government participation. The advantages of conventional over government-backed loans are that conventional loans involve less red tape and shorter processing time. Government loans do not have equivalent flexibility. Buyers can obtain a larger loan amount, and because there are more sources for conventional loans, borrowers have the option of choosing a wide variety of fixed-rate or adjustable-rate loans.

> Conventional loans have no government insurance or guarantee.

Disadvantages of conventional loans in comparison with government-backed loans can include higher down payments and prepayment penalties. Furthermore, private mortgage insurance (PMI) may be required if a purchaser has less than a 20% down payment.

How to Compare Loans

Borrowers should compare loans on the basis of the following:

- LTV (the percentage of the appraised value that the lender will lend determines down payment requirements; loan to value ratio)
- Interest rate and if it can be changed
- Loan costs and fees required
- Prepayment penalties
- Length of loan (longer-term loans result in lower monthly payments)
- Amount of fixed monthly payment
- Initial rate, adjustment period, caps, index, and margin of adjustable-rate loans

GOVERNMENT LOANS

Government Loans

There are several types of government-involved loans, including **FHA-insured loans**, **VA-guaranteed loans**, and **CalVet loans**. There are also California Housing Finance Agency loans. These types of loans are compared in Figure 12.4.

Federal Housing Administration (FHA)

The purposes of the Federal Housing Administration are stated in its preamble: to "encourage improvement in housing standards and conditions, to provide a system of mutual mortgage insurance, and for other purposes."

There are two divisions under which this protection is granted: Title I and Title II. In general, the following types of loans are available:

- Title I—loans for modernization, repairs, or alterations on existing homes

- Title II—loans for purchase or construction of residential structures

FIGURE 12.4:   Government Home Loan Programs

	FHA-Insured	VA-Guaranteed (GI)	CalVet
Who is eligible?	Anyone who qualifies	U.S. veterans	California residents who have met the veteran requirements
Who makes the loans?	Approved lending institutions	Approved lending institutions	Calif. Dept. of Veterans Affairs (mortgage brokers can originate loans)
Type of loan	Insure (up-front insurance premium may be financed)	Guaranteed (see Figure 12.5)	Land contract
Points and fees	Loan fee 1% plus mortgage insurance premium	Negotiable loan fees plus a funding fee (may be financed)	1.25% to 3% (may be financed)
Interest rates	May be negotiated	May be negotiated	Flexible rate based on cost of bonds. Can change annually.
What is the maximum you can pay for a home?	No limit	Loan cannot exceed appraisal	Cannot exceed the CalVet appraisal (certificate of reasonable value [CRV])
Maximum loan allowed	$625,000	No money down, to county limit; loan can't exceed the certificate of reasonable value (CRV)	125% of Fannie Mae maximum
Term	Usually 30 years	Maximum 30 years	30 years
Down payment	Approximately 3.5%	None required for loans up to county limit	0% to 5%
Secondary financing	Not allowed at time of sale, but can be placed later	Generally not allowed at time of sale, but can be placed later	Yes, but the 1st and 2nd cannot exceed 90% of the CalVet appraisal
Prepayment penalty	None	None	None
Assumability	Loans before Dec. 15, 1989, are assumable; subsequent loans assumable with FHA approval	Loans before Mar. 1, 1988, are assumable; subsequent loans require buyer to qualify	Assumable with prior CalVet approval

Section 203(b) of Title II accounts for most loans for 1–4-unit residences. FHA loans provide high LTVs based on appraisal.

The maximum FHA loan amount will vary by region, but the purchaser generally must have a minimum down payment of 3½%.

The down payment may come from a gift, but there is a ban on seller and nonprofit group assistance programs.

The *mortgage insurance premium* (MIP) must be paid at the time of loan origination. Based on the down payment, an MIP is also added to payments for the life of the loan.

Lenders may be authorized to make the underwriting decision that a loan qualifies for FHA insurance. This is known as **direct endorsement**, and it serves to speed up the loan processing time. Because of foreclosure problems, down payment requirements have increased for most other loans. As of January 1, 2009, FHA down payments were increased from 3% to 3.5%. Despite this increase, the low down payment requirement for FHA loans compared with other loans resulted in an increase in FHA loan applications.

A recent rule change allows borrowers who have gone through a foreclosure, bankruptcy, or other adverse events, and who have repaired their credit, to be eligible for an FHA-insured loan after one year. Previously, they had to wait at least three years before they would qualify for a new government-backed loan. To qualify for the shorter period, borrowers must show that their credit problems were caused by job loss or reduction in income beyond their control.

HUD (Department of Housing and Urban Development)

FHA loans are insured by HUD. The insurance protects the lender should the borrower default. Loans insured by HUD must be **qualified mortgages**. To be qualified, the loan must

- be for 30 years or less;
- limit points and fees to 3%;

- have periodic payments without toxic features such as interest only, negative amortization, or balloon payments; and

- have a debt-to-income ratio of no more than 43% of income.

Department of Veterans Affairs (VA)

The Servicemen's Readjustment Act of 1944 (GI Bill) was intended to help veterans to make the necessary readjustments to civilian life, particularly to assist them in the acquisition of homes. The VA does not make loans, but it guarantees a portion of the loan. Figure 12.5 explains the VA-guaranteed loan.

The largest VA loan on which no down payment is required is $729,750 in certain areas, but the VA has suspended zero down loans over $417,000. A 25% down payment is required on amounts over the county no-down-payment limit. VA loans can be used to

- buy or build an owner-occupied home;

- alter, repair, or improve real estate;

- purchase a mobile home; and

- refinance existing mortgage loans for dwellings owned and occupied by veterans.

To qualify for a VA-guaranteed loan, an individual must have had 181 days of active service. An appraiser approved by the VA checks the property.

The loan cannot exceed the appraisal known as the *certificate of reasonable value* (CRV). The certificate of reasonable value is based on a VA appraisal made for insurance purposes. (The loan amount is not regulated, but the guarantee is.)

FIGURE 12.5:   VA Guaranteed Loan (GI)

Loans	Guarantee
Up to 45,000	40% of loan
$45,000 to $144,000	Minimum guarantee of $22,500 Maximum guarantee is 40% of loan up to $36,000
More than $144,000	25% of loan up to a maximum of $60,000

CalVet loans. Under the CalVet loan program (the California Farm and Home Purchase Program), California veterans can acquire a suitable farm or a single-family residence at a low financing cost. The State of California actually takes title to the property and sells it to the veteran under a land contract. Following are some features of the CalVet loan:

- CalVet loans can now be arranged through lenders approved to handle CalVet loans.

- CalVet loans are now processed with DVA guidelines. The loans are available to peacetime as well as wartime veterans and active-duty military. The maximum home loan amount is 125% of the maximum for a Fannie Mae conforming loan; the 2015 limit is $521,250.

- Depending on the type of CalVet loan, the down payment can range from 0 to 5%. The programs with no down payment have a limit of up to $521,250.

- 2015 CalVet loans start at 4.25% interest for a 30-year home loan (higher rate for mobile homes).

- CalVet loans have an origination fee of 1%.

- CalVet loans have a funding fee of 1.25% to 3.30%.

- Mortgage brokers who originate and process CalVet loans receive a $350 processing fee plus a 1% origination fee.

- The state raises the funds for CalVet loans by issuing tax-exempt bonds.

> With a CalVet loan, the veteran is buying under a land contract.

WEB LINK

For more information on CalVet loans, call 1-800-952-5626 or check the website at www.calvet.ca.gov/calvet-programs/home-loans/.

The California Housing Finance Agency (CalHFA). CalHFA is California's self-supporting housing bank that offers fixed-rate conventional and interest-only financing at low rates, and down payment assistance for first-time homebuyers. CalHFA uses no appropriated taxpayer dollars for its programs but utilizes a tax-exempt bond program. Loans are for low-income and moderate-income buyers.

Programs of CalHFA include the following:

- Interest-only programs for the first 5 years of a 35-year fixed-rate mortgage

- Conventional 30-year fixed-rate mortgage

- Down-payment assistance programs for teachers in high-priority schools

- Down-payment assistance for designated high-cost counties

- Down-payment assistance for new homes based on school facility fees paid by the builder

- Down-payment assistance up to 3% to low-income buyers using FHA-insured loans

- Down-payment and closing-cost assistance in community revitalization areas

- Lower interest rates for lower-income disabled purchasers

- Lower interest rates for homebuyers receiving financial assistance from an approved government agency

WEB LINK

@

CalHFA housing programs include mortgage insurance that makes home payments for up to six months if a borrower involuntarily loses her job. Eligibility requirements can be ascertained by visiting the website, www.calhfa.ca.gov.

Because of state budgeting problems, in December 2008, CALHFA suspended its 30-year fixed-rate loan programs, as well as down payment assistance programs.

Other Types of Mortgages and Trust Deeds

Open-end trust deed.   An **open-end trust deed** allows the borrower to receive additional loan money up to an agreed amount, using the same trust deed or mortgage as security. (It is like having a credit card with a set limit.) A home equity line of credit is an example of an open-end loan.

Blanket trust deed.   With a **blanket trust deed**, the borrower uses more than one parcel of property as security. This type of document should contain a **release clause** that allows the partial reconveyance of separate parcels of property on repayment of a portion of the loan.

Construction loan.   This unamortized loan, usually for three years or less, is given until permanent financing is in place.

Take-out loan.   This is permanent financing that takes out (replaces) short-term financing such as gap or construction loans.

Packaged loan.   A loan that includes personal property, as well as real property.

Wraparound trust deed.   A **wraparound trust deed** also is called an *all-inclusive trust deed*. There are times when it is almost impossible for buyers to refinance an existing loan on investment real estate to raise additional capital. With a wraparound mortgage the existing loan is not disturbed. The seller continues the payments on the existing mortgage or trust deed while giving the borrower a new, increased loan, usually at a higher interest rate. The new loan is for the amount due on the existing loan plus the amount of the seller's equity being financed.

Assume a property is being sold for $200,000 with $20,000 down. Also assume that there is a $90,000 trust deed against the property at 7% interest. If the buyer were willing to pay 9% interest, the seller could take advantage of this interest difference with a wraparound loan.

$$\left. \frac{\text{\$90,000 loan} \quad 7\%}{\text{\$90,000 loan} \quad 9\%} \right\} \text{\$180,000 wraparound loan at 9\%}$$

In this case, the seller receives 9% on his equity plus a 2% differential on the 7% being paid on the existing loan. This really gives the seller 11% interest on the equity. In addition, because the seller continues to make the payments on the $90,000 loan, the seller knows that the payments are being made. If the seller had allowed the buyer to assume the existing loan, then the buyer, not the seller, would have taken advantage of the low financing.

To use a wraparound loan, the underlying loan must not have a **due-on-sale clause**. A due-on-sale clause, also known as an alienation clause, accelerates loan payments, making the entire loan amount due upon a sale. These clauses are enforceable by lenders. While a number of ways have been devised to get around the clauses, the methods basically are based on deception. Advocating use of such methods could subject you to liability and disciplinary action, as well as result in a buyer losing a property because of the inability to obtain a new loan. Because of possible problems, legal counsel should be sought before a wraparound loan is used.

Gap loan. These loans are usually short-term loans, such as loans between construction loans and the **take-out loan** (permanent financing) or by buyers who have found a new home but have not yet sold their prior residence. They are also called *swing loans* or *bridge loans*. They generally bear a relatively high rate of interest.

Fixed-rate loans. Lenders will make fixed-rate long-term amortized loans because they must in order to be competitive, but they generally prefer adjustable-rate or shorter-term loans. The reason is that they were hurt in the past by long-term **fixed-rate loans**.

In the late 1970s and early 1980s, many lenders, particularly S&Ls, had a great deal of capital invested in long-term fixed-rate loans. During this period, the United States had great inflation, and interest rates increased dramatically. Lenders had to pay higher interest rates on accounts to attract funds. In many cases, the average yield from their portfolios of loans was less than the average rate they were paying depositors for funds. While relatively short-lived, lenders had been burned and still worry that history could repeat itself.

To encourage borrowers to use other types of loans, lenders offer lower loan costs than for fixed-rate loans and even lower interest rates. With current low index rates, many adjustable-rate loans are pegged so low that lenders are again pushing fixed-rate loans.

15-year vs. 30-year fixed-rate loans. If a buyer is able to pay the additional monthly payment on a 15-year loan, significant savings are possible compared with a 30-year loan.

As an example, at 7½% interest, the monthly payment on a $100,000 loan for 15 years comes to $927.02. For a 30-year loan having the same rate of interest, the monthly payment is $699.22.

For the 30-year loan, total payments equal as follows:

$$12 \text{ (months)} \times 30 \text{ (years)} \times \$699.22 = \$251,719.20$$
or interest of $151,719.20.

For a 15-year loan the total payments are as follows:

$$12 \text{ (months)} \times 15 \text{ (years)} \times \$927.02 = \$166,863.60$$
or interest payments of $66,863.60.

The interest paid on the 30-year loan is more than twice the interest of the 15-year loan, and the payments are only $227.80 higher than the 30-year loan payments.

The savings are likely to be significantly greater than those shown in the example because 15-year loans usually have an interest rate from 0.375% to 0.75% lower than a similar 30-year loan. Lower interest rates are used because shorter-term loans are considered by lenders to present less risk.

40-year loans. To help offset higher home prices that have reduced housing affordability, some lenders may offer 40-year loans. While the payments are reduced by the longer amortization period, making payments for an extra 10 years might not be in the buyer's best long-term interest if the buyer can qualify and make the payments on a 30-year loan. As an example, for a 30-year loan for $300,000 at 6% interest, the monthly payment amounts to $1,798.68. For the same loan at 40 years, the payments would be $1,650.66, or $148.02 less than for the 30-year loan. However, total payments for the 30-year loan would be $647,524, but the 40-year loan total payments would be $792,316, or $144,792 greater. FHA will not insure a loan greater than 30 years.

Interest-only loans. In order to qualify buyers for home loans, many lenders formerly offered **interest-only loans**. These are also known as straight notes. The borrower makes payments of interest only for a set period of time, such as five years. At the end of the period, the borrower must make full amortized payments. As an example, interest only on a 6%, $300,000 loan would be $1,500 per month, which would be $300 less than an amortized payment.

80-20 loans.   For borrowers who didn't have a down payment, 80-20 loans were made before the mortgage meltdown. Eighty percent of the purchase price was made by a conventional lender. Because the loans are for only 80% of value, private mortgage insurance is not required. The balance of the purchase price, 20%, was covered with a second trust deed at a higher rate of interest. The second trust deed was also likely to have higher origination costs.

The 80-20 loans, as well as other low or no down payment loans, were a factor in buyers walking away from their homes when their loans exceeded the value of the homes. The resultant foreclosure sales were a factor in decreasing housing prices in 2008. Because of the foreclosure problems, lenders no longer make 80-20 loans.

Renegotiable-rate   mortgages.   **Renegotiable-rate   mortgages**, also known as rollover loans, usually have payments based on a 30-year amortization. However, they are only partially amortized. Generally, they are due in full in five or seven years. The lender will rewrite the loan at this time at the current interest rate, or the borrower can refinance with another lender.

Because the lender is not locked into the interest rate for a long period, lenders offer these loans for a lower interest rate than for the fixed 30-year rate. Frequently, the rate is about 1% less than fixed-rate loans. Lenders also might offer lower loan origination fees and costs.

Hybrid loans.   Lenders will offer combination fixed–adjustable-rate loans such as a 5–30, where the first 5 years are at a fixed rate and the balance of the loan (25 years) is at an adjustable rate. In order to sell borrowers on the **hybrid loan**, the fixed-rate portion of the loan has an interest rate less than that for a 30-year fixed-rate loan. This allows borrowers to qualify for the loan when they might not qualify for a 30-year fixed-rate loan.

Reverse mortgage (reverse annuity mortgage).   This unusual loan is not for home purchases. A **reverse mortgage** is a loan whereby the lender annuitizes the value of the owner's equity and makes monthly payments to the borrowers based on the equity and the age of the borrowers. The loan is not repaid until the borrowers die or the property is sold. Homeowners must be age 62 or older to qualify for a reverse mortgage.

A normal loan charges simple interest; that is, the interest for the previous month is paid with each payment and is charged on the principal balance only. A reverse mortgage, however, has compound interest (interest is charged on interest). Each month, the interest is greater than the previous month because more principal has been advanced; therefore, the principal balance has increased, and accrued interest also has been added to the principal and has increased the balance due.

Reverse mortgages have higher loan fees than most other loans. Several lenders have agreed to make settlements because of alleged unconscionable loan costs and fees for their reverse mortgages.

Piggyback loan. This is really two loans, first and second, made by a lender at the same time.

Adjustable-rate mortgage (ARM). In contrast to a fixed-rate loan, the interest rate in an **adjustable-rate mortgage** changes periodically, usually in relation to an index, with payments going up or down accordingly. Lenders usually charge lower initial interest rates for ARMs than for fixed-rate loans, which makes the ARM easier on the borrower's pocketbook than a fixed-rate loan for the same amount and also makes it easier for the borrower to qualify for the loan. In addition, it could mean that the borrower could qualify for a larger loan, because lenders sometimes qualify buyers on the basis of current income and the first year's payment. This means the buyer (borrower) could maintain a better lifestyle with an ARM. Moreover, an ARM might be less expensive over a long period than a fixed-rate loan. For example, interest rates may remain at current low rates.

Another advantage of an ARM is that it generally does not have prepayment penalties. Therefore, if the borrower expects to be reselling within a relatively short period, the absence of this penalty could give the ARM a significant advantage over loans requiring prepayment penalties.

To induce borrowers to choose an ARM, lenders may offer lower loan origination costs than for fixed-rate loans. Lower origination costs also make ARMs attractive to borrowers who intend to resell within a few years.

Against these advantages, the buyer must weigh the risk that an increase in interest rates will lead to higher monthly payments in the future. The trade-off with an ARM is that the borrower obtains a lower rate in exchange for assuming more risk. The borrower considering an ARM should envision a worst-case scenario with interest increasing to the set limit to fully understand the degree of risk involved.

Myriad ARMs variations are being offered by financial institutions today. It is important for both the borrower and the agent to learn to ask questions so that they can compare loans adequately. Here are four basic questions the buyer needs to consider:

1. Is my income likely to rise enough to cover higher mortgage payments if interest rates go up, or can I afford the higher payment?

2. Will I be taking on other sizable debts, such as a loan for a car or school tuition, in the near future?

3. How long do I plan to own this home? If I plan to sell soon, rising interest rates may not pose the problem they will if I plan to own the home for a long time.

4. Can my payments increase even if interest rates in general do not increase?

If the buyer can answer these questions satisfactorily, an ARM might be the loan of choice. However, the borrower still has to decide which ARM to take out, which entails obtaining the answers to many more questions.

When discussing an ARM with a borrower, the real estate agent needs to understand and be able to explain certain terms that do not apply to fixed-rate loans. These include *adjustment period, index rate, margin, interest rate cap, overall cap, payment cap, negative amortization, and conversion clause*. The remainder of this section defines these terms and explains the calculations that will enable a borrower to choose the proper ARM for the circumstances.

Adjustment period. The **adjustment period** of an ARM is the period of time between one interest rate and monthly payment change and the next. (Some ARMs have two adjustments: one for the rate, the other for the payment.) This period is different for each ARM; it may occur once a month, every six months, once a year, or even every three years. A loan with an adjustment period of one year is called a *one-year* ARM, and the interest rate can change once each year. Lenders often have a longer adjustment period for the first adjustment. Different lenders use different adjustment periods. Because a single lender might offer four different types of ARMs, each with a different adjustment period, it is important for the borrower to read the loan documents and understand the adjustment period before the loan documents are cut or signed.

Index and margin. Most lenders tie ARM interest-rate changes to changes of an **index rate**. The only requirements a lender must meet in selecting an interest index are as follows:

- The index control cannot be the lender.

- The index must be readily available to and verifiable by the public.

These indexes usually go up and down with the general movement of interest rates. If the index moves up, so does the interest rate on the loan, meaning the borrower will probably have to make higher monthly payments. If the index rate goes down, interest rate and monthly payments may go down as well.

Lenders base ARM rates on a variety of indexes; in fact, the index can be almost any interest rate the lender selects. Also, different lenders may offer a variety of ARMs, and each may have a different index and margin. Among the most common indexes are six-month, three-year, or five-year Treasury securities (T-bills); national or regional cost of funds to savings associations (11th district cost of funds of the Federal Home Loan Bank Board [FHLBB]); and the London InterBank Offering Rate (LIBOR). Borrowers and their agents should ask which index will be used and how often it changes. Also, find out how the index has behaved in the past and where it is published, so the borrower can trace it in the future.

The index rate plus the margin equals the interest rate.

To determine the interest rate on an ARM, lenders add to the index rate a few percentage points (two to three), called the **margin** (also *differential* or *spread*).

index   +   margin   =   ARM interest rate

Elastic, subject to change   Set figure   Limited by caps

The amount of the margin can differ from one lender to another, but it is always constant over the life of the loan. Loans that have lower loan-origination costs tend to have higher margins. Upward adjustments of the ARM interest rate are made at the lender's option, but downward adjustments are mandatory. Actual adjustments to the borrowers' mortgage interest rate can occur only on a predetermined time schedule (the adjustment period, as described). On each loan, the borrowers' terms, including initial rate, caps, index, margin, interest-rate-change frequency, and payment-change frequency, are stated in the note that accompanies the deed of trust. Terms will vary from lender to lender.

In comparing ARMs, look at both the index and the margin for each plan. Some indexes have higher average values, but they are usually used with lower margins. Be sure to discuss the margin with the lender.

In calculating an ARM payment, the first period is calculated in exactly the same way as a fixed-rate loan payment. After the first-period adjustment, it is as if the borrower were starting a new loan: calculations must be made to figure the loan balance and the number of payments left, and the new interest rate must be taken into account. Of course, because no one can anticipate accurately whether interest rates will increase or decrease, in analyzing various ARMs a borrower is considering, the agent can accurately calculate the loan payment for only the first period.

ARM discounts.   Some lenders offer initial ARM rates that are lower than the sum of the index and the margin. Such rates, called *discounted rates*, *introductory rates*, *tickler rates*, or *teaser rates*, are usually combined with loan fees (points) and with higher interest rates after the discount expires. Many lenders offer introductory rates that are significantly below market interest rates. The discount rates may expire after the first adjustment period (for example, after one month, six months, or one year). At the end of the introductory discount rate period, the ARM interest rate automatically increases to the contract interest rate (index plus margin). This can mean a substantial increase in the borrower's interest rate and monthly payment. If the index rate has moved upward, the interest rate and payment adjustment can be even higher. Even if the index rate has decreased, the borrower's interest rate and monthly payment will likely be adjusted upward at the end of the introductory period.

Many lenders use the first year's payment as the basis for qualifying a borrower for a loan. So even if a lender approves the loan based on the low introductory rate, it is the borrowers' responsibility to determine whether they will be able to afford payments in later years, when the discount expires and the rate is adjusted. With a discounted ARM, any savings made during the discounted period may be offset during the life of the loan or be included in the price of the home. In fact, this kind of loan subjects borrowers to greater risk, including that of **payment shock**, which may occur when the mortgage payment rises at the first adjustment.

Whenever the lender's advertised qualifying interest rate is lower than the lender's current ARM index rate plus margin, a below-market rate is being offered. Assume the current index rate is 5% and the margin 2%. That makes the ARM rate 7%. If the advertised qualifying introductory rate is 5%, the introductory rate is 2% below the market rate, making it a discounted rate. Any qualifying rate below 7% in this case is called an *introductory rate* or a *below-market rate*.

Many lenders describe the introductory rate in their documentation as follows: "There is no rate change in the first six months. Thereafter, the interest rate is established by adding a rate differential (margin) to the index provided in the note."

The **annual percentage rate (APR)** gives a more accurate picture of the cost of a loan and must be disclosed by law. The APR differs from the nominal interest rate in that the APR includes the interest as well as the costs associated with obtaining the loan. The APR represents a rate based on a buyer's net loan proceeds, which is the loan amount less the cost of credit. This is outlined in the RESPA letter sent within three days of application for a loan. When calculating the APR, lenders who offer below-market rates must account for the higher index rate that will be charged in the future.

A borrower who chooses an ARM impulsively because of a low initial rate could end up in difficult straits. Agents can help borrowers protect themselves from large increases by looking at a mortgage with certain features that are explained in the next sections. Remember that all loans are different and that many different types of ARMs exist. Agents can help borrowers shop around until they find the loan that will meet their needs with minimal risk.

Caps can limit payment increases and loan interest.

Caps on an ARM.   Most ARMs have caps that protect borrowers from increases in interest rates or monthly payments beyond an amount specified in the note. If loans have no interest rate or payment caps, borrowers might be exposed to unlimited upward adjustments in monthly payments, should interest rates rise.

Caps vary from lender to lender. The borrower needs to check with the lender to determine the cap rates in the loan under consideration. Two types of interest-rate caps are used:

1. A *periodic cap* limits the interest-rate increase or decrease from one adjustment period to the next. These caps are usually 1 percentage point to 2 percentage points or sometimes 7½% of the previous period's payment amount.

2. A *lifetime cap* or overall cap limits the interest-rate increase over the life of the loan. Assume the introductory rate is 4% and is below the market rate and at the first adjustment becomes 5%. The overall cap will be attached to the 5%; thus, a 5% cap could mean an interest rate as high as 10%.

An ARM usually has both a periodic and an overall interest rate cap. A drop in the index does not always lead to an immediate drop in monthly payments. In fact, with some ARMs that have interest rate caps, the monthly payment may increase, even though the index rate has stayed the same or declined. This may happen after an interest rate cap has been holding the interest rate below the sum of the index plus margin. When the next adjustment period comes along and the interest rate stays the same or declines, previous obligations are in arrears and must be paid; thus, the monthly payment will increase.

The rate on a loan can go up at any scheduled adjustment when the index plus margin is higher than the rate before the adjustment. As stated earlier, an ARM usually has an overall interest rate cap. Some ARMs have a stated cap, such as 15%; others specify a percentage over the initial rate, such as an overall interest rate cap of 5%. Again, caps vary from lender to lender and sometimes from loan to loan offered by the same lender. It is important for the borrowers to know what caps are available and what they are obtaining with a loan.

As previously stated, some ARMs include a payment cap that limits the monthly payment increase at the time of each adjustment, usually to a percentage of the previous payment. In other words, if the payment cap is 7½%, a payment of $1,000 could not increase or decrease by more than $75 in the next adjustment period.

Because payment caps limit only the amount of payment increases and not interest-rate increases, payments sometimes do not cover all the interest due on a loan. This is sometimes called **negative amortization** and means the mortgage balance is increasing. The interest shortage in the payment is automatically added to the loan, and interest may be charged on that amount. As of 2010, negative amortization loans were banned in California.

Option ARMs.   Option ARMs are adjustable-rate loans where the borrower has the option of making the payments necessary to amortize the loan or to make a minimum payment that is less than the interest. The result is negative amortization, with the amount due on the principal increasing each month. At a stated future date, such as five years, the borrower must start making payments that will amortize the loan. The low minimum payment of the option ARM allowed borrowers to more easily qualify for a loan. The borrowers hoped that increases in income would allow full payments at the later date and that increased property value would offset the negative amortization. A major California bank indicated in 2005 that 87% of its ARMs were option ARMs. There have been a great many foreclosures in option ARMs when payments increased on homes whose value had decreased. Because of lender risks, option ARMs are likely a thing of the past. In October 2009, then-Governor Schwarzenegger signed emergency legislation banning new negative amortization residential loan originations in California.

Convertible ARMs. Borrowers whose financial circumstances may change at some time during the term of the loan may decide that they do not want to risk any further changes in the interest rate and payment amount; or interest rates may drop, and the borrower might want to lock in the lower rate. In such cases, a conversion clause becomes important. A **convertible ARM** clause is one that allows the borrower to convert the ARM to a fixed-rate loan at designated times. When the borrower converts, the new rate is generally set at the current market rate for fixed-rate loans plus at least 0.375 of 1% as a servicing premium.

Assumable ARMs. Although most ARMs are assumable, lenders normally place conditions on the assumption of the loan. The lender may require that the new borrower supply credit information, complete a credit application, and meet the customary credit standards applied by the lender. In some cases, the lender may charge points or other fees when a loan is assumed.

Some lenders allow only one assumption. Other lenders allow assumption but adjust the overall cap or the margin to the rate in effect at the time of assumption. Some lenders allow assumptions with the original lifetime cap already in effect. Because conditions of assumption vary greatly among lenders, the documentation should be checked for this information.

Figure 12.6 contains a list of questions that a borrower should ask, and the agent or the lender should be able to answer, when the borrower is looking for an ARM.

Loan Costs

In comparing loans, you must also compare loan costs. Lenders break down loan costs so that consumers will understand exactly what they are paying for. No matter what the cost or fee is called, the bottom line is the total of all loan costs. For many loans, these costs can be added to the amount of the loan.

FIGURE 12.6: ARM Checklist

❑ What is the initial (or qualifying) interest rate on the ARM?

❑ How long is this initial rate in effect? When is the first rate and/or payment adjustment?

❑ To what index is the ARM's interest rate tied?

❑ What is the current level of the index?

❑ What margin above the index is used to calculate the actual ARM rate?

❑ How can the index and the margin be used to calculate the mortgage rate initially and at the first adjustment?

❑ What will happen to the interest rate at the first adjustment, assuming the index rate stays the same?

❑ What is the annual percentage rate (APR) of the loan? How does this compare with the APR on other ARMs and that on a fixed-rate loan?

❑ How often is the interest rate on the mortgage adjusted? How often does the monthly payment change?

❑ Does the ARM have a periodic interest rate cap? If so, what is the limit on the increase in the ARM rate at each adjustment? If the index rate increases more than this limit, can the unused change in the index be carried over to the next adjustment period? Does the periodic interest rate cap apply to the first adjustment? Does the periodic rate cap apply to the rate decreases, as well as to any increases?

❑ Does the ARM have an overall cap rate? If so, what are the maximum and minimum rates?

❑ Does the ARM have a payment cap? If so, what is the maximum that the monthly payment can increase at each adjustment? Does the payment cap apply to the first payment adjustment?

❑ Can the borrower convert this ARM to a fixed-rate loan at any time? Does this ARM have an open-end credit feature? What other features does this ARM have?

❑ Is this ARM assumable? Is this assumption feature limited to one time only? What are the qualification features? Will the original caps still be in effect? If not, what are the new caps?

❑ Does the ARM have a loan-to-value ratio greater than 80%? If so, is private mortgage insurance required on the loan?

Calculating Loan Costs

■ An initial application fee

■ A flat fee in addition to loan points

■ Loan points

■ Loan escrow costs (if not a purchase-money loan)

■ Title insurance (if not a purchase-money loan)

■ Document fees

■ Private mortgage insurance

■ A number of charges developed by different lenders, such as processing fees, which are generally fees for miscellaneous lender services (These fees are often called garbage fees.)

CHOOSING AMONG LOAN CATEGORIES

Lenders offer a number of different basic loan classifications, with different lenders offering different variations. Because of differing loan provisions, interest rates, and loan costs, it becomes difficult for borrowers to decide which loan type and lender best meet their particular needs.

Borrowers will find that they must shop for loans the same way they shop for any other large purchase. There are significant variations in costs among lenders. In some cases, loan costs can be negotiated.

Borrowers who believe they will remain in a property for many years likely will want an overall lower interest rate and be willing to pay higher loan-origination costs (including discount points) to obtain that rate.

Borrowers who expect to remain in a property for only a few years likely will want a loan that can be prepaid without a penalty and that has low loan-origination costs. Such borrowers likely will be willing to pay a higher interest rate to obtain the lower origination costs. Generally, lower loan-origination fees mean a higher interest rate.

Borrowers who believe interest rates are about as low as they will go are likely to want a long-term fixed-rate mortgage. Borrowers who believe interest rates are likely to drop probably will want a loan without a prepayment penalty, a short-term loan that can be rewritten at a future interest rate, or an adjustable-rate loan that can be converted to a fixed-rate loan.

Borrowers who have very low down payments would be interested in loans having a high LTV, such as FHA-insured loans, VA-guaranteed loans, and loans with PMI. And if borrowers have a low income for loan-qualifying purposes, they likely will want an ARM with low initial payments, a longer-term loan, or an interest-only loan.

For many buyers, the deciding factor will be the additional improvement in lifestyle afforded by using an ARM. Usually an ARM allows borrowers to buy more home for their money than would be possible with a fixed-rate loan. Assume fixed-rate loans are at 6%, and ARMs have a lower interest rate. If the agent knows how much the buyer can afford for a monthly payment, the agent can calculate the loan amount for which the borrower can qualify. The easiest way to do this is simply to use an amortization table and check the qualifying rate to determine how large a loan that payment will support.

The real estate agent needs to understand the lending business and be willing to communicate with the lender when he does not know why a certain interest rate, point, loan fee, or PMI is required, or does not understand other conditions of the loan.

One of the fundamental misunderstandings about financing arises because real estate buyers and sellers do not realize that money is a commodity. Money is like a loaf of bread, a car, a home, or any other commodity, and it is bought and sold. When it is bought and sold, the lender expects to make a profit on the sale. Some like to compare loaning money to renting. The payment of interest is the cost of renting the money, and points are like first and last months' rent or the security deposit, but unlike security deposits, it is not refundable. Every lender needs to make a profit on the rental of money to stay in business.

If the lender reduces one cost to a borrower in one area, the lender generally will raise it in another area to compensate for the loss. As an example, a lender offering a lower interest rate may charge higher loan costs, as well as a larger prepayment penalty, than a lender offering the higher interest rate. Help your borrower choose the loan that offers the combination of features that best meets that borrower's specific needs.

Computerized Loan Origination

Computerized loan origination (CLO) is now possible on the internet. Various websites provide interest rates, points, and APRs for various types of loans. Agents can complete a loan application on the internet and in many cases have loan approval, subject to verifications, before the client leaves your office.

There are also several large multilender shopping sites for loans that allow a borrower to view loan offerings from a great many lenders on a competitive basis. These sites are updated daily.

A borrower can evaluate loan types, points, costs, and rates to make an informed decision and then be qualified by the selected lender, as well as complete the loan application, all on the internet. The result of competition is often lower loan costs for the borrower. Because of this advantage, many buyers' agents use these shopping sites.

The websites also avoid the possibility that the borrower is being charged an overage. An *overage* is a charge, typically points, by a mortgage banker that exceeds what a lender would charge.

Four of the major loan shopping websites are as follows:

WEB LINK

1. www.eloan.com

2. www.homesadvisor.com

3. www.quickenloans.com

4. www.bankrate.com

We suggest that you gain familiarity with these websites, as well as local mortgage companies, and the process of qualification and loan application. You should also be familiar with the other sites, including local market lenders that are used by your office.

When a real estate agent charges a fee to a borrower for CLO, a disclosure must be provided to the borrower in a format specified by RESPA. The disclosure must inform the borrower that the fee can be avoided by approaching lenders directly.

THE FINANCING PROCESS

The basic steps for obtaining real estate financing are much the same with any type of lender. Figure 12.7 illustrates the following five-step financing process:

1. Qualifying the borrower

2. Qualifying the property

3. Approving and processing the loan

4. Closing the loan

5. Servicing the loan

Qualifying the Borrower

In understanding lender requirements for **qualifying borrowers**, you should realize that lender requirements often are dictated by the secondary mortgage market. Unless a lender expects to hold on to a loan for the life of the loan, the lender wants the loan to meet the requirements of a holder in the secondary market, such as Fannie Mae.

FIGURE 12.7: The Financing Process

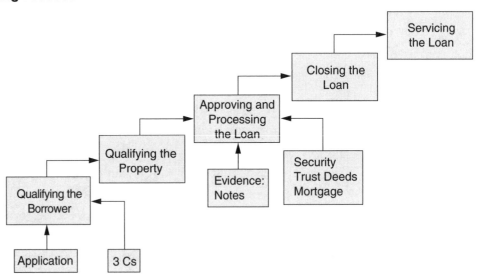

Unit 9 introduced you to lender qualifying requirements in prequalifying prospective purchasers. Lenders first ask prospective borrowers to complete an application form. Most applications are similar to the one in Figure 12.8, which asks for the borrower's employment record, credit references, and a financial statement of assets and liabilities. To verify the accuracy of the information, the loan officer checks with past employers, requests verification of deposits from the bank(s), and contacts references. The loan officer also may obtain a Dun & Bradstreet report (in case of commercial loans) and a credit report by an outside agency, so there is no question of the borrower's ability to repay the loan.

Most lenders use the "three Cs"—*character, capacity,* and *collateral*—as a screening device to determine whether the borrower meets the qualifications set by the lender.

Character.   With regard to prospective borrowers' character, lenders consider their attitude toward financial obligations as evidenced by their track record of borrowing and repaying loans evidenced by credit reports. Lenders also try to ascertain whether borrowers are honest in their dealings.

The desire to pay is very difficult to measure. There are methods used by a lender to determine the borrower's desire to make timely payments, such as **FICO score**. Fair Isaac Co. developed this scoring system used by most lenders. Following are the primary factors used for scoring:

- Late payments

- Negative credit information

- How long credit has been established

- Amount of credit used versus credit available

- Length of time at present residence

- Employment history

Credit scores range from about 300 to 850. Scores above 720 are regarded by lenders as being good and qualify for the lowest rate. Scores above 780 can result in ever lower loan costs as lenders compete for these borrowers.

Traditionally the cut-off point between prime and subprime mortgages was 620, but some mortgage companies now put the line at 680 to 700 with full documentation of an applicant's income and assets. Many lenders are no longer willing to take the risk of 620 FICO scores for nonconforming loans, (loans that are not to be sold to Freddie Mac or Fannie Mae).

FIGURE 12.8:   Uniform Residential Loan Application Form

Uniform Residential Loan Application

This application is designed to be completed by the applicant(s) with the Lender's assistance. Applicants should complete this form as "Borrower" or "Co-Borrower," as applicable. Co-Borrower information must also be provided (and the appropriate box checked) when ☐ the income or assets of a person other than the Borrower (including the Borrower's spouse) will be used as a basis for loan qualification or ☐ the income or assets of the Borrower's spouse or other person who has community property rights pursuant to state law will not be used as a basis for loan qualification, but his or her liabilities must be considered because the spouse or other person has community property rights pursuant to applicable law and Borrower resides in a community property state, the security property is located in a community property state, or the Borrower is relying on other property located in a community property state as a basis for repayment of the loan.

If this is an application for joint credit, Borrower and Co-Borrower each agree that we intend to apply for joint credit (sign below):

Borrower _____   Co-Borrower _____

I. TYPE OF MORTGAGE AND TERMS OF LOAN

Mortgage Applied for:	☐ VA ☐ FHA	☑ Conventional ☐ USDA/Rural Housing Service	☐ Other (explain):	Agency Case Number	Lender Case Number
					Case #6

Amount	Interest Rate	No. of Months	Amortization Type:	Fixed/Other
$ **450,000.00**	**5.000** %	**360**		☑ Fixed Rate ☐ Other (explain): ☐ GPM ☐ ARM (type):

II. PROPERTY INFORMATION AND PURPOSE OF LOAN

Subject Property Address (street, city, state & ZIP) **8709 Grosvenor ST, Silver Spring, MD 20910**	No. of Units **1**
Legal Description of Subject Property (attach description if necessary) **Other; Detached**	Year Built **0**

Purpose of Loan	☑ Purchase ☐ Construction ☐ Other (explain): ☐ Refinance ☐ Construction-Permanent	Property will be: ☑ Primary Residence ☐ Secondary Residence ☐ Investment

Complete this line if construction or construction-permanent loan.

Year Lot Acquired	Original Cost	Amount Existing Liens	(a) Present Value of Lot	(b) Cost of Improvements	Total (a + b)
	$	$	$	$	$

Complete this line if this is a refinance loan.

Year Acquired	Original Cost	Amount Existing Liens	Purpose of Refinance	Describe Improvements ☐ made ☐ to be made
	$	$		Cost: $

Title will be held in what Name(s)	Manner in which Title will be held	Estate will be held in: ☑ Fee Simple ☐ Leasehold (show expiration date)

Source of Down Payment, Settlement Charges, and/or Subordinate Financing (explain)

III. BORROWER INFORMATION

Borrower	Co-Borrower
Borrower's Name (include Jr. or Sr. if applicable) **John Homeowner**	Co-Borrower's Name (include Jr. or Sr. if applicable) **Mary Homeowner**

Social Security Number	Home Phone (incl. area code)	DOB (mm/dd/yyyy)	Yrs. School	Social Security Number	Home Phone (incl. area code)	DOB (mm/dd/yyyy)	Yrs. School
999-40-5000				**500-22-2000**			

☐ Married ☐ Unmarried (include ☐ Separated single, divorced, widowed)	Dependents (not listed by Co-Borrower) no. ages	☐ Married ☐ Unmarried (include ☐ Separated single, divorced, widowed)	Dependents (not listed by Borrower) no. ages

Present Address (street, city, state, ZIP) ☐ Own ☐ Rent **0** No. Yrs. **175 13th Street, Washington, DC, 20013**	Present Address (street, city, state, ZIP) ☐ Own ☐ Rent **0** No. Yrs. **175 13th Street, Washington, DC, 20013**
Mailing Address, if different from Present Address	Mailing Address, if different from Present Address

If residing at present address for less than two years, complete the following:

Former Address (street, city, state, ZIP) ☐ Own ☐ Rent ___ No. Yrs.	Former Address (street, city, state, ZIP) ☐ Own ☐ Rent ___ No. Yrs.

IV. EMPLOYMENT INFORMATION

Borrower		Co-Borrower	
Name & Address of Employer ☐ Self Employed	Yrs. on this job **7.17** Yrs. employed in this line of work/profession	Name & Address of Employer ☑ Self Employed	Yrs. on this job **12.42** Yrs. employed in this line of work/profession
Position/Title/Type of Business	Business Phone (incl. area code)	Position/Title/Type of Business	Business Phone (incl. area code)

If employed in current position for less than two years or if currently employed in more than one position, complete the following:

FIGURE 12.8 (continued):   Uniform Residential Loan Application Form

Borrower		IV. EMPLOYMENT INFORMATION (cont'd)		Co-Borrower	
Name & Address of Employer	☐ Self Employed	Dates (from – to)	Name & Address of Employer	☐ Self Employed	Dates (from – to)
		Monthly Income $			Monthly Income $
Position/Title/Type of Business		Business Phone (incl. area code)	Position/Title/Type of Business		Business Phone (incl. area code)
Name & Address of Employer	☐ Self Employed	Dates (from – to)	Name & Address of Employer	☐ Self Employed	Dates (from – to)
		Monthly Income $			Monthly Income $
Position/Title/Type of Business		Business Phone (incl. area code)	Position/Title/Type of Business		Business Phone (incl. area code)

V. MONTHLY INCOME AND COMBINED HOUSING EXPENSE INFORMATION

Gross Monthly Income	Borrower	Co-Borrower	Total	Combined Monthly Housing Expense	Present	Proposed
Base Empl. Income*	$3,850.00	$4,300.00	$8,150.00	Rent	$2,500.00	
Overtime			$0.00	First Mortgage (P&I)		$2,415.70
Bonuses			$0.00	Other Financing (P&I)		
Commissions	$1,050.00		$1,050.00	Hazard Insurance		$65.00
Dividends/Interest			$0.00	Real Estate Taxes		$300.00
Net Rental Income	$0.00	$0.00	$0.00	Mortgage Insurance		$100.00
Other (before completing, see the notice in "describe other income," below)	0.00	0.00	0.00	Homeowner Assn. Dues		
				Other:		
Total	$4,900.00	$4,300.00	$9,200.00	Total	$2,500.00	$2,880.70

*   **Self Employed Borrower(s) may be required to provide additional documentation such as tax returns and financial statements.**

Describe Other Income

Notice: **Alimony, child support, or separate maintenance income need not be revealed if the Borrower (B) or Co-Borrower (C) does not choose to have it considered for repaying this loan.**

B/C		Monthly Amount
		$

VI. ASSETS AND LIABILITIES

This Statement and any applicable supporting schedules may be completed jointly by both married and unmarried Co-Borrowers if their assets and liabilities are sufficiently joined so that the Statement can be meaningfully and fairly presented on a combined basis; otherwise, separate Statements and Schedules are required. If the Co-Borrower section was completed about a non-applicant spouse or other person, this Statement and supporting schedules must be completed about that spouse or other person also.

Completed ☐ Jointly ☑ Not Jointly

ASSETS	Cash or Market Value	Liabilities and Pledged Assets. List the creditor's name, address, and account number for all outstanding debts, including automobile loans, revolving charge accounts, real estate loans, alimony, child support, stock pledges, etc. Use continuation sheet, if necessary. Indicate by (*) those liabilities, which will be satisfied upon sale of real estate owned or upon refinancing of the subject property.		
Description				
Cash deposit toward purchase held by:	$0.00			
		LIABILITIES	Monthly Payment & Months Left to Pay	Unpaid Balance
List checking and savings accounts below				
Name and address of Bank, S&L, or Credit Union **Savings Account**		Name and address of Company	$ Payment/Months	$
Acct. no.	$18,500.00	Acct. no.		
Name and address of Bank, S&L, or Credit Union **Certificate of Deposit**		Name and address of Company	$ Payment/Months	$
Acct. no.	$40,000.00	Acct. no.		
Name and address of Bank, S&L, or Credit Union **Checking Account**		Name and address of Company	$ Payment/Months	$
Acct. no.	$2,800.00	Acct. no.		

Uniform Residential Loan Application
Freddie Mac Form 65 7/05 (rev. 6/09)

Page 2 of 5

Fannie Mae Form 1003   7/05 (rev.6/09)

FIGURE 12.8 (continued):   Uniform Residential Loan Application Form

VI. ASSETS AND LIABILITIES (cont'd)

Name and address of Bank, S&L, or Credit Union **Money Market Fund**		Name and address of Company	$ Payment/Months	$
Acct. no.	$ 12,000.00	Acct. no.		
Stocks & Bonds (Company name/ number & description)	$0.00	Name and address of Company	$ Payment/Months	$
		Acct. no.		
Life insurance net cash value Face amount: $0.00	$0.00	Name and address of Company	$ Payment/Months	$
Subtotal Liquid Assets	$73,300.00			
Real estate owned (enter market value from schedule of real estate owned)	$0.00			
Vested interest in retirement fund	$0.00			
Net worth of business(es) owned (attach financial statement)	$0.00	Acct. no.		
Automobiles owned (make and year)	$0.00	Alimony/Child Support/Separate Maintenance Payments Owed to:	$0.00	
Other Assets (itemize)	$0.00	Job-Related Expense (child care, union dues, etc.)	$0.00	
		Total Monthly Payments	$0.00	
Total Assets a.	$73,300.00	Net Worth (a minus b) ▶ $ 73,300.00	**Total Liabilities b.**	$0.00

Schedule of Real Estate Owned (If additional properties are owned, use continuation sheet.)

Property Address (enter S if sold, PS if pending sale or R if rental being held for income) ▼	Type of Property	Present Market Value	Amount of Mortgages & Liens	Gross Rental Income	Mortgage Payments	Insurance, Maintenance, Taxes & Misc.	Net Rental Income
		$	$	$	$	$	$
Totals		$0.00	$0.00	$ 0.00	$ 0.00	$0.00	$ 0.00

List any additional names under which credit has previously been received and indicate appropriate creditor name(s) and account number(s):

Alternate Name	Creditor Name	Account Number

VII. DETAILS OF TRANSACTION

a.	Purchase price	$500,000.00
b.	Alterations, improvements, repairs	$0.00
c.	Land (if acquired separately)	$0.00
d.	Refinance (incl. debts to be paid off)	$0.00
e.	Estimated prepaid items	$0.00
f.	Estimated closing costs	$3,500.00
g.	PMI, MIP, Funding Fee	$0.00
h.	Discount (if Borrower will pay)	$0.00
i.	Total costs (add items a through h)	$503,500.00

VIII. DECLARATIONS

If you answer "Yes" to any questions a through i, please use continuation sheet for explanation.

	Borrower		Co-Borrower	
	Yes	No	Yes	No
a. Are there any outstanding judgments against you?	☐	☐	☐	☐
b. Have you been declared bankrupt within the past 7 years?	☐	☑	☐	☑
c. Have you had property foreclosed upon or given title or deed in lieu thereof in the last 7 years?	☐	☑	☐	☑
d. Are you a party to a lawsuit?	☐	☐	☐	☐
e. Have you directly or indirectly been obligated on any loan which resulted in foreclosure, transfer of title in lieu of foreclosure, or judgment?	☐	☐	☐	☐

(This would include such loans as home mortgage loans, SBA loans, home improvement loans, educational loans, manufactured (mobile) home loans, any mortgage, financial obligation, bond, or loan guarantee. If "Yes," provide details, including date, name, and address of Lender, FHA or VA case number, if any, and reasons for the action.)

FIGURE 12.8 (continued):   Uniform Residential Loan Application Form

VII. DETAILS OF TRANSACTION		VIII. DECLARATIONS					
		If you answer "Yes" to any questions a through i, please use continuation sheet for explanation.		Borrower		Co-Borrower	
				Yes	No	Yes	No
j. Subordinate financing	$0.00	f. Are you presently delinquent or in default on any Federal debt or any other loan, mortgage, financial obligation, bond, or loan guarantee?		☐	☐	☐	☐
k. Borrower's closing costs paid by Seller	$3,500.00	g. Are you obligated to pay alimony, child support, or separate maintenance?		☐	☐	☐	☐
l. Other Credits (explain)	$0.00	h. Is any part of the down payment borrowed?		☐	☐	☐	☐
		i. Are you a co-maker or endorser on a note?		☐	☐	☐	☐
m. Loan amount (exclude PMI, MIP, Funding Fee financed)	$450,000.00	---					
		j. Are you a U.S. citizen?		☑	☐	☑	☐
n. PMI, MIP, Funding Fee financed	$0.00	k. Are you a permanent resident alien?		☐	☑	☐	☑
o. Loan amount (add m & n)	$450,000.00	l. **Do you intend to occupy the property as your primary residence?**		☑	☐	☑	☐
		If Yes," complete question m below.					
p. Cash from/to Borrower (subtract j, k, l & o from i)	$50,000.00	m. Have you had an ownership interest in a property in the last three years?		☐	☑	☐	☑
		(1) What type of property did you own—principal residence (PR), second home (SH), or investment property (IP)?		_____		_____	
		(2) How did you hold title to the home— by yourself (S), jointly with your spouse (SP), or jointly with another person (O)?		_____		_____	

IX. ACKNOWLEDGEMENT AND AGREEMENT

Each of the undersigned specifically represents to Lender and to Lender's actual or potential agents, brokers, processors, attorneys, insurers, servicers, successors and assigns and agrees and acknowledges that: (1) the information provided in this application is true and correct as of the date set forth opposite my signature and that any intentional or negligent misrepresentation of this information contained in this application may result in civil liability, including monetary damages, to any person who may suffer any loss due to reliance upon any misrepresentation that I have made on this application, and/or in criminal penalties including, but not limited to, fine or imprisonment or both under the provisions of Title 18, United States Code, Sec. 1001, et seq.; (2) the loan requested pursuant to this application (the "Loan") will be secured by a mortgage or deed of trust on the property described in this application; (3) the property will not be used for any illegal or prohibited purpose or use; (4) all statements made in this application are made for the purpose of obtaining a residential mortgage loan; (5) the property will be occupied as indicated in this application; (6) the Lender, its servicers, successors or assigns may retain the original and/or an electronic record of this application, whether or not the Loan is approved; (7) the Lender and its agents, brokers, insurers, servicers, successors, and assigns may continuously rely on the information contained in the application, and I am obligated to amend and/or supplement the information provided in this application if any of the material facts that I have represented herein should change prior to closing of the Loan; (8) in the event that my payments on the Loan become delinquent, the Lender, its servicers, successors or assigns may, in addition to any other rights and remedies that it may have relating to such delinquency, report my name and account information to one or more consumer reporting agencies; (9) ownership of the Loan and/or administration of the Loan account may be transferred with such notice as may be required by law; (10) neither Lender nor its agents, brokers, insurers, servicers, successors or assigns has made any representation or warranty, express or implied, to me regarding the property or the condition or value of the property; and (11) my transmission of this application as an "electronic record" containing my "electronic signature," as those terms are defined in applicable federal and/or state laws (excluding audio and video recordings), or my facsimile transmission of this application containing a facsimile of my signature, shall be as effective, enforceable and valid as if a paper version of this application were delivered containing my original written signature.

Acknowledgement. Each of the undersigned hereby acknowledges that any owner of the Loan, its servicers, successors and assigns, may verify or reverify any information contained in this application or obtain any information or data relating to the Loan, for any legitimate business purpose through any source, including a source named in this application or a consumer reporting agency.

Borrower's Signature	Date	Co-Borrower's Signature	Date
X		X	

X. INFORMATION FOR GOVERNMENT MONITORING PURPOSES

The following information is requested by the Federal Government for certain types of loans related to a dwelling in order to monitor the lender's compliance with equal credit opportunity, fair housing and home mortgage disclosure laws. You are not required to furnish this information, but are encouraged to do so. The law provides that a lender may not discriminate either on the basis of this information, or on whether you choose to furnish it. If you furnish the information, please provide both ethnicity and race. For race, you may check more than one designation. If you do not furnish ethnicity, race, or sex, under Federal regulations, this lender is required to note the information on the basis of visual observation and surname if you have made this application in person. If you do not wish to furnish the information, please check the box below. (Lender must review the above material to assure that the disclosures satisfy all requirements to which the lender is subject under applicable state law for the particular type of loan applied for.)

BORROWER ☐ I do not wish to furnish this information			**CO-BORROWER** ☐ I do not wish to furnish this information		
Ethnicity: ☐ Hispanic or Latino ☐ Not Hispanic or Latino			**Ethnicity:** ☐ Hispanic or Latino ☐ Not Hispanic or Latino		
Race: ☐ American Indian or Alaska Native ☐ Native Hawaiian or Other Pacific Islander	☐ Asian ☐ White	☐ Black or African American	**Race:** ☐ American Indian or Alaska Native ☐ Native Hawaiian or Other Pacific Islander	☐ Asian ☐ White	☐ Black or African American
Sex: ☐ Female ☐ Male			**Sex:** ☐ Female ☐ Male		

To be Completed by Loan Originator:
This information was provided:
   ☐ In a face-to-face interview
   ☐ In a telephone interview
   ☐ By the applicant and submitted by fax or mail
   ☐ By the applicant and submitted via e-mail or the Internet

Loan Originator's Signature X		Date
Loan Originator's Name (print or type)	Loan Originator Identifier	Loan Originator's Phone Number (including area code)
Loan Origination Company's Name	Loan Origination Company Identifier	Loan Origination Company's Address

Page 4 of 5

Uniform Residential Loan Application
Freddie Mac Form 65   7/05 (rev.6/09)   Fannie Mae Form 1003   7/05 (rev.6/09)

FIGURE 12.8 (continued): **Uniform Residential Loan Application Form**

CONTINUATION SHEET/RESIDENTIAL LOAN APPLICATION		
Use this continuation sheet if you need more space to complete the Residential Loan Application. Mark **B** f or Borrower or **C** for Co-Borrower.	Borrower: **John Homeowner**	Agency Case Number:
	Co-Borrower: **Mary Homeowner**	Lender Case Number: **Case #6**

I/We fully understand that it is a Federal crime punishable by fine or imprisonment, or both, to knowingly make any false statements concerning any of the above facts as applicable under the provisions of Title 18, United States Code, Section 1001, et seq.

Borrower's Signature	Date	Co-Borrower's Signature	Date
X		X	

Uniform Residential Loan Application
Freddie Mac Form 65   7/05 (rev.6/09)

Page 5 of 5

Fannie Mae Form 1003   7/05 (rev.6/09)

FIGURE 12.9:   Qualifying Ratios

Front-End Rate

$$\frac{\text{PITI (Principal, Interest, Taxes, \& Insurance)}}{\text{Borrowers Monthly Gross Income}} = 0.28 \text{ or less}$$

Back-End Rate

$$\frac{\text{Total Loan Obligations}}{\text{Borrowers Monthly Gross Income}} = 0.36 \text{ or less}$$

Capacity.   In considering borrowers' capacity, lenders want to know their ability to repay the debt. Capacity is strengthened by an occupation that ensures a steady income. The level of present debts and obligations also is a factor; too much debt may prevent a borrower from discharging a new obligation.

Lenders will consider second-job income if the applicant has a history of second-job income.

Lending institutions sometimes take overtime wages into consideration. Other lenders will consider both spouses' wages in computing the gross income of the borrower, even if only one spouse is applying for the loan. Occasionally, a lender will request a **cosigner**—a person with additional capital who agrees to share liability for the loan—to strengthen the borrower's application. Lenders also might reduce down payment requirements with a cosigner.

When a lender qualifies a borrower, the lender is attempting to answer two questions:

1. Can the borrower afford the payments?

2. Will the borrower make the payments on time? (This question refers to character.)

To determine whether the borrower has the capacity to make the monthly payments, the lender needs to answer these questions:

- Does the borrower earn enough to make the payments?

- Will the income be a steady source of income?

- Does the borrower have the down payment?

- Can the borrower make the payments on time?

The lender is going to verify the applicant's ability to make timely monthly payments and the applicant's employment history (steady stream of income). The lender will want to know the down payment on the property before determining the loan amount. This information is usually confirmed by the lender through the use of verifications of deposits and employment.

Once the lender knows the loan amount, it can calculate the *principal, interest, taxes, and insurance* (*PITI*) on it. This is the first step in the qualification process. These are qualifying programs available for your smartphone or computer.

> The important qualifying ratios are 28% and 36%.

To qualify the borrower, we examine two ratios (percentages). The **front-end ratio**, also called the *top ratio* (*mortgage payment ratio*), is the mortgage payment (PITI) divided by the borrower's gross income. Conforming loans require that the front-end ratio be approximately 28% or less. The reason it is called the top ratio is because it is at the top of the form (above the bottom ratio). The other ratio is the **back-end ratio**, or *bottom ratio* (*total obligation ratio*). This ratio should be approximately 36% or less to qualify for a conforming loan (see Figure 12.9). Nonconforming loans may have different values for these ratios. The preceding ratios (28% and 36%) are for loans that do not require PMI. For loans with PMI, the ratios might be top equals 33% and bottom equals 38%.

EXAMPLE   Assume the buyers have a gross income of $4,000 per month and wish to buy a home where the principal, interest, and tax payments will amount to $1,100.

$$\frac{1,100\,(\text{PITI})}{4,000\,(\text{gross})} = 0.275 \text{ or } 27.5\%$$

The purchasers would meet the qualifying front-end ratio of 28% or less.

Assume the same purchasers have long-term debt payments of $900 per month, so PITI plus debt payments would mean a total monthly obligation of $2,000.

$$\frac{2,000\,(\text{total payments})}{4,000\,(\text{gross income})} = 0.5 \text{ or } 50\%$$

The buyers would not qualify for the loan. Although the buyers met the front-end ratio of 28% or less, they failed to meet the back-end ratio of 36% or less.

From the **verification of employment** and other financial information, the lender determines the borrower's gross income. Lenders require a signed statement from the borrower to permit a check with the borrower's employer to verify wages and length of employment. *Gross income* is defined as the income made by the borrower before taxes and deductions. For a married couple, the gross income for a loan is generally the total gross income of one spouse plus the total gross income of the other spouse. Employment usually must be verified for two years.

The lender also needs to determine the monthly long-term rotating credit bills owed by the borrower. These include car payments, credit cards, furniture payments, student loans, and other bank or credit union loans, including mortgage loans. If a credit bill will be paid in less than 10 months, it is not included.

Qualifying the Property

Collateral.   After the loan is granted, the lender has to rely for a long time on the value of the security for the loan for the safety of the investment, should the borrower default. For this reason, lenders consider it important to qualify the property, as well as the borrower.

> Collateral refers to the value of the security for the loan.

Because the underlying security for almost every property loan is the property itself, lenders require a careful valuation of the property, the *collateral*. The value depends on the property's location, age, architecture, physical condition, zoning, floor plan, and general appearance. The lender will have an appraisal done by the financial institution's appraiser or by an outside fee appraiser. Brokers who are familiar with lending policies of loan companies are in a good position to make accurate and helpful estimates.

After the S&Ls were deregulated in the 1980s, allowing them to make commercial loans, many made high-value loans at significantly higher interest rates than was possible for residential loans. Competition for many of these loans was intense, and S&Ls did not want to lose choice loan opportunities because of conservative appraisals. They encouraged more liberal appraisals, but appraisers who failed to cooperate found themselves shut out from lucrative business. In the mid-1980s, there was a collapse in the S&L industry with over 500 S&L bankruptcies and a government bailout. Instead of placing the blame on greed of the S&Ls, the blame was placed largely on the appraisers. In 1989, the federal government passed the Financial Institutions Reform, Recovery, and Enforcement Act (FIRREA). Part of the law created the Appraisal Foundation and required state-certified and state-licensed appraisers.

When an appraisal is less than the purchase price, it requires the seller to lower the price or the buyer to come up with a larger down payment because the amount of the loan will be reduced. The purchaser often does not have the resources for the large down payment. In addition, many offers include a contingency that the appraisal will be at least the amount of the purchase price. This provides an avenue of escape for the buyers.

A great many mortgage loan officers are paid by commission. They don't get paid when a loan cannot be funded. Appraisals seldom came in at less than the purchase price. Some appraisals were likely inflated by appraisers in order to gain referrals. This resulted in lenders having insufficient security in case of buyer default.

WEB LINK

@

The Dodd-Frank Wall Street Reform and Consumer Protection Act(Dodd-Frank) (15 USC 1639e) prohibits attempts by lenders or brokers to influence appraisal. (See www.law.cornell.edu/uscode/text/15/1639e.)

The act prohibits the following:

- Withholding or threatening to withhold payments

- Threat of withholding payment

- Promising benefits for higher appraisals

- Basing compensation on appraisal valuation

- Setting predetermined value for appraiser

- Removal of an appraiser from a list of appraisers without evidence of violation of Uniform Standards of Professional Appraisal Practice (USPAP)

- Ordering a second appraisal without evidence an appraisal was flawed

Some **subprime lenders** that specialize in high-risk borrowers made loans for the full appraisal amount, and even loans exceeding the appraisal if the risk factor was sufficiently offset by the higher interest rate.

While competition for loans led to low down and no down financing instruments, losses by lenders have tightened the controls so that few lenders are willing to make no-down-payment loans, even with interest premiums.

Approving and Processing the Loan

Processing involves drawing up loan papers, preparing disclosure forms regarding loan fees, and issuing instructions for the escrow and title companies. Loan papers include the *promissory note* (the evidence of the debt) and the security instruments (the *trust deed* or *mortgage*).

Closing the Loan

Closing the loan involves signing all the loan papers and preparing the closing statements. First-time buyers, especially, are often confused by the various fees involved. Real estate licensees play a vital role in making this transition period smooth.

Servicing the Loan

After the title has been transferred and the escrow closed, the loan-servicing portion of the transaction begins. This refers to the recordkeeping process once the loan has been placed. Some lenders do their own servicing, whereas others use outside sources. The goal of loan servicing is to see that the borrower makes timely payments so that the lender makes the expected yield on the loan, which keeps the cost of the entire package at a minimum.

REGULATION OF REAL ESTATE FINANCING

Because this is a real estate practices text, all references to the regulations governing real estate financing will, of necessity, be brief. For further information relating to this subject, consult a real estate finance book.

Truth in Lending Act

The *Truth in Lending Act* (*Regulation Z*) is a key portion of the federal Consumer Credit Protection Act passed in 1969. The Truth in Lending Act applies to banks, savings associations, credit unions, consumer finance companies, and residential mortgage brokers. This disclosure act requires that lenders reveal to customers, either by delivery or mailing, how much they're being charged for credit in terms of an annual percentage rate (APR). Customers can then make credit cost comparisons among various credit sources. The lender must wait at least seven days after disclosure to consummate the loan.

The act gives individuals seeking credit a right of rescission of the contract. This means that under certain circumstances a customer has the right to cancel a credit transaction up until midnight of the third day after signing. This right of rescission applies to loans that place a lien on the borrower's residence. The rescission rights do not apply to primary financing (first trust deed) to finance the purchase of the borrower's residence (purchase-money loan).

Truth in Savings Act

For savings-type accounts, banks must disclose all fees, costs, and yields (savings, checking, money market, and certificates of deposit). If there are any changes, free checking cannot be claimed. The yield must be expressed as the annual percentage yield (APY).

TILA-RESPA Integrated Disclosure (TRID) Rule

The regulations contained in the **TILA-RESPA Integrated Disclosure (TRID) rule** apply only to first loans on 1–4-unit residential properties. This is another disclosure act. Within three days of the date of the loan application, a lender must furnish the buyer with an itemized list of all closing costs that will be encountered in escrow. This must be a **Loan Estimate** provided to every person requesting credit. Each charge for each settlement service the buyer is likely to incur must be expressed as a dollar amount or range. The lender also must furnish a copy of a special information booklet prepared by the secretary of the Department of Housing and Urban Development (HUD). It must be delivered or placed in the mail to the applicant no later than three business days after the application is received.

The good-faith estimate required by RESPA has been combined with early truth-in-lending disclosures to include the following:

- Estimated monthly payment

- Estimated taxes, insurance, and assessments

- Estimated closing costs and cash required to close

- Services that cannot be shopped for

Figure 12.10 is a sample completed integrated loan estimate prepared by the Consumer Financial Protection Bureau, an independent agency of the U.S. government.

FIGURE 12.10: Loan Estimate

FICUS BANK
4321 Random Boulevard • Somecity, ST 12340

Save this Loan Estimate to compare with your Closing Disclosure.

Loan Estimate

DATE ISSUED	2/15/2013	**LOAN TERM**	30 years
APPLICANTS	Michael Jones and Mary Stone	**PURPOSE**	Purchase
	123 Anywhere Street	**PRODUCT**	Fixed Rate
	Anytown, ST 12345	**LOAN TYPE**	☒ Conventional ☐ FHA ☐ VA ☐ _____
PROPERTY	456 Somewhere Avenue	**LOAN ID #**	123456789
	Anytown, ST 12345	**RATE LOCK**	☐ NO ☒ YES, until 4/16/2013 at 5:00 p.m. EDT
SALE PRICE	$180,000		

*Before closing, your interest rate, points, and lender credits can change unless you lock the interest rate. All other estimated closing costs expire on **3/4/2013** at 5:00 p.m. EDT*

Loan Terms

		Can this amount increase after closing?
Loan Amount	$162,000	**NO**
Interest Rate	3.875%	**NO**
Monthly Principal & Interest *See Projected Payments below for your Estimated Total Monthly Payment*	$761.78	**NO**
		Does the loan have these features?
Prepayment Penalty		**YES** • As high as **$3,240** if you pay off the loan during the first 2 years
Balloon Payment		**NO**

Projected Payments

Payment Calculation	Years 1–7	Years 8–30
Principal & Interest	$761.78	$761.78
Mortgage Insurance	+ 82	+ —
Estimated Escrow *Amount can increase over time*	+ 206	+ 206
Estimated Total Monthly Payment	**$1,050**	**$968**

Estimated Taxes, Insurance & Assessments *Amount can increase over time*	$206 a month	**This estimate includes** ☒ Property Taxes ☒ Homeowner's Insurance ☐ Other: *See Section G on page 2 for escrowed property costs. You must pay for other property costs separately.*	**In escrow?** YES YES

Costs at Closing

Estimated Closing Costs	$8,054	Includes $5,672 in Loan Costs + $2,382 in Other Costs – $0 in Lender Credits. *See page 2 for details.*
Estimated Cash to Close	$16,054	Includes Closing Costs. *See Calculating Cash to Close on page 2 for details.*

Visit **www.consumerfinance.gov/mortgage-estimate** for general information and tools.

LOAN ESTIMATE   PAGE 1 OF 3 • LOAN ID # 123456789

Figure 12.10 (continued):   Loan Estimate

Closing Cost Details

Loan Costs

A. Origination Charges	$1,802
.25 % of Loan Amount (Points)	$405
Application Fee	$300
Underwriting Fee	$1,097

B. Services You Cannot Shop For	$672
Appraisal Fee	$405
Credit Report Fee	$30
Flood Determination Fee	$20
Flood Monitoring Fee	$32
Tax Monitoring Fee	$75
Tax Status Research Fee	$110

C. Services You Can Shop For	$3,198
Pest Inspection Fee	$135
Survey Fee	$65
Title – Insurance Binder	$700
Title – Lender's Title Policy	$535
Title – Settlement Agent Fee	$502
Title – Title Search	$1,261

D. TOTAL LOAN COSTS (A + B + C)	$5,672

Other Costs

E. Taxes and Other Government Fees	$85
Recording Fees and Other Taxes	$85
Transfer Taxes	

F. Prepaids	$867
Homeowner's Insurance Premium (6 months)	$605
Mortgage Insurance Premium (months)	
Prepaid Interest ($17.44 per day for 15 days @ 3.875%)	$262
Property Taxes (months)	

G. Initial Escrow Payment at Closing	$413
Homeowner's Insurance $100.83 per month for 2 mo.	$202
Mortgage Insurance per month for mo.	
Property Taxes $105.30 per month for 2 mo.	$211

H. Other	$1,017
Title – Owner's Title Policy (optional)	$1,017

I. TOTAL OTHER COSTS (E + F + G + H)	$2,382

J. TOTAL CLOSING COSTS	$8,054
D + I	$8,054
Lender Credits	

Calculating Cash to Close

Total Closing Costs (J)	$8,054
Closing Costs Financed (Paid from your Loan Amount)	$0
Down Payment/Funds from Borrower	$18,000
Deposit	– $10,000
Funds for Borrower	$0
Seller Credits	$0
Adjustments and Other Credits	$0
Estimated Cash to Close	$16,054

Figure 12.10 (continued):   Loan Estimate

Additional Information About This Loan

LENDER	Ficus Bank	**MORTGAGE BROKER**	
NMLS/__ LICENSE ID		**NMLS/__ LICENSE ID**	
LOAN OFFICER	Joe Smith	**LOAN OFFICER**	
NMLS/__ LICENSE ID	12345	**NMLS/__ LICENSE ID**	
EMAIL	joesmith@ficusbank.com	**EMAIL**	
PHONE	123-456-7890	**PHONE**	

Comparisons	Use these measures to compare this loan with other loans.	
In 5 Years	$56,582	Total you will have paid in principal, interest, mortgage insurance, and loan costs.
	$15,773	Principal you will have paid off.
Annual Percentage Rate (APR)	4.274%	Your costs over the loan term expressed as a rate. This is not your interest rate.
Total Interest Percentage (TIP)	69.45%	The total amount of interest that you will pay over the loan term as a percentage of your loan amount.

Other Considerations

Appraisal	We may order an appraisal to determine the property's value and charge you for this appraisal. We will promptly give you a copy of any appraisal, even if your loan does not close. You can pay for an additional appraisal for your own use at your own cost.
Assumption	If you sell or transfer this property to another person, we ☐ will allow, under certain conditions, this person to assume this loan on the original terms. ☒ will not allow assumption of this loan on the original terms.
Homeowner's Insurance	This loan requires homeowner's insurance on the property, which you may obtain from a company of your choice that we find acceptable.
Late Payment	If your payment is more than *15* days late, we will charge a late fee of *5% of the monthly principal and interest payment.*
Refinance	Refinancing this loan will depend on your future financial situation, the property value, and market conditions. You may not be able to refinance this loan.
Servicing	We intend ☐ to service your loan. If so, you will make your payments to us. ☒ to transfer servicing of your loan.

Confirm Receipt

By signing, you are only confirming that you have received this form. You do not have to accept this loan because you have signed or received this form.

_____   _____   _____   _____
Applicant Signature   Date   Co-Applicant Signature   Date

A **controlled business arrangement** (CBA) is a situation where a broker offers "one-stop shopping" for a number of broker-controlled services, such as financing arrangements, home inspection, title insurance, property insurance, and escrow. These controlled businesses could be located within the broker's premises. RESPA permits such controlled business arrangements as long as the consumer is clearly informed of the relationship between the broker and the service providers and other providers are available. Fees may not be exchanged between the companies simply for referrals. A broker-controlled mortgage company must have its own employees and cannot contract out its services or it would violate RESPA provisions that prohibit kickbacks for referral services.

It's the position of the attorney general of California that a broker may not pay referral fees to a real estate salesperson for referral to broker-affiliated services.

Fair Credit Reporting Act

The **Fair Credit Reporting Act** affects credit reporting agencies and users of credit information. If a loan is rejected because of information disclosed in a credit report, the borrower must be notified and is entitled to know all the information the agency has in its file on the buyer, as well as the sources and the names of all creditors who received reports within the past six months.

Equal Credit Opportunity Act

The federal **Equal Credit Opportunity Act** prohibits lending discrimination based on an applicant's race, color, religion, national origin, marital status, age, and whether or not the source of income is a public assistance program or Social Security.

Helping Families Save Their Homes Act of 2009

Bankruptcy judges now have the authority to modify mortgages on principal residences. They can order a reduction in the loan interest rate and/or extend the payment period as long as 40 years.

California Homeowners Bill of Rights

The California Homeowner Protection Act set forth the California Homeowners Bill of Rights:

- Dual track foreclosure is not allowed. The foreclosure process cannot be advanced after the homeowners complete an application for loan modification and the application has been fully reviewed.

- Homeowners must have a single point of contact.

- Lenders must verify all documents filed.

- Borrowers can seek redress for material violations of the foreclosure process.

- Tenant lease rights must be honored; if not, a 90-day notice must be given.

- Homeowners can compel owners of foreclosed homes in areas to remedy code violations.

Home Affordable Modification Program (HAMP)

Provides for loan modification of loans guaranteed or insured by Fannie Mae, Freddie Mac, FHA, VA or USDA originated before 2009 if because of financial hardship the borrower cannot make loan payments.

Hope for Homeowners Program (Hope Act)

A HUD program to change variable rate FHA loans to fixed rate.

Service Members Civil Relief Act of 2003

This act applies to citizen military members called to active duty, not career military. The act provides the following:

- A maximum of 6% interest on credit obligations entered into before active duty. Interest above 6% must be forgiven.

- Foreclosures may be postponed by the court until 90 days after active service ceases.

- A court order is required for evictions when rent is $3,329.84 per month or less. (2015 – changes annually.)

- If transferred, service personnel may terminate any lease.

Predatory Lending

California law prohibits predatory lending. Loans made to homeowners by finance companies, real estate brokers, and residential mortgage lenders without considering the borrowers' ability to repay are considered **predatory lending**. Violations subject the lender to civil penalties. This law was enacted because some loans were made where the lenders actually wanted the borrowers to default in order to foreclose on the properties securing the loans.

Some loans had high loan costs that were added to the loan balance. When borrowers had trouble with repayment, they were encouraged to refinance to another loan with high loan costs that offered no economic benefit to the borrower and reduced the borrowers' equity.

Borrowers are protected in the following ways:

- Prepayment penalties for the first 36 months of a loan are strictly limited and not allowed thereafter.

- Loans with terms of five years or less must be amortized.

- Loans other than first trust deeds cannot include negative amortization, and even then it must be properly disclosed.

- Requiring payment advances from loan proceeds are prohibited.

- Interest rates cannot be increased as a result of default.

- The person originating the loan must reasonably believe the borrower will be able to repay the loan from resources other than the borrower's equity in the property.

- Payments made directly to contractors from proceeds of home improvement loans are prohibited. (Payments jointly to the homeowner and the contractor are allowed.)

- Recommending that a consumer default on an existing loan or debt is prohibited.

- Loans with call provisions allowing the lender to accelerate debt at its discretion are generally prohibited.

- Refinancing that does not result in identifiable tangible benefits to the consumer is prohibited.

- Steering or directing a consumer to a loan product with a higher-risk grade than the consumer would otherwise qualify for, or with a higher cost than the consumer would qualify for, is prohibited.

- Structuring a loan as an open line of credit to avoid predatory lending restrictions is prohibited.

- All consumer fraud is prohibited.

See Financial Code 4970-4979.8.

SUMMARY

The Federal Reserve is responsible for monetary policy and has control over the availability and cost of funds by controlling the discount rate charged member banks, by controlling the reserve requirements of banks, and by buying and selling government securities on the open market and controlling the supply of currency. The fiscal policy of the government to raise and lower taxes, as well as to spend, also affects the availability of funds.

While low interest rates increase housing affordability and can lead to a strong market, high rates have an opposite effect.

Whereas primary financing refers to first trust deeds and secondary financing refers to junior liens, the primary and secondary mortgage markets are far different. The primary mortgage market refers to lenders making loans direct to borrowers; the secondary mortgage market refers to the sale of existing loans.

Fannie Mae (the Federal National Mortgage Association) and Freddie Mac (the Federal Home Loan Mortgage Corporation) create a secondary mortgage market by buying FHA, VA, and conforming conventional loans. Conforming loans are loans that meet the standards established by Fannie Mae.

Institutional lenders such as banks, savings associations, and life insurance companies are major sources of primary real estate financing. Noninstitutional lenders include mortgage companies, which originate most real estate loans today. Mortgage companies (mortgage bankers) generally sell loans in the secondary market or act as loan correspondents for other lenders.

Mortgage loan brokers are real estate brokers who serve as middlemen for loans. These loans generally have a high loan cost and bear a higher rate of interest than do loans from institutional lenders. Mortgage loan brokers must provide a Mortgage Loan Disclosure Statement to borrowers. Other noninstitutional lenders include real estate investment trusts, pension funds, and credit unions.

Seller carryback financing is also a source of funding for real estate purchases.

Conventional loans are loans made without any government participation, guarantee, or insurance.

Government participation loans provide for lower down payment requirements and include FHA, VA, and CalVet loans.

The California Housing Finance Agency provides low rates and low down payment loans to first-time homebuyers.

Today, borrowers have a wide choice of types of loans and loan variations, including fixed-rate loans, renegotiable-rate mortgages, reverse mortgages, adjustable-rate mortgages, interest-only loans, 80-20 loans, and 40-year loans. The special features of the loans vary by lender. Buyers must analyze their needs and the important factors of down payment, loan costs, interest, assumability, convertibility, loan term, qualifying rate of interest, and so forth, as they pertain to the borrowers' needs.

The internet provides a convenient and efficient way to shop for loans, as well as to complete and submit loan applications.

The financing process involves qualifying the buyer, using front-end and back-end ratios and FICO scores, qualifying the property, approving and processing the loan, closing the loan, and servicing the loan.

The Truth in Lending Act and the Real Estate Settlement Procedures Act are federal regulations concerning lending activities. The Equal Credit Opportunity Act prohibits lender discrimination based on public assistance programs being the source of income.

The good-faith estimate of loan costs, formerly required by RESPA, has been combined with truth-in-lending disclosures for simplification purposes as mandated by Dodd-Frank.

Brokers and lenders are prohibited from seeking to influence appraisals.

Predatory lending practices are prohibited.

CLASS DISCUSSION TOPICS

1. Using a front-end (top) ratio of 33% and a back-end (bottom) ratio of 38%, qualify a buyer earning $100,000 per year for a 30-year loan of $400,000 with an 8% interest rate. Assume taxes at $5,000 per year and insurance at $1,000 per year. Assume the buyer is making payments on loans of $43,000, and the monthly payments are $2,080.

2. Obtain the ARM terms from three different lenders. Lay them out on paper, showing the differences. Which loan would be best suited for a person having what needs?

3. Discuss prequalification practices of local lenders.

4. Complete a loan application for a fictitious borrower, using realistic income, expense, debt, and savings figures. How large a conforming loan will this fictitious applicant qualify for?

5. Bring to class one current-events article dealing with some aspect of real estate practice.

UNIT 12 QUIZ

1. A loan covering more than one property would be a
    a. compound loan.
    b. blanket encumbrance.
    c. subordinated loan.
    d. reverse mortgage.

2. What type of mortgage has compound interest?
    a. Reverse mortgage
    b. Renegotiable-rate mortgage
    c. Adjustable-rate mortgage
    d. Straight mortgage

3. The difference between the interest rate of an index and the rate charged by a lender under an adjustable-rate mortgage is known as the
    a. discount.
    b. gap.
    c. margin.
    d. cap.

4. A lender who believes interest rates will be rising significantly will be *LEAST* interested in
    a. a hybrid mortgage.
    b. a 30-year fixed-rate mortgage.
    c. a 15-year fixed-rate mortgage.
    d. an adjustable-rate mortgage.

5. A danger that an adjustable-rate mortgage poses to a buyer is
    a. higher payments if interest rates increase.
    b. a longer payment period if interest rates increase.
    c. that the margin will increase.
    d. none of these.

6. An adjustable-rate loan index is 6% at the time a loan is made. The margin for the loan is 2½%. With a 5% lifetime cap, the highest the interest rate could go is
    a. 6%.
    b. 8½%.
    c. 11%.
    d. 13½%.

7. A convertible ARM is a loan that can be changed to
    a. a shorter-term loan.
    b. a fixed-rate loan.
    c. another property.
    d. another borrower.

8. A buyer intends to sell a house within two years. The buyer would prefer
    a. a loan with no prepayment penalty.
    b. a loan with low initial loan costs.
    c. an assumable loan.
    d. all of these.

9. Which loan type is MOST likely to meet all the criteria of question 8?
    a. Renegotiable-rate mortgage
    b. Adjustable-rate mortgage
    c. Fixed-rate mortgage
    d. Reverse mortgage

10. An expansionary policy of the Federal Reserve would be to
    a. lower taxes.
    b. increase the discount rate.
    c. buy government securities.
    d. raise bank reserve requirements.

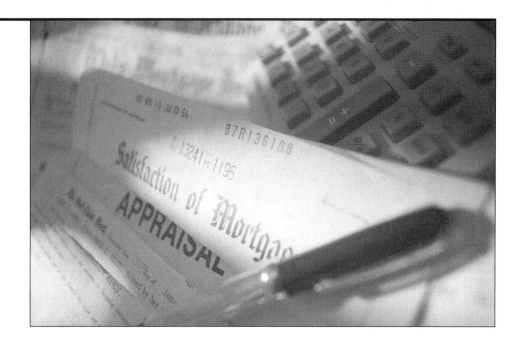

ESCROW AND TITLE INSURANCE

LEARNING OBJECTIVES

When you have completed this unit, you will be able to

- define *escrow* and explain the difference between northern and southern California escrows,

- describe the requirements of an escrow and an escrow's responsibility,

- explain the requirements of escrow licensing and laws governing the escrow,

- describe escrow procedures, and

- explain the role played by title insurance and the difference between standard and extended coverage policies.

KEY TERMS

abstract	deed of reconveyance	preliminary title report
ALTA policy	demand statement	proration
amend the escrow	escrow	rebate law
instructions	escrow agent	recurring costs
beneficiary statement	escrow instructions	special title insurance
closing costs	escrow officer	policies
Closing Disclosure	extended policy	standard policy
CLTA policy	good funds	title insurance
credits	impound account	title plant
debits	marketable title	

ESCROW

The word *escrow* is derived from the French word *escroue*, meaning scroll or roll of writing. An owner of real property executed an instrument in the form of a deed, conveying land to another party on the fulfillment of certain conditions. This instrument, the *escroue*, was given to a third person with instructions that it would take effect as a deed on the performance of an act or the occurrence of an event, such as payment of a designated sum of money. The term was taken in English as **escrow**, meaning "a deed, a bond, money, or a piece of property held in trust by a third party, to be turned over to the grantee only on fulfillment of a condition."

Escrow is the last step in a property transaction. The California Financial Code defines *escrow* as follows:

> Escrow means any transaction wherein one person for the purpose of effecting the sale, transfer, encumbering, or leasing of real or personal property to another person, delivers any written instrument, money, evidence of title to real or personal property or other things of value to a third person to be held by such third person until the happening of a specified event. The performance is then to be delivered by such third person to a grantee, grantor, promisee, promisor, obligee, obligor, bailee, or bailor, or any agent or employee or any of the latter.

This definition has been changed somewhat, and the activities of an escrow agent have been expanded considerably. In brief, an escrow agent is an impartial third party or "stakeholder who receives and disburses documents, money, and papers from every party involved in a transaction, such as a sale of real estate." The escrow operates as a neutral depository.

FIGURE 13.1: Escrow Responsibility

The escrow is an impartial stakeholder.

The business that conducts the escrow is considered the **escrow agent**. The individual who handles the escrow in the office of the escrow agent is the **escrow officer**.

Escrow Requirements

When the buyer offers a sum of money to the seller and the seller's acceptance is transmitted to the buyer, a binding contract is formed. Generally, this is the first requirement for a sales escrow. Escrow is created on the conditional delivery of transfer instruments and monies to a third party.

Although escrows are not generally required by law in California, they have become an almost indispensable mechanism in this state to protect the parties involved in exchanges, leases, and sales of securities, loans, business opportunity sales, mobile home sales, and primarily real property sales.

In some states, the listing real estate office handles escrow functions. In some states, attorneys are used for real estate closings. In some communities, the local lender handles the closing functions. However, closings are primarily handled by either third-party escrows or title companies in California.

Escrow Responsibility

The escrow agent holds all money and documents during the transaction. When conditions agreed upon by the buyer and the seller are met, the deed and the monies involved are disbursed concurrently to the appropriate parties. (See Figure 13.1.) Funds must be **good funds** before they can be disbursed. Good funds include cash, cashier's checks, and personal checks that have cleared.

Broker Responsibility

Once the escrow instructions have been signed, the escrow acts in a dual-agency capacity to carry out the instructions of the buyer and the seller. However, the broker still has agency duties.

The broker should track the escrow to make certain that the escrow is receiving what it requires, when it is required. If there are problems concerning the escrow, the broker should notify the parties and attempt to resolve these problems.

The broker also should monitor the loan application and keep in contact with the lender to avoid or resolve any problems or delays.

Parties to an Escrow

Buyers. When buyers have performed in full (paid the purchase price), they are entitled to a deed transferring title, subject only to encumbrances agreed on by both parties. Buyers do not want to pay sellers until the buyers know they are certain of obtaining title to the property as agreed. While the title search is being conducted, the buyers' deposits are held in escrow.

Sellers. Although sellers may have made a firm contract to sell their real property, they do not want to give up their title until they are certain of receiving their money. They therefore retain legal title to the property as security until they have the money in hand. The sellers' legal title usually is transferred by deed. The title is placed in escrow until buyers have produced the full purchase price for the property. If a seller dies before a transaction has been completed, that seller's right to the unpaid part of the purchase price may pass to the heirs. If a buyer dies, the heirs may be required to continue with the purchase. However, the loan may be affected owing to qualification.

Lenders.   In lending money to buyers to complete a purchase, lenders, like buyers, do not want to commit their funds without assurance that titles to the properties in question are clear. Therefore, impartial third parties (escrow agents) hold money, deeds, and other documents until liens have been paid off and clear titles have been confirmed. Thereafter, it is the escrow agent's responsibility to see that the proper disbursements are made.

The broker is not a party to an escrow.

Brokers.   Real estate agents, unless principals to the transaction, are not parties to the escrow. While the agent is not a party to the escrow, agents should understand escrow procedure so that they can both monitor the escrow to avoid delays and other problems and explain the escrow procedures to their clients and help them comply with escrow requirements. Once the escrow has been opened, the escrow may not make any changes to the escrow instructions based on orders of a real estate agent unless authorized to do so by the principals. However, the escrow instructions might provide for the payment of the commission out of escrow and stipulate that the broker's commission rights cannot be canceled. On a case-by-case basis, the broker can authorize that a commission be paid directly to a salesperson out of broker-entitled funds upon a closing.

Escrow Agents

In California, escrow companies licensed by the California Department of Corporations must be structured as corporations. This includes companies conducting escrows using the internet. Individuals cannot be licensed under the escrow law, but certain organizations and individuals are permitted to act as escrow agents without licensure. These include the following:

Escrows are corporations under the jurisdiction of the Commissioner of Corporations.

- Banks
- Attorneys (to act as an escrow, an attorney must have had a prior client relationship with a party to the escrow)
- Real estate brokers
- Title and trust companies
- Savings associations

In some northern California areas, escrow transactions are handled by title insurance companies; they usually process the escrow and issue the title insurance policy together. In southern California, escrow companies handle most escrow transactions with a title company issuing the title insurance separately. In some northern California areas, there are *separate* (*unilateral*) *escrow instructions* for each of the parties. In southern California, the parties sign *joint* (*bilateral*) *escrow instructions*. There are other regional deviations in the way escrows operate.

In Unit 10, you saw that the purchase agreement can be combined with joint escrow instructions such as the CAR form *California Residential Purchase Agreement and Joint Escrow Instructions*.

Selection of Escrow Holder

The parties to the escrow determine who shall be the escrow holder. In a real estate sales agreement, the buyer will customarily identify the escrow, and the seller, by acceptance of the agreement, agrees to the escrow selected.

Broker as Escrow

The real estate broker exemption from licensing as an escrow is applicable only when the broker represents the buyer or the seller or is a principal in the transaction. The escrow function is therefore incidental to the broker's business and the exemption cannot be a veil through which a primarily escrow business is conducted. The broker may charge for services. Many larger offices have escrow services as a separate profit center for their operations. A number of computer escrow programs are available to aid in this function. Check the website www.softprocorp.com to learn about one such program.

WEB LINK

A broker can act as an unlicensed escrow only if the broker is a principal or represents the buyer or the seller.

While brokers are exempt from the licensing requirements for their own transactions, this exemption applies only to brokers. Brokers cannot delegate escrow duties to others. The exemption is not available to any association of brokers for the purpose of conducting escrows for the group.

Real estate brokers cannot advertise that they conduct escrow business unless specifying that such services are only in connection with the real estate brokerage business. Brokers are also prohibited from using a fictitious or corporate name that contains the word *escrow*. While acting as an escrow, brokers must put aside agency relationships, as well as any special interests, and adopt the position of a neutral depository, the same as any other escrow.

Escrow funds held by a broker must be placed in a special trust account, subject to periodic inspection by the Commissioner of Corporations and, at the broker's own expense, subject to an independent annual audit.

A broker who conducts five or more escrows in a calendar year or conducts escrows totaling $1 million or more must file an annual report with the BRE as to the number of escrows conducted and the dollar amount. The report must be filed within 60 days of end of calendar year. Failure to report as required will result in a penalty of $50 per day for the first 30 days and then $100 per day thereafter, up to $10,000. Failure to pay the penalty can result in suspension or revocation of license (penalties go to the Consumer Recovery Account).

A broker can be licensed separately as an escrow and operate the escrow business in a controlled business arrangement. (See RESPA, Unit 12.)

Requirements for DOC Escrow Licensure

Any corporation applying for a Department of Corporations escrow license under the Escrow Act must

- pay an application fee;
- pass a background check;
- meet minimum financial requirements;
- meet minimum experience requirements (managers must have at least five years of responsible escrow experience);
- furnish a surety bond for $25,000 to $59,000;
- arrange for the fidelity bonding of responsible employees (minimum of $125,000 each);
- be a member of the Escrow Agents' Fidelity Corporation (EAFC);
- set up a trust fund for all monies deposited in escrow;
- keep accurate records, subject to audit at any time by the Commissioner of Corporations and the Bureau of Real Estate; and
- submit to an independent audit annually at its own expense.

Laws Governing Escrow

No escrow licensee may

- disseminate misleading or deceptive statements referring to its supervision by the State of California;

- describe either orally or in writing any transaction that is not included under the definition of escrow in the California Financial Code;

- pay referral fees to anyone except a regular employee of its own escrow company;

- solicit or accept escrow instructions or amended or supplemental instructions containing any blanks to be filled in after the instructions are signed; or

- permit any person to make additions to, deletions from, or alterations of an escrow instruction unless it is signed or initialed by all signers of the original instructions.

Figure 13.2 summarizes legal requirements pertaining to the actions of escrow officers.

FIGURE 13.2:   **Legal Requirements for Escrow Officers**

Officers Must	Officers May Not
act according to issued written instructions.	make a transaction for another officer.
act as a neutral party at all times.	negotiate with the parties separately.
hold monies deposited by parties until disbursed.	suggest that terms or provisions be inserted in the escrow.
follow escrow instructions in every detail unless instructions are in violation of the law.	act as collection agencies to persuade a client to furnish funds.
give to parties only that information that concerns them.	notify parties that they have not ordered a certain document that may be necessary to close an escrow.
make sure that escrow does not close with an unverified check.	

Escrow Procedures

Before closing, the escrow is a dual agent. After closing, the escrow has separate agency duties.

Escrow is a limited agency relationship governed by the content of the escrow instructions, and the escrow holder acts only on specific written instructions of the principals as agent for both parties. When the escrow is closed, the escrow holder becomes agent for each principal with respect to those things in escrow to which the respective parties have become completely entitled. Oral instructions should not be accepted or acted on.

Certain procedures must be followed to fulfill the legal requirements for escrow procedures. The broker needs to provide certain information to the escrow agent. Buyers and sellers must be aware of the responsibilities each must assume in the escrow procedure.

Escrow is a many-faceted procedure and includes but is not limited to the following:

- Order preliminary title report

- Conveying preliminary title report to buyer

- Ordering beneficiary statement or payout demands

- Handle receipt and disbursement of all funds

- Facilitate handling, preparation, and signing of all documents

- Comply with all government regulations

- Act as communicator with parties to the escrow, as well as broker and lender

- Ensure that all conditions of escrow are met

- Satisfy lender conditions and that a clear title will be conveyed to buyer

- Accept fire insurance policy

- Make all payments and fees

- Inform parties when escrow is ready to proceed

- Prepare closing statement

- Authorize the release and recording of all documents and disbursement of funds

- Secure title insurance policy

These duties are in addition to maintaining the highest level of trust and maintaining the confidentiality of the escrow.

FIGURE 13.3: Procedures of an Escrow

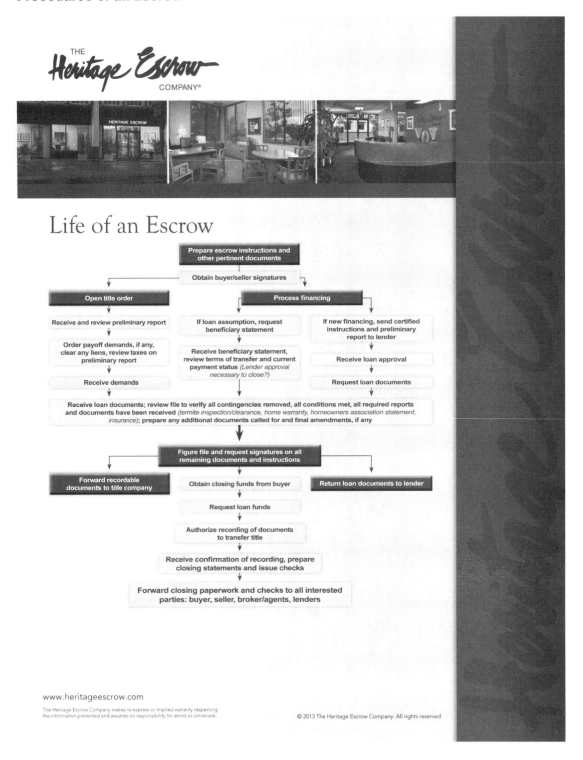

Reprinted with permission.

Advantages of an Escrow

If you decide to buy a television set, you make your purchase from an appliance store. You pay for it by giving cash or adding it to your credit account. You likely would not give a second thought to whether the store has a right to sell the set to you. You probably give no thought at all to whether you need written evidence of your right to own the appliance. It is a simple sales transaction. With the sale of real property, the procedure is much more complicated. The seller could sign a simple deed of conveyance and deliver it to the buyer in exchange for the purchase price. However, neither the buyer nor the seller should agree to such an arrangement, for these reasons:

1. Title to the property may be encumbered. The buyer needs someone to make a title search for the purpose of issuing a title insurance policy.

2. An accurate description of the property is necessary for legal purposes.

3. The seller and the buyer need an experienced person to prepare the instrument of conveyance for their signatures.

4. The buyer and the seller need assurance that their instructions have been carried out and that the deeds will be delivered and any monies transferred only when all terms of the contract have been met.

5. There are distinct advantages to escrow and the use of a neutral third party in the transaction.

6. Escrow provides a custodian of papers, instructions, funds, and documents until the transaction is closed.

7. It makes possible the handling of accounting details in a professional manner.

8. It ensures the validity of a binding contract between participating parties.

9. It is of value to the buyers, assuring them that their monies will not be transferred until the title is conditioned to the specifications of their contract or agreement.

10. It is of value to the sellers, assuring them that the monies have been paid and all other terms and conditions have been met.

Escrow instructions.   **Escrow instructions** are the written directions from the principals to the impartial third party, the escrow agent, to do all the necessary acts to carry out the escrow agreement of the principals. All principals in the escrow agreement (buyers, sellers, lenders, and borrowers) sign identical or conforming instructions that fully set out the understanding of the parties to the transactions. They deliver the signed instructions to the escrow agent.

Figure 10.6 in Unit 10 contains CAR Form RPA-CA, California Residential Purchase Agreement and Joint Escrow Instructions. The form provides that when the purchase offer is accepted, portions of the purchase agreement become the escrow instructions. The wide use of this form has significantly reduced the necessity of escrow instructions being prepared by the escrow holder or agent.

Communities vary in their escrow procedures. However, a title or escrow company would likely use preprinted forms for instructions, whereas a bank or other authorized agent may issue instructions by letter.

When both parties have signed the instructions, the parties are contractually bound to their agreement. If signed separate escrow instructions vary from the purchase agreement, the escrow instructions generally prevail because they most likely were the last agreement signed. In the absence of a purchase contract, the signed escrow instructions become the purchase contract.

Amendments to the escrow instructions must be signed by all parties to the escrow.

Amending the escrow instructions. Once both buyer and seller have signed the escrow instructions, the escrow is bound to carry out their agreement. If any changes are necessary, both buyer and seller must agree to **amend the escrow instructions**. Neither buyer nor seller can unilaterally modify the escrow agreement once it is signed.

Closing the escrow. When the escrow agent has fulfilled all instructions from buyer, seller, and lender; when the remainder of the purchase price has been produced; and when a deed has been signed, the escrow arrangements are complete. The basic steps in closing escrow are as follows:

1. A statement showing the condition of the indebtedness and the unpaid balance of the current loan is requested from the beneficiary, the lender. By law the beneficiary must respond within 21 days of receipt of the request.

2. When the escrow agent has received all funds, documents, and instructions necessary to close the escrow, the escrow agent makes any necessary adjustments and prorations on a settlement sheet.

3. All instruments pertinent to the transaction are then sent to the title insurance company for recording. At this point, time becomes important.

4. The title search runs right up to the last minute of the escrow recording to ensure that nothing has been inserted in the record. If no changes have occurred, the deed and other instruments are recorded on the following morning. Thus, a title policy can be issued with the assurance that no intervening matters of record against the real property have occurred since the last search.

5. On the day the deed is recorded, the escrow agent disburses funds to the parties, according to their signed instructions. These include the following:

   a. Seller's lender—amount of loan(s) and cost(s) remaining at date of recording

   b. Listing and selling brokers' sales commissions

   c. Contractors—termite work, roof repairs, plumbing and/or electrical repairs, and so forth

   d. Other liens against the property

6. After recording, the escrow agent presents closing statements to the parties who should receive them.

7. The title insurance company endeavors to issue a policy of title insurance on the day of recordation.

8. Shortly thereafter, the recorded deed is sent from the county recorder to the customer.

Failed escrow.   If an escrow cannot be completed, the parties must agree to the release of funds (less costs and fees). If a party refuses to agree to the release of funds when there is not a good-faith dispute as to who is entitled to the funds, that party can be liable for treble damages but not less than $100 or more than $1,000 (CC1057.3(b)). A buyer's deposit may be released only if the parties agree. The matter is settled in arbitration or a judgment is rendered regarding the dispute.

Terms Used in Escrow Transactions

Recurring costs.   Impound account costs for taxes and insurance are called **recurring costs**.

Impound account.   When a real estate loan is made, monthly payments for taxes and fire insurance often are required. The lender estimates the funds needed for taxes and insurance, which vary from year to year. These funds are placed in a special reserve trust fund called an **impound account**. When the sale of the property is final and the loan is paid off, the seller is entitled to the unused portion of the impound account, as well as any interest earned.

Beneficiary statement. If an existing loan is to be paid or assumed by the buyer, the escrow agent will obtain a **beneficiary statement** showing the exact balance due from the one holding the deed of trust.

Demand statement. The **demand statement** indicates the amount due to the lender from escrow if the loan is to be paid off. It could include a prepayment penalty. (It is different from the beneficiary statement, which shows balance and condition of loan.)

Reconveyance. If the seller has a loan that is not being assumed by the buyer, the loan must be paid off to clear the title. The seller instructs the escrow agent to pay off the loan, for which the seller receives a **deed of reconveyance**. A *reconveyance fee* is charged the seller for this service. The sum due the lender is entered in the seller's escrow instructions as an estimate. The total figure will not be known until the final computations are made by the escrow officer at the time of closing.

Closing costs. The sum that the seller and the buyer have to pay beyond the purchase price is called the **closing costs**. Closing costs consist of fees charged for the mortgage loan, title insurance, escrow services, reconveyances, recording of documents, and transfer tax, among others. Amounts vary, depending on the particular locale involved and the price of the property. Figure 13.4 shows a sample of the customary seller's closing costs, but these costs vary regionally. Costs also vary, not only from area to area but also from institution to institution within an area. Some costs change with fluctuations in the economy. Figure 13.5 lists those items that are the buyer's responsibility.

As indicated in these lists, certain costs are customarily charged to the buyer and others to the seller. However, the two parties may agree to share some costs. Who pays closing costs is a negotiable item, unless required by a government-backed loan. Adapt this division of charges to your area. For actual fees, obtain copies of fee schedules from an escrow or title company in your area.

Prorations

The adjustment and distribution of costs to be shared by buyer and seller is called **proration**. Costs typically prorated include interest, taxes, insurance, and in the event that income property is involved, prepaid rents. Costs are prorated in escrow as of the closing of escrow or an agreed-upon date. Who is responsible for the day of closing may vary by local custom, although this can be changed by agreement. Generally, the buyer is responsible for the day of closing. Proration of taxes in California is generally based on a 30-day month and a 360-day year, known as a *banker's year*. In some other states, proration is based on the actual number of days. Mortgage interest is charged on a true per diem basis and is not rounded to a 30-day month.

Property taxes.   Property taxes are levied annually (July 1 to June 30 is the tax year) and are paid in two installments. Taxes often require proration. If, for example, the sellers had paid the first installment of a given year's taxes but completed the sale before that tax period was over, they would receive a credit for the remainder of that period's taxes. If, on the other hand, the sellers retained the property through part of the second tax period but had not yet paid taxes for that period, the amount due would be prorated between the sellers and the buyers, with the sellers having to pay for the portion of the tax period during which they still owned the property.

FIGURE 13.4: Closing Costs Customarily Paid by the Seller

Legal Closing

1. Owner's title policy

2. Escrow services (generally shared by buyer and seller)

3. Drawing deed

4. Obtaining reconveyance deed

5. Notary fees (typically, signing party pays to notarize)

6. Recording reconveyance

7. Documentary transfer tax (provided county and/or city has adopted this tax), $0.55 for each $500 or fractional part thereof (Check your local area for differences in rates and requirements for transfer taxes.)

8. Other agreed charges

Financial Closing

1. Mortgage discounts (points)

2. Appraisal charge for advance loan commitment

3. Structural pest control report or structural repair (if any needed). Typically, inspections are paid for by the buyer, and the structural pest report is provided by seller. Buyer and seller may negotiate who pays for inspection fees.

4. Interest on existing loan from last monthly payment to closing date

5. Beneficiary statement (balance on existing loan)

6. Loan payoff (first trust deed and/or any junior trust deed)

7. Prepayment penalty

8. Other agreed charges

Adjustments between Seller and Buyer (depend on closing or other date agreed on)

1. Pay any tax arrears in full

2. Pay any improvement assessment arrears (assessment may have to be paid in full)

3. Pay any other liens or judgments necessary to pass clear title

4. Pay broker's commission

5. Reimburse buyer for prepaid rents and deposits and adjust taxes, insurance, and interest as required

6. Occupancy adjustments

Source: *California Department of Real Estate Reference Book*, 1989–1990 Edition.

Insurance.   Fire insurance is normally paid for one year in advance. If the buyer assumes a fire insurance policy that has not yet expired, the seller is entitled to a prorated refund of the unused premium. (Assumption may not be allowed since insurance is a personal contract.)

Interest.   If a loan of record is being taken over by the buyer, interest will be prorated between buyer and seller. Because interest is normally paid in arrears, if a closing is set for the 15th of the month and the buyer assumes a loan with payments due on the 1st of the month, the seller owes the buyer for one-half-month's interest.

Rents.   Prepaid rents will be prorated in cases involving income-producing properties. Rents are generally prorated on an actual day basis (calendar year) using 365 or 366 days.

FIGURE 13.5:   Closing Costs Customarily Paid by the Buyer

Legal Closing

1. Standard or owners policy in some areas (usually a negotiable charge)
2. ALTA policy and inspection fee, if ordered
3. Escrow services (generally shared by buyer and seller)
4. Drawing second mortgage (if used)
5. Notary fee (typically, signing party pays to notarize)
6. Recording deed (person receiving deed pays to record)
7. Other agreed charges

Financial Closing

1. Loan origination fee
2. Appraisal fee
3. Credit report
4. Drawing up note(s) and trust deed(s)
5. Notary fees
6. Recording trust deed
7. Tax agency fee
8. Termite inspection fee (if Section 2)
9. Interest on new loan (from date of closing until first monthly payment due)
10. Assumption fee
11. Other agreed charges
12. New fire insurance premium one year prepaid, if applicable
13. For new FHA-insured loan, mortgage insurance premium

Adjustments between Seller and Buyer (depend on closing or other date agreed on)

1. Reimburse seller for prepaid taxes
2. Reimburse seller for prepaid insurance
3. Reimburse seller for prepaid improvement assessment
4. Reimburse seller for prepaid impounds (in case buyer is assuming an existing loan)
5. Other occupancy adjustments

Reserves (Impounds) Limitations by Real Estate Settlement Procedures Act (RESPA)—Variations

1. Any variation from custom in closing a transaction should be agreed on in advance. Some times through sheer bargaining power one party can demand relief from and be relieved of all or some of the customary charges and offsets generally assessed. The financial aspects of each transaction differ and should always be negotiated by the parties.
2. Accruals: Unless agreed on in advance, interest-bearing debts are accrued up to date of settlement and constitute a charge against the seller.

Source: *California Department of Real Estate Reference Book*, 1989–1990 Edition.

Closing Disclosure

Procedure for closing disclosure.   Closing statements do not follow usual bookkeeping formulas. In a normal accounting situation, such as balancing a checkbook, all the credits (deposits to the account) are added. Then all the debits (checks written) are totaled and deducted from the credits, and the remainder is the balance.

At a closing, separate statements are issued for the buyer and the seller. Each settlement sheet includes **debits** (amounts owed) and **credits** (amounts entitled to receive). In contrast to usual accounting procedures, on the seller's settlement sheet all the credits to the seller are added (selling price of the property, prorations, etc.). Any debits owed by the seller are then totaled and deducted from the credits. The difference is entered as a cash credit (usually) to the seller, and the escrow agent forwards a check for this amount at the close of escrow.

On the buyer's settlement sheet, the buyer is charged (debited) with the purchase price of the property. The loans the buyer has obtained are credited to the buyer. Cash is credited, prorations may be debited or credited (as the case warrants), and escrow fees and closing costs are debited. The difference between the total debits and credits usually is required in cash by the escrow agent. The cash payment into escrow becomes an additional credit and forces the account to balance. Because of the forced balances, the totals on the buyers' and sellers' statements will be different from each other and from the purchase price.

Dodd-Frank simplified closing disclosure requirements of the Truth in Lending Act and RESPA. The Closing Disclosure includes a detailed accounting of the mortgage transaction, including a breakdown of closing costs paid by the buyer, the seller and others. The new closing form replaces the HUD-1 Settlement Statement. The Closing Disclosure form must be in the hands of the borrower at least three business days before closing. A copy must also be provided to the seller no later than the day of closing, Figure 13.6 is a completed sample Closing Disclosure prepared by the Consumer Financial Protection Bureau, an independent agency of the U.S. government.

If information on the closing statement becomes inaccurate before closing, a corrected statement must be provided at least one business day before closing. Material changes requiring corrections include

- changes in the type of loan,

- a difference in the APR, and

- addition of a prepayment penalty.

Broker's Added Responsibility

Despite the care taken in escrow, mistakes can be made. The real estate broker's final duties are to meet with the buyers or the sellers and explain the closing statement, to help them understand all charges and credits on the statement, and to verify that they have received the correct amount from escrow or paid the correct amount into escrow.

IRS reporting. Cash payments of over $10,000 must be reported to the IRS on IRS Form 8300. Gross proceeds to the seller are reported on IRS Form 1099S.

When Is Escrow Complete?

Escrow is complete when the following actions have been taken:

- The escrow officer sends the deed and deeds of trust to the recorder's office to be recorded. This offers protection of the title to the buyer and of the lien to the lender. The broker's responsibility is to confirm the recordation and inform the clients.

- The escrow agent sends to the seller and the buyer the closing statements showing the disbursement of funds.

- The escrow agent forwards the title policy, assuring the buyer of marketable title, except for certain items; the agent sends the original copy to the buyer.

Liability of an Escrow

Escrow could be held liable for its negligence or breach of duty. However, escrow companies do not have any duty to warn a party of possible fraud or point out any detrimental fact or risk of a transaction. If, however, the escrow was a broker, the broker would have these disclosure obligations.

FIGURE 13.6:   Closing Disclosure

Closing Disclosure

This form is a statement of final loan terms and closing costs. Compare this document with your Loan Estimate.

Closing Information		Transaction Information		Loan Information	
Date Issued	4/15/2013	Borrower	Michael Jones and Mary Stone	Loan Term	30 years
Closing Date	4/15/2013		123 Anywhere Street	Purpose	Purchase
Disbursement Date	4/15/2013		Anytown, ST 12345	Product	Fixed Rate
Settlement Agent	Epsilon Title Co.	Seller	Steve Cole and Amy Doe		
File #	12-3456		321 Somewhere Drive	Loan Type	☒ Conventional ☐ FHA
Property	456 Somewhere Ave		Anytown, ST 12345		☐ VA ☐ _____
	Anytown, ST 12345	Lender	Ficus Bank	Loan ID #	123456789
Sale Price	$180,000			MIC #	000654321

Loan Terms

		Can this amount increase after closing?
Loan Amount	$162,000	**NO**
Interest Rate	3.875%	**NO**
Monthly Principal & Interest *See Projected Payments below for your Estimated Total Monthly Payment*	$761.78	**NO**

		Does the loan have these features?
Prepayment Penalty		**YES** • As high as **$3,240** if you pay off the loan during the first 2 years
Balloon Payment		**NO**

Projected Payments

Payment Calculation	Years 1-7	Years 8-30
Principal & Interest	$761.78	$761.78
Mortgage Insurance	+ 82.35	+ —
Estimated Escrow *Amount can increase over time*	+ 206.13	+ 206.13
Estimated Total Monthly Payment	**$1,050.26**	**$967.91**

Estimated Taxes, Insurance & Assessments *Amount can increase over time* *See page 4 for details*	$356.13 a month	**This estimate includes** ☒ Property Taxes ☒ Homeowner's Insurance ☒ Other: Homeowner's Association Dues *See Escrow Account on page 4 for details. You must pay for other property costs separately.*	**In escrow?** YES YES NO

Costs at Closing

Closing Costs	$9,712.10	Includes $4,694.05 in Loan Costs + $5,018.05 in Other Costs – $0 in Lender Credits. *See page 2 for details.*
Cash to Close	$14,147.26	Includes Closing Costs. *See Calculating Cash to Close on page 3 for details.*

CLOSING DISCLOSURE   PAGE 1 OF 5 • LOAN ID # 123456789

FIGURE 13.6 (continued): Closing Disclosure

Closing Cost Details

Loan Costs	Borrower-Paid		Seller-Paid		Paid by Others
	At Closing	Before Closing	At Closing	Before Closing	
A. Origination Charges	**$1,802.00**				
01 0.25 % of Loan Amount (Points)	$405.00				
02 Application Fee	$300.00				
03 Underwriting Fee	$1,097.00				
04					
05					
06					
07					
08					
B. Services Borrower Did Not Shop For	**$236.55**				
01 Appraisal Fee to John Smith Appraisers Inc.					$405.00
02 Credit Report Fee to Information Inc.		$29.80			
03 Flood Determination Fee to Info Co.	$20.00				
04 Flood Monitoring Fee to Info Co.	$31.75				
05 Tax Monitoring Fee to Info Co.	$75.00				
06 Tax Status Research Fee to Info Co.	$80.00				
07					
08					
09					
10					
C. Services Borrower Did Shop For	**$2,655.50**				
01 Pest Inspection Fee to Pests Co.	$120.50				
02 Survey Fee to Surveys Co.	$85.00				
03 Title – Insurance Binder to Epsilon Title Co.	$650.00				
04 Title – Lender's Title Insurance to Epsilon Title Co.	$500.00				
05 Title – Settlement Agent Fee to Epsilon Title Co.	$500.00				
06 Title – Title Search to Epsilon Title Co.	$800.00				
07					
08					
D. TOTAL LOAN COSTS (Borrower-Paid)	**$4,694.05**				
Loan Costs Subtotals (A + B + C)	$4,664.25	$29.80			

Other Costs					
E. Taxes and Other Government Fees	**$85.00**				
01 Recording Fees Deed: $40.00 Mortgage: $45.00	$85.00				
02 Transfer Tax to Any State			$950.00		
F. Prepaids	**$2,120.80**				
01 Homeowner's Insurance Premium (12 mo.) to Insurance Co.	$1,209.96				
02 Mortgage Insurance Premium (mo.)					
03 Prepaid Interest ($17.44 per day from 4/15/13 to 5/1/13)	$279.04				
04 Property Taxes (6 mo.) to Any County USA	$631.80				
05					
G. Initial Escrow Payment at Closing	**$412.25**				
01 Homeowner's Insurance $100.83 per month for 2 mo.	$201.66				
02 Mortgage Insurance per month for mo.					
03 Property Taxes $105.30 per month for 2 mo.	$210.60				
04					
05					
06					
07					
08 Aggregate Adjustment	– 0.01				
H. Other	**$2,400.00**				
01 HOA Capital Contribution to HOA Acre Inc.	$500.00				
02 HOA Processing Fee to HOA Acre Inc.	$150.00				
03 Home Inspection Fee to Engineers Inc.	$750.00			$750.00	
04 Home Warranty Fee to XYZ Warranty Inc.			$450.00		
05 Real Estate Commission to Alpha Real Estate Broker			$5,700.00		
06 Real Estate Commission to Omega Real Estate Broker			$5,700.00		
07 Title – Owner's Title Insurance (optional) to Epsilon Title Co.	$1,000.00				
08					
I. TOTAL OTHER COSTS (Borrower-Paid)	**$5,018.05**				
Other Costs Subtotals (E + F + G + H)	$5,018.05				

J. TOTAL CLOSING COSTS (Borrower-Paid)	**$9,712.10**				
Closing Costs Subtotals (D + I)	$9,682.30	$29.80	$12,800.00	$750.00	$405.00
Lender Credits					

FIGURE 13.6 (continued): Closing Disclosure

Calculating Cash to Close

Use this table to see what has changed from your Loan Estimate.

	Loan Estimate	Final	Did this change?
Total Closing Costs (J)	$8,054.00	$9,712.10	YES · See **Total Loan Costs (D)** and **Total Other Costs (I)**
Closing Costs Paid Before Closing	$0	− $29.80	YES · You paid these Closing Costs **before closing**
Closing Costs Financed (Paid from your Loan Amount)	$0	$0	NO
Down Payment/Funds from Borrower	$18,000.00	$18,000.00	NO
Deposit	− $10,000.00	− $10,000.00	NO
Funds for Borrower	$0	$0	NO
Seller Credits	$0	− $2,500.00	YES · See Seller Credits in **Section L**
Adjustments and Other Credits	$0	− $1,035.04	YES · See details in **Sections K and L**
Cash to Close	$16,054.00	$14,147.26	

Summaries of Transactions

Use this table to see a summary of your transaction.

BORROWER'S TRANSACTION

K. Due from Borrower at Closing	$189,762.30
01 Sale Price of Property	$180,000.00
02 Sale Price of Any Personal Property Included in Sale	
03 Closing Costs Paid at Closing (J)	$9,682.30
04	
Adjustments	
05	
06	
07	
Adjustments for Items Paid by Seller in Advance	
08 City/Town Taxes to	
09 County Taxes to	
10 Assessments to	
11 HOA Dues 4/15/13 to 4/30/13	$80.00
12	
13	
14	
15	

L. Paid Already by or on Behalf of Borrower at Closing	$175,615.04
01 Deposit	$10,000.00
02 Loan Amount	$162,000.00
03 Existing Loan(s) Assumed or Taken Subject to	
04	
05 Seller Credit	$2,500.00
Other Credits	
06 Rebate from Epsilon Title Co.	$750.00
07	
Adjustments	
08	
09	
10	
11	
Adjustments for Items Unpaid by Seller	
12 City/Town Taxes 1/1/13 to 4/14/13	$365.04
13 County Taxes to	
14 Assessments to	
15	
16	
17	

CALCULATION	
Total Due from Borrower at Closing (K)	$189,762.30
Total Paid Already by or on Behalf of Borrower at Closing (L)	− $175,615.04
Cash to Close ☒ From ☐ To Borrower	**$14,147.26**

SELLER'S TRANSACTION

M. Due to Seller at Closing	$180,080.00
01 Sale Price of Property	$180,000.00
02 Sale Price of Any Personal Property Included in Sale	
03	
04	
05	
06	
07	
08	
Adjustments for Items Paid by Seller in Advance	
09 City/Town Taxes to	
10 County Taxes to	
11 Assessments to	
12 HOA Dues 4/15/13 to 4/30/13	$80.00
13	
14	
15	
16	

N. Due from Seller at Closing	$115,665.04
01 Excess Deposit	
02 Closing Costs Paid at Closing (J)	$12,800.00
03 Existing Loan(s) Assumed or Taken Subject to	
04 Payoff of First Mortgage Loan	$100,000.00
05 Payoff of Second Mortgage Loan	
06	
07	
08 Seller Credit	$2,500.00
09	
10	
11	
12	
13	
Adjustments for Items Unpaid by Seller	
14 City/Town Taxes 1/1/13 to 4/14/13	$365.04
15 County Taxes to	
16 Assessments to	
17	
18	
19	

CALCULATION	
Total Due to Seller at Closing (M)	$180,080.00
Total Due from Seller at Closing (N)	− $115,665.04
Cash ☐ From ☒ To Seller	**$64,414.96**

FIGURE 13.6 (continued): **Closing Disclosure**

Additional Information About This Loan

Loan Disclosures

Assumption

If you sell or transfer this property to another person, your lender

☐ will allow, under certain conditions, this person to assume this loan on the original terms.

☒ will not allow assumption of this loan on the original terms.

Demand Feature

Your loan

☐ has a demand feature, which permits your lender to require early repayment of the loan. You should review your note for details.

☒ does not have a demand feature.

Late Payment

If your payment is more than *15* days late, your lender will charge a late fee of *5% of the monthly principal and interest payment.*

Negative Amortization (Increase in Loan Amount)

Under your loan terms, you

☐ are scheduled to make monthly payments that do not pay all of the interest due that month. As a result, your loan amount will increase (negatively amortize), and your loan amount will likely become larger than your original loan amount. Increases in your loan amount lower the equity you have in this property.

☐ may have monthly payments that do not pay all of the interest due that month. If you do, your loan amount will increase (negatively amortize), and, as a result, your loan amount may become larger than your original loan amount. Increases in your loan amount lower the equity you have in this property.

☒ do not have a negative amortization feature.

Partial Payments

Your lender

☒ may accept payments that are less than the full amount due (partial payments) and apply them to your loan.

☐ may hold them in a separate account until you pay the rest of the payment, and then apply the full payment to your loan.

☐ does not accept any partial payments.

If this loan is sold, your new lender may have a different policy.

Security Interest

You are granting a security interest in

456 Somewhere Ave., Anytown, ST 12345

You may lose this property if you do not make your payments or satisfy other obligations for this loan.

Escrow Account

For now, your loan

☒ will have an escrow account (also called an "impound" or "trust" account) to pay the property costs listed below. Without an escrow account, you would pay them directly, possibly in one or two large payments a year. Your lender may be liable for penalties and interest for failing to make a payment.

Escrow		
Escrowed Property Costs over Year 1	$2,473.56	Estimated total amount over year 1 for your escrowed property costs: *Homeowner's Insurance Property Taxes*
Non-Escrowed Property Costs over Year 1	$1,800.00	Estimated total amount over year 1 for your non-escrowed property costs: *Homeowner's Association Dues* You may have other property costs.
Initial Escrow Payment	$412.25	A cushion for the escrow account you pay at closing. See Section G on page 2.
Monthly Escrow Payment	$206.13	The amount included in your total monthly payment.

☐ will not have an escrow account because ☐ you declined it ☐ your lender does not offer one. You must directly pay your property costs, such as taxes and homeowner's insurance. Contact your lender to ask if your loan can have an escrow account.

No Escrow		
Estimated Property Costs over Year 1		Estimated total amount over year 1. You must pay these costs directly, possibly in one or two large payments a year.
Escrow Waiver Fee		

In the future,

Your property costs may change and, as a result, your escrow payment may change. You may be able to cancel your escrow account, but if you do, you must pay your property costs directly. If you fail to pay your property taxes, your state or local government may (1) impose fines and penalties or (2) place a tax lien on this property. If you fail to pay any of your property costs, your lender may (1) add the amounts to your loan balance, (2) add an escrow account to your loan, or (3) require you to pay for property insurance that the lender buys on your behalf, which likely would cost more and provide fewer benefits than what you could buy on your own.

FIGURE 13.6 (continued):   Closing Disclosure

Loan Calculations

Total of Payments. Total you will have paid after you make all payments of principal, interest, mortgage insurance, and loan costs, as scheduled.	$285,803.36
Finance Charge. The dollar amount the loan will cost you.	$118,830.27
Amount Financed. The loan amount available after paying your upfront finance charge.	$162,000.00
Annual Percentage Rate (APR). Your costs over the loan term expressed as a rate. This is not your interest rate.	4.174%
Total Interest Percentage (TIP). The total amount of interest that you will pay over the loan term as a percentage of your loan amount.	69.46%

Questions? If you have questions about the loan terms or costs on this form, use the contact information below. To get more information or make a complaint, contact the Consumer Financial Protection Bureau at **www.consumerfinance.gov/mortgage-closing**

Other Disclosures

Appraisal
If the property was appraised for your loan, your lender is required to give you a copy at no additional cost at least 3 days before closing. If you have not yet received it, please contact your lender at the information listed below.

Contract Details
See your note and security instrument for information about
 • what happens if you fail to make your payments,
 • what is a default on the loan,
 • situations in which your lender can require early repayment of the loan, and
 • the rules for making payments before they are due.

Liability after Foreclosure
If your lender forecloses on this property and the foreclosure does not cover the amount of unpaid balance on this loan,

☒ state law may protect you from liability for the unpaid balance. If you refinance or take on any additional debt on this property, you may lose this protection and have to pay any debt remaining even after foreclosure. You may want to consult a lawyer for more information.

☐ state law does not protect you from liability for the unpaid balance.

Refinance
Refinancing this loan will depend on your future financial situation, the property value, and market conditions. You may not be able to refinance this loan.

Tax Deductions
If you borrow more than this property is worth, the interest on the loan amount above this property's fair market value is not deductible from your federal income taxes. You should consult a tax advisor for more information.

Contact Information

	Lender	Mortgage Broker	Real Estate Broker (B)	Real Estate Broker (S)	Settlement Agent
Name	Ficus Bank		Omega Real Estate Broker Inc.	Alpha Real Estate Broker Co.	Epsilon Title Co.
Address	4321 Random Blvd. Somecity, ST 12340		789 Local Lane Sometown, ST 12345	987 Suburb Ct. Someplace, ST 12340	123 Commerce Pl. Somecity, ST 12344
NMLS ID					
ST License ID			Z765416	Z61456	Z61616
Contact	Joe Smith		Samuel Green	Joseph Cain	Sarah Arnold
Contact NMLS ID	12345				
Contact ST License ID			P16415	P51461	PT1234
Email	joesmith@ ficusbank.com		sam@omegare.biz	joe@alphare.biz	sarah@ epsilontitle.com
Phone	123-456-7890		123-555-1717	321-555-7171	987-555-4321

Confirm Receipt

By signing, you are only confirming that you have received this form. You do not have to accept this loan because you have signed or received this form.

_____   _____
Applicant Signature   Date   Co-Applicant Signature   Date

CLOSING DISCLOSURE   PAGE 5 OF 5 • LOAN ID # 123456789

TITLE INSURANCE

In a number of states, **marketable title** is shown by an **abstract**. An *abstract of title* is a recorded history of a property. It includes a summary of every recorded document concerning the property. An attorney reads the abstract and gives an opinion of title based on what the abstract reveals. A problem with using abstracts to verify title is that the records of recordation do not reveal title defects, such as a forged instrument in the chain of title, unknown spousal interests, incapacity of a grantor, an illegal contract, or failure of delivery. These risks and more are covered by title insurance, which explains why the use of title insurance has been expanding.

Title insurance insures the ownership of real property (land, buildings, and minerals below the surface) against any unknown encumbrances and other items that may cloud the title. These are primarily claims that might be made by a third party against the property. Buyers are assured that a thorough search has been made of all public records affecting the property being purchased and that the buyers have a marketable title.

Title insurance is paid for once, at the time title passes from one owner to another, and it remains in effect until the property is sold again, at which time title passes to the new owner. If a property owner dies, title insurance continues to protect the owner's heirs.

If a buyer does not elect to buy title insurance protection, that buyer is not protected, even though a prior owner had title insurance.

Both the lender and the buyer should benefit from and have title insurance—the buyer to ensure clear title, and thus protect her investment, and the lender to protect his interest in the property.

For years, title insurance companies had similar rates. It is now possible to obtain title insurance at significant savings online. Entitle Direct, www.entitledirect.com, is one such company. It is rated "A Prime" by Demotech, Inc., which rates insurer financial stability.

The two basic types of policies are the California Land Title Association (CLTA) policy and the American Land Title Association (ALTA) policy.

In 1987, the title insurance industry issued a new set of policies with new coverages and exclusions.

Standard Policy

The policy usually used by the buyer in California is the **CLTA policy**. This policy is called a **standard policy**. The standard policy of title insurance covers matters of record, if not specifically excluded from coverage, as well as specified risks not of record, such as the following:

- Forgery

- Lack of capacity of a grantor

- Undisclosed spousal interests (a grantor who claimed to be single had a spouse with community property interests)

- Failure of delivery of a prior deed

- Federal estate tax liens

- Deeds of a corporation whose charter has expired

- Deeds of an agent whose capacity has terminated

Excluded from coverage by a standard policy of title insurance are the following:

- Defects known by the insured and not disclosed to the title insurer

- Zoning (although a special endorsement is possible that a current use is authorized by current zoning)

- Mining claims (filed in mining districts; legal descriptions are not required)

- Taxes and assessments that are not yet liens

- Easements and liens not a matter of record (such as prescriptive easements and rights to a mechanic's lien)

- Rights of parties in possession (unrecorded deeds, leases, options, etc.)

- Matters not a matter of record that would be disclosed by checking the property (such as encroachment)

■ Matters that would be revealed by a correct survey

■ Water rights

■ Reservations in government patents

A title insurance policy may include an exception to a particular problem so that the policy will not cover a loss resulting from that problem.

> A standard CLTA policy protects the buyer as to matters of record and specified risks.

Generally, in southern California the seller pays for the standard policy of title insurance. In some northern California communities, the buyer pays for this coverage. Any agreement of the parties as to who pays takes precedence over local custom. (In some areas of California, the escrow and title insurance functions are joined in a single firm, while in other areas the functions are separate.)

ALTA Policy

An **ALTA extended policy** is generally purchased for the benefit of the lender. The buyer pays for this lender protection. It insures that the lender has a valid and enforceable lien, subject to only the exclusions from coverage noted in the exception schedule of the policy. It insures the lender for the amount of the loan, not the purchase price of the property. There are three basic ALTA policies—one deals with homes described by lot, block, and tract; one deals with homes described by either the metes-and-bounds or government survey system; and one deals with construction loans.

> While ALTA covers the United States, CLTA only covers California. An ALTA lender policy provides extended coverage to the lender, not the buyer.

The extended coverage lender policy protects the lender only, not the purchaser, from the risks covered. Buyers who desire extended protection must pay for that protection. An owner's policy that offers this extended protection is available. (Both CLTA and ALTA have homeowner extended coverage policies.)

In addition to the coverage offered by the standard policy, the extended coverage policy of title insurance includes the following:

■ Unrecorded liens

■ Off-record easements

- Rights of parties in physical possession, including tenants and buyers under unrecorded instruments

- Rights and claims that a correct survey or physical inspection would disclose

- Mining claims

- Water rights

- Lack of access

Insurers might require a survey before they issue an extended coverage policy of title insurance. The extended coverage policy does not cover the following:

- Matters known by the insured but not conveyed to the insurer

- Government regulations, such as zoning

- Liens placed by the insured

- Eminent domain

- Violations of the map act

The coverage of standard and extended coverage policies can be seen in Figure 13.7.

There are also special construction loan title insurance policies, policies that guarantee trustee sales, bankruptcy guarantees, boundary line agreement guarantees, and special policies for unimproved land. California Title Company publishes a summary of California endorsement to title policies. Information on the endorsements offered can be obtained from California Title Company at www.caltitle.com.

WEB LINK

@

FIGURE 13.7: Owner's Title Insurance Policy

Standard Coverage

1. Defects found in public records
2. Forged documents
3. Incompetent grantors
4. Incorrect marital statements
5. Improperly delivered deeds

Extended Coverage

Standard Coverage plus defects discoverable through:

1. Property inspection, including unrecorded rights of persons in possession
2. Examination of survey
3. Unrecorded liens not known of by policyholder

Not Covered by Either Policy

1. Defects and liens listed in policy
2. Defects known to buyer
3. Changes in land use brought about by zoning ordinances

The premiums paid reflect the work that goes into the issuance of a title policy, not the amount paid in claims. Typically, less than 5% of premium dollars is paid out by a title insurer in claims.

Preliminary Title Report

> The preliminary title report does not provide any insurance.

Before a policy of title insurance is issued, the issuer issues a **preliminary title report**. This report is designed to provide an interim response to an application for title insurance. It is also intended to facilitate the issuance of a particular type of policy. The preliminary report identifies the title to the estate or interest in the prescribed land. It also contains a list of the defects, liens, encumbrances, and restrictions that would be excluded from coverage if the requested policy were to be issued as of the date of the report.

Licensees often will obtain a copy of the preliminary report in order to discuss the matters set forth in it with their clients. Thus, a preliminary report provides the opportunity to seek the removal of items referenced in the report that are unacceptable to the prospective insured. Such arrangements can be made with the assistance of the escrow office.

With respect to preliminary reports, the title industry has been making a concerted effort to improve communications with agents representing sellers and buyers. The latest forms are distinguished from early versions in that the printed encumbrances and exclusions are set forth verbatim and not incorporated by reference. Consequently, the preliminary report now constitutes a more complete communication of the offer to issue a title insurance policy.

In fact, preliminary reports are just one of the steps in the risk elimination process. Risk elimination includes the maintenance and collection of title records (known as the **title plant**), the searching and examination of the records, and the underwriting standards of each title insurance company.

The preliminary report does not necessarily show the condition of the title; it merely reports the current vesting of title and the items the title company will exclude from coverage if the policy should be issued later. The elements of this definition are threefold:

1. A preliminary report is an offer.

2. It is *not* an abstract of title reporting a complete chain of title.

3. It is a statement of the terms and conditions of the offer to issue a title policy.

The title insurer customarily makes a last-minute check to ensure there are no new recordings concerning a property's title before issuing its policy of insurance.

Special Policies

There are a number of **special title insurance policies**, such as construction lender policies and policies for vendees (purchasers under real property sales contracts), policies insuring leasehold interest, and even policies for oil and gas interests. Special coverage policy amendments also can be purchased.

Policy Interpretation

Title insurance policies are interpreted in accordance with the reasonable expectations of the insured. In the event of ambiguities, they normally would be resolved against the insurer.

Rebate Law (RESPA)

Title insurance companies are precluded by law from providing kickbacks to brokers for referral of business. They must charge brokers the same as other customers and make a sincere effort to collect any premiums due. The **rebate law** extends to escrows, as well as to title insurers. Besides being grounds for disciplinary action, receiving a rebate from a title insurer is considered commercial bribery and could subject a licensee to up to one year in jail and a $10,000 fine for each transaction.

SUMMARY

An escrow is a third-party stakeholder who receives and disburses documents and funds in a real property transaction. The escrow is usually selected by the buyer and the seller in the purchase agreement. The escrow cannot be completed until all conditions are met. The escrow basically has agency duties to both buyer and seller. There may be duties to a lender as well. The broker is not a party to the escrow, and the escrow agent has no duty to obey instructions of the broker after the escrow instructions have been signed.

Escrows must be corporations and licensed as escrow. An exception is that a broker can act as an escrow without a license if the broker was a principal to the transaction or represented either the buyer or the seller. Aside from the broker, the lender, and attorney exemptions, an escrow must be a corporation and must meet strict licensing requirements.

An escrow is opened with the parties signing escrow instructions. A valid escrow consists of a signed agreement and conditional delivery of transfer documents to the escrow. The delivery is conditioned on the buyer's fully meeting obligations. Once escrow instructions have been signed by both buyer and seller, any change to the instructions requires the signatures of both buyer and seller.

When the escrow disburses funds and records the deed, the escrow is considered closed. A Closing Disclosure is issued by the escrow showing the debits and the credits of the transaction. Rents, taxes, interest, and insurance are likely to be prorated by the escrow. Proration is based on a 30-day month and a 360-day year. After escrow closes, the broker should make certain the client fully understands the disclosure statement.

Escrow companies are liable for their negligence, but they are not liable for failure to warn a party of possible fraud or to point out a detrimental fact or risk of a transaction.

An abstract shows only the recorded history of a property. A title opinion based on an abstract does not reveal defects such as forgery, lack of capacity, unknown spousal interests, and so forth. These and other risks are covered by a standard policy of title insurance, which also covers risks of record. Greater coverage for lenders can be obtained with an ALTA extended coverage policy. If buyers want this protection for themselves, they have to buy an extended coverage owners policy.

The preliminary title report is an offer to insure and does not give the buyer any protection unless a policy of title insurance is purchased. There are special title insurance policies for specific needs.

The rebate law prohibits title insurance carriers and escrows from rebating fees for referrals or otherwise providing special advantages or deals to brokers.

CLASS DISCUSSION TOPICS

1. Which offices and developments in your area handle their own escrows? Why?

2. In your area, are escrow instructions separate for buyer and seller or are the instructions a single agreement?

3. What are typical escrow costs for the sale of a $600,000 residence in your area?

4. What does it cost for a standard policy of title insurance for a $600,000 home in your area?

5. What does it cost for a $600,000 extended coverage policy of title insurance for lender protection?

6. What does it cost for a preliminary title report on a $600,000 home sale?

7. How does a preliminary title report differ from a property profile provided by a title insurer?

8. Bring to class one current-events article dealing with some aspect of real estate practice for class discussion.

UNIT 13 QUIZ

1. A broker can act as an escrow when the broker
   a. represents the buyer in the transaction.
   b. represents the seller in the transaction.
   c. is a principal in the transaction.
   d. is any of these.

2. An escrow company is prohibited from
   a. paying referral fees to anyone other than an employee of the escrow company.
   b. bonding employees.
   c. both of these.
   d. neither of these.

3. To determine the balance due on a loan, escrow requests
   a. a closing statement.
   b. a beneficiary statement.
   c. a reconveyance.
   d. an impound statement.

4. Which is a debit to the seller on a seller's closing statement?
   a. Selling price
   b. Prepaid taxes
   c. First trust deed to be assumed by buyer
   d. All of these

5. Which is a credit to the buyer on the buyer's closing statement?
   a. Purchase price
   b. Escrow costs
   c. Title insurance
   d. First trust deed assumed

6. An escrow company has a duty to
   a. warn parties if the escrow knows of possible fraud.
   b. suggest changes when one party is not being adequately protected.
   c. do both of these.
   d. do neither of these.

7. A standard policy of title insurance is used to show
   a. that there are no encumbrances against a property.
   b. that the seller has a marketable title.
   c. both of these.
   d. neither of these.

8. Which of the following is covered by the CLTA standard policy of title insurance?
   a. Easements not a matter of public record
   b. Rights of a party in possession
   c. Unknown spousal interests
   d. Encroachment

9. Which is *NOT* covered by an ALTA extended coverage policy of title insurance?
   a. Mining claims
   b. Liens placed by the insured
   c. Water rights
   d. Off-record easement

10. Title insurance companies may
    a. give rebates to brokers for referrals.
    b. give brokers preferential rates on their own purchases.
    c. charge brokers the same as others but make no effort to collect.
    d. do none of these.

TAXATION

LEARNING OBJECTIVES

When you have completed this unit, you will be able to

■ explain why taxes play an important role in real estate ownership and investment;

■ describe statutory exemptions on property taxation; and

■ understand tax shelters, probate, and living trusts.

KEY TERMS

acquisition indebtedness	home improvements	realized gain
adjusted basis	homeowner's exemption	recognized gain
ad valorem taxes	installment sale	reverse exchange
basis	investment property rule	sale-leaseback
boot	like-kind rule	special assessments
capital gain	living trust	stepped-up basis
capital loss	no-choice rule	supplemental tax bill
deferred gain	no-loss rule	tax-deferred exchange
depreciable basis	original basis	1031 exchange
depreciation	primary personal residence	Urban Agriculture Incentive Zone Act
entity rule	probate	veteran's exemption
equity indebtedness	Proposition 13	Williamson Act
estate tax	Proposition 58	
excluded gain	Proposition 60	
Foreign Investment in Real Property Tax Act	Proposition 90	

REAL PROPERTY TAXES

Real Property Tax Calendar

> Real property taxes are based on value.

Real property taxes are **ad valorem taxes**. *Ad valorem* is a Latin expression that means "according to value." Real estate tax rates are a percentage of the property's "full cash value." The concept is not new; throughout history, people's wealth has been determined largely by the amount of real property they own. Landowners almost always have been taxed on the basis of their property holdings. Governments favor real estate taxation because it is the one form of taxation that cannot be evaded. If a taxpayer fails to pay taxes, the levying body can foreclose on its tax lien to satisfy the taxpayer's obligations. In the United States, property taxes are fully deductible on a homeowner's income tax return. However, special assessments for improvements generally are not considered a tax-deductible expense. They do, however, increase the cost basis.

The levying of real property taxes profoundly affects the real estate market. If taxes are high, potential customers may hesitate to involve themselves with such an expense by purchasing property. On the positive side, revenues from property taxes are a vital source of government income on the local level, enabling local government to provide for the health, education, safety, and welfare of the citizenry.

A basic understanding of real property taxes in California begins with knowing the chronological order for processing real property taxes.

Taxes are assessed and paid based on a fiscal year (July 1 through June 30). Taxes may be paid in two equal installments. The acronym *NDFA* (No Darn Fooling Around) is a memory tool for understanding the dates of these two payments:

N – November 1, first installment due

D – December 10, first installment becomes delinquent

F – February 1, second installment due

A – April 10, second installment becomes delinquent

Billing

If taxes are to be paid through a lending agency, the county sends a tax bill to that agency and a copy of it to the owner. The owner's copy states that it is for information only. If the owner is to pay the taxes, the original bill is sent directly to the owner for payment. The tax bill includes any special assessments. Unpaid taxes become delinquent, and a penalty is charged even if the taxpayer never received a notice of taxes due. It is the taxpayer's responsibility to make sure that tax payment deadlines are met.

Figure 14.1 shows a sample tax bill.

Typical California Tax Bill

A typical California tax bill includes the following information:

- An identifying parcel number, with reference to the map page and property number or other description
- A breakdown between land assessments and improvement assessments
- Tax exemptions such as homeowner's exemption
- A breakdown of the bonded indebtedness or special assessments
- The full amount of the tax
- Itemized or perhaps separate payment cards with the full tax equally divided into first and second installments

The supplemental tax bill covers the difference between the seller's assessed valuation and the new valuation based on the sales price.

Supplemental tax bill.   A recent homebuyer may come into an agent's office and say, "I paid my property tax, and a month later I received a new assessment for almost the same amount. How much are my taxes on this property?" Before the property is purchased, the agent should explain to buyers that in the first year of ownership, they will receive two or three tax bills: the regular tax bill and one or two **supplemental tax bills**. Supplemental tax bills are issued because property is reassessed as of the sale date. A change of ownership statement must be filed in the county assessor's office within 45 days of the transfer. The sale will generally trigger a reassessment.

Property taxes are billed and paid for the fiscal year of July 1 through June 30. When a buyer purchases a new home, it takes time to notify the tax collector's office of the sale of property and for the tax collector's office to issue the new property tax bill based on the new assessed value. The county assessor is directed to put new values on a supplemental assessment roll from the completion date of construction or the change of ownership date (for example, a sale). If the new value is higher than the current assessed value, a supplemental tax bill is sent to the property owner that reflects the higher valuation for the remainder of the tax year.

FIGURE 14.1: Sample Tax Bill

RIVERSIDE COUNTY SECURED PROPERTY TAX BILL
For Fiscal Year July 1, 2015 through June 30, 2016

Offices in Riverside, Palm Desert and Temecula
Visit our website: www.countytreasurer.org
IMPORTANT INFORMATION ON REVERSE SIDE

10

DON KENT, TREASURER 058342
4080 Lemon St (1st Floor) Riverside, California
(P.O. Box 12005, Riverside, CA 92502-2205)

Telephone: (951) 955-3900
or, from area codes 951 and 760 only
toll free: 1 (877) RIVCOTX (748-2689)

Property
Data   752250035-1 LOT 41 MB 275/097 TR 28926

Address
Owner,   12345 ADAMS STREET PALM SPRINGS 92262
JANUARY 1, 2015   DOE, JOHN Q & MARY S

DOE, JOHN Q & MARY S
12345 ADAMS STREET
PALM SPRINGS, CA 92262-2515

ASSESSMENT NUMBER

752250035-1

Tax Rate Area	Bill Number
075-004	000473330

O   09/18/2015
All questions about ownership, values or
exemptions must be directed to the
Riverside County Assessor at (951) 955-6200.

UNPAID PRIOR-YEAR TAXES
(See Item #6 on reverse)

NONE

Tax bill requested by	Loan Identification	Multiple Bills

CHARGES LEVIED BY TAXING AGENCIES (See Item #4 on reverse)		AMOUNT
1% TAX LIMIT PER PROP 13		3954.46
DESERT SANDS UNIFIED SCHOOL	(760) 771-8516	431.62
DESERT COMMUNITY COLLEGE	(760) 773-2513	82.52
COACHELLA VALLEY WATER DISTRICT	(760) 398-2661	395.44
COACHELLA VALLEY MOSQUITO & RIFA	(866) 807-6864@	6.06
AD COACHELLA VALLEY RC/PK 93-1	(866) 807-6864@	9.90
CVWD SEWER SERVICE CHARGE ID81	(760) 391-9600@	331.80

LAND	137,907
STRUCTURES	264,539
TRADE FIXTURES	
TREES & VINES	
BUSINESS PERSONAL PROPERTY	

FULL VALUE		402,446
EXEMPTIONS	HOX	7,000
NET VALUE		395,446
TAX RATE PER $100 VALUE		1.23002
TAXES		$4,864.06
Special Assessments & Fixed Charges		$347.76
TOTAL AMOUNT If over $50,000, see Item #1 on reverse		$5,211.82

$2,605.91	$2,605.91
Add 10% penalty after 12/10/2015	Add 10% penalty plus cost after 04/10/2016
$2,605.91	$2,605.91

PLEASE KEEP TOP PORTION FOR YOUR RECORDS
(NO RECEIPTS WILL BE ISSUED - YOUR CANCELLED CHECK IS YOUR RECEIPT)

EXAMPLE Mr. and Mrs. Newly Boute purchased a home on January 2 of this year for $300,000. Assume no bond issues or assessment other than the basic levy of 1%. The new property tax will be $3,000 (1% of $300,000). The old assessment on the home was $100,000. Therefore, the property tax on the home was $1,000 for the fiscal year from July 1 of last year to June 30 of this year. So, when the Boutes purchased their home, their tax bill for the second installment of the fiscal year would be $500 (half of $1,000) due February and delinquent April 10, which is the old bill. The Boutes should be paying $1,500 on the new tax bill (half of $3,000). Because they paid $500 on the old bill, they will have to pay a supplemental tax bill of $1,000 ($1,500 − $500). See the following chart.

	FISCAL YEAR	
	July 1 Last Year Jan. 1	This Year June 30
Old	$500	$ 500
Assessed Value		
$100,000 × 0.01 = $1,000		
Property Tax		
New		
Assessed value		
$300,000 × 0.01 × 0.5 = $3,000		
($1,500 for 6 months)		
Property tax (for only half a year)		$ 1,500
Since they paid $500		
Supplemental bill will be for $1,000		$ 1,000
Total paid for year		$ 1,500

Special Assessments

Cities, counties, and special districts may, by a two-thirds vote of the electors of the district, impose special taxes on such districts. These **special assessments** are levied for specified local improvements, such as streets, sewers, irrigation, drainage, flood control, and special lighting. This voter-approved bonded indebtedness varies from county to county and within each county.

Proposition 13

Proposition 13 was enacted in 1978. It states basically that newly acquired real estate or new construction will be assessed according to the fair market value (FMV) and taxed at a maximum tax rate of 1% (called the *basic* levy). In addition, the assessed values of properties acquired before 1978 will be reduced to the amount shown on the 1975 tax roll. Because different areas of a county have different bond issues or special assessments for that particular area, additional monies up to 1% are added to the basic levy (Proposition 13), causing the tax rate for these areas to range from 1% to more than 2%, depending on the area.

E X A M P L E   Your client, Mr. Bior, purchased a home this year for $300,000. Because of Proposition 13, the property taxes will be $3,000 ($300,000 × 0.01). Mr. Bior's area could have an additional assessment of 0.5%. Therefore, for his particular area, his property taxes could be $4,500 ($300,000 × 0.015).

> Proposition 13 limits annual increases in assessed valuation to 2 percent.

One additional aspect of Proposition 13 is that the assessment value may be increased by up to 2% each year, as long as the Consumer Price Index (CPI) is not exceeded. The CPI measures inflation. This 2% increase in the assessed value represents the maximum amount the county assessor may increase the property's value each fiscal year.

E X A M P L E   Mr. Bior purchased a home for $300,000 and paid $4,500 ($300,000 × 0.015) in property taxes the first year. For the second year, the assessed value of the property will be $306,000 ($300,000 × 1.02). Presumably, the tax rate of 1.5% remains the same. Thus, Mr. Bior's property tax bill will be $4,590 ($306,000 × 0.015) for the second year. The property tax bill can be calculated in the same manner for each subsequent year of ownership.

One of the objectives of Proposition 13 is to keep property taxes as low as possible. According to Proposition 13, certain transfers of title (such as a sale) will cause a reassessment of the property, which will increase the property taxes. Transfers changing the form of ownership (changing from joint tenancy to community property), creation of revocable living trusts, and cosigners for loan qualification and transfers of a principal residence from parent to child or child to parent are exempt from reassessment.

Proposition 58

> Proposition 58 allows transfers without reassessment to a spouse or children.

Proposition 58 provides that transfers of real property between spouses or domestic partners and transfers of the principal residence and the first $1,000,000 of other real property between parent and child are exempt from reassessment. The code defines a *child* as a natural child (any child born of the parents), any stepchild or spouse of that stepchild when the relationship of stepparent and stepchild exists, a son-in-law or daughter-in-law of the parent(s), or a child who was adopted by the age of 18. (Note that Proposition 193 subsequently extended the exemption from reassessment to persons who inherit property from a grandparent when both parents of the grandchild are deceased. The grandchild can therefore keep the grandparent's assessment for property taxes.)

To receive this exclusion, a claim must be filed with the county assessor. The claim must contain a written certification by the transferee made under penalty of perjury that the transferee is a parent or child of the transferor. This statement must also state whether the property is the transferor's principal residence. If the property is not the transferor's principal residence and the full cash value of the real property transferred (the taxable value on the roll just prior to the date of transfer) exceeds the allowable exclusion ($1,000,000), the eligible transferee must specify the amount and allocation of the exclusion on the claim. The $1,000,000 exemption can be doubled by both parents combining their $1,000,000 exemptions to transfer $2,000,000 in property to a child without an increase in tax assessment.

Proposition 60

Proposition 60 allows homeowners over 55 years of age to transfer their assessed valuation to a new residence in the same county.

The purpose of **Proposition 60** was to encourage older people to move to less-expensive housing without having to pay higher taxes because of reassessment on a new home. Proposition 60 provides that qualified homeowners aged 55 or over, as well as taxpayers who are severely and permanently disabled, may transfer the current base-year value of their present principal residence to a replacement (that is, sell their old home and buy a new home), with the following conditions:

- Both properties must be in the same county.

- The transferor must be at least 55 years old as of the date of transfer (sale). (If married, only one spouse needs to be at least 55 but must reside in the residence; if co-owners, only one co-owner needs to be at least 55 and must reside in the residence.)

- The original residence must be eligible for a homeowner's exemption at the time of sale (transfer).

- The new home must be of equal or lesser value than the old residence.

Proposition 90

Proposition 90 is an extension of Proposition 60. Proposition 60 limits the purchase of the new home to the same county. Proposition 90 allows the purchase of the new home in a different county in California. However, the county the homeowner is planning to move into may reject Proposition 90. The only counties that have accepted Proposition 90 are Alameda, Los Angeles, Orange, Santa Clara, San Diego, Riverside, San Bernardino, San Mateo, Eldorado and Ventura. To qualify, a homeowner must meet all the requirements for Proposition 60.

Change-in-Ownership Statement

Any person acquiring an interest in property subject to local taxation must notify the county assessor by filing a *change-in-ownership statement* within 45 days of the date of recording or, if the transfer is not recorded, within 45 days of the date of transfer. Failure to do so will result in a penalty. In practice, escrow typically handles this task.

Exemptions

Some of the numerous properties that are assessed are partially or wholly tax exempt. For example, many nonprofit charitable organizations, churches, all government, and several nonprofit educational institutions are entirely exempt. Other relief is available in various forms for homeowners, veterans, senior citizens, and renters.

Homeowner's exemption. Each residential property that is owner-occupied is entitled to an annual tax **homeowner's exemption** of $7,000 from the "full cash value." The homeowner needs to apply only once for this homeowner's exemption if from year to year there is no change in the ownership of and residency on the property. A homeowner must have been the owner of record on or before January 1 (apply by February 15) and actually have occupied the property to claim this exemption for the upcoming tax year beginning July 1. A homeowner is allowed only one exemption at a time. Once this exemption has been filed, it remains in effect until terminated. The assessor must be notified of a termination, or an assessment plus 25% penalty may be made.

Veteran's exemption. California's war veterans may receive a $4,000 **veteran's exemption** on the full cash value of their homes. Because a person cannot take both the homeowner's and the veteran's exemptions, a person would not apply for the basic veteran's exemption if eligible for the higher homeowner's exemption. A totally disabled veteran or the veteran's surviving spouse may be eligible for a higher exemption. The exemption increases with inflation. In 2016, the exemption applies for disabled veterans on their personal residence property valued up to $191,266 and for disabled veterans who possess income limited to $57,258or less.

Senior citizen's property tax postponement. Another form of relief is the *senior citizen's property tax postponement*. Homeowners who are at least 62 years old with household income of $35,500 or less and who have a 40% home equity may be eligible to have the State of California pay all or part of the real property tax on their home. Persons of any age who are blind or totally disabled and meet the income requirement are also eligible. The taxes are postponed and not repaid until the property is sold or the claimant no longer occupies the property. The program was discontinued because of budgetary problems but will be reinstated in 2016. Taxes are secured by a lien against the home in favor of the State of California.

Lower assessment for agriculture. The Urban Agricultural Incentive Zone Act provides tax incentives for urban farms from 0.1 acre to 3 acres. The Williamson Act allows local governments to tax land based upon agriculture use rather than land value if the owner contracts to keep it in agriculture use for a specified period.

Documentary transfer tax. Counties may adopt a documentary transfer tax of 55 cents for each $500 or fraction thereof of consideration. Cities in counties that have adopted the tax may add an additional tax. As an example, the City of Berkeley has a $15 per $1,000 property transfer tax, making the total city and county tax $16.10. Most cities with transfer taxes have set them at half the county rate or 55 cents per $500.

Parties can negotiate as to who pays the tax, but generally the seller pays in southern California and the buyer pays in northern California. In central California, it can be a combination of both.

The county recorder will not accept taxable conveyance for recording without a Documentary Transfer Tax Declaration. Documents subject to the tax must show the amount of tax paid on its face, it cannot be hidden.

INCOME TAXES

> Real estate licensees should not advise a buyer or a seller as to income tax matters. Questions should be directed to an accountant or a tax attorney.

Today, income taxes play an important role in real estate owners' decisions, from buying or selling their personal residences to decisions involving the most exotic real investment properties. Because the tax laws are always changing, it is important for the real estate agent to stay abreast of them. Agents should advise buyers and sellers to seek professional advice from an accountant or tax attorney if the situation indicates a possible problem. Because of significant liability issues, the agent should refrain from providing tax advice.. We will discuss income taxes as they relate to business and investment property, as well as to a personal residence.

While rental income is taxed at regular tax rates, capital gains are taxed at preferential rates in order to encourage investments. A capital gain is the gain on the sale of a capital asset. Capital assets include real estate.

Capital Gains

Before the 1997 Taxpayer Relief Act, capital gains were taxed at a 28% maximum tax rate if the capital assets were held more than one year. The 1997 act reduced the rate to 20% for long-term capital gains.

The 2003 Jobs & Growth Tax Relief Reconciliation Act cut the long-term capital gains to a maximum of 15% for gains from the sale of assets held for more than 12 months. (Gains from the sale of assets held for one year or less are taxed as regular income.) Except for high-income taxpayers, who will have long-term capital gains taxed at 20%, the capital gains tax will remain at 15% for 2013.

In California, the state income tax on capital gains is the same as for other income (no special treatment).

For taxpayers in the 10% and 15% tax brackets, the long-term gain was cut to 5%. In 2008, the long-term capital gains tax for these lower income brackets was reduced to zero.

Under the American Taxpayer Relief Act of 2012, as of 2013, the capital gains rate has been permanently increased to 20% for single filers with incomes above $400,000 and married couples filing jointly with incomes exceeding $450,000.

In addition, there is a 3.8% Medicare surcharge applied to net investment income for taxpayers whose threshold income exceeds $200,000 for single filers and $250,000 for married couples filing jointly. Therefore, higher-income taxpayers could be paying 23.8% tax on capital gains, the 20% rate plus the surcharge.

Business and Investment Property

Property held for business and investment has some distinct differences in federal income tax treatment from property used as a personal residence. We will begin with the concept of depreciation.

Depreciation

The two most obvious and important characteristics of real estate invest-ments are income and expenses. Real estate is one of those assets that benefit from a special accounting device for a special kind of expense called **depreciation**.

Land may not be depreciated.

Depreciation is a method of accounting for the wear that results from the use of a capital good. A capital good, such as a piece of equipment or a build-ing, does not last forever. As it is used, it wears out or becomes obsolete; at some point, the owner must replace it or substantially repair it. Deprecia-tion is used to reflect this replacement cost. The main reasons depreciation is allowed are to encourage investment in real estate and to reflect, in accounting terms, the real costs of property ownership. Only investment or income property may benefit from depreciation. Only improvements to land may be depreciated. Land is never depreciated.

For depreciation purposes, real estate can be divided into two categories:

1. Residential property

2. Nonresidential property

> The depreciation period is 27½ years for residential property and 39 years for nonresidential property. Landing is never depreciated.

Residential property is where people live—for example, single-family residences, duplexes, triplexes, fourplexes, and multiunit apartments. A personal residence may not be depreciated. Nonresidential property is property that is not residential in nature—for example, industrial, commercial, office buildings, and other similar types of properties. Since January 1, 1987, all real property must use the straight-line method of depreciation where the value of the property is depreciated in equal annual amounts over the depreciable life of the property.

Generally, residential rental property must use a useful life of 27½ years and nonresidential property must use a useful life of 39 years. Either residential or nonresidential property may elect to use 40 years.

Basis

To explore the tax implications of investment properties, the agent must understand the concept of **basis** and know how to correctly compute the original basis, depreciable basis, and adjusted basis. The **original basis** (OB) is used to determine the depreciable basis and adjusted basis. The **depreciable basis** (DB) is used to determine the amount of allowable depreciation. The **adjusted basis** (AB), which changes as time progresses, is required to calculate the gain on the disposition of a property.

> Original basis is purchase price plus buying expenses.

Original basis.   The *original basis* of a property is the sum of its *purchase price* (PP) and the *buying expenses* (BE) on acquisition (OB = PP + BE). When a client purchases a property, the escrow statement includes the sale price and a listing of other costs and expenses. These amounts can be classified into four basic groups:

1. Purchase price (PP)

2. Operating expenses (OE)

3. Buying expenses (BE) (nonrecurring closing costs associated with the purchase)

4. Nondeductible items (ND), such as impound accounts

Depreciable basis. The *depreciable basis* is defined as the original basis minus the value of the land:

It is the cost basis of the improvements.

$$\text{depreciable basis} = \text{original basis} - \text{land value}$$

There are three methods for determining the value attributable to the land: the assessed value method, the appraisal method, and the contract method.

Assessed value method. The county assessor's property tax statement now lists the full cash value of both the land and the improvements. The value of the improvements for depreciation purposes is thus the assessor's determination of the part of the purchase price that represents the value of the improvements.

Appraisal method. The property owner may secure the services of a professional appraiser to appraise the building and the land. The appraisal method may give either a more or a less favorable ratio than the assessed value method. The taxpayer should compare the ratios from the two methods to verify which is more advantageous.

Contract method. One other method of determining the percentage of improvements is the contract method. With this method, the buyer and the seller determine the relative values of the improvements and land and designate these values in the contract, deposit receipt, or escrow instructions. Note that the determination must be at arm's length and reasonable. Before using this method, we strongly suggest that the owner obtain professional help. The owner should be prepared to justify value in the event of an IRS audit.

Adjusted basis.   The *adjusted basis* of a property is the amount that the client has invested in the property for tax purposes. In other words, the adjusted basis is equal to original basis, plus capital improvements made, less all depreciation taken:

adjusted basis = original basis + improvements − depreciation

It is extremely important that the homeowner or investor understand the relationship between the basis and the final sales price of the property, because basis is the beginning point for calculating the amount of gain or loss on the sale. Calculation of the basis is affected by how the property originally was acquired.

- *Basis by purchase* is the price paid for the property, as described.

- *Basis by gift* is the donor's (gift giver's) adjusted basis plus the gift tax paid, not to exceed the fair market value at the time of the gift.

- *Basis by inheritance* generally is the fair market value at the time of the owner's death.

Computing gain.   The basis is the beginning point for computing the gain or the loss on the sale, but numerous adjustments to the basis always are made during the ownership period. Some of the costs that increase the basis are title insurance, appraisal fees, legal fees, cost of capital improvements, and sales costs on disposition. Accrued (past) depreciation is deducted from the basis. The result is the adjusted basis.

The gain (or loss) is the difference between the adjusted basis and the sales price. An example may clarify this:

$80,000	Purchase price
+ 800	Cost associated with purchase
+ 3,000	Capital improvements
$83,000	
− 12,500	Accumulated depreciation
$71,300	Adjusted cost basis
$100,000	Sales price
− 4,000	Sales cost
− 71,300	Adjusted cost basis
$24,700	Total gain

Computing Depreciation

To compute the depreciation, follow these six steps:

1. Compute the original basis

2. Determine allocation between land and building

3. Compute the depreciable basis

4. Determine whether the property is residential or nonresidential (If residential, you must use the 27½-year table for residential property. If nonresidential, you must use the 39-year table.)

5. Divide the depreciable basis by 27.5 (residential) or 39 (nonresidential).

6. This will give you the annual straight-line depreciation.

E X A M P L E

$\underline{\$100,000}$ depreciable basis = $3,636.36 annual depreciation
27.5 (residential)

$\underline{\$100,000}$ depreciable basis = $2,564.10 annual depreciation
39 (nonresidential)

For the year of the sale, the depreciation would be determined by multiplying the percentage shown in Figure 14.2 times the depreciable basis.

FIGURE 14.2: Depreciation of Real Property

—General Depreciation System				Method: Straight Line				Recovery Period: 27.5 years			
The month in the 1st recovery year the property is placed in service:											
Year	1	2	3	4	5	6	7	8	9	10	11	12
1	3.485%	3.182%	2.879%	2.576%	2.273%	1.970%	1.667%	1.364%	1.061%	0.758%	0.455%	0.152%
2–27.5	3.636%	3.636%	3.636%	3.636%	3.636%	3.636%	3.636%	3.636%	3.636%	3.636%	3.636%	3.636%

The month in the 1st recovery year the property is placed in service:											
—General Depreciation System				Method: Straight Line				Recovery Period: 39 years			
1	2.461%	2.247%	2.033%	1.819%	1.605%	1.391%	1.177%	0.963%	0.749%	0.535%	0.321%	0.107%
2–39	2.564%	2.564%	2.564%	2.564%	2.564%	2.564%	2.564%	2.564%	2.564%	2.564%	2.564%

Capital Gains Due to Depreciation

The capital gains tax rate for gains attributable to depreciation is the rate for regular income, with a maximum of 25%. As an example:

Property cost	$300,000
Depreciation taken	− 100,000
Adjusted cost basis	$200,000

If the property were sold at $500,000, there would be a $300,000 gain; $200,000 of the gain would be taxed at the 15% rate, but the $100,000 of the gain that is attributable to the depreciation that was taken would likely be taxed at the 25% rate.

Mortgage Foreclosure Debt Relief Act of 2007

A person relieved of debt receives an IRS Form 1099C from the lender. Because debt relief is considered taxable income, this amount is ordinarily taxed. However, the Mortgage Foreclosure Debt Relief Act of 2007 provides that debt forgiveness on the principal residence resulting from loan restructuring, short sale, or foreclosure be excluded from income. Although the act expired at the end of 2013, the IRS, as well as California, has ruled that a short sale of 1-4 residential units will not be taxed on unpaid debt.

1031 Exchanges

- The **1031 exchange** is part of federal tax law—Internal Revenue Code Section 1031 (the State of California has a similar code section). Section 1031 allows for exchange of personal property, as well as real property. Many of the concepts for 1031 **tax-deferred exchanges** come from court cases and IRS regulations and revenue rulings and from Section 1031.

Because of depreciation taken, as well as appreciation of property, many property owners do not want to sell and be required to pay the high taxes. An exchange allows the owner to delay taxes and thus have more money to invest in a new property. Because of refinancing, many owners are in a position where their equity is not sufficient to cover their tax liability. An exchange allows them to defer tax liability.

EXAMPLE   A woman owns a 10-unit apartment house she wants to dispose of, and she plans to buy a 20-unit apartment building. The 10-unit building would sell for $1,000,000, with selling costs of $50,000 and an adjusted basis of $275,000. Her taxable gain would be as follows:

Sales price	$1,000,000
Selling costs	– 50,000
Net sales price	$950,000
Adjusted basis	– 275,000
Taxable gain	$675,000

If the woman sells the property, she will have to pay federal and state taxes on the gain. She would be taxed at the 15% federal capital gains rate, possibly a 3.8% surcharge, a 25% rate for the portion of the gain attributable to depreciation, as well as having California regular tax liability on the gain. These taxes will have to be paid out of the proceeds from the sale. If she exchanged rather than sold, she would have her entire equity to invest in the new property and could defer any tax liability.

When a client becomes involved in a 1031 exchange, two questions must be answered:

1. Does the transaction qualify for a 1031 exchange?

2. What are the mathematics of the exchange?

   — How are equities balanced?

   — Who is giving or receiving boot? (Boot is unlike property that does not qualify for a tax-deferred exchange.)

   — Is the exchange partially or totally tax deferred, and what is the basis in the new property?

This section discusses the transactions that qualify for a 1031 tax-deferred exchange.

Tax-deferred exchanges involve at least three parties.   Most agents think of A exchanging with B. While this is essentially what happens, more often three parties are involved. The most widely used exchange is the *buy-sell exchange*, sometimes called a *three-corner exchange* or *three-legged exchange*. The three people involved are the exchanger (person wanting to exchange), the seller (a person who wants to sell property and doesn't want to retain any property), and the buyer (a person who wants the property of the exchanger).

In a three-legged exchange, the buyer offers to purchase the exchanger's property, but the buyer does not have any property to exchange. So the exchanger needs to find another property ("up-leg"), the property the exchanger wants to acquire. When the exchanger finds the up-leg, the buyer buys this property from the seller. Now the buyer has a property to exchange with the exchanger. Note that if the exchanger sold her property to the buyer and then bought the seller's property, this transaction would be a purchase and a sale. To satisfy the IRS, the buyer will buy the seller's property and exchange with the exchanger, and this is all done in escrow in a matter of minutes. A general rule of exchanging is that any person can be the center (hub) of the exchange except the person wanting the exchange. Sometimes this procedure is called the *flashing of mirrors*.

EXAMPLE   Here is an example of improper escrow instructions. E wants to complete a 1031 tax-deferred exchange, and S and B agree to cooperate in completing the exchange. E will transfer his property to B, and S will transfer his property to E to complete the exchange. Here is the diagram for this transaction.

$$S \rightarrow E \rightarrow B$$

E is the hub of the exchange; hence, the exchange is invalid. If the escrow instructions were to read, "S will transfer his property to B, B will transfer S's property to E, and E will transfer his property to B," then the following diagram would apply:

$$E \overset{\leftarrow}{\rightarrow} B \leftarrow S$$

The latter would be a valid exchange.

When a client wants a 1031 tax-deferred listing, a statement that the client wants to make a 1031 tax-deferred exchange should be on the listing and in the multiple listing service. This statement helps convince the IRS that the client intends to make a 1031 exchange from the beginning of the transaction.

The buy-up rule. With the *buy-up rule*, to qualify for a totally tax-deferred exchange, the exchanger needs to trade up in value and put all equity dollars into the new property or properties.

Trade up means the new property must be equal to or greater in value than the old property. If the exchanger withdraws any cash, the cash withdrawn will be taxable. Withdrawing cash will not disallow the exchange—an exchange may be partial—but the client will not have a totally tax-deferred exchange.

EXAMPLE E wants to complete a 1031 tax-deferred exchange. The FMV of his property is $350,000; therefore, the property he is trading for must be valued at $350,000 or more. If E trades for property and $50,000 cash, he will pay taxes on $50,000 only, and the $300,000 he put into the new property will be deferred.

The entity rule. Three basic entities can hold property: individuals, partnerships, and corporations. The **entity rule** can be stated as follows: The way the exchanger holds property going into an exchange is the way the exchanger must hold the property coming out of the exchange. As an example, two partners cannot trade a partnership property for two properties, each of which would be separately owned by the partners.

The investment property rule. The **investment property rule** comes from Internal Revenue Code (IRC) Section 1031(a)(1):

> In general—no gain or loss shall be recognized on the exchange of property held for productive use in a trade or business or for investment if such property is exchanged solely for property of like kind which is to be held either for productive use in a trade or business or for investment.

Personal residence does not qualify for a tax deferred exchange.

Note: A personal residence is not held for productive use in a trade or business or for investment. Therefore, a person cannot have a tax-deferred exchange of his personal residence for business or investment property. (Like-kind property is discussed later in the unit.) By turning a personal residence into a rental or to a property for a trade or business, the former personal residence could be eligible for a tax deferred exchange.

Like-kind rule.   Exchanges of property must observe the **like-kind rule**. In exchanging, property is categorized as either personal or real property. Personal property and real property are not like kind.

For personal property, like-kind property must be exactly the same in character or have the same nature, and this sometimes is very difficult to determine.

For real property, like-kind property is simply any piece of real property exchanged for any other piece of real property:

What Is Real Property?

Real property includes the following:

■   Vacant land (unimproved real estate)

■   Improved real estate, such as farms, buildings, orchards, and so on

■   Leases that have a remaining term at the time of the exchange of 30 years or more (the 30 years may include all options)

■   Mineral and water rights (if they are considered real property by the state, they are included)

Source: Critchton 122 F.2d 181 (1941), Rules, 55-749 and 68-3331

Therefore, the general rule for real property is that any piece of real property may be exchanged for any other piece of real property (like-for-like), except for inventory and personal residences.

The no-choice rule.   If an exchange qualifies as an exchange, it must be treated as an exchange. If the real estate transaction was structured as an exchange, the gain must be deferred (postponed).

The no-loss rule.   In conjunction with the no-choice rule is a rule called the **no-loss rule**. If a real estate transaction qualifies as an exchange, a loss cannot be recognized. Losses must be deferred along with gains. The no-loss rule comes from IRC Section 1031(a)(1).

To be a valid 1031 exchange, the exchanger cannot have control of the buyer's money.

Money control.   An *accommodating party* is a third party who has control of buyers' money in a delayed exchange.

At no time can the exchanger have control of the buyer's money. This point was emphasized by the *June P. Carlton* case. Carlton owned ranch land and wished to structure a 1031 exchange. The agreement was to sell property to General Development Corporation (GDC) if a suitable replacement property (up-leg) could be found. Two suitable parcels of land were found by Carlton: property belonging to Lyons and Fernandez (sellers). Carlton gave an option to GDC, and GDC advanced $50,000 to Carlton. Carlton thought that this would be a 1031 exchange.

The IRS argued, and the court agreed, that Carlton had sold the ranch land to General Development Corporation. Because Carlton had received $50,000 in her hands, the $50,000 did not go directly to the sellers, Lyons and Fernandez. One of the essences of an exchange is the transferring of property, and the mark of a sale is the receipt of cash. This case points out the extreme importance of proper procedure: the exchanger can never receive cash or even the right to cash. —*June P. Carlton v. Comm.* 385 F.2d 238 (5th Cir., 1967)

Delayed exchange.   IRC Section 1031(a)(3) allows a delayed exchange with the following characteristics:

> For a deferred exchange, the property must be identified within 45 days and the exchange completed within 180 days of transfer of the exchanged property.

REQUIREMENT THAT PROPERTY BE IDENTIFIED WITHIN 45 DAYS AND THAT EXCHANGE BE COMPLETED NOT MORE THAN 180 DAYS AFTER TRANSFER OF EXCHANGED PROPERTY—For purposes of this subsection, any property received by the taxpayer shall be treated as property which is not like-kind property if—

(A)   such property is not identified as property to be received in the exchange on or before the day which is 45 days after the date on which the taxpayer transfers the property relinquished in the exchange, or

(B)   such property is received after the earlier of—

   (i)   the day which is 180 days after the date on which the taxpayer transfers the property relinquished in the exchange, or

   (ii)   the due date (determined with regard to extension) for the transferor's return of the tax imposed by this chapter for the taxable year in which the transfer of the relinquished property occurs.

Properties purchased and closed within the 45-day period qualify as an identification.

Reverse exchange.   In a **reverse exchange**, the replacement property is acquired before the property owner gives up her property. An exchange accommodation titleholder takes title to the property the exchanger wishes to acquire and holds the title until the sale of the exchange property can be arranged. This type of exchange removes the problem of acquiring property within a prescribed time period of the delayed exchange. However, the sale must be within 180 days.

WEB LINK

For information on reverse exchange, as well as other forms of exchanges, visit the Federation of Exchange Accommodators website at www.1031.org.

Boot.   Unlike property in an exchange is called **boot**. In many exchanges, some property will be given in an exchange that is boot. Boot is taxable to the person receiving it. It is important to understand that the property needs to qualify as like kind only to the person seeking the tax-deferred exchange.

Boot is defined as all other unlike properties: cash, paper (trust deeds or notes), and personal properties (cars, boats, planes, paintings, jewels, etc.).

> Boot is cash received, unlike property or debt relief.

Boot may be classified as cash boot or mortgage boot. *Cash boot* is a result of the balancing of equities, which must be done in every exchange. *Mortgage boot* is the difference between the loans on the conveyed property and the loans on the acquired property. This is also called *debt relief*. If the client assumes a mortgage larger than the one that he conveys, then he has paid mortgage boot. However, if he assumes a mortgage that is less than the one that he conveys, then he has received mortgage boot (debt relief).

E X A M P L E   If I traded my real property for your real property and $20,000, the $20,000 I received would be taxable boot. If you gave me your new car as part of the trade for my property, then the value of the car would be taxable boot.

Assume we traded properties without boot but your property was free and clear of debt while my property was mortgaged and you assumed the mortgage. I would be taxed on the amount of the mortgage (debt relief).

Installment Sales

By using an **installment sale**, the investor can spread the tax gain on a sale over two or more years. The following guidelines concern the use of the installment method of reporting deferred-payment sales:

In an installment sale, the gain is taxed in the year it is received.

- The total tax to be paid in any one year may be reduced by spreading the payment amount, and thus the gain, over two or more tax years.

- The seller pays tax in future years with cheaper, inflated dollars.

- The seller does not pay the entire tax until after receiving the entire amount of the purchase price. A provision of the previous law stating that no more than 30% of the sales could be received in the taxable year of the sale to qualify for installment sales treatment has been eliminated.

- The installment sales method is automatic unless the taxpayer elects not to have the installment sale treatment apply.

Sale-Leaseback

Buyers and sellers can derive tax advantages through an arrangement in which property is sold with provisions for the seller to continue occupancy as a lessee. This form of transaction is called a **sale-leaseback**, *purchase-lease, sale-lease, lease-purchase*, or *leaseback*.

In a sale-leaseback, the seller benefits from capital being freed and rent that is a fully tax-deductible expense.

With a sale-leaseback, seller/lessees gain the advantages of getting property exactly suited to their needs without tying up working capital in fixed assets. Often, more capital can be raised this way than by borrowing. In addition, because leases are not considered long-term liabilities, rent is totally tax deductible. Frequently, writing off total lease payments is better than depreciation, for the land portion of property cannot be depreciated. If a property has a significant mortgage, a sale-leaseback would remove debt from a balance sheet, which would present a positive impression to lenders and purchasers of the corporate stock.

Often, only the land is sold and leased back because rent on land is a deductible expense, and improvements can be written off with depreciation deductions.

For companies working under government contracts that pay cost plus a fixed fee, rent is an allowable expense item, but mortgage payments are not. This is why many aircraft, electronics, and other defense plants are leased rather than owned.

Buyer/lessors gain the advantage of obtaining a long-term carefree investment and appreciation in the value of the property, as well as having the convenience of a built-in tenant. Usually, the yield on a sale-leaseback is higher than on a mortgage.

The lease payments will pay off the original investment, and the lessor still will have title to the property. The investment will not be paid off prematurely (as mortgages often are through refinancing), so the investor will not have to go out seeking another good investment to replace the one prematurely paid off. In addition, the lease terms often give the lessor a claim against other assets of the lessee in the event of a default, which is better security protection than a trust deed affords.

Principal Residence

Real estate that constitutes a homeowner's personal residence receives special tax treatment. The term *personal residence* is generally understood to refer to the taxpayer's **primary personal residence**, the dwelling in which a taxpayer lives and which the taxpayer occupies most of the time. A taxpayer may have only one principal residence at a time, and it may be as follows:

- Single-family house
- Houseboat
- Mobile home
- Motor home
- Trailer
- Condominium
- Cooperative housing

If you live in one unit of a multiple-unit dwelling, that unit will be considered your principal residence.

Primary or secondary residence.   The taxpayer's primary residence is the place occupied more often than any other. All other residences are termed *secondary residences*. One secondary residence will receive favorable income tax treatment, but unlike a primary residence, a secondary residence does not qualify for universal exclusion treatment.

Land.   The term *residence* includes not only the improvements but also the land [Rev. Rul. 56 420, 1956 2 (CD 519)]. However, vacant land cannot be considered a personal residence. When a principal residence is located on a large tract of land, the question arises as to just how much of the land is included with the principal residence. There is no clear-cut answer to this question, but the courts have made the determination based on the use and the intent of the taxpayer rather than on the amount of land involved.

> The universal exclusion requires two years' occupancy and can be taken every two years.

Universal exclusion for gain on sale of principal residence.   A seller of any age who has owned and used the home as a principal residence for at least two years of the five years before the sale can exclude from income up to $250,000 of gain ($500,000 for joint filers meeting conditions). In general, the exclusion can only be used once every two years.

Married couples filing jointly in the year of sale may exclude up to $500,000 of home-sale gain if either spouse owned the home for at least two of the five years before the sale. Both spouses must have used the home as a principal residence for at least two of the five years before the sale.

One spouse's inability to use the exclusion because of the once-every-two-years rule won't disqualify the other spouse from claiming the exclusion. However, the other spouse's exclusion cannot exceed $250,000.

EXAMPLE   Mary sells her principal residence in December 2010 at a $100,000 gain. She is single at that time, and qualifies for and claims the home sale exclusion. She marries Abel in May 2011 and moves into the home that has been his principal residence for the 20 years of his bachelorhood. If Abel sells the home the following July, up to $250,000 of his profit is tax free.

The two-year occupancy need not be continuous. For example, a person could have occupied the property as a principal residence for 6 months and then rented it for a year but later moved back for an 18-month occupancy.

If the total occupancy is 24 months during a five-year period, then the occupancy requirement will have been fully met.

California has adopted the federal universal exclusion of $250,000/$500,000. If a sale gain meets the federal criteria for exclusion, it would also be excluded from California income taxation.

Tax Benefits

Taxpayers are eligible for certain income tax write-offs while they own their homes. The general rule for income tax purposes is that ownership transfers when the title is transferred (a deed given) or when the buyer is given the rights of possession (the benefits and burdens of ownership), whichever occurs first. To be eligible for these tax deductions, a taxpayer must be the legal owner or equitable owner of the home.

Note: When the property is purchased on a land contract, the owner has equitable title. According to tax law, a buyer who has possession of the property (equity) owns the property and receives all the tax deductions of the property.

During ownership, owners taking itemized deductions may write off real estate taxes and mortgage interest in the year they are paid. Note that paying monies into an impound account is not the same as paying them to the agency to which they are owed. Monies paid into an impound account are not deductible. Only the money paid from the impound account to the proper authority can be deducted.

Home interest and property taxes are deductible.

Home interest. Interest on a primary residence and second home will be treated as home mortgage interest on mortgage amounts of up to $1 million, whereas interest on additional secondary homes will be treated as personal interest. Personal interest does not qualify as a deductible expense.

For homes that qualify as either a primary home or a second home, the interest is called *home mortgage interest* or *qualified residence interest*. There are two types of home interest: acquisition indebtedness and home equity indebtedness (or equity indebtedness).

Acquisition indebtedness interest. Taxpayers may deduct interest on home acquisition debt of $1,000,000 or less (first and second home).

EXAMPLE A man purchased a home for $10,000,000 with a $9,000,000 purchase money loan. He is limited in his interest deductions to the interest on $1,000,000 only.

Home equity debt interest. Taxpayers may deduct interest on up to $100,000 of home equity debt (money borrowed on property to use for other purposes).

Home Improvements

Systematically recording amounts spent for **home improvements** and retaining any and all receipts are of great importance to the homeowner. Unfortunately, they are often neglected. Many homeowners are completely unaware of the ultimate tax implications of the home improvements or capital improvements that are added to their properties through the years. These improvements may be added to the homeowner's basis, making the adjusted basis greater and reducing the gain at the time of sale. The adjusted basis (AB) is equal to the original basis (OB) plus home improvements (HI):

$$AB = OB + HI$$

adjusted basis = original basis + home improvements

There is a great deal of misunderstanding about what items are classified as home improvements. The IRS defines improvements differently for homes than it does for rental property. Examples of home improvements include the following:

- Electrical wiring (new, replacement, rearrangement)
- Floors
- Heating units
- Partitions (including removal)
- Pipes and drainage (including replacement)

- Roof (new or reshingling over old shingles)

- Walls (plastering, strengthening)

- Room additions

- Patios

- Pools

- Fencing

- Landscaping (trees, shrubbery, grass seed, etc.)

- Sprinkler systems

Maintenance items are not home improvements. Some examples are as follows:

- Painting

- Papering

- Carpeting

- Drapes

- Furniture

- Replacement of built-in appliances (stoves, ovens, dishwashers, etc.)

Relief for "forced" sales.   A relief provision may apply to some taxpayers who sell their principal residence but fail to meet the once-every-two-years rule for use of the exclusion. If the taxpayer's failure to meet the rule occurs because the home must be sold due to a change in the place of employment, health status, or—to the extent provided by regulations—other unforeseen circumstances, then the taxpayer may be entitled to a partial exclusion. Under these circumstances, the excludable portion of the gain that would have been tax-free had the requirements been met is computed proportionately.

EXAMPLE   A woman sells her principal residence because she has a new job in another city. On the date of the sale, she has used and owned her principal residence for the past 18 months. She has never excluded gain from another home sale. If she had used her principal residence for two years, the entire amount of the gain ($250,000) would be excluded. Although the woman fails to meet the use and ownership requirements for the full exclusion, because the sale is forced by employment, she is entitled to a partial exclusion. The amount of gain excluded by this seller cannot exceed the amount determined by the following computation (computed using months; see the observation above): the woman occupied her home for 18 of the 24 months required for the full exclusion. Therefore, she is entitled to a 75% exclusion from her gain (18/24 = 0.75). As a result, the woman may exclude $187,500 (250,000 × 0.75 = $187,500) of her gain on the sale of her principal residence.

Capital loss.   A taxpayer may use a capital loss to offset a capital gain in the year of the loss. If a taxpayer lost $100,000 on one capital sale but made $100,000 on another capital sale in the same year, there would be no capital gain tax. If, however, the taxpayer made $50,000 on the profitable sale, the taxpayer would have a $50,000 loss carryover. The taxpayer can take $3,000 of the carryover loss and use it as a deduction against income each year. To take advantage of a capital loss, a taxpayer should consider selling another capital asset where a profit would be made in the same year as the property loss.

FIRPTA

Before 1985, a foreigner (a person who is neither a U.S. citizen nor a U.S. resident alien) could purchase property in this country and later sell it, and then move back to her homeland and not pay income taxes on the sale of the property. Because it is very difficult, if not impossible, to collect delinquent taxes from such an individual, the U.S. Congress passed the **Foreign Investment in Real Property Tax Act (FIRPTA)**. The State of California passed a similar law. To distinguish between federal and California law, the federal law will be called *FED-FIRPTA* and the state law *CAL-FIRPTA*.

Federal Withholding

FED-FIRPTA generally requires that a buyer withhold estimated taxes equal to 10% of the sale price in transactions involving real property in the United States sold or exchanged by a foreign person. In addition, CAL-FIRPTA requires that a buyer withhold estimated taxes equal to one-third of the amount required to be withheld under FED-FIRPTA (31/3% of the sales price). The 10% estimated withholding must be reported and paid to the Internal Revenue Service within 10 days after the close of escrow. If the buyer fails to withhold the estimated taxes, and the seller fails to pay taxes on the sale, the buyer is subject to a penalty equal to 10% of the purchase price or the seller's actual tax liability plus interest and penalties, whichever is less.

For personal residences, FED-FIRPTA applies only to sales prices of $300,000 or more. When a buyer signs a certification (Figure 14.3) stating that he plans to use the property as a personal residence and the purchase price is less than $300,000, the buyer is relieved of withholding estimated taxes.

All other property—investment, rental, commercial, land, and so forth—requires withholding when a foreign person sells the property. If a foreign person owns a five-unit apartment building and sells it for $600,000, $60,000 will have to be withheld for the federal government and $20,000 for the State of California.

If more than one person owns the property and some are U.S. citizens and some are foreign, the amount of withholding must be prorated on the basis of the capital invested. If a married couple own property and one spouse is a citizen and the other is not, withholding is prorated 50/50.

Withholding under section 1.1445(a) may be reduced or eliminated pursuant to a withholding certificate issued by the Internal Revenue Service in accordance with the rules of this section. (It usually takes six to eight weeks to receive the certificate from the IRS.)

EXAMPLE   A foreign person is selling her personal residence to buy a new home of more value. Assuming that this transaction is not taxable, does the buyer of the old property need to withhold?

Yes. If the foreign person does not want the buyer to withhold, she will have to file for a withholding certificate from the IRS.

How is the buyer to know if the seller is a foreign person? The burden falls on the buyer, and there are only a few measures that will relieve the buyer of the obligation to withhold. In one such case, the seller must provide the buyer with an affidavit of nonforeign status. The seller also must provide a U.S. taxpayer identification number and state, under penalty of perjury, that he is not a foreign person.

As previously stated, California has adopted its own law covering real property sales by foreign persons who are defined as nonresidents of California.

California Withholding

As of 2003, buyers of property, other than the seller's personal residence, must withhold 31/3% of the net proceeds of the sale and remit them to the Franchise Tax Board at close of escrow. Besides the seller's personal residence, the following are other exclusions:

- Property sold for less than $100,000

- Property sold at a loss

- Property involved in a tax-deferred exchange

- Involuntary conversion (foreclosure sale)

TAX SHELTER

Because depreciation is shown as an expense for income tax purposes, it can reduce the tax liability of a real estate investor and could result in a paper loss, even though cash receipts exceed cash expenses.

Taxpayers can use real estate operating losses (passive losses) to offset real estate income without limit. Real estate losses also can be used, with limitations, to offset active income such as wages.

FIGURE 14.3:   Seller's Federal Residency Declarations

FEDERAL RESIDENCY DECLARATIONS
Citizen Status (Internal Revenue Code §1445)

| Prepared by: Agent_____ | Phone_____ |
| Broker_____ | Email_____ |

| NOTE: If the declarations differ for individual sellers, then each seller must fill out a separate form. |

DATE: _____, 20_____, at _____, California.

Items left blank or unchecked are not applicable.

FACTS:

1. This declaration complies with Section 1445 of the United States Internal Revenue Code regarding Seller's status as a citizen or resident of the United States or otherwise, and is for reliance by Broker and any buyer.

    1.1 Seller _____

        U.S. Tax Identification Number (or Social Security Number) _____

    1.2 Seller _____

        U.S. Tax Identification Number (or Social Security Number) _____

2. Regarding the proposed sale of real estate referrred to as _____
_____.

SELLER'S DECLARATIONS:

3. Seller hereby declares:

    3.1 ☐ I am a citizen of the United States of America;

    3.2 ☐ I am a resident alien of the United States of America; my resident status is established by the following:

        a. ☐ I have been declared a permanent legal resident of the United States by the U.S. Immigration and Naturalization Service. Resident Alien registration number _____, or;

        b. ☐ I have resided at least 31 days in the United States during the current calendar year, and my days of residence in the United States over the last three years are as follows:

            Current calendar year. . . . . _____ X 1 = _____

            Last calendar year . . . . _____ X 0.334 = 0.00

            Second preceding year. . . . . _____ X 0.167 = 0.00

                        TOTAL DAYS = 0.00

        Since the total days equals or exceeds 183 days, I meet the substantial presence test of Internal Revenue Code §7701(b)(3).

> **Exclusions:**
> Residency does not include days during which Seller:
> *   remained in the U.S. due to a medical condition which arose while he was visiting;
> *   was in transit between two points outside the U.S.;
> *   worked for an agency of a foreign government;
> *   was a teacher, trainee, or student; or participated as a professional athlete

4. ☐ I am neither a United States citizen nor a resident alien as defined in item 3, above; and

    4.1 Unless I obtain a "qualifying statement" [IRC §1445(b)(4)], or other special permission from the Internal Revenue Service, I authorize Buyer of the above-referenced real estate to deduct and withhold 10% of the sales price for the federal government. I further authorize Escrow-holder to deduct these amounts from funds due me at close of escrow, and to deposit it as a tax deposit in an authorized commercial bank.

5. I consent to the reliance on this declaration of the Brokers, Agents, Escrow-holder, and Buyer in any transaction regarding this real estate.

6. **Note:** This transaction is exempt from IRC §1445 withholding if the sales price is $300,000 or less and Buyer will use the real estate as his residence.

BUYER'S ACKNOWLEDGMENT:

7. I have read and received a copy of this Seller's Residency Declaration.

8. ☐ I hereby declare I will use the real estate as my residence. If the final sales price is $300,000 or less, I consent to reliance on this declaration by Brokers, Agents, Escrow-holder and the nonresident alien Seller.

I declare under penalty of perjury that the foregoing is true and correct.	**I declare under penalty of perjury that the foregoing is true and correct.**
Date: _____, 20_____	Date: _____, 20_____
Seller: _____	Buyer: _____
Seller: _____	Buyer: _____

FORM 301 03-11 ©2011 **first tuesday**, P.O. BOX 20069, RIVERSIDE, CA 92516 (800) 794-0494

©2015 **RPI — Realty Publications, Inc.**, P.O. BOX 5707, RIVERSIDE, CA 92517

Taxpayers with an adjusted gross income of less than $100,000 can use real estate losses (which are considered passive losses) to shelter up to $25,000 of their active income. Taxpayers whose adjusted gross income is between $100,000 and $150,000 lose $1 of this $25,000 maximum for each $2 that their adjusted gross income exceeds $100,000.

> Taxpayers with adjusted gross income less than $100,000 can shelter up to $25,000 of active income with passive losses.

If investors do not actively manage their property (active management includes hiring a property manager), then the taxpayer is precluded from sheltering active income. Because investors have no management responsibilities in investments such as limited partnerships, the investor cannot use such losses to shelter active income.

Real estate professionals can use passive losses from investment property to offset other income without any limitations if they meet specific criteria, which include devoting at least 750 hours during the tax year to property management activities.

Estate Tax

Death is a tax shelter in that it avoids capital gains tax on the increased value of assets of the deceased. However, the assets may be subject to an estate tax. For persons dying in 2015, the estate tax exclusion for an individual is $5.43 million (adjusted annually for inflation). The maximum estate tax rate is 40%.

Inherited property receives a stepped-up basis, meaning that the property is valued at the time of decedent's death. This means the asset is shielded from any capital gains based on appreciation in value that occurred before to the decedent's death.

If a decedent gifted property prior to death, then the recipient would retain the cost basis of the grantor and a subsequent sale could subject the grantee to substantial capital gain taxation.

California no longer has an estate tax, although several states do tax estates. Differences in estate taxation, as well as income tax rates, have caused some wealthy individuals to make economic decisions as to where their residence should be.

Federal Gift Tax

The federal gift tax is taxed to the donor. The annual exemption is $14,000 per donee. A married couple with three children could give each child $14,000 each year, making total gifts of $84,000 each year that are tax exempt.

PROBATE AND LIVING TRUSTS

Probate is the court-approved procedure to pay off the just debts of a deceased person and to distribute the assets according to a will or intestate succession. There are three reasons for probate avoidance:

- The cost of probate

- Reduction of possible estate taxation

- Time

In California, a $1,000,000 estate could be subject to a $23,000 attorney fee plus $23,000 for an executor fee, for a total of $46,000. There are also finding fees of approximately $400, as well as appraisal costs.

Probate may be avoided by use of a joint tenancy, community property, or a revocable living trust.

With a *living trust*, trustors transfer their property to their trust but retain absolute control and serve as trustee. Upon death, a successor trustee distributes the estate without probate expenses.

For larger estates, it is possible for married couples to double the size of their exemption. Assume a couple has an estate worth over $5,430,000 and the current exemption from estate taxation is $5,430,000. They could have two trusts, known as an A-B trust. If one spouse dies, the spouse could give $5,430,000, the exempt amount, to the trust for the benefit of the successors. The balance of the trust would go to the A portion of the trust for the benefit of the other spouse. Since estate taxes are not levied on gifts to a spouse, the first death is not subject to estate taxation. When the surviving spouse dies, that estate goes to the B trust, but the one portion that is subject to estate taxation would be the portion in excess of $5,000,000. The B trust, which is distributed to the successors (heirs), therefore, will have received a $10,860,000 exemption from estate taxation rather than $5,430,000.

SUMMARY

Real estate taxes are ad valorem taxes. Property is reassessed when sold, and property is taxed for the basic levy at a maximum rate of 1% of the fair market value (Proposition 13). The tax rate cannot increase more than 2% per year. Additional special assessments can be added, up to 1% of the fair market value. The homeowner's exemption is $7,000 from the assessed valuation. There is also a veteran's exemption of $4,000. In 2015, the exemption for a totally disabled veteran was $126,380.

Tax transfers between family members may be exempt from reassessment. For taxpayers older than 55, a sale and repurchase of a principal residence within the same county may allow the taxpayer to keep the old assessed valuation if the new purchase is at the same price as or less than the sales price of the old residence. For residents over 55 years of age, the transfer of assessed value can extend to other counties if the other county has agreed to it (Proposition 90).

For some senior citizens (low income or disabled), a postponement of taxes is possible until the claimant no longer occupies the property.

Capital gains are sale gains on the sale of capital assets. A long-term gain, over 12 months, is currently taxed at a maximum of 15%, except the rate is 20% for high-income taxpayers. There is also a 3.8% Medicare surcharge for high-income taxpayers.

Depreciation is a noncash expense for tax purposes that applies to improvements to income, business, and investment property. It is a return on the investment. Any gain on sale is taxed from the basis adjusted by adding buying expenses and capital improvements to the purchase price, then deducting the accumulated depreciation (adjusted cost basis). For residential property, a 27½-year life is used for depreciation purposes. For nonresidential property, a 39-year life is used.

A taxpayer can defer gains on the sale of business or investment property by use of a 1031 exchange. The property must be like-for-like (real property for real property), and the taxpayer would be taxed only on boot received. Boot is unlike property received, as well as debt relief. A delayed tax-deferred exchange is possible if the taxpayer identifies the property within 45 days of a transfer and closes escrow within 180 days of the transfer.

Installment sales allow a taxpayer to spread a gain over the years in which the gain is received. This could mean a lower tax rate.

A sale-leaseback allows a seller to gain operating capital, reduce debt, and have the 100% tax deduction of business rent.

Residential property owners have a tax advantage for interest payments on $1,000,000 in acquisition indebtedness (for primary and secondary residences), as well as up to $100,000 in equity indebtedness.

A homeowner's gain on the sale of a residence is determined by deducting the adjusted cost basis (cost plus improvements) and the selling expenses from the selling price. The Taxpayer Relief Act of 1997 made some significant changes to tax law regarding gains on the sale of real estate. These changes include a once-every-two-year exclusion from taxation for gains on the sale of a principal residence that has been occupied by the sellers for at least two years during the prior five-year period. This exclusion from taxation is as follows:

- Married couples, $500,000

- Single persons, $250,000

When a property is sold by a foreign national, it is the buyer's responsibility to withhold 10% of the price for federal income taxes and 31/3% for state income taxes, unless the transaction is exempt from such withholding. The state withholding applies to all nonresidents of California.

Depreciation is a paper expense that can be used to shelter up to $25,000 in active income from taxation (The maximum amount is reduced by $1 for every $2 in income over $100,000).

Death results in a stepped-up cost basis that is based on value at the time of the decedent's death. There is a federal estate tax but no California estate tax. By using a living trust, a couple can double the amount of their estate tax exemption.

CLASS DISCUSSION TOPICS

1. A buyer of an apartment building has $60,000 annual rent, total cash expenses of $52,000, and depreciation of $9,000. What are the investor's benefits, if any?

2. A person renting a home pays $1,200 per month in rent. The owner offers it for sale to the tenant at a price of $240,000. The tenant is offered a $200,000, 7%, 30-year loan; PITI payments will come to $1,650 per month.

3. Although the tenant has $40,000 for the down payment, she concludes that she cannot afford the house and will continue to rent it. Discuss the wisdom of her decision. What assumptions would be necessary to arrive at any conclusion?

4. Diagram a three-party exchange.

5. Compute the adjusted basis when the original basis was $137,500, improvements to the property totaled $31,650, and depreciation taken was $11,436.

6. Bring to class one current-events article dealing with some aspect of real estate practice for class discussion.

UNIT 14 QUIZ

1. The MOST difficult tax to avoid is the
   a. sales tax.
   b. real property tax.
   c. income tax.
   d. estate tax.

2. The months of November, December, February, and April relate to
   a. real property taxes.
   b. income taxes.
   c. estate taxes.
   d. sales taxes.

3. What did Proposition 13 provide for?
   a. It set a maximum tax rate.
   b. It set assessments for property acquired before 1978 back to the value on the 1975 tax roll.
   c. The tax can be increased 2% per year.
   d. All of these.

4. The proposition that allows a tax assessment for certain homeowners to be transferred from one county to another is Proposition
   a. 13.
   b. 58.
   c. 60.
   d. 90.

5. The homeowner's property tax exemption is
   a. $50,000 for a single person.
   b. $4,000 from assessed valuation.
   c. $7,000 from assessed valuation.
   d. the first $100,000 of assessed valuation.

6. Depreciation for a residential property uses
   a. the straight-line method.
   b. a 27½-year table.
   c. a 39-year table.
   d. both a and b.

7. To have a tax-deferred delayed exchange, which of the following is required?
    a. The exchange property must be identified within 45 days after the taxpayer relinquishes his property.
    b. The sale must be completed within 180 days after the taxpayer relinquishes his property.
    c. Both of these.
    d. Neither of these.

8. To have a 1031 tax-deferred exchange, you need all of the following *EXCEPT*
    a. like-for-like properties.
    b. to receive boot rather than pay it.
    c. a trade of investment real property for investment real property.
    d. to hold property after the exchange in the same manner as you held property going into the exchange.

9. Albert wants to exchange property with Baker. Which would be boot to Albert in the exchange?
    a. Cash given by Albert to balance equities
    b. Cash received by Albert to balance equities
    c. Acceptance of a greater debt by Albert
    d. Both a and c

10. A homeowner can receive preferential tax treatment by
    a. an interest deduction.
    b. use of the universal exclusion.
    c. a property tax deduction.
    d. all of these.

UNIT FIFTEEN

PROPERTY MANAGEMENT AND LEASING

LEARNING OBJECTIVES

When you have completed this unit, you will be able to

- describe the variety of positions, duties, and responsibilities available within the property management field;

- explain the different types of properties managed and how each affects the manager's activities;

- name the types of leases and their provisions;

- explain landlord and tenant responsibility; and

- describe how a tenant can be evicted.

KEY TERMS

Accredited
  Management
  Organization
Accredited Resident
  Manager
assignment
Certified Property
  Manager
condominium
  association
  management
Costa-Hawkins Rental
  Housing Act
effective rent
estate at sufferance

estate at will
estate for years
exculpatory clause
gross lease
habitability
Help Families Save
  Their Home Act
holdover clause
Institute of Real Estate
  Management
late charge
management
  agreement
net lease
percentage lease

periodic tenancy
Protecting Tenants at
  Foreclosure Act of
  2009
recapture clause
rent schedule
resident manager
scheduled rent
security deposit
step-up lease
sublease
30-day notice
three-day notice
trust ledger
unlawful detainer

THE PROPERTY MANAGEMENT FIELD

Property management is not a new field of specialization. In biblical days, owners employed "overseers" who supervised the running of estates. In colonial America, English companies that had land charters, such as the Virginia Company, employed managers to run their operations.

Most properties were managed by owners. The growth of the modern property management profession was facilitated by two factors:

1. The invention of the electric elevator and the use of structural steel, which allowed for highrise construction, starting in the late 1800s. Highrise construction allows a property owner to have more tenants with a smaller construction footprint. The large number of tenants creates a greater responsibility for a landlord. These huge structures generally were owned by large companies or groups of investors, who had to hire managers for their operations.

2. The Great Depression of the 1930s, which resulted in lenders accumulating vast inventories of property because of foreclosures. To maximize the income and protect the property, these lenders required property managers.

Professionalism

The number of people involved in property management increased rapidly. However, because many of these managers lacked reasonable qualifications due to limited knowledge and abilities, there were many failures within the property management field.

In 1933, to slow down this failure trend and to improve the professional standing of this management group, approximately 100 companies met and formed the **Institute of Real Estate Management (IREM)**, a subdivision of the National Association of REALTORS® (NAR). These companies certified that they would

- refrain from commingling their clients' funds with personal funds,

- bond all employees handling client funds, and

- disclose all fees, commissions, or other payments received as a result of activity relating to the client's property.

This move improved the situation, but after several years it became apparent that the companies were not meeting the standards set, mainly because of constant personnel changes.

In 1938, the IREM changed its policy and developed the designation **Certified Property Manager (CPM)** to certify individual managers rather than the companies that employed them. The concept has been successful. IREM's certification requirements are designed to ensure that managers have the general business and industry-specific experience necessary to maintain high standards within the profession. To earn the CPM designation, an individual must

- actively support the institute's rules and regulations;

- demonstrate honesty, integrity, and the ability to manage real estate, including at least three years' experience in a responsible real estate management position; and

- be a member of a local real estate board and a member of the National Association of REALTORS®.

IREM also has the designation **Accredited Resident Manager (ARM)** for residential managers. **Accredited Management Organization (AMO)** is a designation given by IREM to a company. To receive this designation, a company must

- have at least one CPM in charge,

- have property management as a primary activity,

- follow minimum standards and the rules of IREM, and

- renew its accreditation yearly.

There are several other professional property management organizations. They include the Real Estate Management Broker's Institute of the National Association of Real Estate Brokers, the Apartment Owners and Managers Association of America, the Building Owners and Managers Association International (BOMA), and the National Society of Professional Resident Managers. These organizations produce publications, conduct seminars, and award professional designations.

Kinds of Property Managers

There are three basic kinds of managers: licensee/property managers, individual property managers, and resident managers.

> A person working under direct supervision of a licensed property manager need not be licensed.

Licensee/property manager. A licensee/property manager is a licensee of a real estate office or agency that manages a number of properties for various owners. Such a manager may be a member of the firm who spends full time in management, may be self-employed as a managing agent, or may be one of several managers in the management department of a large real estate company. Persons working under the direct supervision of a licensed property manager need not be licensed to show property, accept preprinted rental applications, provide information on rental terms, and accept signed leases and deposits.

Individual property manager. An *individual property manager* manages a single property for the owner and may or may not possess a real estate license. This person usually is employed on a straight salary basis.

Resident manager.   A **resident manager**, as the title implies, lives on the property and may be employed by the owner or by a managing agent. The resident manager does not require a real estate license. A resident manager usually is qualified for this assignment by previous management experience or by special training. Personality is critical to success; specifically, the manager should exhibit the following:

- The merchandising ability to contact, show, and close the rental of a unit

- A high degree of self-confidence and willingness to take charge

- Accuracy in handling money, checks, bank deposits, and other bookkeeping duties

- Awareness of and sensitivity to the events occurring on and around the property

- Orderliness and legibility in keeping records and meticulousness in filing, cataloging, and making reports

- Computer skills, such as the ability to access and interpret data

- The ability to select residents on the basis of economic capability and credit references

- The diligence to maintain the property (The amount of maintenance will vary with the size of the property and the policies of management)

State law requires a resident manager for property containing 16 or more units and specifies that the resident manager must be a "responsible person." Mobile home parks having more than 50 units must have a resident manager.

Functions of a Property Manager

The author of the following statement is unknown, but the words give a splendid overview of the making of a property manager:

The past is his experience, and with its valuable ramifications, he is helped immeasurably to mold the plans for his future. During his years of experience, he has built and sold houses, appraised property, dealt in long-term commercial and industrial leases, made many complicated and intricate transactions, bought and sold hotels—in short, has had a long experience with the public, including businessmen, husbands and wives, doctors and lawyers, engineers and financiers, yes, with gamblers, beggars and thieves, mothers-in-law, fanatics, the feebleminded, strong and weak characters of every type and description, politicians too, and with this experience has automatically been turned out a well-rounded, socially conscious, alert, and aggressive person— in short, a skillful businessman, and when he has reached this point, he has automatically qualified for the job of property management.

Depending on the complexity of the property, the property manager's duties and responsibilities are many and varied. Inherent in these duties is the dual role of an administrator for the owner and an advocate for the resident.

The property manager's responsibility is to understand and communicate with both parties. The astute property manager is in an ideal position to both represent the owner and work with the residents with procedures that are fair and equitable. The manager should recognize that the owner wants a fair return on investment and that the resident wants decent housing or space that is properly maintained.

Administrator for the owner. As the administrator for the owner, the property manager must recognize that the owner is interested primarily in the following:

- The highest return from the property, realizing its highest and best use

- The enhancement or preservation of the physical value of the property

Specific duties of a property manager. Under the property management system, the owner is relieved of all executive functions as well as of all details connected with the operation or physical upkeep of the property.

A conscientious manager realizes the following:

- Renters need to know what is expected of them and what they can expect from the owner. (This should be stated in writing.)

- Residents' questions should be handled properly and promptly.

- If any request is denied, the manager should state why and avoid pointless arguing.

- The owner, manager, and employees should guard against the attitude that all tenants are unreasonable. However, it would be disastrous to adopt the principle that the customer is always right. The resident is, of course, always entitled to fair and sympathetic treatment.

- The property manager must make certain that tenants' and prospective tenants' legal rights are protected.

As an agent, the property manager must show good faith and loyalty to her principal (the owner); perform her duties with skill, care, and due diligence; fully disclose all pertinent facts; avoid commingling funds; and refrain from personal profits without the principal's full knowledge and consent.

State-defined responsibilities.   In addition to the general responsibilities described here, the California Bureau of Real Estate has prepared a list of specific duties:

- Establish the rental schedule that will bring the highest yield consistent with good economics

- Merchandise the space and collect the rents

- Create and supervise maintenance schedules and repairs

- Supervise all purchasing

- Develop a policy for tenant-resident relations

- Develop employee policies and supervise employees' operations

- Maintain proper records and make regular reports to the owner

- Qualify and investigate prospective tenants' credit

- Prepare and execute leases

- Prepare decorating specifications and secure estimates

- Hire, instruct, and maintain satisfactory personnel to staff the building(s)

- Audit and pay bills

- Advertise and publicize vacancies through selected media and broker lists

- Plan alterations and modernizing programs

- Inspect vacant space frequently

- Keep abreast of economic conditions and posted competitive market conditions

- Pay insurance premiums and taxes and recommend tax appeals when warranted

Basic Responsibilities

The principal functions of a property manager can be summarized as seven basic responsibilities:

1. Marketing space by advertising and securing desirable tenants

2. Collecting rents

3. Handling tenant complaints and physically caring for the premises

4. Purchasing supplies and equipment and paying for repairs

5. Hiring needed employees and maintaining good public relations

6. Keeping proper records and preparing required reports

7. Making recommendations to the owner on matters of improvements, changes in use and insurance coverage, and operational changes requiring owner approval

Establishing rent schedules. Rent schedules are the rents to be asked for and set forth in the lease. **Effective rent** is often less than **scheduled rent** if inducements are provided to the tenant, such as one month's free rent for a one-year lease. If the scheduled rent were $1,200 a month, the effective rent in this case would only be $1,100 per month ($1,200 × 11 months = $13,200 for the year or $1,100 per month). *Rent levels* usually are determined on the premise of scarcity and comparability of values in the area. How much rent is charged will affect the cost and time required to rent the unit, the length of each tenant's stay, decorating costs between tenants, and overall vacancy rate. To set up proper **rent schedules**, the manager must make a skilled and thorough analysis of the neighborhood. This analysis will include but not be limited to the following:

- The character of the immediate neighborhood

- The economic level and size of families

- Trends in population growth and occupants per unit

- Directional growth of the community and expansion and growth of local industries

- Availability of transportation, recreation, shopping, churches, and schools

- The condition of the housing market versus population growth trends

- Current area vacancy factors

- Similarly desirable rental units currently available

The objective of the analysis is to set up a rental schedule commensurate with the findings.

WEB LINK

@

There are internet sites that provide data on comparable properties. They are very helpful in setting rent schedules. Two such websites are www.rentometer.com and www.zilpy.com.

The objective of good property management is to achieve the combination of rent and vacancy that provides the owner with the greatest net. Conducting surveys and establishing rental schedules are very important. Statistics show that uncollected rent is worse than a vacancy, because the property suffers wear and tear from the occupant and the opportunity to place a desirable tenant in the unit is lost. In establishing rent levels, the property manager should realize that a vacant unit is not in competition with units already rented. The only competition is with other vacant units.

KNOWING THE LAW

The property manager must know the legal rights of tenants and legal procedures to take in notices and evictions. The manager must be aware of federal and state antidiscrimination statutes. The manager must also understand what actions could be construed as sexual harassment. Knowledge of local and state building health and safety codes, as well as any rent control restrictions, is also necessary as they relate to management duties.

The Occupational Safety and Health Act (OSHA) is important to property managers who are hiring seven or more employees. The law requires compliance with safety standards, recordkeeping, and reporting. It covers equipment condition, maintenance, and safety precautions. The maximum penalty OSHA can assess for a single violation is $7,000. The amount of $70,000 can be assessed for repeated or willful violations. California has passed its own Cal OSHA provisions.

TYPES OF PROPERTY MANAGED

Properties requiring management include office buildings, apartment buildings and other residential properties, commercial structures, shopping centers, distribution centers, public buildings, recreation centers, hotels, motels, industrial facilities, restaurants, and theaters. Recently, other properties have joined the list and are rapidly gaining in importance and popularity. These include the following:

- Condominium associations
- Industrial parks
- Mobile home parks
- Miniwarehouses
- Marinas
- Airports

A few of these are described in more detail in this section.

Professional Qualifications of a Property Manager

What kind of person is qualified to be not only a human relations specialist but also a detail manager? Such a person must be able to play the following roles:

- ■ Merchandising specialist. The property manager must be able to advertise and to sell prospective tenants on the merits of a building.

- ■ Leasing expert. Being well informed on all types of leases assists a manager in determining the most beneficial lease for a particular client.

- ■ Accounting specialist. The law requires that certain records be kept and reports made.

- ■ Maintenance supervisor. Preventive and corrective maintenance will prevent expensive repairs at some future date.

- ■ Purchasing supervisor. The manager must keep up with all current technological advances in building in order to be able to recommend needed replacements for obsolete installations.

- ■ Credit specialist. Credit ratings are extremely important. Knowing whether a tenant can live up to the terms of a lease is vital.

- ■ Insurance adviser. Understanding the various types of policies available and the extent of coverage can save both the owner and the tenant time and money.

- ■ Tax interpreter. A manager must be well versed in property taxes and their effect on the property being managed. The manager should be cognizant of the relationship of depreciation to the income and profit of the property.

- ■ Psychology expert. This capacity is crucial to day-to-day communication.

- ■ Budget manager. A property manager must be able to maintain and operate within the budget established for the property.

Residential Properties

Residential properties are by far the most numerous of the properties subject to professional management. There are approximately 133 million occupied housing units in the United States (Census Bureau 2013 estimate).

The housing market is stratified, meaning that the marketplace behaves differently based on price range. There may be a high vacancy rate at one rental range and a severe housing shortage at another range. Nevertheless, a general nationwide housing shortage has resulted in a rapid rise in rental rates. Three million new housing starts each year would be required merely to replace end-of-the-line units that should be demolished.

Residential property managers should be familiar with local rent control ordinances to make certain that rents and rent increases charged are not in violation of the law. Rent control restrictions vary significantly by community.

Allowable rental increases are also subject to different restrictions. Under the **Costa-Hawkins Rental Housing Act**, landlords who are subject to rent control are free to establish new base rents for new tenants, as well as for sublessees and assignees when landlord consent is required for the sublease or assignment.

Residential managers also must fully understand their obligations under state and federal fair housing legislation, as well as under the Real Estate Commissioner's Regulations dealing with fair housing. (See Unit 2 for specific requirements.)

Residential managers of lower-priced units should be familiar with Section 8 housing. This is a rental program under which all or part of a low-income tenant's rent is paid through the county. County administrators must inspect the property for eligibility, and tenants must meet stated criteria and be approved by the county.

Condominiums. Individual ownership of condominiums generally involves property management. Condominiums and cooperatives are similar from the standpoint of management duties.

A growing segment in the property management field is **condominium association management**. This type of management is often heavy on the accounting aspects. The duties of the condominium association manager likely would include the following:

- Collecting fees and assessments from members

- Issuing financial statements to the association

- Ensuring that homeowners associations provide members an annual financial statement and the Assessment and Reserve Funding Disclosure Summary form, which spells out current assessments, additional scheduled assessments reserve account balance, and obligations

- Contracting for or hiring for all maintenance and repairs

- Enforcing covenants, conditions, and restrictions (CC&Rs)

- Handling tenant interpersonal disputes and/or complaints

- Filing tax returns (if applicable), as well as handling workers' compensation, unemployment compensation, insurance, and so forth

- Seeing that the property is insured as to damage and owner liability

- Making suggestions to the board of directors

- Attending directors' meetings

In condominium associations, property managers don't make policy; they merely carry out policy as directed by the board of directors and the covenants, conditions, and restrictions in each deed. A condominium association manager must understand that different board members have different personal agendas. For example, some members may be primarily focused on security, while others are interested in keeping assessments to a minimum. A property manager must avoid becoming involved in the politics of the homeowners association and must focus on the instructions of the board. However, the manager does have a duty to make informed recommendations to the board.

A number of computer programs designed for condominium association management provide financial records, spreadsheets, work orders, and even much of the routine correspondence of the association.

Mobile home parks.   Management of a mobile home park is a specialty field involving the following:

- Park development

- Public amenities

- Enforcement of park rules

- Approval of lease assignments on sale of units

The tenant in a mobile home park is entitled to a 12-month lease on request.

In parks where the individual lots are owned by the mobile-unit owners, the mobile home park management duties become similar to the duties of a condominium association manager. However, the park manager should be aware that the laws governing evictions from rental space parks are much more restrictive for park owners than for other residential landlords. The park manager must give tenants a 12-month lease on request at current rent and must furnish tenants with an annual copy of the current California Civil Code covering mobile home parks, so that tenants understand their rights and responsibilities. The management of a mobile home park cannot require a homeowner to use a specific broker when replacing a unit in a rental park.

Multifamily units.   Residential property bought for investment is the most common professionally managed property. Statistics indicate that multiple-family units account for approximately 30% of residential housing in the United States.

The more problems a property has, the more it needs professional management. Because properties that have had a troubled history can take a great deal of a property manager's time, the manager's fee scale is generally higher for such properties.

Public housing.   Ownership of public housing is important to property management. The largest single landlord in the United States is the collective 3,300 public housing authorities. More than 1.2 million units are controlled by public housing authorities. A great many property managers are employed by federal, state, and local housing authorities.

Traditionally, management of public housing has almost exclusively concentrated on the physical and financial aspects of the projects. Management is beginning to realize the importance of social aspects of public housing management.

Single-family homes.   Besides homes purchased for rental, there are many instances requiring single-family home management for absentee owners. In resort areas, many owners use property management to care for their properties and, in some cases, to handle short-term rentals. Property management might also be required for property in probate and for lenders who have foreclosed. Generally, because single-family units require more management time per unit than multifamily units, management charges tend to reflect this greater effort.

Office Buildings

Office buildings are the major commercial property. Office space requirements, as well as available inventory, are directly related to the local economy. The larger users of office space, such as banks, savings associations, and insurance companies, often build for their own use but also provide a large amount of excess of space for leasing purposes.

Overbuilding of office structures intensified the need for professional management because owners didn't want to give any advantage to other owners: Competition for lessees can be heated.

Most areas of California now have a glut of office space. In such areas, concessions are necessary to attract tenants. In some instances, property managers agree to assume a tenant's current lease to encourage the tenant to take a larger space under a long-term lease. The agent then has the job of marketing the "trade-in" space.

Specialized offices, such as medical or legal offices, have special problems.

Merchandising office space.   Rental or lease of office space can be tied to the following criteria:

- Appearance of surroundings

- Transportation facilities

- Prestige and image of area

- Proximity to clients

- Building appearance

- Lobby appearance

- Elevator appearance and condition

- Corridor appearance

- Office interiors

- Tenant services offered

- Management

- Other tenants

Advertising is an essential part of conducting an aggressive leasing campaign for office space. Such publicity ideas as the following can be most helpful:

- Groundbreaking ceremonies

- Signs

- Brochures

- Newspaper ads

- Website (referenced in ads and brochures)

- Mailing lists of professional groups, including attorneys, doctors, and CPAs

- Personal solicitation

- Use of a model office

- Communication with other leasing agents

- Making technical data readily available, including floor plans, available space, and space arrangements

Maintenance. The manager of an office building must handle maintenance or service problems unique to this type of operation. This job includes such activities as the following:

- Servicing all operating equipment and public facilities, such as lobbies, lights, and washrooms

- Maintaining elevators, which are indispensable in a highrise (usually involves an elevator maintenance contract)

- Cleaning (usually done at night)

- Other routine maintenance, including window cleaning, waste removal, light bulb replacement, heating, ventilation, and air-conditioning

- Preparing and updating a maintenance operations manual that shows a list of all equipment with the vital information concerning each piece of equipment

- Compliance with health and fire codes, as well as the Americans with Disabilities Act.

Protection. Protection of the premises is a management function. It includes such vital items as these:

- Key control

- Alarm systems

- Lighting

- Security guard employment

- Fire-prevention techniques

Retail Space

Management of retail space requires many of the same skills and concerns as office management. In multiunit commercial properties, the manager should consider the effect a prospective tenant will have on the business of other tenants. Managers will often seek out particular tenants or businesses in order to contribute to the overall operation of the property.

Industrial Management

Industrial management is rather specialized because of the skills required. Industrial managers must have knowledge in many areas, including the following:

- Fire-suppression systems (sprinklers) and water capacity and pressure for various uses

- Floor and ceiling load capacities

- Hazardous and toxic substances (use and storage), as well as underground tanks

- Air- and water-quality control

- Loading dock requirements

- Electrical capacity and three-phase wiring

- Reading blueprints for modification

- Specific zoning regarding uses allowed

- Special insurance requirements

- Security and security systems

- Large cooling, heating, and ventilation systems

Industrial managers might manage specific property or an entire industrial park. The industrial property manager's duties primarily relate to renting, but they also involve common area maintenance and protecting the property and the owners from liability.

SECURITY

Security is of prime importance to lessors and lessees for all types of property. It applies to personal security of tenants, employees, and guests as well as security for the lessee's property.

Because no property can be absolutely safe, a property manager should never indicate to tenants that a property is safe or secure. This could be seen by the court as a warranty as to safety. Nevertheless, your best efforts should be used to make the premises as safe as is reasonably possible.

A property manager should consider, as applicable to a property, the following:

- *Emergency evacuation plan*—In light of 9/11, such a plan is extremely important for large structures. Evacuation plans for earthquakes are also very important in California.

- *Properly marked exits*—This may require going beyond bare legal requirements.

- *Appropriate landscaping*—Remove any trees or shrubbery around entrances and walkways that could conceal a person.

- *Exterior lighting*—Take special care in entryways, walkways, and parking areas. Perimeter areas could be lighted by motion sensor lighting. Having well-lit property is a cost-effective way to reduce crime.

- *Interior lighting*—Light all hallways and public areas (use fluorescent and LED bulbs that are unlikely to be removed). Battery-operated emergency lighting that is kept charged by the electrical service but goes on when service is cut should be considered.

- *Circuit breaker box*—This should be locked or in a locked room.

- *Exterior and unit doors*—All should be solid core rather than hollow core. Steel doors should be considered. Apartment doors should have peepholes and a security chain with screws at least 2½ inches long.

- *Door locks*—Do not use key-in-knob locks; they are easy to pry off. Do not use mortised locks because they create a very weak spot in the door. Use a dead bolt and a strike plate held in place by screws three inches or longer. The more tumblers a lock has, the harder it is to pick.

- *Window locks*—Use security latches on windows. Tenants must be able to easily open windows in an emergency.

These are just a few of the security measures you should consider. Hiring security consultants who can analyze your property could be dollars well spent.

Liability of Manager

Managers have been held liable for failure to comply with health and safety ordinances, as well as for building code violations. If funds are not available for compliance, it would be in the manager's best interest to give up management.

Managing for Foreign Owners

Property managers who remit rent payments to a foreign owner must withhold 30%, unless exempt by tax treaty. Failure to comply can result in manager liability for 30% of gross rent plus penalties and interest.

MANAGEMENT AGREEMENT

It makes no difference whether the property involved is an office building, a residential property, or a shopping center; the responsibilities assumed by the manager are so important that they warrant a written agreement. The **management agreement** formalizes the relationship between the owner and the manager and points out the rights, and duties of each party. The forms used for this purpose may vary, but regardless of the property involved, certain basic points must be included:

- Identification of the parties

- Sufficient identification of the property

- The contract period, including the beginning and the termination dates

- Management's and owner's responsibilities

- Management fees—the amount, when it is to be paid, and the manner of payment

- Provision for management accounting, including records to be kept and reports to be made

> Management fees are usually a percentage of the gross, not the net.

Management fees can cover one or a combination of the following:

- Flat fees

- Minimum fee

- Minimum plus percentage of the gross (very common compensation)

- Leasing fee (flat fee or a percentage of the lease rental; generally a higher percentage for the first year and a lower percentage for subsequent years)

- Additional fees or percentages for special services, such as drafting leases, supervising repairs, remodeling, handling evictions, overseeing contracts, and collecting delinquent accounts of former tenants

In addition, management contracts provide for reimbursement of costs, which may or may not include such items as advertising. Generally, the more management problems a property has, the higher the management fee percentage. Larger properties tend to be managed at lower percentages.

Figure 15.1 is the Property Management Agreement Form 590 prepared by RPI — Realty Publications, Inc., This excellent form is self-explanatory.

FIGURE 15.1:   Property Management Agreement

PROPERTY MANAGEMENT AGREEMENT

NOTE: This form is used by a licensed broker or their agent when entering into an employment to act as a property manager for an owner's rental property, to document the employment and set forth the rights, responsibilities and expectations of the property manager and the landlord, including authorized activities, performance standards and expense limitations.

DATE: _____, 20_____, at _____, California.

Items left blank or unchecked are not applicable.

1. **RETAINER PERIOD:**

   1.1   Owner hereby retains and grants Broker the exclusive right to lease, rent, operate and maintain the property as Property Manager, commencing _____, 20_____, and continuing for one year and thereafter until terminated.

2. **RECEIPT OF SECURITY DEPOSITS:**

   2.1   Owner hands $_____ to Broker for deposit into the trust account towards Owner's security deposit obligation to Tenants.

3. **RECEIPT OF CASH RESERVE:**

   3.1   Owner hands $_____ to Broker as a deposit towards Owner's obligation under the agreement.

   3.2   Owner to maintain a minimum cash reserve, in addition to any security deposits, in the amount of $_____. On request from Broker, Owner will advance additional funds to maintain this minimum balance.

   3.3   The cash reserve may be used to pay costs diligently incurred by Broker or due Broker in fulfilling Broker's obligations.

4. **BROKERAGE FEE:**

   NOTICE: The amount or rate of real estate fees is not fixed by law. They are set by each Broker individually and are negotiable between Owner and Broker.

   4.1   Broker compensation to be:

   a.   _____% of all rents collected and deposited by Broker during the month, except for any first month's rent for which a Broker fee is paid under §4.1 b as follows,

   b.   _____% of the first month's rent collected and deposited under ☐ rental agreements, and ☐ leases,

   c.   All sums remaining from credit check fees in excess of credit report expenses, and

   d.   ☐ Late payment charges and returned check charges paid by a tenant.

5. **TRUST ACCOUNT:**

   5.1   Broker will place Owner's deposit for costs and security deposits into

   ☐ Broker's trust account, or ☐ separate trust account for Owner, maintained with

   _____ at their _____ branch

   a.   This account will be ☐ non-interest bearing, or ☐ interest bearing.

   5.2   All funds received by Broker for the account of Owner will be placed in the trust account.

   5.3   Amounts to pay and satisfy the obligations incurred by Broker may be disbursed from the account after payment is due.

   5.4   On termination of this agreement, Broker will return to Owner all remaining trust funds belonging to Owner.

6. **PERIODIC ACCOUNTING:**

   6.1   Within ten days after each calendar ☐ month, or ☐ quarter, and on termination of this agreement, Broker will deliver to Owner a Statement of Account for all receipts and expenditures, together with a check to Owner for any funds in excess of minimum reserves under §3.2.

   6.2   Amounts to compensate Broker under §4 may be withdrawn from the trust account.

   6.3   Each Statement of Account delivered by Broker will include no less than the following information for the period:

   a.   Amount of security deposits received or refunded.

   b.   Amount of rent or receipts, itemized by unit.

   c.   An itemized description of disbursements.

   d.   End of month balance of the income, expense and security deposit trust accounts.

   6.4   ☐ Broker to reserve and disburse from the trust account any property and employee taxes, special assessments, insurance premiums, loan payments and other payments required to be made by the owner.

   6.5   Advertising costs incurred to locate new tenants to be paid ☐ by Owner, or ☐ by Broker.

FIGURE 15.1 (continue): Property Management Agreement

7. **TITLE CONDITION AND LOANS:**

7.1 The property is referred to as _____

_____

_____

_____.

7.2 Owner's interest in the property is:

☐ Fee simple, ☐ _____

7.3 Loan payments are to be timely disbursed by Broker to:

a. Lender _____

Address _____

_____

_____

Phone _____

Payment of $_____, due on the _____ day and delinquent on the _____ day of each month.

b. Lender _____

Address _____

_____

_____

Phone _____

Payment of $_____, due on the _____ day and delinquent on the _____ day of each month.

8. **BROKER AGREES TO:**

8.1 Use diligence in the performance of this employment.

8.2 Continuously maintain a California real estate broker's license.

8.3 Collect all rents, security deposits or other charges and expenses due Owner, and timely refund tenants' security deposits, less allowable deductions and including any interest due tenants.

8.4 Prepare and place advertisements for prospective tenants.

8.5 Show property to prospective tenants, obtain credit reports and confirm creditworthiness of tenants before executing rental or lease agreements.

8.6 Execute, renegotiate or cancel rental or lease agreements with tenants.

No lease to exceed _____ months.

8.7 Serve rent collection and other notices, file unlawful detainer and money damage actions, recover possession of premises or settle with delinquent tenants.

8.8 Inspect the property monthly and each unit when tenants vacate.

8.9 Maintain and periodically confirm the inventory of personal property on premises.

8.10 Evaluate rental and lease agreements periodically for income, expense and provision updates.

8.11 Contract for utilities, services and equipment to operate and maintain the property and safeguard the tenants.

8.12 Contract for any repairs, maintenance or improvements needed to rent or lease the property.

a. Owner to approve all repairs in excess of $_____.

8.13 Obligate Owner to no unauthorized agreement or liability.

8.14 Protect and enhance the goodwill of Owner's rental business and keep confidential and secure any knowledge of Owner's business activities acquired during this employment.

8.15 Hire, supervise and discharge ☐ a resident manager, and ☐ an assistant resident manager.

8.16 Inspect and take any action necessary to comply with federal, state, county or municipal safety and building codes affecting the property.

8.17 Notify Owner of any potential hazards to the tenants or property, and Owner to respond within seven (7) days. Should an emergency situation arise placing the tenants or property in jeopardy, Broker may immediately remedy the situation without further authority from Owner.

9. **OWNER AGREES TO:**

9.1 Hand Broker all keys and entry codes to the property, and copies of rental and lease agreements with existing tenants.

9.2 Hand Broker (if Broker is to disburse) loan payment coupons/envelopes, property tax bills, insurance premium billings and _____.

9.3 Indemnify Broker for the expense of any legal action arising out of Broker's proper performance of this agreement.

FIGURE 15.1 (continue):   **Property Management Agreement**

9.4   Provide public liability, property damage and workers' compensation insurance sufficient in amount to protect Broker and Owner, naming Broker as an additional insured.

9.5   Owner's insurance agent is _____

10. TERMINATION:

10.1   This agreement will continue until terminated by mutual written agreement or until either party, for legally justifiable cause, serves a written Notice of Termination. [See **RPI** Form 590-2]

10.2   Owner may terminate this agreement at any time during the initial one-year term by paying Broker a fee equal to three times Broker's management fee earned during the month preceding termination.

10.3   On termination, Owner will assume the obligation of any contract entered into by Broker under this agreement.

11. GENERAL PROVISIONS:

11.1   Broker is authorized to place a For Rent/Lease sign on the property and publish and disseminate property information.

11.2   Owner authorizes Broker to cooperate with other brokers and divide with them any compensation due.

11.3   The authorized agent-for-service is ☐ Broker, ☐ Owner, ☐ _____

11.4   Broker may have or will contract to represent Owners of comparable properties or represent Tenants seeking comparable properties during the retainer period. Thus, a conflict of interest exists to the extent Broker's time is required to fulfill the fiduciary duty owed to others he now does or will represent.

11.5   Before any party to this agreement files an action on a dispute arising out of this agreement which remains unresolved after 30 days of informal negotiations, the parties agree to enter into non-binding mediation administered by a neutral dispute resolution organization and undertake a good faith effort during mediation to settle the dispute.

11.6   The prevailing party in any action on a dispute will be entitled to attorney fees and costs, unless they file an action without first offering to enter into mediation to resolve the dispute.

11.7   If this agreement authorizes Property Manager to execute and negotiate lease terms greater than one year, Landlord acknowledges receipt of the Agency Law Disclosure. [See **RPI** Form 305]

11.8   ☐ See attached addendum(s) for additional terms. [See **RPI** Form 250]

11.9   _____
_____
_____

Broker:	**Owner:**
I agree to render services on the terms stated above.	**I agree to employ Broker on the terms stated above.**
☐ See attached Signature Page Addendum. [**RPI** Form 251]	☐ See attached Signature Page Addendum. [**RPI** Form 251]
Date: _____, 20_____	
Broker's Name: _____	Date: _____, 20_____
Broker's CalBRE #: _____	Owner: _____
Agent: _____	Signature: _____
Agent's CalBRE #: _____	Owner: _____
Signature: _____	Signature: _____
Address: _____	Address: _____
_____	_____
Phone: _____ Cell: _____	Phone: _____ Cell: _____
Email: _____	Email: _____

FORM 590	11-15	©2015 **RPI — Realty Publications, Inc.**, P.O. BOX 5707, RIVERSIDE, CA 92517

ACCOUNTING RECORDS

Although the number of bookkeeping records needed depends on the type of property managed and the volume of business involved, the selection and maintenance of an adequate trust fund accounting system is essential in property management because of the fiduciary nature of the business. The responsibility for trust fund records is placed with the property management broker. The trust fund requirements set forth in Unit 3 are applicable to property managers and must be complied with. It is further recommended that an outside accountant be employed to review and audit the accounting system.

Reasons for Accounting Records

There are a number of basic reasons for keeping orderly records in property management:

- The law states that a separate record must be kept for each managed property.

- The fiduciary relationship between the owner and the manager dictates full disclosure.

- Contractual relationships call for an accounting of all funds.

- Records are needed for income tax purposes.

- It may be necessary to satisfy third parties who have an interest in the property.

- Accurate records serve as controls in evaluating income and expenses, analyzing costs, and preparing budgets.

- Records provide the broker with a source of information when inquiries are made or problems arise.

In the days before computers, property managers relied on file systems for each property, with file cards for each tenant. The only time the manager really understood the operating conditions of a property was when the monthly account was tabulated to show income received and disbursements. Computer programs now provide property managers with instant access to property data on one property, on a group of properties, or even on one tenant. These programs have reduced the paperwork of property management.

Computer programs for property management range in cost from only a few hundred dollars to around $10,000. Most computer companies offer free demonstration disks so you can see what a program can do. The following are just a few of the firms offering programs that are likely to meet your property management needs:

- Yardi   www.yardi.com

- AppFolio   www.appfolio.com

- Buildium   www.buildium.com

WEB LINK

@

An unusual program is the Yield Star Price Optimizer (www.realpage .com/yieldstar/price-optimizer-difference/). It allows property managers to update pricing based on real-time information as to leasing and availability of units. According to Camden Property Trust, one of the nation's largest residential REITs, it allows higher rents faster than competitors in a rising market and faster adjustments in a down market.

Today, to operate a property management firm without computer assistance would be like running a brokerage office without the internet. It is possible, but it is not very efficient.

Some Property Management Tasks That Can Be Performed by Computer

- Trust journals
- Security deposit registries
- Monthly, quarterly, semiannual, and annual financial reports
- Accounts payable ledger
- Accounts receivable ledger
- Operating account deposits
- Tenant registries
- Vacancies
- Rental analysis
- Rental summary
- Rent increase calendar
- Automatic billing
- Late charges
- Late-charge reports
- Late letters
- Notices and unlawful detainer
- Market rent variances
- Rent receipts
- Property fees
- Payment histories
- Owner's checks and/or billing
- Owner's ledger
- Owner's income/loss
- Bad-check report
- Tenant data
- Check registry
- Check writing
- Insurance register
- Lease expiration register
- Mortgage check register
- Comparative lease analysis
- Inactive property files
- Repair orders
- Lease abstracts
- Vendor lists
- Vendor history (by vendor)
- Insurance expiration data
- Tickler files (scheduling payments)
- Association fees
- Owner's 1099s
- Hold-back (reserves) register
- Checkbook reconciliation
- Budgets (monthly and annual)
- Maintenance history
- Repetitive correspondence

Trust Ledger

Section 2830 of the commissioner's regulations requires that a **trust ledger** for property management accounts be established. As rents come in, they are posted to the owner's account. Also recorded in the trust ledger is the money paid out on behalf of the owner. This includes any repair costs, payments of encumbrances, and payments for utilities or commissions. These expenses are charged against the income of the property, and the manager sends a statement to the owner at the end of each month. Again, trust records today generally are kept using computer software.

IRS Reporting

Any person who receives rental income must provide IRS Form 1099 for all service providers of $600 or more.

LEASEHOLD ESTATES

One of the responsibilities of a property manager involves leasing the property or acting as a consultant when drawing up the terms of the lease.

A leasehold estate arises when an owner or a property manager acting as the owner's agent grants a tenant the right to occupy the owner's property for a specified period for a consideration. The *lessor* is the owner and the *lessee* is the tenant.

Basic Types of Leasehold Estates

There are four basic types of leasehold estates, based on the length and nature of their duration: the estate for years, the estate from period to period, the estate at sufferance, and the estate at will.

> An estate for years has a definite termination date.

Estate for years.   An estate that continues for a definite fixed period of time is an **estate for years**. The lease may be for any specified length of time, even for less than a year, measured in days, weeks, or months. Professional property managers will generally insist on an estate for years.

Estate from period to period.   An estate from period to period is commonly called a **periodic tenancy**. The lease continues from period to period (either year to year, month to month, or week to week), as designated. The most common periodic tenancy is month to month.

A periodic tenancy can be ended by a notice for the length of the rent-paying period but for no more than 30 days (60 days for mobile homes). However, if a residential tenant has lived on the premises for at least 12 months, a landlord must provide a 60-day notice to terminate the tenancy.

If a tenant is under a rental agreement with a government agency, in certain Section 8 housing situations, a 90-day notice must be given to terminate.

The lessor can change lease terms on a periodic tenancy by providing a tenant a 30-day written notice; however, if the rent is increased more than 10% during a 12-month period, then a 60-day notice is required.

Estate at sufferance. An **estate at sufferance** is created when a tenant obtains possession of property legally but then remains on the property without the owner's consent, such as a holdover tenant after the expiration of the leasehold interest. A tenant at sufferance would need to be evicted from the property and cannot simply be ejected as a trespasser would. If the lessor accepts rent, the estate then becomes a periodic tenancy based on the rent-paying period.

Estate at will. An **estate at will** has no specified time limit. Possession is given with permission, but no agreement is made as to rent. As an example, possession is given to a prospective tenant before the lease terms are agreed to. In California, such an estate requires a **30-day notice** to terminate.

Types of Leases

The three basic lease forms the property manager will be expected to work with are the gross lease, the net lease, and the percentage lease.

Gross lease. Under a **gross lease**, the tenant pays a fixed rental and the owner pays all other expenses for the property. Most residential leases and small commercial leases on office buildings are gross leases. As an example, the typical month-to-month lease is for a gross amount.

To keep a tenant on a gross lease from holding over at the end of the term, the lease might include a **holdover clause**, which materially raises the rent when the lease period expires. This encourages the tenant to either sign a new lease or vacate the premises.

Net lease means the owner gets a net amount and property expenses are paid by the tenant. Payments are similar to an annuity.

Net lease. Under the terms of a **net lease**, besides a basic rent, building expenses are passed on to the tenant. There are three types of net leases:

- Single net lease—The tenant pays the taxes and the base rent.

- Double net lease—The tenant pays for the insurance, as well as taxes and base rent.

- Triple net lease—In addition to taxes, insurance, and base rent, the tenant is responsible for all property maintenance and repairs.

The term *net lease* is generally used in reference to a triple net lease.

Net leases are generally long-term leases and often are found in sale-lease-backs and where buildings are constructed for a particular tenant. The buyer (investor) wants a stated return. To keep the same relative purchasing power, the lessor on a net lease generally wants the net amount tied to an inflationary index, such as the Consumer Price Index.

Percentage lease.   A **percentage lease** generally provides for a stated percentage of the gross receipts of a business to be paid as rent. Generally, the percentage lease is tied in with a minimum rent and a covenant to remain in business. The percentage lease also might include hours of operation and a prohibition against the lessee's conducting offsite "warehouse" sales.

Percentage leases are typically used in shopping centers, where each business aids other businesses. Shopping center leases may have a requirement that a separate percentage of the gross be used for cooperative advertising in newspaper supplements or on radio or TV.

In addition, a percentage lease may include a **recapture clause**, which provides that should a tenant not obtain a desired gross, then the lessor has the right to terminate the lease.

Leases may combine features; for example, a basic gross lease plus a percentage of the gross. What can be done with leases is limited only by the imagination of the parties.

Figure 15.2 shows typical percentages charged for different businesses having percentage leases. In determining the percentage of gross sales that must be paid by the lessee, the greater the tenant's markup, the higher the percentage on the lease (e.g., 50% on a parking lot rental and 2% on a supermarket rental). Percentages will vary based on vacancy factors, alternative locations, quality of goods sold, traffic count, et cetera.

A tenant having a higher percentage markup on sales should be able to pay a higher percentage of sales as rent.

Various professional associations publish average percentages currently being charged for different types of businesses. Lessors, of course, want the maximum percentage possible that will still allow the business to remain a viable entity. Typically, a percentage lease will include an audit provision that allows a landlord the ability to periodically audit the books of a tenant to determine whether they are reporting all their income to the landlord.

Step-up lease. A **step-up lease** has a fixed rent like a gross lease, but it provides for increases at set periods. Increases may be predetermined or according to a definite formula. For example, a 10-year lease at $2,000 per month could provide for a $100 monthly increase in rent every two years, so that the rent would be $2,400 for the last two years of the lease. As an alternative, the lease could provide that the rent increase would be made annually based on the percentage increase in the consumer price index.

RESIDENTIAL LEASING

Most rentals are residential, and most property managers are primarily involved in residential leases. The property manager has a duty to the owner to use care in the selection of tenants. The most important decision any property manager makes is, *Who do I rent to?* A tenant who has no desire to pay rent or is destructive, or both, is worse than having no tenant at all. As protection, property managers should not allow occupancy to a prospective tenant until that person is cleared as being a desirable tenant for the property and the deposit and rent checks have cleared.

FIGURE 15.2: Typical Lease Percentages Charged

Type of Business	Percentage of Gross Sales
Liquor stores	1.5–5
Card and gift	3–6
Drugstores	2.5–4
Jewelry	7 and up
Pet stores	5–8
Restaurants	4–7
Grocer and supermarkets	1–2

Rental Application

Figure 15.3 is an Application to Rent by RPI — Realty Publications, Inc. You can see that the application requires personal information, as well as financial data and employment information.

Many lessors also require a copy of the prospective lessee's last pay stub, which serves to verify income. As a minimum, the lessor should verify the present employment and length of employment with the present employer, as well as check with present or prior landlords regarding any problems they may have had. Keep in mind that you must similarly check all tenants, or you could be in violation of one or more of the fair housing laws.

It is also a good practice to see and make a copy of the prospective tenant's driver's license. This will show you that the applicant is who he claims to be, as well as provide you with a previous address.

Although the civil rights law prohibits discrimination for reasons of race, sex, age, national origin, and so forth (Unit 2), there are valid reasons for discrimination. You can discriminate against a tenant who has had problems with other tenants at a previous rental, was late in making payments, broke rules, damaged the property, left owing rent, or generally has had a poor work or credit history. You don't have to accept a problem tenant. It is a lot easier to refuse a rental than it is to rectify a mistake once it is made.

Lease Provisions

A landlord may charge a nonrefundable screening fee.

You are allowed to charge a nonrefundable screening fee of up to a certain maximum amount. The maximum fee is adjusted each year based on changes in the Consumer Price Index since January 1, 1998, when the fee was $35. The change is indexed for inflation. (The fee is adjusted annually to reflect the cost of living index.) This fee is to cover the costs of obtaining and gathering information to make an acceptance or rejection decision regarding a tenant. The fee is adjusted annually for inflation (Civil Code 1950.6).

Civil Code Section 2924.85, requires rental applicants be given notice that an owner has received a notice of default and that there is a pending foreclosure.

Even though you are renting on a month-to-month basis, you should nevertheless use a written rental agreement that clearly sets forth lessor and lessee duties and obligations. If you have apartment rules or regulations, they should be attached to the lease or rental agreement and signed by the tenant.

Don't try to draft a lease or use sections from a number of leases for a "cut and paste" lease. You could be personally liable for errors or omissions, and it also could be considered the unauthorized practice of law. If a simple form lease, such as the short term Residential Lease Agreement published by RPI—Realty , (Figure 15.4), is not appropriate, consult an attorney. You will note that the lease form provides for some of the disclosures covered in Unit 3. When the appropriate block is checked, this form can be used for a month-to-month rental or a lease with a definite termination date.

If a lease is negotiated in Spanish, Chinese, Tagalog, Vietnamese, or Korean, the lease (as well as other contracts) must include a translation in the language in which it was negotiated.

Name of parties.   Any lease should include the full names of all parties. If any person is younger than 18, you ordinarily would need a cosigner unless the underage party qualifies as an emancipated minor by reason of marriage, is an active military service member, or has been declared emancipated by a court. In signing the lease, the parties should sign "jointly and severally," so it is clear that each signer is liable for the entire rent and you can go to one or to all tenants for the rent.

FIGURE 15.3:   Application to Rent

APPLICATION TO RENT

| Prepared by: Agent _____ | Phone _____ |
| Broker _____ | Email _____ |

DATE: _____, 20_____, at _____, California.

THIS CREDIT APPLICATION is for payment of monthly rent in the amount of $_____.

Property address: _____

Received from Applicant(s) $_____, ☐ cash, or ☐ check, for a consumer credit report which is a non-refundable cost and not a deposit.

Received from Applicant(s) $_____, ☐ cash, or ☐ check, as a deposit toward the first month's rent on Landlord's acceptance of the applicant's creditworthiness.

Applicant(s):

Applicant One _____ Date of Birth ____/____/_____
(Name)

    Social Sec. # _____ Drivers Lic. # _____ State___

    Phone _____ Cell _____ Email _____

Applicant Two _____ Date of Birth ____/____/_____
(Name)

    Social Sec. # _____ Drivers Lic. # _____ State___

    Phone _____ Cell _____ Email _____

Additional Occupant(s): Name _____

                          Name _____

Rental History: Have you ever been party to an eviction? ☐ Yes ☐ No   Filed bankruptcy? ☐ Yes ☐ No

Present Address _____

    City _____ Zip _____

    Length of Residency _____ Monthly Rent $_____

    Landlord/Agent _____ DRE # _____

    Address _____

    Phone _____ Cell _____ Email _____

    Reason for Moving _____ Moving Date ____/____/_____

Previous Address _____

    City _____ Zip _____

    Length of Residence _____ Monthly Rent $_____

    Landlord/Agent _____ DRE # _____

    Address _____

    Phone _____ Cell _____ Email _____

Employment:

Applicant One

    Employer _____

    Address _____

    Phone _____ Cell _____ Email _____

    Length of Employment _____ Position _____ Wages _____

    Pay Period _____ Union _____

    Previous Employer _____

    Address _____

    Phone _____ Cell _____ Email _____

Applicant Two

    Employer _____

    Address _____

    Phone _____ Cell _____ Email _____

    Length of Employment _____ Position _____ Wages _____

    Pay Period _____ Union _____

— — — — — — — — — — — — — *PAGE ONE OF TWO — FORM 553* — — — — — — — — — — — — —

FIGURE 15.3 (continued): Application to Rent

— — — — — — — — — — — — — — — PAGE TWO OF TWO — FORM 553 — — — — — — — — — — — — — — — —

Previous Employer _____

Address _____

Phone _____ Cell _____ Email _____

Additional Income Amount $_____ Source _____

Recipient _____

General Credit Information:

Automobile One: Make _____

    Year _____ Model _____ Lic. #/State _____

    Lender _____

Automobile Two: Make _____

    Year _____ Model _____ Lic. #/State _____

    Lender _____

Bank/branch _____

    Check Acc. # _____ Savings Acc. # _____

Bank/branch _____

    Check Acc. # _____ Savings Acc. # _____

Credit References:

    1. _____

    Address _____

    Account # _____ Balance due $_____ Phone _____

    2. _____

    Address _____

    Account # _____ Balance due $_____ Phone _____

Personal Reference _____

    Address _____

    Phone _____ Cell _____ Email _____

Personal Reference _____

    Address _____

    Phone _____ Cell _____ Email _____

Nearest Relative (name/relationship) _____

    Address _____

    Phone _____ Cell _____ Email _____

Emergency Contact (name/relationship) _____

    Address _____

    Phone _____ Cell _____ Email _____

I/We declare all information given in this application is true and correct. I/We authorize your credit reporting agency to obtain and verify a complete consumer report and supply the information obtained to you. This information is not privileged.

Date: _____, 20_____

Name: _____

Signature: _____
                         (Applicant 1)

Name: _____

Signature: _____
                         (Applicant 2)

I acknowledge receipt of this credit application and accompanying payment.

Landlord: _____

Signature: _____

Phone: _____

Email: _____

FORM 553   **02-14**   © 2014 **first tuesday**, P.O. Box 5707, RIVERSIDE, CA 92517 (800) 794-0494

FIGURE 15.4: Residential Lease Agreement

THIS FORM FOR USE
IN CALIFORNIA ONLY

Real Estate Forms
Since 1966

RESIDENTIAL LEASE-RENTAL AGREEMENT
AND DEPOSIT RECEIPT

AGENCY RELATIONSHIP CONFIRMATION. The following agency relationship is hereby confirmed for this transaction and supersedes any prior agency election (If no agency relationship insert "NONE"):

LISTING AGENT: _____ is the agent of (check one):

(Print Firm Name)

☐ **the Owner exclusively; or** ☐ **both the Tenant and the Owner.**

LEASING AGENT: _____ (if not the same as the Listing Agent) is the agent of (check one):

(Print Firm Name)

☐ **the Tenant exclusively; or** ☐ **the Owner exclusively; or** ☐ **both the Tenant and the Owner.**

Note: This confirmation DOES NOT take the place of the AGENCY DISCLOSURE form (such as P.P. Form 110.42 CAL) required by law if the term exceeds one year.

RECEIVED FROM _____, hereinafter referred to as Tenant,
the sum of $_____ (_____
dollars), evidenced by _____, as a deposit. Upon acceptance of this Agreement, the Owner of the premises, will apply the deposit as follows:

	TOTAL	RECEIVED	BALANCE DUE PRIOR TO OCCUPANCY
Rent for the period from _____ to _____ .	$_____	$_____	$_____
Security deposit (not applicable toward last month's rent)	$_____	$_____	$_____
Other _____	$_____	$_____	$_____
TOTAL	$_____	$_____	$_____

In the event this Agreement is not accepted by the Owner, **within** _____ **days**, the total deposit received will be refunded.

Tenant offers to rent from the Owner the premises situated in the City of _____,
County of _____, State of California, commonly known as _____
_____,

upon the following **terms and conditions:**

1. **TERM.** The term will commence on _____, and continue (**check one of the two following alternatives**):
   ☐ LEASE until _____, for a total rent of $_____ (_____
   _____ dollars).
   ☐ RENTAL on a month-to-month basis, until either party terminates this Agreement by giving the other party written notice as required by law.

2. **RENT.** Rent will be $_____, per month, payable in advance by personal check, cashier's check, cash or money order, on the _____ day of each calendar month to Owner or his or her authorized agent, by mail or personal delivery to the following address:
   _____
   or at such other place as may be designated by Owner in writing from time to time. Payment by personal delivery may be made (check one): ☐ Monday through Friday, 9:00 a.m. to 5:00 p.m., or ☐ at the following times: _____
   _____. In the event rent is not received by Owner in full **within** ____ **days** after due date, Tenant agrees that it would be impracticable or extremely difficult to fix the actual damages to Owner caused by that failure, and Tenant agrees to pay a **late charge** of $_____. Tenant further agrees to pay $ 25.00 for each dishonored bank check. All late fees and returned check fees will be considered additional rent. The late charge period is not a grace period, and Owner is entitled to make written demand for any rent if not paid when due and to collect interest thereon. Any unpaid balance including late charges, will bear interest at 10% per annum, or the maximum rate allowed by law, whichever is less.

3. **MULTIPLE OCCUPANCY.** It is expressly understood that this Agreement is between the Owner and each signatory jointly and severally. Each signatory will be responsible for timely payment of rent and performance of all other provisions of this Agreement.

4. **UTILITIES.** Tenant will be responsible for the payment of all utilities and services, except: _____
   _____, which will be paid by Owner.

5. **USE.** The premises will be used exclusively as a residence for no more than _____ persons. Guests staying more than a total of _____ days in a calendar year without written consent of Owner will constitute a violation of this Agreement. Tenant shall park operable automobiles in assigned spaces only. Trailers, boats, campers, and inoperable vehicles are not allowed without the written consent of Owner. Tenant may not repair motor vehicles on the leased premises.

6. **ANIMALS.** No animals will be brought on the premises without the prior consent of the Owner; except _____.

7. **RULES AND REGULATIONS.** In the event that the premises is a portion of a building containing more than one unit, or is located in a common interest development, Tenant agrees to abide by all applicable rules, whether adopted before or after the date of this Agreement, including rules with respect to noise, odors, disposal of refuse, animals, parking, and use of common areas. Tenant will

Tenant [_____] [_____] [_____] [_____] has read this page.

Page 1 of 4
FORM 105.1 CAL (10-2012) COPYRIGHT BY PROFESSIONAL PUBLISHING LLC, NOVATO, CA

Form generated by: TrueForms™ www.TrueForms.com 800-499-9612

PROFESSIONAL PUBLISHING

FIGURE 15.4 (continue):   Residential Lease Agreement

Property Address _____

pay any penalties , including attorney fees, imposed by homeowners' association for violations by tenant or tenant's guests.

8. **ORDINANCES AND STATUTES.** Tenant will comply with all statutes, ordinances, and requirements of all municipal, state and federal authorities now in force, or which may later be in force, regarding the use of the premises. Tenant will not use the premises for any unlawful purpose including, but not limited to, using, storing or selling prohibited drugs. If the premises are located in a rent control area, the Tenant should contact the Rent and Arbitration Board for his or her legal rights.

9. **ASSIGNMENT AND SUBLETTING.** Tenant will not assign this Agreement or sublet any portion of the premises without prior written consent of the Owner.

10. **MAINTENANCE, REPAIRS, OR ALTERATIONS.** Tenant acknowledges that, unless the Owner is notified immediately upon occupancy, the premises, including the furniture, furnishings and appliances, including all electrical, gas and plumbing fixtures, are in good working order and repair. Tenant will keep the premises in a clean and sanitary condition, and will immediately notify Owner of any damage to the premises or its contents, or any inoperable equipment or appliances. Tenant will surrender the premises, at termination, in as good condition as received, normal wear and tear excepted. Tenant will be responsible for any damage, repairs or replacements, caused by Tenant's negligence and that of the tenant's family, invitees, and guests, except ordinary wear and tear. **Verification of the working order (using the "test" button) and the maintenance of both the smoke detector(s) and carbon monoxide detector(s) is the responsibility of the Tenant.** Tenant will not commit any waste upon the premises, or any nuisance or act which may disturb the quiet enjoyment of any neighbors. Tenant will not paint, paper or otherwise redecorate or make alterations to the premises without the prior written consent of the Owner. Tenant will irrigate and maintain any surrounding grounds, including lawns and shrubbery, if they are for the Tenant's exclusive use. **It is understood that Owner's insurance does not cover Tenant's personal property.**

11. **INVENTORY.** Any furnishings and/or equipment to be furnished by Owner will be listed in a special inventory. The inventory will be signed by both Tenant and Owner concurrently with this Lease. Tenant will keep the furnishings and equipment in good condition and repair, and will be responsible for any damage to them other than normal wear and tear. Tenant acknowledges receipt of _____ sets of keys, _____ garage door openers, other: _____

12. **DAMAGES TO PREMISES.** If the premises are damaged by fire, earthquake or other casualty which renders the premises totally or partially uninhabitable, either party will have the right to terminate this Agreement as of the date on which the damage occurs. Written notice of termination will be given to the other party **within fifteen (15) days after occurrence** of such damage. Should such damage or destruction occur as the result of the negligence of Tenant, or his or her invitees, then only the Owner will have the right to terminate. Should this right be exercised by either Owner or Tenant, rent for the current month will be prorated between the parties as of the date the damage occurred. Any prepaid rent and unused security deposit will be refunded to Tenant. If this Agreement is not terminated, Owner will promptly repair the premises and there will be a proportionate reduction of rent until the premises are repaired and ready for Tenant's occupancy. The proportionate reduction will be based on the extent which repairs interfere with Tenant's reasonable use of the premises.

13. **ENTRY AND INSPECTION.** Owner and owners agents will have the right to enter the premises: (a) in case of emergency; (b) to make necessary or agreed repairs, decorations, alterations, improvements, supply necessary or agreed services, inspect the condition of the property, show the premises to prospective or actual purchasers, lenders, tenants, workers, or contractors; (c) when tenant has abandoned or surrendered the premises. Except under (a) and (c), entry may be made only during normal business hours, and with at least 24 hours prior written notice to Tenant including the date, approximate time, and purpose of entry.

   If the purpose of the entry is to exhibit the dwelling unit to prospective or actual purchasers, the notice may be given orally, in person or by telephone, if the owner or his or her agent has notified the tenant in writing within 120 days of the oral notice that the property is for sale. At the time of entry, the Owner or agent shall leave written evidence of the entry inside the unit.

14. **INDEMNIFICATION.** Owner will not be liable for any damage or injury to Tenant, or any other person, or to any property, occurring on the premises, or in common areas, unless such damage is the legal result of the negligence or willful misconduct of Owner, his or her agents, or employees. Tenant agrees to hold Owner harmless from any claims for damages, no matter how caused, except for injury or damages caused by negligence or willful misconduct of Owner, his or her agents or employees.

15. **PHYSICAL POSSESSION.** If Owner is unable to deliver possession of the premises at the commencement date set forth above, Owner will not be liable for any damage caused, nor will this Agreement be void or voidable, but Tenant will not be liable for any rent until possession is delivered. Tenant may terminate this Agreement if possession is not delivered **within _____ days** of the commencement of the term in Item 1.

16. **DEFAULT.** If Tenant fails to pay rent when due, or perform any provision of this Agreement, after not less than **three (3) days written notice** of such default given in the manner required by law, the Owner, at his or her option, may terminate all rights of Tenant, unless Tenant, within said time, cures such default. If Tenant abandons or vacates the property while in default of the payment of rent, Owner may consider any property left on the premises to be abandoned and may dispose of the same in any manner allowed by law. In the event the Owner reasonably believes that such abandoned property has no value, it may be discarded. All property on the premises will be subject to a lien for the benefit of Owner securing the payment of all sums due, to the maximum extent allowed by law.

   In the event of a default by Tenant, Owner may elect to: (a) continue the lease in effect and enforce all his rights and remedies, including the right to recover the rent as it becomes due, provided that Owner's consent to assignment or subletting by the Tenant will not be unreasonably withheld; or (b) at any time, terminate all of Tenant's rights and recover from Tenant all damages he or she may incur by reason of the breach of the lease, including the cost of recovering the premises, and including the worth at the time of such termination, or at the time of an award if suit be instituted to enforce this provision, of the amount by which the unpaid rent for the balance of the term exceeds the amount of such rental loss which the Tenant proves could be reasonably avoided.

Tenant [_____] [_____] [_____] [_____] has read this page.

Page 2 of 4
FORM 105.2 CAL (10-2012) COPYRIGHT BY PROFESSIONAL PUBLISHING LLC, NOVATO, CA

PROFESSIONAL PUBLISHING

Form generated by: **TrueForms**™   **www.TrueForms.com**   800-499-9612

FIGURE 15.4 (continue):   **Residential Lease Agreement**

Property Address _____

17. SECURITY. The security deposit will secure the performance of Tenant's obligations. Owner may, but will not be obligated to, apply all portions of said deposit on account of Tenant's obligations. Any balance remaining will be returned to Tenant, together with an accounting of any disbursements, **21 calendar days** after the Tenant has vacated the premises, or earlier if required by law. Tenant will not have the right to apply the security deposit in payment of the last month's rent. No interest will be paid to Tenant on account of the security deposit, unless required by local ordinance.

18. WAIVER. Failure of Owner to enforce any provision of this Agreement will not be deemed a waiver. The acceptance of rent by Owner will not waive his or her right to enforce any provision of this Agreement.

19. NOTICES. Unless otherwise provided, any notice which either party may give or is required to give, must be in writing, may be given personally or by mailing the same, postage prepaid, to Tenant at the premises or to Owner or Owner's authorized agent at the address shown in the signature block or at such other places as may be designated by the parties from time to time. Notice will be deemed effective three (3) days after mailing, or on personal delivery, or when receipt is acknowledged in writing.

20. HOLDING OVER. Any holding over after expiration of this Agreement will be (check one):

☐ with the consent of Owner, a month-to-month tenancy at a monthly rent equal to the rent for the month immediately preceding the expiration date, or such other amount as agreed upon by Owner and Tenant. The monthly rent shall be payable in advance and the occupancy subject to all of the other terms and conditions set forth in this Agreement, until either party terminates the tenancy by giving the other party **thirty (30) days (or longer if required by law) written notice**; or

☐ the property is subject to a local rent control ordinance and the holding over will be a month-to-month tenancy with the rent and termination provisions as mandated by the ordinance.

21. TIME. Time is of the essence of this Agreement.

22. ATTORNEY'S FEES. In any action or proceeding involving a dispute between Tenant and Owner arising out of the execution of this Agreement, whether for tort or for breach of contract, and whether or not brought to trial or final judgment, the prevailing party will be entitled to receive from the other party a reasonable attorney fee, expert witness fees, and costs to be determined by the court or arbitrator(s).

23. SUBROGATION. To the maximum extent permitted by insurance policies which may be owned by the parties, Lessor and Lessee waive any and all rights of subrogation against each other which might otherwise exist.

24. FAIR HOUSING. Owner and Tenant understand that the state and federal housing laws prohibit discrimination in the sale, rental, appraisal, financing or advertising of housing on the basis of race, color, religion, sex, sexual orientation, marital status, national origin, ancestry, familial status, source of income, age, mental or physical disability, immigration or citizenship status. In addition, California Civil Code §1940.3 prohibits a landlord from making any inquiry regarding the immigration or citizenship status of any tenant or prospective tenant.

25. SMOKING RESTRICTIONS. Check box: Landlord ☐ does allow smoking, as follows: ☐ in the unit and/or ☐ on the premises, including exterior and common areas. Landlord ☐ does NOT allow smoking in the unit but does allow smoking in exterior areas, but ☐ not including common areas. This applies to tobacco and all other substances. If smoking is further regulated by local laws, tenant agrees to comply. Tenant will inform guests of any smoking restrictions to insure their cooperation.

26. ADDITIONAL TERMS AND CONDITIONS.

_____
_____
_____
_____
_____
_____
_____
_____
_____
_____
_____

27. ☐ This unit is subject to rent control and the agency responsible to adjudicate claims is: _____

28. ENTIRE AGREEMENT. The foregoing constitutes the entire agreement between the parties and may be modified only in writing signed by all parties. This Agreement and any modifications, including any photocopy or facsimile, may be signed in one or more counterparts, each of which will be deemed an original and all of which taken together will constitute one and the same instrument. The following addenda, if checked, have been made a part of this Agreement before the parties' execution:

☐ Addendum _____ : Lead-Based Paint Disclosure (Required by Law for Rental Property Built Prior to 1978)
☐ Addendum _____ : Regarding Mold Contamination and Agreement to Maintain Premises
☐ Addendum _____ : _____
☐ Addendum _____ : _____

NOTICE: Pursuant to Section 290.46 of the Penal Code, information about specified registered sex offenders is made available to the public via an Internet Web site maintained by the Department of Justice at http://www.meganslaw.ca.gov. Depending on an offender's criminal history, this information will include either the address at which the offender resides or the community of residence and ZIP Code in which he or she resides.

Tenant [_____] [_____] [_____] [_____] has read this page.

CAUTION: The copyright laws of the United States forbid the unauthorized reproduction of this form by any means including scanning or computerized formats.

FIGURE 15.4 (continue): **Residential Lease Agreement**

Property Address _____

Tenant _____
(Signature)

_____
(Please Print Name)

Date _____ Telephone _____

Address _____

_____

Email _____

Tenant _____
(Signature)

_____
(Please Print Name)

Date _____ Telephone _____

Address _____

_____

Email _____

Tenant _____
(Signature)

_____
(Please Print Name)

Date _____ Telephone _____

Address _____

_____

Email _____

Tenant _____
(Signature)

_____
(Please Print Name)

Date _____ Telephone _____

Address _____

_____

Email _____

The undersigned Owner accepts the foregoing offer and agrees to lease the premises on the terms and conditions set forth above.

Owner _____
(Signature of Owner or Authorized Agent)

_____
(Please Print Name)

Date _____

Telephone _____ Fax _____

Address _____

_____

Email _____

Owner _____
(Signature)

_____
(Please Print Name)

Date _____

Telephone _____ Fax _____

Address _____

_____

Email _____

Receipt for deposit acknowledged by _____ Date _____

Tenant acknowledges receipt of a copy of the accepted lease on (date) _____

[_____] [_____] [_____] [_____]
initials

CAUTION: The copyright laws of the United States forbid the unauthorized reproduction of this form by any means including scanning or computerized formats.

Page 4 of 4
FORM 105.4 CAL (10-2012) COPYRIGHT BY PROFESSIONAL PUBLISHING LLC, NOVATO, CA

Form generated by: TrueForms™   www.TrueForms.com   800-499-9612

PROFESSIONAL PUBLISHING

Reprinted with permission, Professional Publishing. Endorsement not implied.

Description of premises.   The premises should be described in such a manner that there is no ambiguity. If a parking space or a garage is included, it should be specified.

Dates.   An estate for years must have a beginning date and an ending date. A periodic tenancy would have a beginning date and length of period.

Rent and late charge.   The rent amount or rental formula should be clearly stated, as well as where and when the rent is due. Landlords may not require rent payments be made in cash unless the tenant has previously attempted to pay rent with a check drawn on insufficient funds or has instructed a bank to stop payment on a rent check. Consider late charges for late payments. Keep in mind that if the late charge is too high, a court could determine it to be a penalty and declare it unenforceable.

Pets.   Pet agreements are common in residential leases. Lessors may require an additional deposit and also charge additional rent or limit the size and type of pet allowed. Pet deposits are refundable except for damage amounts. All security deposits cannot exceed California limits.

Water beds.   Common water-bed agreements require the tenant to have a liner on any water bed and to pay for a policy of water-bed insurance, should the water bed cause damage to the premises.

Inspection.   Some leases provide for pre-tenancy walk-through inspections. Deficiencies should be noted on a form provided for this purpose, which should be signed by tenant and landlord. (See Figure 15.5.)

Cleaning and security deposits.   A controversial item in leases and rental agreements is the **security deposit**. The security deposit functions as a form of insurance for the landlord in case the rental premises are left damaged or dirty or rent is owed. According to the law, the amount of the security deposit that may be demanded or received is limited to an amount equal to two months' rent, in the case of unfurnished residential property, and to three months' rent for furnished residential property. Nonrefundable deposits, such as *cleaning deposits*, are not allowed.

FIGURE 15.5: **Condition of Premises Addendum**

CONDITION OF PREMISES ADDENDUM

Prepared by: Agent _____ Phone _____
Broker _____ Email _____

DATE: _____, 20_____, at _____, California.

Items left blank or unchecked are not applicable.

FACTS:

1. This is an addendum to the following agreement:

☐ Lease agreement
☐ Rental agreement
☐ Occupancy agreement

1.1 ☐ of same date, or dated _____, 20_____, at _____, California,
1.2 entered into by _____, as the Landlord, and
1.3 _____, as the Tenant,
1.4 regarding real estate referred to as _____
_____.

AGREEMENT:

2. Landlord and Tenant have jointly inspected the premises and common areas and agree the premises and unchecked items such as fixtures, appliances and furnishings are in a satisfactory and sanitary condition.
3. Check only those items which are unsatisfactory and state why in "REMARKS."

4. **EXTERIOR/COMMON AREAS:**

☐ Garage/parking lot	☐ Garbage facilities	☐ Storage area	☐ TV antenna
☐ Pool/spa	☐ Satellite dish	☐ Patio/decks	☐ CATV hookup
☐ Stairs/railings	☐ Garage door opener(s)	☐ Hallway/lobby	☐ Laundry area
☐ Fencing	☐ Roof	☐ Exterior lighting	☐ Eaves/gutters
☐ Sprinklers/hose	☐ Mailbox	☐ Walkways	☐ _____

5. **ENTRY:**

☐ Door	☐ # of keys _____	☐ Doorbell/knocker	☐ Closet
☐ Intercom/security	☐ Shelves	☐ Locks	☐ _____

6. **KITCHEN:**

☐ Range	☐ Trash compactor	☐ Oven	☐ Water purifier
☐ Refrigerator	☐ Counters/laminate	☐ Garbage disposal	☐ Cabinets/drawers
☐ Exhaust fan(s)	☐ Pantry/shelves	☐ Dishwasher	☐ Tile/linoleum
☐ Microwave	☐ Sink/faucets		

7. **BATHROOM:**

☐ Sink	☐ Tile/linoleum	☐ Faucets/hardware	☐ Closets/shelves
☐ Toilet	☐ Exhaust fan(s)	☐ Shower	☐ Shower enclosure
☐ Tub	☐ Medicine cabinet		

8. **ELECTRICAL:**

☐ Outlets	☐ Lighting	☐ Switchplates	☐ Thermostat
☐ Fixtures	☐ Furnace	☐ Smoke detectors	☐ Ventilation
☐ Air conditioning	☐ _____		

9. **PLUMBING:**

☐ Water heater	☐ Washer	☐ Hot/cold water	☐ Dryer
☐ Gas hookups	☐ _____		

— — — — — — — — — — — — — PAGE ONE OF TWO — FORM 560 — — — — — — — — — — — — — —

©2015 RPI — Realty Publications, Inc., P.O. BOX 5707, RIVERSIDE, CA 92517

FIGURE 15.5 (continued):   Condition of Premises Addendum

— — — — — — — — — — — — — — — — *PAGE TWO OF TWO — FORM 560* — — — — — — — — — — — — — — — — —

10. INTERIOR:

☐ Wall coverings	☐ Floor coverings	☐ Ceilings	☐ Walls
☐ Draperies	☐ Rods/tracks	☐ Glass doors	☐ Windows
☐ Doorknobs	☐ Fireplace	☐ Wood doors	☐ Paint
☐ Floors	☐ Baseboards/trim	☐ Hardware/fittings	☐ Shades
☐ Closets	☐ Screens	☐ Sills/jambs	☐ Kickplates/stops
☐ Chimney/flue			

11. REMARKS:

_____

_____

_____

_____

_____

_____

_____

_____

_____

_____

_____

_____

_____

_____

_____

_____

_____

_____

_____

_____

12. REPAIRS PROMISED:

12.1   _____

_____

Completion date _____

12.2   _____

_____

Completion date _____

I agree to the terms stated above.	**I accept the premises as stated above.**
☐ See attached Signature Page Addendum. [ft Form 251]	☐ See attached Signature Page Addendum. [ft Form 251]
Date: _____, 20_____	Date: _____, 20_____
Landlord/Manager: _____	Tenant: _____
Signature: _____	Signature: _____
Address: _____	Tenant: _____
_____	
Phone: _____Cell: _____	Signature: _____
Fax: _____	Address: _____
Email: _____	_____
	Phone: _____Cell: _____
	Fax: _____
	Email: _____

FORM 560   03-11   ©2011 **first tuesday**, P.O. BOX 20069, RIVERSIDE, CA 92516 (800) 794-0494

Landlords must notify a departing tenant of the tenant's right to be present at a pre-vacancy inspection of the tenant's rental unit. The purpose is to allow the tenant to correct any deficiencies noted.

Nonrefundable tenant deposits are forbidden.

At the termination of the tenancy, the landlord is permitted to retain only that portion of the security deposit reasonably necessary to remedy tenant defaults. The landlord must notify the lessee in writing as to the retention of any portion of the security deposit unless the expenses were less than $125. Copies of receipts for labor and material must be included for amounts deductible from the security deposit. If the landlord must return any portion of the deposit to the tenant, it must be returned within three weeks after tenancy is terminated (60 days for nonresidential tenants). The bad-faith failure to return the security deposit will subject the landlord to actual damages plus a penalty of up to two times the amount of the security deposit. If the landlord defaults on this obligation, the tenant may initiate legal action through an attorney or small-claims court or file a complaint with the Consumer Protection Bureau.

Lease-option arrangement. With a lease-option, usually used when loans are not easily available or the lessor lacks the required down payment, the purchaser leases the property desired with an option to purchase at a later date. A portion of the amount paid as rent usually will be applied against the purchase price. (Options also can be for lease extensions.)

Exculpatory clauses are invalid for residential leases.

Exculpatory clause (hold-harmless clause). Leases frequently contain an **exculpatory clause**, whereby the tenant agrees to relieve the landlord from all liability for injury or property damage resulting from the condition of the property or the negligence of the owner. Many residential leases contain these clauses, but the clauses are invalid for residential leases. Even though the tenant has agreed, the tenant has not given up her rights under the law.

Right of entry. A lease may provide the landlord the right to check the property for specific purposes. In the absence of any agreement, the landlord can enter residential property only under the following circumstances:

■ An emergency requires entry.

■ The tenant consents to an entry.

- The entry is during normal business hours after a reasonable notice (24 hours is considered reasonable) to make necessary or agreed repairs, alterations, or improvements, or to show the property to prospective or actual purchasers, mortgagees, tenants, workers, or contractors; landlord can enter without a 24-hour notice to make repairs requested by the tenant.

- The tenant has abandoned or surrendered the premises.

- The landlord has obtained a court order to enter.

Landlord Disclosures

Residential landlords in California must make the following disclosures to tenants:

- Existence of registered sexual offender database (Megan's Law)

- Presence of known lead-based paint

- Pesticides used

- Any asbestos discovered on property

- Known carcinogenic material (if landlord has 10 or more employees)

- Methamphetamines contamination

- Application for demolition permit

- That the building is within one mile of a closed military base where explosives were stored

- If a previous tenant died on the premises within the past three years

- If the unit is in a condominium conversion project

Landlord's Responsibilities

A residential lease has an **implied warranty of habitability**. This duty does not extend to cases in which the problem is one of tenant cleanliness. The landlord must assume at least that the

- plumbing is in proper working order;

- the heat, lights, and wiring work and are safe;

- the floors, stairways, and railings are in good condition;

- when rented, the premises are clean and free of pests;

- areas under lessor control are maintained; and

- the roof does not leak and no doors or windows are broken.

If a landlord demands or collects rent for an untenable dwelling, the lessor is liable for actual damages sustained by the tenant and special damages of not less than $100 or more than $5,000. The tenant can also raise the defense of habitability against any eviction action.

Tenant's Responsibilities

If a landlord fails to take corrective action within a reasonable time of notice when a repair is the landlord's responsibility, the tenant has the following four options:

1. The tenant may abandon the property and not be held liable for back rents or an unfulfilled lease.

2. The tenant may refer the problem to a mediator, an arbitrator, or in serious circumstances, the small-claims court.

3. The tenant may notify the owner in writing of an emergency situation that must be taken care of. If the owner does not respond, the tenant may call in a professional repairman and offset the cost of repair with up to one month's rent on the next rent check. However, tenants may do this only twice in each year of tenancy.

4. The tenant can remain in possession and pay a reduced rent based on reduction of usefulness of the premises when the landlord fails to maintain a habitable dwelling.

The tenant cannot be prohibited from installing a satellite dish within the area under tenant control.

The landlord must allow the installation of a electric vehicle charging station, as long as station meets minimum standards.

The landlord must allow tenant agriculture in potable containers that meet minimum standards.

The California Civil Code states that the tenant is obligated to do the following:

- Keep the living unit clean and sanitary
- Dispose of garbage and other waste sanitarily
- Use all utility fixtures properly, keeping them clean and sanitary
- Avoid defacing or damaging property
- Use property only for its intended lawful purpose
- Pay rent on time
- Abide by rules and regulations
- Give 30-day notice when vacating (month-to-month lease)
- Return door and mailbox keys when vacating
- Leave the unit in a clean condition when vacating

Assignment vs. Sublease

Provided that the terms of the lease do not prohibit such activity, a tenant has the right to assign or sublet her interest in the property.

In an assignment, the assignee is a tenant of the landlord. In a sublease, the sublessee is the tenant of the sublessor.

Assignment transfers the entire leasehold rights to a third party. The third party, the assignee, pays rent directly to the original lessor. While the assignee becomes primarily liable on the lease, the original lessee retains secondary liability (if assignee defaults).

A **sublease** of property transfers only a part of the tenant's interest. The sublessee pays rent to the original lessee, who in turn is responsible to the lessor. The original lessee is said to have a *sandwich lease*.

The lease should clearly indicate if it may be assigned or subleased. Lessors frequently provide that assignment or subleasing be allowed only with the approval of the lessor; however, this approval must not be unreasonably withheld.

Some leases provide that if the premises are sublet at a rent higher than the lessee is paying the lessor, the higher portion will be split between the lessor and the lessee. This encourages tenants to try to sublet for a maximum amount and also allows the lessor to share in the increased rent. (See Figure 15.6 for the difference between assignments and subleases.)

Airbnb Inc., www.airbnb.com, allows apartment dwellers to market rental units or rooms through a global website. They can rent a room or their unit on short-term rental, often overnight, much as a hotel room. Airbnb violates many leases in that leases usually require landlord approval to sublease. Therefore, these unauthorized rentals could be cause for eviction. Because Airbnb takes a percentage of the rent, many large apartment owners now want a cut of the revenue ($340 million revenue reported by Airbnb in the third quarter of 2015). Airbnb has indicated they are negotiating with landlords for a sharing arrangement to legitimize their rental operation. Some cities are concerned that Airbnb will turn many apartments into hotels, which will deplete the stock of affordable housing.

TERMINATION OF LEASE

A tenancy for a specified period, as in an estate for years, requires no notice for termination because the date has already been specified. Other than by expiration of the lease term, termination may be made by the following:

- The tenant for violation of the landlord's duty to place the tenant in quiet possession
- The tenant, if a victim of domestic violence
- The tenant for the landlord's failure to repair
- The tenant on eviction by the landlord
- Either party on destruction of the premises
- The landlord on use of the premises for unauthorized purposes or on abandonment of the premises by the tenant
- Either party on breach of a condition of the lease
- The tenant for the landlord's breach of the implied warranty of habitability

Landlords cannot terminate or refuse to renew a lease because the tenant was the victim of domestic violence. Protection is waived if the victim allows the perpetrator to visit the property. The landlord must rekey at the tenant's request within 24 hours of written proof that a court protection order is in effect.

A residential landlord can prohibit smoking of tobacco products in the premises if it's stated in the lease. For existing tenants, a notice of change of terms of tenancy must first be given.

FIGURE 15.6:   Assignment vs. Subletting

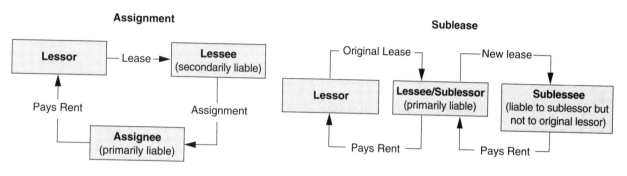

Protecting Tenants at Foreclosure Act of 2009

Before this act, foreclosure of a prior lien would nullify a residential tenant lease. Now the lease survives foreclosure and the tenant is allowed to remain in possession until the lease term expires. However, if the buyer at foreclosure intends to occupy the property, the lease may be terminated with 90 days' notice.

In case of a month-to-month lease, the tenant is entitled to 90 days' notice to vacate.

Tenants in foreclosed properties must be given notice of their rights.

Evictions and Unlawful Detainer

A landlord may evict tenants and bring an **unlawful detainer** action against them for failure to pay rent when due, violation of provisions contained in the lease or rental agreement, or failure to vacate the premises after termination of 30-day or 60-day written notice. The process of removing a tenant for being behind in rent follows:

1. The landlord serves the tenant with a **three-day notice** to quit or pay rent.

2. If the tenant fails to heed the notice, the landlord files an unlawful detainer action in court.

3. If the landlord wins, the court awards the landlord a judgment. The landlord then asks for a writ of possession authorizing the sheriff to evict the tenant.

4. The sheriff sends the tenant an eviction notice. If the tenant fails to leave, the sheriff then physically removes the tenant.

Because of drug-related crime, the legislature has authorized several city attorney and prosecutor offices to bring unlawful detainer actions to abate drug-related nuisances (the landlord will be charged fees and costs).

Property managers frequently bring action against tenants and former tenants in small-claims courts for back rent or for damages to the premises. Attorneys are not allowed in small-claims courts. The maximum amount of the suit is $5,000 by a business ($10,000 for individuals). The procedure is simple and informal:

1. Determine the full legal name and address of the person(s) you are suing.

   This will help you decide where you must file your claim.

2. Visit the clerk of the small-claims court and fill out the form after paying a small fee.

3. Arrange for the order to be served on the defendant (but not by yourself). The clerk will mail it for a fee, or you may authorize someone to serve it personally.

4. While waiting for the trial, gather all important documents and have them ready. Contact all potential witnesses and arrange for them to come with you to the trial, or obtain a subpoena from the clerk for any witness who will not come voluntarily. If you need an

interpreter, find out if one is available at small-claims court; otherwise, bring your own.

5. Come to the court building early and ask the clerk where your case is being heard. When you reach the courtroom, check the calendar to see that your case is listed.

6. When your case is called, give your testimony, presenting only the facts.

   Be brief. Submit all papers and documents you think will help your case.

7. If you win, ask the defendant for the money awarded you in the judgment.

8. If you have difficulties in collecting your money, ask the clerk to assist you.

9. As plaintiff, you are not allowed to appeal if you lose (unless you must pay as the result of a counterclaim).

Retaliatory Eviction Menace

A landlord cannot decrease services, increase rent, or evict a tenant within 180 days after the tenant exercises a right protected under the law, including the following:

- Complaining to the landlord about the habitability of the premises

- Complaining to a public agency about defects

- Lawfully organizing a tenant association

Tenants cannot waive their rights against retaliatory eviction.

Prohibition of retaliatory eviction is a defense against eviction. If a landlord is shown to have acted maliciously, the tenant will be entitled to actual damages plus $100 to $2,000 in punitive damages.

The landlord is subject to $2,000 in damages for threatening a residential tenant to vacate by force or by other menacing conduct.

SUMMARY

Property management, an ancient field of real estate specialization, is on the cutting edge of technology today. Property management has made rapid strides in professionalism, and besides the Institute of Real Estate Management (IREM), there are a number of other professional organizations.

Real estate managers fall into the following three general categories:

1. Licensee/property manager, who generally works out of a property management office handling numerous properties

2. Individual property manager, who handles just one property and who usually is an employee of an owner

3. Resident property managers

Property managers' duties vary with the type of property, but basically the manager has two main duties:

1. Strive for that rent/vacancy combination that will maximize the net earnings

2. Protect the property

To accomplish these duties, a property manager needs expertise in a variety of fields, from marketing to maintenance. The property manager, as a professional, has a duty to advise the owner in the operation of the property.

While most property management is residential, residential is broken down into specialized areas, such as mobile home parks and condominium associations. Property management also can involve commercial and industrial property and even public buildings, marinas, and so forth.

Commercial and industrial property management requires special lease knowledge, as well as technical knowledge of buildings and tenant requirements.

The property manager has a management contract similar to a sale listing that provides for a management fee and a leasing fee. Fees are based on complexity of the management and the rent received. The manager is responsible for trust records and owner accounting. Many other accounting records can also aid a property manager. Computer software is available to fulfill almost all needs of the property manager.

Leases are gross, net, percentage, or a combination of all three. Generally, net and percentage leases are found in connection with commercial rentals. To protect the owner in residential leasing, a rental application allows the owner to check out a tenant before committing to the tenant. Leases should be used for all tenancies, even month-to-month agreements, because they spell out rights and obligations of the parties.

In a lease assignment, all of the tenants' interests are transferred. In a sublease, the sublessor remains on the lease and the sublessee is the tenant's tenant.

Leases may be terminated for a number of reasons. If a tenant has breached a lease, the owner can sue for damages. The owner also may evict a tenant for breach of a material provision of the lease or if the tenant fails to leave after proper notice.

Residential landlords have disclosure requirements that relate to health and safety.

Residential landlord responsibilities include keeping the plumbing and other systems in operating order and keeping the structure safe and tight from the elements and free of pests. Residential tenant duties include keeping the unit clean; disposing of garbage properly; avoiding damaging the premises, systems, or appliances; paying rent on time; and leaving the unit clean when vacating.

A landlord may not evict a tenant (retaliatory eviction) because the tenant complained to the landlord or a public agency about the condition of the premises, or because the tenant lawfully organized a tenant group.

The Protecting Tenants at Foreclosure Act of 2009 allows residential tenants to remain in possession until the end of their lease. Month-to-month tenants are entitled to a 90-day notice to vacate.

CLASS DISCUSSION TOPICS

1. A particular percentage lease provides that after a tenant reaches a specific gross annual amount, the percentage decreases. Why was this written into the lease?

2. Identify property in your geographic area that you feel needs professional property management. Why?

3. Which offices in your area have separate property management departments?

4. Which properties in your area do you think would require the greatest management effort? Why?

5. Identify a nonresidential property in your community that has been vacant for a long time. What type of tenant would the property be suited for, and how would you market the property?

6. Do you know of any property where you feel the security is inadequate? If so, why? What could be done to provide better security?

7. Bring to class one current-events article dealing with some aspect of real estate practice for class discussion.

UNIT 15 QUIZ

1. The term CPM refers to
   a. California Property Manager.
   b. Certified Property Manager.
   c. Certified Professional Manager.
   d. none of these.

2. Which of the following statements regarding a property manager's compensation is *TRUE*?
   a. Compensation is generally a percentage of the gross.
   b. As the income of properties managed increases, the percentage fee charged tends to increase.
   c. Both of these.
   d. Neither of these.

3. Property managers can be protected against receiving no fees when managing a vacant property they are unable to rent by a
   a. holdover clause.
   b. recapture clause.
   c. minimum fee.
   d. separate leasing fee.

4. A lease for 30 months would be described as
   a. an estate at sufferance.
   b. an estate at will.
   c. an estate for years.
   d. a periodic tenancy.

5. A lease under which the tenant is to pay $500 per month for three years is a
   a. gross lease.
   b. net lease.
   c. percentage lease.
   d. month-to-month lease.

6.   A lease that contains a minimum rent and a covenant to remain in business is
    a.   a percentage lease.
    b.   a net lease.
    c.   a gross lease.
    d.   none of these.

7.   Which business would likely pay the highest percentage on a percentage lease?
    a.   Parking lot
    b.   Supermarket
    c.   Clothing store
    d.   Restaurant

8.   Which business is likely to pay the lowest percentage on a percentage lease?
    a.   Sporting goods store
    b.   Music shop
    c.   Supermarket
    d.   Clothing store

9.   A valid two-year lease need *NOT*
    a.   have parties capable of contracting.
    b.   contain a legal description of the property.
    c.   contain the amount of rent and manner of payment.
    d.   be a written agreement.

10.   Which statement regarding security deposits is *TRUE*?
    a.   Nonrefundable cleaning deposits are not allowed.
    b.   Deposits for furnished rentals can't exceed three months' rent.
    c.   Security deposits for unfurnished rentals can't exceed two months' rent.
    d.   All of these.

INTERNET SITES FOR REAL ESTATE PROFESSIONALS

The following is a partial listing of thousands of real estate–related sites. Neither the authors nor the publisher recommend any particular sites, but we have included these for your own evaluation.

APARTMENTS FOR RENT

www.apartments.com
www.apartment finder.com
www.apartment list.com
www.homeaway.com
www.homes.com (plus mortgage center)
www.nestigator.com
www.onradpad.com
www.trulia.com
www.move.com/apartments/
www.nestigaor.com
www.rent.com
www.homeaway.com
www.rentals.com

ASSOCIATIONS

Association of Real Estate License Law Officials
www.arello.org
Building Owners and Managers Association
www.boma.org
California Association of REALTORS®
www.car.org
California Community Colleges Real Estate Education Center
http://cccreec.org

California Real Estate Education Association

www.creea.org

Federation of Exchange Accommodators

www.1031.org

Institute of Real Estate Management

www.irem.org

International Association of Home Staging Professionals

www.iahsp.com

NAR Code of Ethics

www.realtor.org/code-of-ethics/

National Apartment Association

www.naahq.org

National Association of Real Estate Brokers

www.nareb.com

National Association of Real Estate Investment Trusts (REITs)

www.reit.com/nareit

National Association of REALTORS®

www.realtor.org

Real Estate Educators Association

www.reea.org

Real Estate Staging Association

www.realestatestagingassociation.com

BOOKS

www.dearborn.com/products/bookstore/

www.nolo.com

CAN-SPAM (EMAIL SOLICITATIONS)

www.ftc.gov/tips-advice/business-center/guidance/
can-spam-act-compliance-guide-business

CHOOSING A BROKER

www.homegain.com (Homeowners post their property and desired form of representation and brokers send their proposals. This site also includes homeowner and homebuyer information.)

CREDIT REPORTS

www.annualcreditreport.com

DO-NOT-CALL REGISTRY

www.donotcall.gov

DO-IT-YOURSELF FORMS

www.legalzoom.com

ENVIRONMENTAL LAW

http://resources.ca.gov/ceqa/ (an information site developed by the California Natural Resources Agency that includes a database containing California environmental law with links to federal law)

ENVIRONMENTAL PROTECTION AGENCY SITE

www.epa.gov

FORMS

California Association of REALTORS® (CAR)
www.car.org/legal/standard-forms/
First Tuesday
www.firsttuesday.us

GOVERNMENT-RELATED SITES

California Bureau of Real Estate
www.bre.ca.gov
California Department of Fair Employment and Housing
www.dfeh.ca.gov
California Department of Finance
www.dof.ca.gov
California Department of Housing and Community Development
www.hcd.ca.gov
California Department of Justice
www.meganslaw.ca.gov (listing of names, addresses and zip codes of registered sex offenders)
California Office of Real Estate Appraisers
www.orea.ca.gov
Consumer Price Index
www.bls.gov/cpi/
Department of Housing and Urban Development (HUD)
www.hud.gov
Department of Veterans Affairs
www.va.gov
Environmental Protection Agency
www.epa.gov
Fair Housing (HUD)
www.hud.gov/fairhousing/
Fannie Mae
www.fanniemae.com
Farmer Mac
www.farmermac.com
Federal Reserve Bank of San Francisco
www.frbsf.org
Freddie Mac
www.freddiemac.com
Ginnie Mae
www.ginniemae.gov
Government websites (search engine)
www.usa.gov
National Flood Insurance Program
www.fema.gov/national-flood-insurance-program/

FORECLOSURES

www.realtytrac.com

FOR SALE BY OWNER

www.craigslist.com
www.forsalebyowner.com
www.owners.com
www.FSBO.com
www.homepoint.com
www.homesbyowner.com

HOME PRICES (VALUE)

www.realtytrac.com (recent home prices by area)
www.homes.com/homeprices/
www.zillow.com

LISTINGS OF PROPERTY FOR SALE

www.ca-homes.com
www.californiarealestate.com
www.century21.com www.coldwellbanker.com
www.coldwellbankerpreviews.com www.craigslist.org
www.era.com www.forsalebyowner.com
www.homefinder.com
www.homes.com
www.homeseekers.com
https://homes.yahoo.com
www.househunt.com
http://newhomes.move.com
www.oodle.com
www.owners.com
www.realtor.com

www.realtyexecutives.com
www.remax.com www.trulia.com
www.zillow.com

Note: Most of the listed sites also provide for loan prequalification and application.

LOANS

www.bankofamerica.com
www.bankrate.com
www.eloan.com
www.greenlightloans.com
www.lendingtree.com
www.loantek.com
www.mortgageloan.com
www.quickenloans.com
www.wellsfargo.com

MORTGAGE CALCULATIONS

www.homefair.com
www.interest.com
www.mortgage-calc.com

PROFESSIONAL INFORMATION

Federation of Exchange Accommodators
www.1031.org
Inman News
www.inman.com
The Real Estate Library
www.relibrary.com
The Real Estate Professional magazine
www.therealestatepro.com
RealtyNow
www.realtynow.com

RealtyTimes
www.realtytimes.com
RISMedia (Real Estate Magazine)
www.rismedia.com

REAL ESTATE ATTORNEYS

www.lawyers.com
www.martindale.cm
http://real-estate-law.freeadvice.com/real-estate-law/

RENTAL COMPARABLES

www.rentometer.com

VIRTUAL HOME TOURS

www.abirdseye.com
www.easypano.com
www.ipix.com
www.paradym.com
www.spotlighthometours.com/

GLOSSARY

abstract of title. A summary or digest of all recorded transfers, conveyances, legal proceedings, and any other facts relied on as evidence of title to show continuity of ownership and indicate any possible impairments to title.

acceleration clause. A provision in a real estate financing instrument that allows the lender to declare the remaining indebtedness due and payable on the occurrence of certain conditions, such as the sale of the property or the borrower's default in payment.

acceptance. Indication by the person to whom an offer is made (the offeree) of agreement to the terms of the offer. If the offer requires a writing, the acceptance also must be in writing.

accession. The process of manufactured or natural improvement or addition to property.

accommodating party. Third party who has control of funds in delayed exchange.

accretion. Accession by natural forces, such as alluvion.

acknowledgment. A formal declaration made before an authorized person by a person who has executed a written instrument, stating that the execution of the instrument is the person's own act.

acquisition cost. For FHA-insured loans, the price to procure property, including purchase price and all nonrecurring closing costs, including discount points, FHA application fee, service charge and credit report, FHA appraisal, escrow, document preparation, title insurance, termite inspection, reconveyance, and recording fees.

acre. A measure of land equaling 160 square rods, 4,840 square yards or 43,560 square feet, or a tract about 208.71 feet square.

action for declaratory relief. Legal proceeding brought to determine the respective rights of the parties before a controversy arises.

action to quiet title. A court proceeding brought to establish title to real property.

actual age. The number of years since completion of a building; also called *historical* or *chronological age.*

actual authority. The authority agents have because it is specified in the agency agreement or that the agents believes they have because of an unintentional or careless act of the principal.

administrator/administratrix. Personal representative of the estate of a decedent, appointed by the probate court. *See also* **executor/executrix**.

ad valorem. A Latin phrase meaning "according to value," used to describe a tax charged in relation to the value of the property taxed.

adverse possession. A method of acquiring title to real property by occupying the property against the interests of the true owner and fulfilling other statutory requirements.

affordability index. An NAR index that measures the ability of median family income to support a mortgage for the median-priced home. An index of 100 means that the median income is equal to the amount necessary to afford the median-priced home.

after-acquired title. If title is acquired by a grantor only after a conveyance to a grantee, the deed to the grantee becomes effective at the time the grantor actually receives title.

agency. The relationship between a principal and the agent of the principal that arises out of a contract, whether express or implied, written or oral, by which the agent is employed by the principal to do certain acts dealing with a third party.

agent. One who acts for and with authority from another person, called the principal; a special agent is appointed to carry out a particular act or transaction, and any other agent is a general agent.

air rights. The real property right to the reasonable use of the airspace above the surface of the land.

alienation. The transferring of property to another.

all-inclusive trust deed. *See* **wraparound mortgage or trust deed**.

alluvion. Alluvium; the increase of soil along the bank of a body of water by natural forces.

Americans with Disabilities Act. Federal law prohibiting discrimination that would deny the equal enjoyment of goods, services, facilities, and accommodations in any existing place of public accommodation, based on an individual's physical or mental disabilities. .

amortization. The payment of a financial obligation in installments; recovery over a period of time of cost or value. An amortized loan includes both principal and interest in approximately equal payments, usually due monthly, resulting in complete payment of the amount borrowed, with interest, by the end of the loan term. A loan has negative amortization when the loan payments do not cover all the interest due, which then is added to the remaining loan balance.

annual percentage rate (APR). The relative cost of credit as determined in accordance with Regulation Z of the Board of Governors of the Federal Reserve System for implementing the federal Truth in Lending Act.

anticipation, principle of. Expectation that property will offer future benefits, which tends to increase present value.

apparent authority. Authority to act as an agent that someone appears to have but does not actually have, which will place no obligation on the party the agent claims to represent if that party is in no way responsible for the representation.

appraisal. An estimate of a property's monetary value on the open market; an estimate of a property's type and condition, its utility for a given purpose, or its highest and best use.

appropriation, right of. *See* **right of appropriation**.

appurtenance. Anything affixed (attached) to or used with land for its benefit and that is transferred with the land.

APR. *See* **annual percentage rate**.

area. Measure of the floor or ground space within the perimeter of a building or land parcel.

arm's-length transaction. A transaction in which neither party acts under duress and both have full knowledge of the property's assets and defects, the property involved has been on the market a reasonable length of time, there are no unusual circumstances, and the price represents the normal consideration for the property sold without extraordinary financing.

assessed valuation. A valuation placed on a piece of property by a public authority as a basis for levying taxes on that property.

assessor. The official responsible for determining assessed values.

assumption. An undertaking or adoption of a debt or an obligation resting primarily on another person.

attachment. The process by which the real or personal property of a party to a lawsuit is seized and retained in the custody of the court; intended to compel an appearance before the court or to furnish security for a debt or costs arising out of the litigation.

attorney-in-fact. An agent who has been granted a power of attorney by a principal.

avulsion. The tearing or washing away of land along the bank of a body of water by natural forces.

balance, principle of. The combination of land uses that results in the highest property values overall.

balloon payment. An installment payment on a promissory note—usually the final payment—that is significantly larger than the other installment payments.

bankruptcy. A federal court proceeding in which the court takes possession of the assets of an insolvent debtor and sells the nonexempt assets to pay off creditors on a pro rata basis; title to the debtor's assets is held by a trustee in bankruptcy.

base lines. Imaginary lines that run east-west and intersect meridians that run north-south to form the starting point for land measurement using the rectangular survey system of land description.

basis. Cost basis is the dollar amount assigned to property at the time of acquisition under provisions of the Internal Revenue Code for the purpose of determining gain, loss, and depreciation in calculating the income tax to be paid on the sale or exchange of the property; adjusted cost basis is derived after the application of certain additions, such as for improvements, and deductions, such as for depreciation.

beneficiary. One on whose behalf a trustee holds property conveyed by a trustor; the lender under a deed of trust.

bequest. Transfer of property, particularly personal property, called a *legacy*, by will. *See also* **devise**.

bill of sale. Written instrument that conveys title to personal property.

blanket mortgage. A loan covering more than one property.

blind ad. An ad that fails to indicate that the advertiser is an agent.

blockbusting. The practice on the part of unscrupulous speculators or real estate agents of inducing panic selling of homes at prices below market value, especially by exploiting the prejudices of property owners in neighborhoods in which the racial makeup is changing or appears to be on the verge of changing.

bond. An obligation; a real estate bond is a written obligation issued on security of a mortgage or trust deed.

book value. The current value for accounting purposes of an asset expressed as original cost plus capital additions minus accumulated depreciation.

breach. The failure of a duty imposed by law or by contract, either by omission or commission.

building code. Standards for building, planning, and construction established by state law and local ordinance.

bundle of rights. The legal rights of ownership of real property, including the rights of possession, use, disposition, and exclusion of others from the property.

Bureau of Real Estate. California agency that administers the real estate law, including the licensing of real estate brokers and salespeople; headed by the real estate commissioner, who is appointed by the governor and presides over the Real Estate Advisory Commission (whose 10 members are appointed by and serve at the commissioner's discretion).

business opportunity. The assets of an existing business enterprise, including its goodwill.

buyer's market. Real estate marketplace that has more sellers than buyers.

CalVet loan. Home or farm loan procured through the California Veterans Farm and Home Purchase Program.

capital assets. Assets of a permanent nature used in the production of income, such as land, buildings, machinery, and equipment; usually distinguishable under income tax law from "inventory," assets held for sale to customers in the ordinary course of the taxpayer's trade or business.

capital gain. The amount by which the net resale proceeds of a capital item exceed the adjusted cost basis of the item.

capitalization rate. The rate of interest that is considered a reasonable return on an investment, used in the process of determining value based on net operating income; the yield necessary to attract investment.

capitalization recapture. The return of an investment; an amortization rate based on the right of the investor to get back the purchase price at the end of the term of ownership or over the productive life of the improvements; computed by straight-line depreciation, by using Inwood tables or Hoskold tables. (Students should refer to a real estate appraisal text for further explanation.)

cash flow. The net income generated by a property before depreciation and other noncash expenses.

CC&Rs. Covenants, conditions, and restrictions; limitations on land use imposed by deed, usually when land is subdivided, as a means of regulating building construction, density, and use for the benefit of other property owners; may be referred to simply as *restrictions*.

certificate of reasonable value. Property appraisal required for a VA-guaranteed loan.

certificate of redemption. Issued by the county tax collector when all past due amounts have been paid.

certificate of sale. Document received by the buyer at an execution or a judicial foreclosure sale; replaced by a sheriff's deed if the debtor fails to redeem the property during the statutory redemption period.

certificate of title. Statement of a property's owner of record as well as any existing encumbrances.

chain of title. The history of the conveyances and encumbrances affecting the present owner's title to property, as far back as records are available.

change, principle of. Effect on property value of constantly varying physical, economic, social, and political forces.

chattel mortgage. Use of personal property to secure or guarantee a promissory note.

chattel real. An estate related to real estate, such as a lease of real property.

chattels. Personal property; any property that is not real property.

Civil Rights Act of 1866. The first U.S. civil rights act. It applied to race only and had no exceptions.

Civil Rights Act of 1968. This comprehensive act is known as the Fair Housing Act.

closing. The completion of a real estate transaction, at which point required documents are transmitted and funds are transferred.

Closing Disclosure. New form mandated by the TILA-RESPA rule that helps consumers to understand all the costs of the transaction. It must be provided to consumers three business days before closing.

cloud on the title. Any claim, condition, or encumbrance that impairs title to real property.

coastal zone. An area of about 1,800 square miles that runs the length of the state from the sea inland about 1,000 yards, with wider spots in coastal estuarine, habitat, and recreational areas; any development or improvement of land within the coastal zone must meet local requirements for coastal conservation and preservation of resources, as authorized by the Coastal Zone Conservation Act.

codicil. Written amendment to a will, made with the same legal formalities.

color of title. A claim of possession to real property based on a document erroneously appearing to convey title to the claimant.

commingling. Mixing broker and principal funds.

commission. An agent's compensation for performing the duties of the agency; in real estate practice, typically a percentage of the selling price of property, rentals, or other property value.

common law. The body of law from England based on custom, usage, and court decisions.

community apartment project. A form of subdivision in which the owner has an individual interest in the land and exclusive right of occupancy of an apartment on the land.

community property. All property acquired by husband and wife during marriage except that qualifying as separate property.

community redevelopment agency (CRA). An agency authorized by state law but formed by a local governing body to provide low-and moderate-income housing and employ low-income persons by rehabilitating existing structures and/or bringing new development.

competition, principle of. Business profits encourage competition, which ultimately may reduce profits for any one business.

comparative market analysis. Informal estimate of market value performed by a real estate agent for either seller or buyer, utilizing the sales history of nearby properties; usually expressed as a range of values that includes the probable market value of the subject property.

compound interest. Interest paid on original principal and also on the accrued and unpaid interest that has accumulated as the debt matures.

concurrent ownership. Ownership of property by more than one person, not necessarily in equal shares.

condemnation. *See* **eminent domain**.

condition. A qualification of an estate granted that can be imposed only in a conveyance; it can be a condition precedent or a condition subsequent. *See also* **CC&Rs**.

condition precedent. A qualification of a contract or transfer of property providing that unless and until the performance of a certain act, the contract or transfer will not take effect.

condition subsequent. A stipulation in a contract or transfer of property that already has taken effect that will extinguish the contract or defeat the property transfer.

condominium. A subdivision providing an exclusive ownership (fee) interest in the airspace of a particular portion of real property, as well as an interest in common in a portion of that property.

conforming loan. Loan that meets Fannie Mae and Freddie Mac purchase criteria.

conformity, principle of. Holds that property values are maximized when buildings are similar in design, construction, and age, particularly in residential neighborhoods.

consideration. Anything of value given or promised by a party to induce another to enter into a contract; may be a benefit conferred on one party or a detriment suffered by the other.

constructive eviction. Interference by the landlord in a tenant's legitimate use of leased property, such as by making unwarranted alterations to the property.

contract. A written or oral agreement to do or not to do certain things. There may be an express agreement of the parties, or a contract may be implied by their conduct. A unilateral contract imposes an obligation on only one of the parties, whereas both parties to a bilateral contract have an obligation to perform. A contract is executory when a contract obligation is to be performed in the future, and executed when all obligations have been performed and the contract transaction has been completed. A real estate contract must be a signed writing made by competent parties, for valuable consideration, with an offer by one party that is accepted by the other.

contribution, principle of. A component part of a property is valued in proportion to its contribution to the value of the entire property, regardless of its separate actual cost.

conventional loan. A loan secured by a mortgage or trust deed that is made without governmental underwriting (FHA-insured or VA-guaranteed).

cooperative apartment. *See* stock cooperative.

corporation. A legal entity that acts through its board of directors and officers, generally without liability on the part of the person or persons owning it. A domestic corporation is one chartered in California— any other corporation is a foreign corporation in California.

correction lines. Guide meridians running every 24 miles east and west of a meridian, and standard parallels running every 24 miles north and south of a base line, used to correct inaccuracies in the rectangular survey system of land description caused by the earth's curvature.

Costa-Hawkins Rental Housing Act. Statute that allows landlords of rent-controlled property to set new base rents for new tenants.

cost approach. Appraisal method in which site value is added to the present reproduction or replacement cost of all property improvements, less depreciation, to determine market value.

covenant. An agreement or a promise to do or not to do a particular act, usually imposed by deed. *See also* **CC&Rs.**

covenant of quiet enjoyment. Promise of a landlord, implied by law, not to interfere in the possession or use of leased property by the tenant.

covenant to repair. Express or legally implied obligation of the landlord to make necessary repairs to leased premises.

declaration of homestead. *See* homestead.

dedication. The giving of land by its owner for a public use, and the acceptance of the land for such use by the appropriate government officials.

deed. Written instrument that, when properly executed and delivered, conveys title to real property from a grantor to a grantee.

deed in lieu of foreclosure. A deed to real property accepted by a lender from a defaulting borrower to avoid the necessity of foreclosure proceedings by the lender.

deed of trust. *See* trust deed.

defendant. A person against whom legal action is initiated for the purpose of obtaining criminal sanctions (in a case involving violation of a penal statute) or damages or other appropriate judicial relief (in a civil case).

deficiency judgment. A judgment given by a court when the value of security pledged for a loan is insufficient to pay off the debt of the defaulting borrower.

demand statement. Statement requested by escrow as to amount due lender at close of escrow to pay off loan and any charges.

depreciation. Decrease in value of an asset that is allowed in computing property value for tax purposes; in appraising, a loss in the value of a property improvement from any cause; depreciation is *curable* when it can be remedied by a repair or an addition to the property, and it is incurable when there is no easy or economic way to cure the loss. *See also* **physical deterioration, functional obsolescence,** and **external obsolescence.**

designated agent. In some states one agent in an office can be the seller's agent and another agent in the same office can be the buyer's agent.

devise. Transfer of title to property by will. *See also* **bequest.**

devisee. Person receiving title to property by will. *See also* **legatee.**

devisor. One who wills property to another.

direct endorsement. A lender who is authorized to determine if a loan qualifies for FHA insurance.

discount points. *See* **points.**

discount rate. Interest rate charged member banks by Federal Reserve Banks.

documentary transfer tax. A tax applied on all transfers of real property located in a county where the county is authorized by the state to collect; notice of payment is entered on the face of the deed or on a separate paper filed with the deed.

Dodd-Frank Act. The Dodd-Frank Wall Street Reform and Consumer Protection Act signed into law in 2010.

dominant tenement. *See* **easement.**

donee. One who receives a gift.

donor. One who makes a gift.

dual agency. An agency relationship in which the agent represents two principals in their dealings with each other.

due-on-sale clause. An acceleration clause in a real estate financing instrument granting the lender the right to demand full payment of the remaining indebtedness on a sale of the property.

easement. The right to a specific use of or the right to travel over the land of another. The land being used or traveled over is the servient tenement; the land that is benefited by the use is the dominant tenement. An easement appurtenant is a property interest that belongs to the owner of the dominant tenement and is transferred with the land; an easement in gross is a personal right that usually is not transferable by its owner.

easement by prescription. Acquiring a specific use of or the right to travel over the land of another by statutory requirements similar to those for adverse possession.

economic life. The period of time over which an improved property will yield a return on investment over and above the return attributable solely to the land.

economic obsolescence. *See* **external obsolescence**.

economic rent. The reasonable rental expectancy if the property were available for renting at the time of its valuation.

effective gross income. Property income from all sources, less allowance for vacancy and collection losses.

effective rent. Scheduled rent adjusted for rental incentives given.

elder abuse law. Requirement that realty agents and others report elder financial abuse, fraud, or undue influence.

emblements. Crops produced annually by labor and industry, as distinguished from crops that grow naturally on the land.

eminent domain. The right of the government to acquire title to property for public use by condemnation; the property owner receives compensation—generally fair market value. *See also* **inverse condemnation**.

encroachment. The unlawful intrusion of a property improvement onto adjacent property.

encumbrance. Anything that affects or limits the fee simple title to or affects the condition or use of real estate.

environmental impact report (EIR). Evaluation of effects on the environment of a proposed development; may be required by local government.

environmental obsolescence. *See* **external obsolescence**.

e-PRO certification. NAR professional designation of an internet professional.

Equal Credit Opportunity Act. Act that prohibits lender discrimination against a borrower based on the fact that the source of income is public assistance.

Equator Platform. A system for obtaining short sale approval.

equity of redemption. The right to redeem property during the foreclosure period, or during a statutorily prescribed time following a foreclosure sale.

escalator clause. Provision in a lease agreement for an increase in payments based on an increase in an index, such as the Consumer Price Index.

escheat. The reverting of property to the state when there are no heirs capable of inheriting.

escrow. The deposit of instruments and/or funds (with instructions) with a neutral third party to carry out the provisions of an agreement or a contract.

escrow agent. Escrow holder; the neutral third-party company holding funds or something of value in trust for another or others.

escrow offices. The employee of the escrow agent who handles the escrow.

estate. The interest held by the owner of property.

estate at sufferance. The occupancy of a tenant after the lease term expires.

estate at will. A tenancy in which the tenant's time of possession is indefinite.

estate for years. A tenancy for a fixed term.

estate from period to period. Periodic tenancy; a tenancy for a fixed term, automatically renewed for the same term unless the owner or the tenant gives the other written notice of intention to terminate the tenancy.

eviction. Dispossession by process of law.

exchange. A means of trading equities in two or more real properties, treated as a single transaction through a single escrow.

exclusive-agency listing. A listing agreement employing a broker as sole agent for a seller of real property under the terms of which the broker is entitled to compensation if the property is sold through any other broker, but not if a sale is negotiated by the owner without the services of an agent.

exclusive-authorization-and-right-to-sell listing. A listing agreement employing a broker as agent for a seller of real property under the terms of which the broker is entitled to compensation if the listed property is sold during the duration of the listing, whether by the listing agent, another agent, or the owner acting without the services of an agent.

executor/executrix. Personal representative of the estate of a decedent, named in the decedent's will. *See also* **administrator/administratrix**.

express agreement. An agreement established by a deliberate act of the parties that both parties acknowledge as their intention.

external obsolescence. Economic or environmental obsolescence; loss in value due to outside causes, such as changes in nearby land use.

Fair Employment and Housing Act. *See* Rumford Act.

Fannie Mae (Federal National Mortgage Association). Now a private corporation dealing in the secondary mortgage market.

Farmer Mac (Federal Agricultural Mortgage Corporation). Now a private corporation providing a secondary mortgage market for farms and rural housing.

fee simple absolute. A fee simple estate with no restrictions on its use.

fee simple defeasible. An interest in land, such as a fee simple conditional or fee simple with special limitation, that may result in the estate of ownership being defeated.

fee simple estate. The greatest interest in real property one can own, including the right to use the property at present and for an indeterminate period in the future.

fee simple qualified. A fee simple estate with some restrictions on the right of possession.

feng shui. Laws governing orientation and spatial relationship in regard to the flow of energy.

fiduciary. A person in a position of trust and confidence who owes a certain loyalty to another, such as an agent to a principal.

final subdivision map. *See* tentative subdivision map.

fiscal year. A business or an accounting year as distinguished from a calendar year.

fixture. Anything permanently attached to land or improvements so as to become real property.

foreclosure. Sale of real property by mortgagee, trustee, or other lienholder on default by the borrower. *See also* **judicial foreclosure action**.

form appraisal report. A short report, typically two pages plus addenda, using a preprinted form to summarize the data contributing to an appraiser's conclusion of value.

fraud. The intentional and successful use of any cunning, deception, collusion, or artifice to circumvent, cheat, or deceive another person, so that the other person acts on it to the loss of property and legal injury; actual fraud is a deliberate misrepresentation or a representation made in reckless disregard of its truth or falsity, the suppression of truth, a promise made without the intention to perform it or any other act intended to deceive; constructive fraud is any misrepresentation made without fraudulent intent (the deliberate intent to deceive). Fraud is affirmative when it is a deliberate statement of a material fact that the speaker knows to be false and on which the speaker intends another person to rely, to the speaker's detriment. Fraud is negative when it is a deliberate concealment of something that should be revealed.

Freddie Mac (Federal Home Loan Mortgage Corporation). Now a private secondary mortgage corporation.

freehold estate. An estate in land in which ownership is for an indeterminate length of time, as in a fee simple or life estate.

front foot. Property measured by the front linear foot on its street line, each front foot extending the depth of the lot.

functional obsolescence. Loss in value due to adverse factors within a structure that affect its marketability, such as its design, layout, or utility.

general partnership. An association of two or more persons to carry on a business as co-owners for profit.

general plan. Master plan; includes a statement of policy of the development and land uses within a city or county and a program to implement that policy.

gift deed. A deed for which the only consideration is "love and affection."

Ginnie Mae (Government National Mortgage Association). A government corporation that provides assistance to federally related housing projects. Funds are raised by selling securities backed by pools of mortgages.

goodwill. An intangible but salable asset of a business derived from the expectation of continued public patronage.

grant deed. A limited warranty deed using a granting clause—the word *grant* or words to that effect—assuring the grantee that the estate being conveyed is free from encumbrances placed on the property by the present owner (the grantor) and that the grantor has not previously conveyed the property to anyone else.

grantee. A person to whom property is transferred by grant.

grantor. A person conveying property to another by grant.

gross income. Total property income from all sources before any expenses are deducted.

gross income multiplier. Gross rent multiplier; a number derived by dividing the sales price of a comparable property by the income it produces, which then is multiplied by the gross income produced by the subject property to derive an estimate of value.

gross lease. Provides for the tenant to pay a fixed rental over the lease term, with the landlord paying all expenses of ownership, such as taxes, assessments, and insurance.

ground lease. An agreement for the use of land only, sometimes secured by improvements placed on the land by the user.

ground rent. Earnings of improved property credited to earnings of the ground itself after allowance is made for earnings of improvements.

guarantee of title. Guarantee of title as determined from examination of the public records and described in the guarantee document.

guide meridians. *See* **correction lines**.

hard money loans. Cash loans made by individual investors.

highest and best use. In appraising real estate, the most profitable, physically possible, and legally permissible use for the property under consideration.

holder in due course. Someone who takes a negotiable instrument for value, in good faith and without notice of any defense against its enforcement that might be made by any person.

holdover tenancy. Possession of property by a tenant who remains in possession after the expiration or termination of the lease term.

holographic will. A will written entirely in the testator's handwriting, signed and dated by the testator.

homestead. A statutory exemption of real property used as a home from the claims of certain creditors and judgments up to a specified amount; requires a declaration of homestead to be completed and filed in the county recorder's office.

implied warranties. Warranties by grantor to grantee that will be implied by law, even if not mentioned in the deed; the grantor warrants that he has not already conveyed the property and that there are no encumbrances on the property brought about by the grantor or any person who might claim title from the grantor.

income capitalization approach. Appraisal method in which the actual or likely net operating income of property is divided by its expected rate of return (capitalization rate) to arrive at an estimate of market value. *See also* **capitalization rate**.

independent contractor. A person employed by another who has almost complete freedom to accomplish the purposes of the employment.

index method. Way of estimating building reproduction cost by multiplying the original cost of the subject building by a factor that represents the percentage change in construction costs, generally from the time of construction to the time of valuation.

inherent authority. The authority of an agent to perform activities that are not specifically mentioned in the agency agreement but are necessary or customary to carry out an authorized act.

injunction. A writ or an order issued by a court to restrain one or more parties to a suit or proceeding from doing an act deemed to be inequitable or unjust in regard to the rights of some other party or parties in the suit or proceeding.

installment sales contract. *See* **sales contract**.

institutional lenders. A financial intermediary or depository, such as a savings association, commercial bank, or life insurance company, that pools the money of its depositors and then invests funds in various ways, including trust deeds and mortgage loans.

interest. A portion, share, or right in something; partial ownership; the charge in dollars for the use of money for a period of time.

interest rate. The percentage of a sum of money borrowed that is charged for its use.

interim loan. A short-term temporary loan used until permanent financing is available, typically during building construction.

interpleader. A court proceeding that may be brought by someone, such as an escrow agent, who holds property for another, for the purpose of deciding who among the claimants is legally entitled to the property.

intestate succession. Statutory method of distribution of property that belonged to someone who died intestate (without having made a valid will).

inverse condemnation. A legal action brought by the owner of land when government puts nearby land to a use that diminishes the value of the owner's property.

joint tenancy. Ownership of property by two or more co-owners, each of whom has an equal share and the right of survivorship.

joint venture. Two or more individuals or firms joining together on a single project as partners, typically with a lender contributing the necessary funds and the other partner(s) contributing their expertise.

judgment. The final determination of a court of competent jurisdiction of a matter presented to it; may include an award of money damages.

judicial foreclosure action. Proceeding in which a mortgagee, a trustee, or another lienholder on property requests a court-supervised sale of the property to cover the unpaid balance of a delinquent debt.

land. The earth's surface, including substances beneath the surface extending downward to the center of the earth and the airspace above the surface for an indefinite distance upward.

land contract. *See* **sales contract.**

landlord. Lessor; one who leases property to another.

lateral support. The support that the soil of an adjoining owner gives to a neighbor's land.

lease. A contract between a property owner, called *lessor* or *landlord*, and another, called *lessee* or *tenant*, conveying and setting forth the conditions of occupancy and use of the property by the tenant.

leaseback. *See* sale-leaseback.

leasehold estate. A tenant's right to occupy real estate during the term of the lease; a personal property interest.

legacy. Property, usually personal property, transferred by will.

legal description. A land description used to define a parcel of land to the exclusion of all others that is acceptable by a court of law.

legatee. Person who receives property, called a legacy, by bequest. *See also* devisee.

letter of opinion. A letter from appraiser to client presenting only the appraiser's conclusion of value, with no supporting data.

leverage. Use of debt financing to purchase an investment, thus maximizing the return per dollar of equity invested; enables a purchaser to obtain possession for little or no initial cash outlay and relatively small periodic payments on the debt incurred.

lien. An encumbrance that makes property security for the payment of a debt or discharge of an obligation; a voluntary lien is one agreed to by the property owner, such as a deed of trust; an involuntary lien exists by operation of law to create a burden on property for certain unpaid debts, such as a tax lien.

life estate. An interest in real property conveying the right to possession and use for a term measured by the life or lives of one or more persons, most often the holder of the life estate.

limited equity housing cooperative. A stock cooperative financed by the California Housing Finance Agency.

limited partnership. Partnership of one or more general partners, who run the business and are liable as partners, and limited partners, investors who do not run the business and are liable only up to the amount invested.

liquidated damages. An amount agreed on by the parties to be full damages if a certain event occurs.

listing agreement. Authorization by the owner of property, acting as principal, for a real estate broker to act as the agent of the principal in finding a person to buy, lease, or rent property; may be used to employ a real estate broker to act as agent for a person seeking property to buy, lease, or rent.

Loan Estimate. New form mandated by the TILA-RESPA rule that helps consumers to understand the key features, costs, and risks of a mortgage loan. It must be provided to consumers no later than three business days after they submit a loan application.

lot and block system. Subdivision system; method of legal description of land using parcel maps identified by tract, block, and lot numbers.

marker. *See* **metes and bounds**.

marketable title. Title that a reasonably prudent purchaser, acting with full knowledge of the facts and their legal significance, would be willing and ought to accept.

market comparison approach. *See* **sales comparison approach**.

market data approach. *See* **sales comparison approach**.

market value. The most probable price a property would bring in an arm's-length transaction under normal conditions on the open market. *See also* **arm's-length transaction**.

material fact. A fact that would be likely to affect the judgment of a person to whom it is known, such as information concerning the poor physical condition of a building that is for sale.

mechanic's lien. A statutory lien against real property in favor of persons who have performed work or furnished materials for the improvement of the property.

Mello-Roos bonds. Improvement bonds that place offsite improvement costs on the home purchaser rather than on the developer.

meridians. Imaginary lines that run north to south and intersect base lines that run east to west to form the starting point for land measurement using the rectangular survey system of land description.

metes and bounds. Method of legal description of land using distances (called metes) measured from a point of beginning and using natural or artificial boundaries (called bounds), as well as single objects (called monuments or markers) as points of reference.

minor. A person younger than 18 years of age.

mobile home. A structure transportable in one or more sections, designed and equipped to contain no more than two dwelling units, to be used with or without a foundation system; does not include a recreational vehicle.

mobile home park. Any area or tract of land where two or more mobile home lots are rented, leased, or held out for rent or lease.

monument. *See* metes and bounds.

mortgage. A legal instrument by which property is pledged by a borrower, the mortgagor, as security for the payment of a debt or an obligation owed to a lender, the mortgagee.

Mortgage Loan Disclosure Statement. The statement on a form approved by the real estate commissioner that is required by law to be furnished by a mortgage loan broker to the prospective borrower of a loan of a statutorily prescribed amount before the borrower becomes obligated to complete the loan.

multiple listing clause. Clause in a listing agreement, usually part of an exclusive authorization and right-to-sell listing, taken by a member of a multiple listing service, providing that members of the multiple listing service will have the opportunity to find a ready, willing, and able buyer for the listed property.

multiple listing service (MLS). An organization of real estate agents providing for a pooling of listings and the sharing of commissions on transactions involving more than one agent.

narrative appraisal report. The longest and most thorough appraisal report, containing a summary of all factual materials, techniques, and appraisal methods used in setting forth the appraiser's conclusion of value.

negotiable instrument. An instrument, such as a promissory note, that is capable of being assigned or transferred in the ordinary course of business.

net listing. A listing agreement providing that the agent may retain as compensation for services all sums received over and above a net price to the owner.

net, net, net lease. *See* triple net lease.

net operating income. Profit; the money remaining after expenses are deducted from income.

niche marketing. Specialization in an area, type of property, and/or category of buyer.

nonexclusive listing. *See* open listing.

notice. Knowledge of a fact; actual notice is express or implied knowledge of a fact; constructive notice is knowledge of a fact that is imputed to a person by law because of the person's actual notice of circumstances and the inquiry that a prudent person would have been expected to make; legal notice is information required to be given by law.

novation. The substitution or exchange of a new obligation or contract for an old one by mutual agreement of the parties.

null and void. Of no legal validity or effect.

observed condition method. Breakdown method; depreciation computed by estimating the loss in value caused by every item of depreciation, whether curable or incurable.

one hundred percent commission. An office where salespersons pay broker fees but keep commissions earned.

open listing. Nonexclusive listing; the nonexclusive right to secure a purchaser, given by a property owner to a real estate agent; more than one agent may be given such authorization, and only the first to procure a ready, willing, and able buyer— or an offer acceptable to the seller—will be entitled to compensation.

opinion of title. An attorney's written evaluation of the condition of the title to a parcel of land after examination of the abstract of title.

option. A right given for a consideration to purchase or lease property on specified terms within a specified time, with no obligation on the part of the person receiving the right to exercise it.

option ARM. Adjustable-rate mortgage where the buyer has the option of making a minimum payment.

overriding trust deed. *See* wraparound mortgage or trust deed.

ownership in severalty. Separate ownership; ownership of property by one person only.

participation loan. A loan where the lender takes an equity position in the property, as well as interest for the loan.

partition action. Court proceeding by which co-owners may force a division of the property or its sale, with co-owners reimbursed for their individual shares.

partnership. *See* general partnership.

percentage lease. Provides for rent as a percentage of the tenant's gross income, usually with a minimum base amount; the percentage may decrease as the tenant's income increases.

personal property. All property that is not real property.

physical deterioration. Loss in value brought about by wear and tear, disintegration, use and action of the elements.

piggyback loan. A second mortgage taken out at the same time as the first mortgage to reduce down payment requirements and/or avoid the need for private mortgage insurance.

plaintiff. The person who sues in a court action.

planned unit development (PUD). A land-use design that provides intensive utilization of the land through a combination of private and common areas with prearranged sharing of responsibilities for the common areas; individual lots are owned in fee with joint ownership of open areas; primarily residential but may include commercial and/or industrial uses.

planning commission. An agency of local government charged with planning the development, redevelopment, or preservation of an area.

plottage. Assemblage; an appraisal term for the increased value of two or more adjoining lots when they are placed under single ownership and available for use as a larger single lot.

pocket listing. A listing not provided to other brokers.

points. One point represents one percentage point of a loan amount; may be charged by lenders at the time of loan funding to increase the loan's effective interest rate.

police power. The right of government to enact laws and enforce them to benefit the public health, safety, and general welfare.

power of attorney. A written instrument authorizing an agent to act in the capacity of the principal; a general power of attorney provides authority to carry out all of the business dealings of the principal; a special power of attorney provides authority to carry out a specific act or acts.

power of sale. The power that may be given by a promissory note to a trustee, a mortgagee, or another lienholder to sell secured property without judicial proceedings if the borrower defaults.

predatory lending. Making loans without regard to payment ability of borrower in order to obtain the security by foreclosure.

primary mortgage market. Composed of lenders that deal directly with borrowers. *See also* **secondary mortgage market.**

prime rate. Interest rate that banks charge their most favorably rated commercial borrowers.

principal. The employer of an agent; one of the parties to a transaction; the amount of money borrowed.

private mortgage insurance (PMI). Mortgage guaranty insurance available to conventional lenders on the high-risk portion of a loan, with payment included in the borrower's loan installments.

probate. Court proceeding by which the property of a decedent is distributed according to the decedent's will or, if the decedent died intestate (without a will), according to the state law of intestate succession.

procuring cause. The cause originating a series of events that lead directly to the intended objective; in a real estate transaction, the procuring cause is the real estate agent who first procures a ready, willing, and able buyer.

progression, principle of. The worth of a less-valuable building tends to be enhanced by proximity to buildings of greater value.

promissory note. A written promise to repay a loan under stipulated terms; establishes personal liability for payment by the person making the note.

property management. A branch of the real estate business involving the marketing, operation, maintenance, and other day-to-day requirements of rental properties by an individual or a firm acting as agent of the owner.

proration. Adjustment of interest, taxes, insurance, and other costs of property ownership on a pro rata basis as of the closing or agreed-upon date; usually apportions those costs based on seller's and buyer's respective periods of ownership.

puffing. Exaggerating the attributes or benefits of property as an inducement to purchase.

purchase money mortgage or trust deed. Trust deed or mortgage given as part or all of the purchase consideration for real property.

qualified mortgage. Loans that meet standards for HUD insurance.

quantity survey method. Way of estimating building reproduction cost by making a thorough itemization of all construction costs, both direct (material and labor) and indirect (permits, overhead, profit), then totaling those costs.

quiet title. *See* action to quiet title.

quitclaim deed. A deed that conveys any interest the grantor may have in the property at the time of the execution of the deed, without any warranty of title or interest.

ranges. In the rectangular survey system of land description, townships running east and west of a meridian.

ratification. The adoption or approval of an act by the person on whose behalf it was performed, as when a principal ratifies conduct of an agent that was not previously authorized.

ready, willing, and able buyer. A buyer who wants and is prepared to purchase property, including being able to finance the purchase, at the agreed price and terms.

real estate. Real property; land; includes the surface of the earth, the substances beneath the surface, the airspace above the surface, fixtures, and anything incidental or appurtenant to the land.

real estate board. A local organization whose members consist primarily of real estate brokers and salespeople.

real estate broker. A person employed for a fee by another to carry on any of the activities listed in the real estate law definition of a broker.

Real Estate Education and Research Fund. California fund financed by a fixed portion of real estate license fees, designed to encourage research in land use and real estate development.

real estate investment trust (REIT). Way for investors to pool funds for investments in real estate and mortgages, with profits taxed to individual investors rather than to the corporation.

real estate salesperson. A person licensed under the provisions of the real estate law to act under the control and supervision of a real estate broker in carrying on any of the activities listed in the license law.

real estate syndicate. An organization of real estate investors, typically in the form of a limited partnership.

real property. *See* **real estate.**

reconciliation. In appraising, the final step, in which the estimates of value reached by each of the three appraisal approaches (sales comparison, cost, and income capitalization) are weighed in light of the type of property being appraised, the purpose of the appraisal, and other factors, to arrive at a final conclusion of value.

reconveyance deed. Instrument by which the trustee returns title to the trustor after the debt underlying a deed of trust is paid.

recovery account. State fund financed by real estate license fees and intended to help compensate victims of real estate licensee fraud, misrepresentation, deceit, or conversion of trust funds, when a court-ordered judgment cannot be collected.

rectangular survey system. Section and township system; U.S. government survey system; method of legal description of land using areas called townships measured from meridians and base lines.

recurring costs. Impound costs for taxes and insurance.

red flag. A physical indication of a possible problem with a property.

redlining. An illegal lending policy of denying real estate loans on properties in older, changing urban areas (usually with large minority populations) because of alleged higher lending risks, without due consideration of the individual loan applicant.

reformation. An action to correct a mistake in a contract, a deed, or another document.

regression, principle of. A building's value will decline if the buildings around it have a lower value.

release. Removal of part of a contract obligation, for consideration, by the party to whom the obligation is owed; removal of part of a property from a lien on payment of part of the debt owed.

reliction. The increase of a landowner's property by the receding of an adjacent body of water.

remainder. The right of future possession and use that will go to someone other than the grantor upon termination of a life estate.

rent. The consideration paid for possession and use of leased property.

rent control. A regulation imposed by a local governing body as a means of protecting tenants from relatively high rent increases over the occupancy period of a lease; if a law provides for vacancy decontrol, when a unit becomes vacant, there is no restriction on the rent set for a new tenant.

REO's. Foreclosure real estate owned by lender.

repair and deduct. Tenant's remedy when landlord is on notice of and fails to make necessary repairs to leased premises; a tenant may spend up to one month's rent on repairs, but no more than twice in any 12-month period.

replacement cost. The cost of a new building using modern construction techniques, design, and materials but having the same utility as the subject property.

reproduction cost. The cost of a new building of exactly the same design and materials as the subject property.

rescission. The cancellation of a contract and restoration of the parties to the same position they held before the contract was formed.

restraint on alienation. An illegal condition that would prohibit a property owner from transferring title to real estate.

restriction. A limitation on the use of real property; public restrictions imposed by government include zoning ordinances; private restrictions imposed by deed may require the grantee to do or refrain from doing something. *See also* **CC&Rs**.

reverse exchange. Delayed exchange where the property desired is acquired prior to sale of exchanger's property.

reverse mortgage. Mortgage where the borrower receives payments and does not repay loan until the property is sold or the borrower dies.

reversion. The right of future possession and use retained by the grantor of a life estate.

right of appropriation. Right of government to take, impound, or divert water flowing on the public domain from its natural course for some beneficial purpose.

right of entry. The right of the landlord to enter leased premises in certain circumstances.

right of survivorship. The right of surviving cotenants to share equally in the interest of a deceased cotenant; the last surviving cotenant is sole owner of the property.

riparian rights. The right of a landowner whose property borders a lake, river, or stream to the use and enjoyment of the water adjacent to or flowing over the property, provided the use does not injure other riparian landowners.

Rumford Act. California's fair housing law. Also called the Fair Employment and Housing Act.

safety clause. A clause that protects the broker's commission when a sale is consummated after a listing expires to a buyer procured by the broker.

sale-leaseback. A transaction in which, at the time of sale, the seller retains occupancy by concurrently agreeing to lease the property from the purchaser.

sales comparison approach. Market comparison approach; market data approach; appraisal method in which the sales prices of properties that are comparable in construction and location to the subject property are analyzed and adjusted to reflect differences between the comparables and the subject.

sales contract. Land contract; installment sales contract; a contract used in a sale of real property whereby the seller retains title to the property until all or a prescribed part of the purchase price has been paid, but no earlier than one year from the date of possession.

salvage value. In computing depreciation for tax purposes under all but the declining balance method, the reasonably anticipated fair market value of the property at the end of its useful life.

sandwich lease. A leasehold interest between the primary lease and the operating lease.

satisfaction. Discharge of an obligation before the end of its term by payment of the total debt owed.

scheduled rent. Rent charged, not adjusted for rental incentives.

secondary financing. A loan secured by a second (or subsequent) mortgage or trust deed on real property.

secondary mortgage market. Investment opportunities involving real property securities, other than direct loans from lender to borrower; loans may be bought, sold, or pooled to form the basis for mortgage-backed securities.

section. A standard land area of one mile square, containing 640 acres, used in the rectangular survey system of land description.

section and township system. *See* **rectangular survey system**.

security deposit. An amount paid at the start of a lease term and retained by the landlord until the tenant vacates the premises, all or part of which may be kept by the landlord at that time to cover costs of any default in rent payments or reasonable costs of repairs or cleaning necessitated by the tenant's use of the premises.

security instrument. A written document executed by a debtor that pledges the described property as the lender's assurance that the underlying debt will be repaid.

seller's market. Real estate market with more buyers than sellers.

separate property. Property owned by a married person other than community property, including property owned before marriage, property acquired by gift or inheritance, income from separate property, and property acquired with the proceeds of separate property.

servient tenement. *See* **easement**.

set-back ordinance. An ordinance requiring improvements built on property to be a specified distance from the property line, street or curb.

severalty, ownership in. *See* **ownership in severalty**.

sheriff's deed. Deed given to the purchaser at a court-ordered sale to satisfy a judgment, without warranties.

short sale. A sale for less than is owed on a loan where the lender agrees to accept sale proceeds to extinguish the debt.

sick building syndrome. Illness attributed to a sealed structure; believed related to ventilation.

simple interest. Interest computed on the principal amount of a loan only. *See* **compound interest.**

sinking fund. Fund set aside from the income from property that, with accrued interest, eventually will pay for replacement of the improvements.

sole proprietor. Only owner of a business.

special limitation. A limiting condition specified in a transfer of fee simple ownership that, if not complied with, will immediately and automatically extinguish the estate and return title to the grantor.

special studies zone. One of the areas, typically within a quarter-mile or more of an active earthquake fault, requiring a geologic report for any new project involving improvements or structures initiated after May 4, 1975; the report may be waived by the city or county if the state geologist approves.

special warranty deed. A deed in which the grantor warrants or guarantees the title only against defects arising during the grantor's ownership of the property and not against defects existing before the time of the grantor's ownership.

specific performance. Action to compel a breaching party to adhere to a contract obligation, such as an action to compel the sale of land as an alternative to money damages.

specific plan. Formulated after adoption of a general plan by a city or a county to give further details of community development, including projected population density and building construction requirements.

square-foot method. Way of finding reproduction cost by multiplying the current cost per square foot of a comparable building by the number of square feet in the subject building.

staging. Preparing a home for sale showings.

standard parallels. *See* **correction lines.**

statute of frauds. A state law requiring that certain contracts be in writing and signed before they will be enforceable, such as a contract for the sale of real estate.

statute of limitations. Law that stipulates the specific time period during which a legal action must be brought following the act that gives rise to it.

statutory warranty deed. A short-term warranty deed that warrants by inference that the seller is the undisputed owner, has the right to convey the property, and will defend the title if necessary; if the seller does not do so, the new owner can defend against said claims and sue the former owner.

steering. The illegal act of directing prospective homebuyers to or from a particular residential area on the basis of the homebuyer's race or national origin.

step-up lease. Lease with set rent that provides for periodic rent increases.

stock cooperative. A form of subdivision, typically of an apartment building, in which each owner in the stock cooperative is a shareholder in a corporation that holds title to the property, each shareholder being entitled to use, rent, or sell a specific apartment unit. *See also* **limited equity housing cooperative**.

straight-line method. Depreciation computed at a constant rate over the estimated useful life of the improvement.

straight note. A note in which a borrower repays the principal in a lump sum at maturity, with interest due in installments or at maturity.

subdivision. The division of real property into separate parcels or lots for the purpose of sale, lease, or financing.

subdivision public report. Issued by the real estate commissioner after a subdivision developer has met the requirements of the Subdivided Lands Law; provides details of the project and financing, and a copy must be given to all prospective purchasers; sales may begin on the basis of an approved preliminary public report, but no sales can be closed or transactions completed until the final public report is received.

subject to. When a grantee takes title to real property "subject to" a mortgage or a trust deed, the grantee is not responsible to the holder of the promissory note for the payment of any portion of the amount due, and the original maker of the note retains primary responsibility for the underlying debt or obligation.

sublease. A lease given by a lessee (tenant).

subordination agreement. An agreement by the holder of an encumbrance against real property to permit that claim to take an inferior position to other encumbrances against the property.

subprime lender. A lender who will take loans that are considered too risky by other lenders. Subprime loans bear a higher rate of interest.

substitution, principle of. Market value tends to be set by the present or recent cost of acquiring an equally desirable and valuable property, comparable in construction and/or utility.

supply and demand, principle of. Takes into account the effect on market value of the relationship between the number of properties on the market at a given time and the number of potential buyers.

survey. The process by which a parcel of land is measured and its area ascertained.

syndicate, real estate. *See* real estate syndicate.

take-out loan. The loan arranged by the owner or builder developer for a buyer; the permanent financing that pays off and replaces the interim loan used during construction.

tax deed. Deed issued by the county tax collector when property is sold at public auction because of nonpayment of taxes.

tenancy in common. Co-ownership of property in equal or unequal shares by two or more persons, each holding an undivided interest without right of survivorship.

tenancy in partnership. The ownership by two or more persons, acting as partners, of property held for partnership purposes.

tenant. Lessee under a lease; one who has the legal right to possession and use of property belonging to another.

tentative subdivision map. The initial or tentative map required of subdividers by the Subdivision Map Act, submitted to the local planning commission, which notes its approval or disapproval; a final map embodying any changes requested by the planning commission also must be submitted.

testator. A person who makes a will.

third-party originator. A party who prepares loan applications for borrowers and submits the loan package to lenders.

tiers. In the rectangular survey system of land description, townships running north and south of a base line.

time-share estate. A right of occupancy in a time-share project (subdivision) coupled with an estate in the real property.

time-share project. A form of subdivision of real property into rights to the recurrent, exclusive use or occupancy of a lot, parcel, unit, or segment of the property on an annual or other periodic basis, for a specified period.

time-share use. A license or contractual or membership right of occupancy in a time-share project that is not coupled with an estate in the real property.

title insurance. Insurance to protect a real property owner or a lender up to a specified amount against certain types of loss affecting title or marketability.

tort. Any wrongful act, other than a breach of contract, for which a civil action may be brought by the person wronged.

township. A standard land area of six miles square, divided into 36 sections of one mile square each, used in the rectangular survey system of land description.

toxic mold. Usually a greenish black mold that causes respiratory problems. It usually grows on material with a high cellulose content.

trade fixtures. Articles of personal property that are annexed by a business tenant to real property that are necessary to the carrying on of a trade and are removable by the tenant.

triple net lease. Guarantees a specified net income to the landlord, with the tenant paying that amount, plus all operating and other property expenses, such as taxes, assessments, and insurance.

trust account. An account separate from a broker's own funds (business and personal) in which the broker is required by law to deposit all funds collected for clients before disbursement.

trust deed. A deed issued by a borrower of funds (the trustor) conveying title to a trustee on behalf of a lender, the beneficiary of the trust; the trust deed authorizes the trustee to sell the property to pay the remaining indebtedness to the beneficiary if the trustor defaults on the underlying obligation.

trustee. One who holds property conveyed by a trustor on behalf of (in trust for) the beneficiary, to secure the performance of an obligation.

trustee in bankruptcy. *See* bankruptcy.

trustee's deed. Deed given to the purchaser at a foreclosure sale by the trustee acting under a deed of trust.

trustor. One who conveys property to a trustee to hold on behalf of (in trust for) a beneficiary to secure the performance of an obligation; borrower under a deed of trust.

Truth in Lending Act. Federal act requiring loan term disclosures, as well as advertising disclosures.

undue influence. Use of a fiduciary or confidential relationship to obtain a fraudulent or an unfair advantage over another person because of that's person's weakness of mind, distress, or necessity.

Uniform Commercial Code. Establishes a unified and comprehensive method for regulation of security transactions in personal property, superseding the existing statutes on chattel mortgages, conditional sales, trust receipts, assignments of accounts receivable, and others in this field.

unit-in-place method. Way of estimating building reproduction cost by adding the construction cost per unit of measure of each of the component parts of the subject property; each unit cost includes material, labor, overhead, and builder's profit.

unlawful detainer. The legal action that may be brought to evict a tenant who is in unlawful possession of leased premises.

Unruh Act. California's antidiscrimination act that applies to businesses.

upside-down loan. A loan that exceeds the fair market value of a property.

useful life. The period of years in which a property improvement may be used for its originally intended purpose.

U.S. government survey system. *See* rectangular survey system.

usury. The charging of a rate of interest on a loan that is greater than the rate permitted by law.

vacancy decontrol. *See* rent control.

vacancy factor. The percentage of a building's space that is unrented over a given period.

value in use. The subjective value of property to its present owner, as opposed to market value, which should be objective.

vicarious liability. A principal is liable for wrongful and negligent acts of the agent within the scope of the agency.

void. To have no force or effect; that which is unenforceable.

voidable. That which can be adjudged void but is not void unless action is taken to make it so.

waiver. The giving up of a right or privilege voluntarily.

warranties, implied. *See* implied warranties.

warranty deed. A deed that expressly warrants that the grantor has good title; the grantor thus agrees to defend the premises against the lawful claims of third persons.

warranty of habitability. Legally implied obligation of a landlord to meet minimal housing and building standards.

will. A written, legal declaration of a person called a *testator*, expressing the testator's desires for the disposition of the testator's property after death.

wraparound mortgage or trust deed. Overriding or all-inclusive trust deed; a financing device in which a lender assumes payments on an existing mortgage or trust deed and takes from the borrower a junior mortgage or trust deed with a face value in an amount equal to the amount outstanding on the old instrument and the additional amount of money borrowed.

writ of execution. Court order directing the sheriff or another officer to satisfy a money judgment out of the debtor's property, including real estate not exempt from execution.

writ of possession. Order issued by the court directing the sheriff or the marshal to take all legal steps necessary to remove the occupant(s) from the specified premises.

yield. Profit; return; the interest earned by an investor on an investment or by a bank on the money it has loaned.

zoning. An act of city or county government specifying the possible uses of property in a particular area.

ANSWER KEY

Unit 1

1. **(b)** The real estate marketplace could best be described as being stratified based on price. Demand and supply could vary in different price ranges. p. 8

2. **(a)** Most real estate agents are primarily involved in residential property sales because most properties sold are residential. p. 14

3. **(b)** Real estate salespersons will be treated by the IRS as independent contractors if: the salesperson's reimbursement is based solely on sales, not hours worked; there is a written contract stating that the salesperson shall be treated as an independent contractor for tax purposes; and the salesperson is licensed as a real estate agent. Merely representing oneself as an independent contractor would be a violation of disclosure requirements and is not considered to be an IRS criteria. p. 17

4. **(b)** A broker is ordinarily liable to salespersons for workers' compensation which covers work-related injuries. p. 21

5. **(c)** When choosing a broker, a new licensee should remember that training is more important than commission split for new licensees. p. 26

6. **(d)** The best way to learn is to use the ideas you observe or read about. By using ideas, they become yours. p. 34

7. **(d)** Role-playing situations are only limited by imagination and can be verbalized or nonverbalized. They can also involve more than one person. p. 36

8. **(c)** Exact goals are measurable, such as setting a number of calls you plan to make or appointment for showings to make. p. 39

9. **(c)** It is important to make goals attainable, based on what you want, and exact. Goals should also be shared so you are accountable for making them. When no one knows the goals, it is easier to abandon them. p. 39

10. **(d)** Proper daily planning should: increase "A" Time activities, and place more emphasis on probabilities than possibilities. p. 40

Unit 2

1. **(a)** If a group of brokers agree to not allow another broker to show any of their listings, this is called a group boycott and is prohibited by the Sherman Act. p. 81

2. **(b)** What is legal but unethical is likely to become illegal. p. 63

3. **(d)** All of the following phrases indicate a discriminatory preference: "Christian family," "Prefer working married couple," and "Just two blocks to St. Michael's." p. 71

4. **(b)** If an employer widens the doorway to a restroom to allow wheelchair access, this is considered reasonable accommodation for handicapped and complies with the Americans with Disabilities Act (ADA). p. 73

5. **(d)** The Civil Rights Act of 1866 covers racial discrimination and originally gave rights to former slaves. p. 68

6. **(d)** If a broker specifically shows prospective buyers homes based on racial make-up, this is illegal, unethical, and known as steering. It is specifically prohibited by Civil Rights Act of 1968. p. 71

7. **(c)** A broker can only refuse to show a property to a prospective buyer if the development has an age exemption because all occupants are 55 years of age or older. This is an exception to Fair Housing Act. p. 72

8. **(d)** A landlord cannot refuse to rent to protected classes. p. 72

9. **(a)** The state act that specifically prohibits discrimination in business establishments is the Unruh Act. p. 76

10. **(d)** Placing trust funds in the personal care of a bonded employee is a violation of the law. pp. 82–83

Unit 3

1. **(d)** In a real estate transaction, the agent has a fiduciary duty to their principal, must disclose any known detrimental information to a buyer (even if representing the seller), and must disclose any material facts to their principal. pp. 107–109

2. **(b)** Agency disclosure applies to commercial and residential units and listing agent can only be seller's agent or dual agent. pp. 112–113

3. **(d)** The confirmation of agency must be in writing, the three steps of the disclosure process are disclose, elect, and confirm, and the selling agent must confirm the agency prior to the buyer making an offer. pp. 116–117

4. **(b)** A seller of a 4-unit apartment building must provide a Real Estate Transfer Disclosure Statement. pp. 118–120

5. **(c)** An agent's duty of inspection and disclosure covers a visual inspection only of readily accessible areas. p. 124

6. **(a)** Earthquake safety disclosure only applies to 1–4-unit residential properties. p. 129

7. **(a)** The buyer must sign to acknowledge receipt of a booklet relating to environmental hazards. There is also a booklet Residential Guide to Earthquake Safety for which the buyer also signs a receipt. pp. 129–130

8. **(b)** Brownfields is a term used to describe contaminated soil. p. 137

9. **(c)** The purpose of the Subdivided Lands Law is to protect purchasers from fraud. p. 141

10. **(a)** The right of rescission is provided by law for purchase agreements involving time-shares and undivided interest subdivisions. pp. 153–154

Unit 4

1. **(b)** The CAN-SPAM Act puts control on unsolicited misleading emails. p. 193

2. **(c)** Unlicensed party is limited to introduction and may not engage in any sales activities. p. 209

3. **(d)** Direct mail solicitation for listings is more effective if you indicate you will be contacting them. This forces the recipient to think about your call. You must consider the do-not-call register. p. 214

4. **(d)** Under do-not-call regulations, it would be proper to make a call for survey purposes or as an agent of a prospective buyer. p. 190

5. **(d)** Owners of single housing units would often rather sell than rent. p. 198

6. **(d)** A notice of vacancy is not a legal action. Notices of eviction, foreclosure, and probate are all legal notices and can provide good leads for listings. pp. 199–200

7. **(d)** A high vacancy rate, tenant evictions, and code violations are all indications that an owner might be interested in selling an income property. pp. 199–200

8. **(b)** Endless chain refers to obtaining additional prospects from every lead. p. 207

9. **(d)** The real estate term farming refers to working or prospecting a geographic are or special interest area for buyers and sellers. p. 213

10. **(d)** A nongeographic farm would be specialization in mobile homes, income property, or lots. p. 215

Unit 5

1. **(c)** A comparative market analysis (CMA) shows comparable sale prices and is used to estimate value for listing purposes. p. 222

2. **(c)** The most important portion of your analysis is the prices of comparable properties that have sold since it shows the reality of the marketplace. p. 223

3. **(c)** For data used on the CMA, the older the data, the less reliable and sales prices that seem unusually high or low are often the result of market imperfections. p. 223

4. **(c)** Owners must be made to realize that the higher they price their home over fair market value, the longer it will take to sell and the lower the likelihood of a sale during the listing period. The agent is not doing the seller a favor by taking a listing over market value. pp. 224–225

5. **(c)** A recommended list price below what the CMA indicates is in an owner's best interest when the seller must sell quickly. pp. 224–225

6. **(d)** What a seller receives in hand from a sale is the seller's net proceeds. p. 231

7. **(b)** The principal reason owners try to sell their homes without an agent is to save the commission. Even when not specifically stated, it is frequently the reason an owner wants to try to sell without an agent. p. 235

8. **(d)** Your listing presentation book material should be organized to follow your listing presentation, should not be used in lieu of a verbal presentation, and can be helpful in selling an owner on the concept of listing in general and listing with your firm in particular. p. 231

9. **(d)** When selling the benefits of listing with a small office, the best approach would be to emphasize that you specialize in a small number of select properties. p. 244

10. **(d)** The shorter time to sell is positive while a percentage of success indicates a percentage of failure. pp. 252–254

Unit 6

1. **(d)** A valid exclusive listing requires a lawful purpose, mutual consent, and consideration. p. 263

2. **(d)** A verbal listing is unenforceable. p. 263

3. **(b)** If an open listing is sold by any other party, the listing broker is not entitled to any compensation. This makes it least attractive to a broker and the least likely to be advertised. pp. 264–265

4. **(c)** A listing under which the owner can sell the listed property without paying a commission but the agent is nevertheless an exclusive agent is an exclusive agency listing. p. 272

5. **(a)** Would be entitled to commission if there was a valid listing. p. 272

6. **(d)** An exclusive-right-to-sell listing likely includes an agency relationship disclosure, an attorney fee provision, and an arbitration agreement. p. 266

7. **(d)** In an exclusive-right-to-sell listing, escrow does not have to close for an agent to be entitled to a commission. Additionally, it must have a termination date for the agent to collect a commission, and the agent must give the owner a copy of the listing when the owner signs. It is not true that the agent is precluded from working with other agents to sell the property. p. 266

8. **(c)** The type of listing that has the greatest likelihood of resulting in a sale is an exclusive-right-to-sell listing as it has the best outcome for the agent's work. p. 266

9. **(d)** If an owner tells you that another agent told them that they could get far more for the property than your CMA indicated, your best response would be to state that your CMA covers all recent comparables and clearly shows the market value. Asking to see the CMA prepared by the other agent would be a good idea. p. 285

10. **(d)** By taking a listing at a low fee that will result in a less than normal fee for any cooperating brokers you are not benefiting your office, the selling office, or the owner. p. 288

Unit 7

1. **(b)** The most likely reason why an expired listing was not extended with the original listing office is dissatisfaction with communications. p. 300

2. **(a)** Agent advice to owners on showing their home could include cleaning instructions, landscaping instructions, and repair instructions. However, having the owners present for an open house would probably not be encouraged because buyers are less likely to feel at ease and will not openly discuss their feelings when owners are present. p. 301

3. **(a)** If there has been little or no interest in a property, the agent should convey this information to the sellers. pp. 300, 307

4. **(c)** Standard system used by many lenders. p. 332

5. **(b)** It is good to get neighborhood information from owners to give your listings a competitive advantage. p. 334

6. **(c)** An owner should understand that a list price above the CMA is merely a hope unsupported by fact. Adjusting a price gives nothing away because there is no buyer, and without a buyer there is only an offering price. pp. 312–313

7. **(c)** Placing a rider strip on your listing to show positive features not readily seen such as "4 bedrooms". p. 314

8. **(b)** A property brief should not be used as a substitute for other types of advertising. They are, however, great for a handout at open houses, a handout at caravans, and as a mailing piece in response to enquiries. pp. 318–319

9. **(a)** A broker open house is of greatest value when it is in a large market because many agents may miss the caravan. p. 326

10. **(d)** Advantages of open houses include pleasing owners because they indicate activity, they locate buyers for other properties, and they can obtain leads for listings. They also assist in marketing the property that is open for inspection. p. 327

Unit 8

1. **(b)** The AIDA approach includes: attention, interest, desire, and action. p. 343

2. **(d)** Personal advertising includes name tags, calling cards, blogs and car signs. pp. 346–347

3. **(b)** The term logo refers to an identifying design or symbol. p. 347

4. **(c)** Blind ads fail to include broker identification. p. 351

5. **(b)** The most cost-effective advertising medium for selling a home would be the internet. p. 362

6. **(a)** Classified ads are different from most other forms of real estate advertising because they are actually sought out by the reader. pp. 351–352

7. **(d)** Real estate professionals know that ads that tell about the problems of the property are often very effective, attracting bargain hunters, flippers, and do-it-yourself buyers. p. 352

8. **(c)** An advertiser with an extremely low advertising budget would most likely avoid billboards. Press releases, For Sale signs, and the internet are relatively low- or no-cost. pp. 358–359

9. **(d)** Capital letters are not easier to read than lowercase letters. However, it is true that readers' eyes tend to move from upper left to lower right, one large picture is generally more effective than several smaller ones, and short words are easier to read than long ones. p. 357

10. **(c)** In preparing display ads, a good advertiser should use no more than two typefaces per ad. p. 357

Unit 9

1. **(d)** Callers from a For Sale sign are likely to be satisfied with the area and with the general exterior appearance, or they would not have called. pp. 383–384

2. **(c)** In general, callers from signs are more likely to end up buying homes that cost less than the home they called about and callers from ads are more likely to end up buying homes that cost more than the home they called about. pp. 383–384

3. **(d)** There is duty to attempt to best meet needs of buyers. pp. 394–395

4. **(d)** In showing property, you should adjust to needs of purchaser and show properties based on needs. pp. 394–395

5. **(d)** The qualifying period includes discovering the buyers' motivation, needs, and interests, as well as a down payment they can make and the amount they can finance. p. 397

6. **(a)** The front-end qualifying ratio is the ratio of gross housing cost to gross income. p. 397

7. **(b)** The back-end qualifying ratio refers to the ratio of total housing expense plus long-term debt to gross income. p. 397

8. **(c)** You need information to sell and open-end questions elicit information. p. 394

9. **(d)** All reduce likelihood of becoming a victim. p. 393

10. **(c)** If another agent is showing a home when you arrive for a showing, you should wait inconspicuously until the other agent completes the showing and leaves. p. 418

Unit 10

1. **(d)** A good salesperson does not use technical terms to impress buyers, does not speak fast to reach closing, and does not approach each customer in the same way. pp. 427–428

2. **(d)** A love of family, comfort and convenience, and security are all buying motives. pp. 432–436

3. **(d)** Disadvantages of home ownership include increase in expenses, risk, and a lack of liquidity. p. 438

4. **(d)** Buying signals could include whispering with a spouse, pacing off a room, or seeming reluctant to leave a property. pp. 437–438

5. **(d)** Asking a question is the best response to, "The price is too high." "Why?" would have been the appropriate first question. pp. 438–439

6. **(d)** A professional salesperson knows that it is more effective to ask than tell, it is good to appeal to emotions, and it is not recommended to be assertive with a cautious buyer. pp. 438–442

7. **(b)** When asking a prospective buyer whether he would prefer one of a range of dates, you are using the positive choice closing technique. p. 444

8. **(a)** The paragraph in the purchase contract referring to the intent to occupy is important because it relates to liquidated damages. p. 465

9. **(d)** The buyer and seller by mutual agreement can modify an accepted offer to purchase. p. 467

10. **(b)** The buyer is responsible for the damage to the air conditioning unit based on the California Residential Purchase Agreement and Joint Escrow Instructions. p. 468

Unit 11

1. **(b)** The three separate sales involved in selling real estate are: obtaining the listing, obtaining the offer, and gaining acceptance of the offer. p. 478

2. **(c)** When you receive two offers on a listed property, you should present the offers at the same time and in a nonprejudicial manner, no matter the source of the offers. pp. 480–481

3. **(a)** It would be most difficult to persuade an owner to accept a reasonable offer received three days after listing the property. p. 483

4. **(c)** When presenting an offer on your listing for less than list price, it is good policy to recommend that the sellers counter or reject offers when acceptance is not in their best interest. pp. 495–496

5. **(c)** The common buyer apprehension felt after placing an offer is known as buyer's remorse. p. 487

6. **(b)** Once a counteroffer is not accepted, the owner does not have the option of accepting the original offer. Question asks, "Not True." p. 493

7. **(a)** If an offer received on your listing contains the word "subordination," you should be wary. p. 488

8. **(c)** Rent skimming is a buyer's failure to apply rents to loans that were assumed. p. 489

9. **(d)** If a reasonable, but lower than listing price, offer is received, you should recommend to the owners that they accept the offer. p. 487

10. **(d)** After an offer is accepted, the listing agent should keep track of the escrow progress, make certain all papers are signed by the parties, and make certain that conditions are being met. pp. 499–500

Unit 12

1. **(b)** A loan covering more than one property would be a blanket encumbrance. p. 532

2. **(a)** A reverse mortgage has compound interest. p. 536

3. **(c)** The difference between the interest rate of an index and the rate charged by the lender under an ARM is known as the margin. p. 539

4. **(b)** A lender who believes that interest rates will rise significantly will be least interested in a 30-year fixed-rate mortgage, although a borrower might prefer it. pp. 533–534

5. **(a)** A danger that ARMs pose to buyers is the threat of higher payments if interest rates increase. p. 537

6. **(d)** With an adjustable-rate loan index at 6% at the time the loan is made, a margin for the loan at 2-1/2%, and a 5% lifetime cap, the highest the interest rate could go is 13-1/2%. p. 538

7. **(b)** A convertible ARM is a loan that can be changed to a fixed-rate loan. p. 543

8. **(d)** A buyer who intends to sell a house within two years would prefer a loan with no prepayment penalty, a loan with low initial loan costs, and an assumable loan. pp. 545–546

9. **(b)** An adjustable-rate mortgage is most likely to meet all the criteria of a buyer who intends to sell a house within two years (no prepayment penalty, low initial loan costs, and assumable). p. 545–546

10. **(c)** An expansionary policy of the Federal Reserve would be to buy government securities putting more money into the economy. p. 509

Unit 13

1. **(d)** A broker can act as an escrow when the broker is a principal or represents the buyer or seller in the transaction. pp. 578–579

2. **(a)** An escrow company is prohibited from paying referral fees to anyone other than an employee of the escrow company. p. 580

3. **(b)** To determine the balance due on a loan, escrow requires a beneficiary statement. p. 586

4. **(c)** First trust deed to be assumed by the buyer is a debit to the seller on the seller's closing statement. p. 588

5. **(d)** First trust deed assumed is a credit to the buyer on the buyer's closing statement. Purchase price, escrow costs, and title insurance are debits. p. 588

6. **(d)** An escrow company does not have a duty to warn parties of possible fraud or suggest changes when one party is not being adequately protected. p. 592

7. **(b)** A standard policy of title insurance is used to show that the seller has marketable title. It ensures against undisclosed encumbrances. pp. 599–600

8. **(c)** Unknown spousal interests are covered by the CLTA standard policy of title insurance. p. 599

9. **(b)** Liens placed by the insured are not covered by an ALTA extended policy of title insurance. However, mining claims, water rights, and off-record easements are. pp. 600–601

10. **(d)** Title insurance companies do not give rebates to brokers for referrals, do not give brokers preferred rates on their own purchases, and cannot charge brokers the same as others but make no effort to collect. p. 604

Unit 14

1. **(b)** The most difficult tax to avoid is the real property tax because it cannot be hidden. p. 610

2. **(a)** The months of November, December, February, and April relate to real property taxes. p. 611

3. **(d)** Proposition 13 provided for a maximum tax rate, it set assessments for property acquired before 1978 back to the value on the 1975 tax roll, and allowed for a 2% per year tax increase. pp. 614–615

4. **(d)** Proposition 90 provided for a tax assessment for certain homeowners to be transferred from one county to another. p. 617

5. **(c)** The homeowner's property tax exemption is $7,000 from assessed value. p. 617

6. **(d)** Depreciation for a residential property uses the straight-line method and a 27-1/2-year table. p. 624

7. **(c)** To have a tax-deferred delayed exchange, the exchange property must be identified within 45 days and must be completed within 180 days of the taxpayer relinquishing their property. p. 630

8. **(b)** To have a 1031 tax-deferred exchange, you need to have like-for-like properties, have a trade of investment real property for investment real property, and must hold property after the exchange in the same manner as you held property going into the exchange. pp. 625–630

9. **(b)** If Albert wants to exchange property with Baker, cash received by Albert to balance equities would be boot to Albert in the exchange. Debt relief would also be boot. p. 631

10. **(d)** A homeowner can receive preferential tax treatment by an interest deduction, use of the universal exclusion, and a property tax deduction. pp. 634–635

Unit 15

1. **(b)** The term *CPM* refers to Certified Property Manager of IREM. p. 651

2. **(a)** Compensation is generally a percentage of the gross. Percentage is lower for higher income properties. p. 668

3. **(c)** A property manager can be protected against receiving no fees when managing a vacant property they are unable to rent by a minimum fee. p. 668

4. **(c)** A lease for 30 months would be described as an estate for years because it is a definite fixed period. p. 675

5. **(a)** A lease under which the tenant is to pay $500 per month for three years is a gross, or flat, lease (fixed rent). p. 676

6. **(a)** A lease that contains a minimum rent and a covenant to remain in business is a percentage lease. p. 677

7. **(a)** A parking lot would likely pay the highest percentage on a percentage lease. p. 678

8. **(c)** A supermarket would likely pay the lowest percentage on a percentage lease. p. 678

9. **(b)** A valid two-year lease need not contain a legal description of the property. pp. 680, 687–690

10. **(d)** Regarding security deposits, the following is true: nonrefundable cleaning deposits are not allowed, deposits for furnished rentals cannot exceed three months' rent, and security deposits for unfurnished rentals cannot exceed two months' rent. p. 687

INDEX

Notes

Notes

Notes

Notes

Notes

Notes

Notes

Notes

Notes

Notes

Notes

Notes

Notes